Culpeper's
Complete Herbal

Culpeper's Complete Herbal

_

A book of natural remedies
for ancient ills

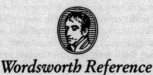

Wordsworth Reference

Culpeper's

ORIGINAL EPISTLE TO THE READER

Take Notice, That in this Edition I have made very many Additions to every sheet in the book: and, also, that those books of mine that are printed of that Letter the small Bibles are printed with, are very falsely printed: there being twenty or thirty gross mistakes in every sheet, many of them such as are exceedingly dangerous to such as shall venture to use them: And therefore I do warn the Public of them: I can do no more at present; only take notice of these Directions by which you shall be sure to know the *True one* from the *False*.

The first Direction.—The true one hath this Title over the head of every Book, THE COMPLETE HERBAL AND ENGLISH PHYSICIAN ENLARGED. The small Counterfeit ones have only this Title, THE ENGLISH PHYSICIAN.

The second Direction.—The true one hath these words, GOVERNMENT AND VIRTUES, following the time of the Plants flowering, &c. The counterfeit small ones have these words, VIRTUES AND USE, following the time of the Plants flowering.

The third Direction.—The true one is of a larger Letter than the counterfeit ones, which are in *Twelves*, &c., of the Letter small Bibles used to be printed on. I shall now speak something of the book itself.

All other Authors that have written of the nature of Herbs, give not a bit of reason why such an Herb was appropriated to such a part of the body, nor why it cured such a disease. Truly my own body being sickly, brought me easily into a capacity, to know that health was the greatest of all earthly blessings, and truly he was never sick that doth not believe it. Then I considered that all medicines were compounded of Herbs, Roots, Flowers, Seeds, &c., and this first set me to work in studying the nature of simples, most of which I knew by sight before; and indeed all the Authors I could read gave me but little satisfaction in this particular, or none at all. I cannot build my faith upon Authors' words, nor believe a thing because they say it, and could wish every body were of my mind in this,—to labour to be able to give a reason for every thing

v

they say or do. They say Reason makes a man differ from a Beast; if that be true, pray what are they that, instead of reason for their judgment, quote old Authors? Perhaps their authors knew a reason for what they wrote, perhaps they did not; what is that to us ? Do we know it ? Truly in writing this work first, to satisfy myself, I drew out all the virtues of the vulgar or common Herbs, Plants, and Trees, &c., out of the best or most approved authors I had, or could get; and having done so, I set myself to study the reason of them. I knew well enough the whole world, and every thing in it, was formed of a composition of contrary elements, and in such a harmony as must needs show the wisdom and power of a great God. I knew as well this Creation, though thus composed of contraries, was one united body, and man an epitome of it: I knew those various affections in man, in respect of sickness and health, were caused naturally (though God may have other ends best known to himself) by the various operations of the Microcosm; and I could not be ignorant, that as the cause is, so must the cure be; and therefore he that would know the reason of the operation of the Herbs, must look up as high as the Stars, astrologically. I always found the disease vary according to the various motions of the Stars; and this is enough, one would think, to teach a man by the effect where the cause lies. Then to find out the reason of the operation of Herbs, Plants, &c., by the Stars went I; and herein I could find but few authors, but those as full of nonsense and contradiction as an egg is full of meat. This not being pleasing, and less profitable to me, I consulted with my two brothers, DR. REASON and DR. EXPERIENCE, and took a voyage to visit my mother NATURE, by whose advice, together with the help of DR. DILIGENCE, I at last obtained my desire; and, being warned by MR. HONESTY, a stranger in our days, to publish it to the world, I have done it.

But you will say, *What need I have written on this Subject, seeing so many famous and learned men have written so much of it in the English Tongue, much more than I have done?*

To this I answer, neither GERRARD nor PARKINSON, or any that ever wrote in the like nature, ever gave one wise reason for what they wrote, and so did nothing else but train up young novices in Physic in the School of tradition, and teach them just as a parrot is taught to speak; an Author says so, therefore it is true; and if all that Authors say be true, why do they contradict one another ? But in mine, if you view it with the eye of reason, you shall see a reason for everything that is written, whereby you may find the very ground and foundation of Physic; you may know what you do, and wherefore you do it; and this shall call me Father, it being (that I know of) never done in the world before.

I have now but two things to write, and then I have done.

 1. *What the profit and benefit of this Work is.*

 2. *Instructions in the use of it.*

The profit and benefit arising from it, or that may occur to a wise man from it are many; so many that should I sum up all the particulars, my Epistle would be as big as my Book; I shall quote some few general heads.

First. The admirable Harmony of the Creation is herein seen, in the influence of Stars upon Herbs and the Body of Man, how one part of the Creation is subservient to another, and all for the use of Man, whereby the infinite power and wisdom of God in the creation appear; and if I do not admire at the simplicity of the Ranters, never trust me; who but viewing the Creation can hold such a sottish opinion, as that it was from eternity, when the mysteries of it are so clear to every eye? but that Scripture shall be verified to them, *Rom.* i. 20: "*The invisible things of him from the Creation of the World are clearly seen, being understood by the things that are made, even his Eternal Power and Godhead; so that they are without excuse.*"—And a Poet could teach them a better lesson:

 "*Because out of thy thoughts God shall not pass,*
 His image stamped is on every grass."

This indeed is true, God has stamped his image on every creature, and therefore the abuse of the creature is a great sin; but how much the more do the wisdom and excellency of God appear, if we consider the harmony of the Creation in the virtue and operation of every Herb!

Secondly, Hereby you may know what infinite knowledge *Adam* had in his innocence, that by looking upon a creature, he was able to give it a name according to its nature; and by knowing that, thou mayest know how great thy fall was and be humbled for it even in this respect, because hereby thou art so ignorant.

Thirdly, Here is the right way for thee to begin at the study of Physic, if thou art minded to begin at the right end, for here thou hast the reason of the whole art. I wrote before in certain Astrological Lectures, which I read, and printed, intituled, *Astrological Judgment of Diseases*, what planet caused (as a second cause) every disease, how it might be found out what planet caused it; here thou hast what planet cures it by *Sympathy* and *Antipathy*; and this brings me to my last promise, *viz.*

 Instructions for the right use of the book.

And herein let me premise a word or two. The Herbs, Plants, &c. are now in the book appropriated to their proper planets. Therefore,

First, Consider what planet causeth the disease; that thou mayest find it in my aforesaid Judgment of Diseases.

Secondly, Consider what part of the body is afflicted by the disease, and whether it lies in the flesh, or blood, or bones, or ventricles.

Thirdly, Consider by what planet the afflicted part of the body is governed: that my Judgment of Diseases will inform you also.

Fourthly, You may oppose diseases by Herbs of the planet, opposite to the planet that causes them: as diseases of *Jupiter* by herbs of *Mercury*, and the contrary; diseases of the *Luminaries* by the herbs of *Saturn*, and the contrary; diseases of *Mars* by herbs of *Venus*, and the contrary.

Fifthly, There is a way to cure diseases sometimes by *Sympathy*, and so every planet cures his own disease; as the *Sun* and *Moon* by their Herbs cure the Eyes, *Saturn* the Spleen, *Jupiter* the Liver, *Mars* the Gall and diseases of choler, and *Venus* diseases in the instruments of Generation.

NICH. CULPEPER

from
my house in
SPITALFIELDS
next door to
THE RED LION
5th September
1653

Mrs. Alice Culpeper

MY DEAREST,

THE works that I have published to the world (though envied by some illiterate physicians) have merited such just applause, that thou mayest be confident in proceeding to publish anything I leave thee, especially this master-piece: assuring my friends and countrymen, that they will receive as much benefit by this, as by my *Dispensatory*, and that incomparable piece called *Semiotica Uranica* enlarged, and *English Physician*.

These are the choicest secrets, which I have had many years locked up in my own breast. I gained them by my constant practice, and by them I maintained a continual reputation in the world, and I doubt not but the world will honour thee for divulging them; and my fame shall continue and increase thereby, though the period of my Life and Studies be at hand, and I must now bid all things under the sun farewell. Farewell, my dear wife and child; farewell, Arts and Sciences, which I so dearly loved; farewell, all worldly glories; adieu, readers,

NICHOLAS CULPEPER

✦ ✦ ✦

NICHOLAS CULPEPER, the Author of this Work, was son of Nicholas Culpeper, a Clergyman, and grandson of Sir Thomas Culpeper, Bart. He was some time a student in the university of Cambridge, and soon after was bound apprentice to an Apothecary. He employed all his leisure hours in the study of Physic and Astrology, which he afterwards professed, and set up business in Spital-fields, next door to the Red Lion, (formerly known as the Half-way House between Islington and Stepney, an exact representation of which we have given under our Author's Portrait), where he had considerable practice, and was much resorted to for his advice, which he gave to the poor gratis. Astrological Doctors have always been highly respected; and those celebrated Physicians of the early times, whom our Author seems to have particularly studied, Hippocrates, Galen, and Avicen, regarded those as homicides who were ignorant of Astrology. Paracelsus, indeed, went farther; he declared, a Physician should be predestinated to the cure of his patient; and the horoscope should be inspected, the plants gathered at the critical moment, &c.

Culpeper was a writer and translator of several Works, the most celebrated of which is his Herbal, "being an astrologo-physical discourse of the common herbs of the nation; containing a complete Method or Practice of Physic, whereby a Man may preserve his Body in Health, or cure himself when sick, with such things only as grow in England, they being most fit for English Constitutions."

This celebrated and useful Physician died at his house in Spitalfields, in the year 1654. This Book will remain as a lasting monument of his skill and industry.

> "Culpeper, the man that first ranged the woods and
> climbed the mountains in search of medicinal
> and salutary herbs, undoubtedly merited
> the gratitude of posterity"
>
> DR. JOHNSON

The English Physician

Enlarged

AMARA DULCIS

CONSIDERING divers shires in this nation give divers names to one and the same herb, and that the common name which it bears in one county, is not known in another; I shall take the pains to set down all the names that I know of each herb: pardon me for setting that name first, which is most common to myself. Besides Amara Dulcis, some call it Mortal, others Bitter-sweet; some Woody Night-shade, and others Felon-wort.

Descript.] It grows up with woody stalks even to a man's height, and sometimes higher. The leaves fall off at the approach of winter, and spring out of the same stalk at spring-time: the branch is compassed about with a whitish bark, and has a pith in the middle of it: the main branch branches itself into many small ones with claspers, laying hold on what is next to them, as vines do: it bears many leaves, they grow in no order at all, at least in no regular order; the leaves are longish, though somewhat broad, and pointed at the ends: many of them have two little leaves growing at the end of their foot-stalk; some have but one, and some none. The leaves are of a pale green colour; the flowers are of a purple colour, or of a perfect blue, like to violets, and they stand many of them together in knots: the berries are green at first, but when they are ripe they are very red; if you taste them, you shall find them just as the crabs which we in Sussex call Bitter-sweet, *viz.* sweet at first and bitter afterwards.

Place.] They grow commonly almost throughout England, especially in moist and shady places.

Time.] The leaves shoot out about the latter end of March, if the temperature of the air be ordinary; it flowers in July, and the seeds are ripe soon after, usually in the next month.

Government and virtues.] It is under the planet Mercury, and a notable herb of his also, if it be rightly gathered under his influence. It is excellently good to remove witchcraft both in men and beasts, as also all sudden diseases whatsoever. Being tied round about the neck, is one of the most admirable remedies for the vertigo or dizziness in the head; and that is the reason (as Tragus saith) the people in Germany commonly hang it about their cattle's necks, when they fear any such evil hath betided them. Country people commonly take the berries of it, and having bruised them, apply them to felons, and thereby soon rid their fingers of such troublesome guests.

We have now showed you the external use of the herb; we shall speak a word or two of the internal, and so conclude. Take notice, it is a Mercurial herb, and therefore of very subtile parts, as indeed all Mercurial plants are; therefore take a pound of the wood and leaves together, bruise the wood (which you may easily do, for it is not so hard as oak) then put it in a pot, and put to it three pints of white wine, put on the pot-lid and shut it close; and let it infuse hot over a gentle fire twelve hours, then strain it out, so have you a most excellent drink to open obstructions of the liver and spleen, to help difficulty of breath, bruises and falls, and congealed blood in any part of the body, it helps the yellow jaundice, the dropsy, and black jaundice, and to cleanse women newly brought to bed. You may drink a quarter of a pint of the infusion every morning. It purges the body very gently, and not churlishly as some hold. And when you find good by this, remember me.

They that think the use of these medicines is too brief, it is only for the cheapness of the book; let them read those books of mine, of the last edition, *viz. Reverius, Veslingus, Riolanus, Johnson, Sennertus,* and *Physic for the Poor.*

ALL-HEAL

It is called All-heal, Hercules's All-heal, and Hercules's Woundwort, because it is supposed that Hercules learned the herb and its virtues from Chiron, when he learned physic of him. Some call it Panay, and others Opopane-wort.

Descript.] Its root is long, thick, and exceeding full of juice, of a hot and biting taste, the leaves are great and large, and winged almost like ash-tree leaves, but that they are something hairy, each leaf consisting of five or six pair of such wings set one against the other upon foot-stalks, broad below, but narrow towards the end; one of the leaves is a little deeper at the bottom than the other, of a fair yellowish fresh green colour: they are of a bitterish taste, being chewed in the mouth; from among these rises up a stalk, green in colour, round in form, great and strong in magnitude, five or six feet in altitude, with many joints, and some leaves thereat; towards the top come forth umbels of small yellow flowers, after which are passed away, you may find whitish, yellow, short, flat seeds, bitter also in taste.

Place.] Having given you a description of the herb from bottom to top, give me leave to tell you, that there are other herbs called by this name; but because they are strangers in England, I give only the description of this, which is easily to be had in the gardens of divers places.

Time.] Although Gerrard saith, that they flower from the beginning of May to the end of December, experience teaches them that keep it in their gardens, that it flowers not till the latter end of the summer, and sheds its seeds presently after.

Government and virtues.] It is under the dominion of Mars, hot, biting, and choleric; and remedies what evils Mars inflicts the body of man with, by sympathy, as vipers' flesh attracts poison, and the loadstone iron. It kills the worms, helps the gout, cramp, and convulsions, provokes urine, and helps all joint-aches. It helps all cold griefs of the head, the vertigo, falling-sickness, the lethargy, the wing cholic, obstructions of the liver and spleen, stone in the kidneys and bladder. It provokes the terms, expels the dead birth: it is excellent good for the griefs of the sinews, itch, stone, and toothache, the biting of mad dogs and venomous beasts, and purges choler very gently.

ALKANET

BESIDES the common name, it is called Orchanet, and Spanish Bugloss, and by apothecaries, Enchusa.

Descript.] Of the many sorts of this herb, there is but one known to grow commonly in this nation; of which one take this description. It hath a great and thick root, of a reddish colour, long, narrow, hairy leaves, green like the leaves of Bugloss, which lie very thick upon the ground; the stalks rise up compassed round about, thick with leaves, which are less and narrower than the former; they are tender, and slender, the flowers are hollow, small, and of a reddish colour.

Place.] It grows in Kent near Rochester, and in many places in the West Country, both in Devonshire and Cornwall.

Time.] They flower in July and the beginning of August, and the seed is ripe soon after, but the root is in its prime, as carrots and parsnips are, before the herb runs up to stalk.

Government and virtues.] It is an herb under the dominion of Venus, and indeed one of her darlings, though somewhat hard to come by. It helps old ulcers, hot inflammations, burnings by common fire, and St. Anthony's fire, by antipathy to Mars; for these

uses, your best way is to make it into an ointment; also, if you make
a vinegar of it, as you make vinegar of roses, it helps the morphew
and leprosy; if you apply the herb to the privities, it draws forth
the dead child. It helps the yellow jaundice, spleen, and gravel in
the kidneys. Dioscorides saith it helps such as are bitten by a
venomous beast, whether it be taken inwardly, or applied to the
wound; nay, he saith further, if any one that hath newly eaten it,
do but spit into the mouth of a serpent, the serpent instantly dies.
It stays the flux of the belly, kills worms, helps the fits of the mother.
Its decoction made in wine, and drank, strengthens the back, and
eases the pains thereof. It helps bruises and falls, and is as gallant
a remedy to drive out the small pox and measles as any is; an ointment made of it, is excellent for green wounds, pricks or thrusts.

ADDER'S TONGUE OR SERPENT'S TONGUE

Descript.] This herb has but one leaf, which grows with the stalk
a finger's length above the ground, being flat and of a fresh green
colour; broad like Water Plantain, but less, without any rib in it;
from the bottom of which leaf, on the inside, rises up (ordinarily)
one, sometimes two or three slender stalks, the upper half whereof
is somewhat bigger, and dented with small dents of a yellowish
green colour, like the tongue of an adder serpent (only this is as
useful as they are formidable). The roots continue all the year.

Place.] It grows in moist meadows, and such like places.

Time.] It is to be found in May or April, for it quickly perishes
with a little heat.

Government and virtues.] It is an herb under the dominion of the
Moon and Cancer, and therefore if the weakness of the retentive
faculty be caused by an evil influence of Saturn in any part of the
body governed by the Moon, or under the dominion of Cancer,
this herb cures it by sympathy. It cures these diseases after specified,
in any part of the body under the influence of Saturn, by antipathy.

It is temperate in respect of heat, but dry in the second degree.
The juice of the leaves, drank with the distilled water of Horse-tail,
is a singular remedy for all manner of wounds in the breast, bowels,
or other parts of the body, and is given with good success to those
that are troubled with casting, vomiting, or bleeding at the mouth
or nose, or otherwise downwards. The said juice given in the
distilled water of Oaken-buds, is very good for women who have
their usual courses, or the whites flowing down too abundantly.
It helps sore eyes. Of the leaves infused or boiled in oil, omphacine
or unripe olives, set in the sun four certain days, or the green leaves
sufficiently boiled in the said oil, is made an excellent green balsam,

not only for green and fresh wounds, but also for old and inveterate ulcers, especially if a little fine clear turpentine be dissolved therein. It also stays and refreshes all inflammations that arise upon pains by hurts and wounds.

What parts of the body are under each planet and sign, and also what disease may be found in my astrological judgment of diseases; and for the internal work of nature in the body of man; as vital, animal, natural and procreative spirits of man; the apprehension, judgment, memory; the external senses, *viz*. seeing, hearing, smelling, tasting and feeling; the virtuous, attractive, retentive, digestive, expulsive, &c. under the dominion of what planets they are, may be found in my *Ephemeris* for the year 1651. In both which you shall find the chaff of authors blown away by the fame of Dr. Reason, and nothing but rational truths left for the ingenious to feed upon.

Lastly. To avoid blotting paper with one thing many times, and also to ease your purses in the price of the book, and withal to make you studious in physic; you have at the latter end of the book, the way of preserving all herbs either in juice, conserve, oil, ointment or plaister, electuary, pills, or troches.

AGRIMONY

Descript.] This has divers long leaves (some greater, some smaller) set upon a stalk, all of them dented about the edges, green above, and greyish underneath, and a little hairy withal. Among which arises up usually but one strong, round, hairy, brown stalk, two or three feet high, with smaller leaves set here and there upon it. At the top thereof grow many small yellow flowers, one above another, in long spikes; after which come rough heads of seed, hanging downwards, which will cleave to and stick upon garments, or any thing that shall rub against them. The knot is black, long, and somewhat woody, abiding many years, and shooting afresh every Spring; which root, though small, hath a reasonable good scent.

Place.] It grows upon banks, near the sides of hedges.

Time.] It flowers in July and August, the seed being ripe shortly after.

Government and virtues.] It is an herb under Jupiter, and the sign Cancer; and strengthens those parts under the planet and sign, and removes diseases in them by sympathy, and those under Saturn, Mars and Mercury by antipathy, if they happen in any part of the body governed by Jupiter, or under the signs Cancer, Sagitarius or Pisces, and therefore must needs be good for the gout, either used outwardly in oil or ointment, or inwardly in an electuary, or syrup, or concerted juice: for which see the latter end of this book.

It is of a cleansing and cutting faculty, without any manifest heat, moderately drying and binding. It opens and cleanses the liver, helps the jaundice, and is very beneficial to the bowels, healing all inward wounds, bruises, hurts, and other distempers. The decoction of the herb made with wine, and drank, is good against the biting and stinging of serpents, and helps them that make foul, troubled or bloody water.

This herb also helps the cholic, cleanses the breast, and rids away the cough. A draught of the decoction taken warm before the fit, first removes, and in time rids away the tertian or quartan agues. The leaves and seeds taken in wine, stays the bloody flux; outwardly applied, being stamped with old swine's grease, it helps old sores, cancers, and inveterate ulcers, and draws forth thorns and splinters of wood, nails, or any other such things gotten in the flesh. It helps to strengthen the members that be out of joint: and being bruised and applied, or the juice dropped in it, helps foul and imposthumed ears.

The distilled water of the herb is good to all the said purposes, either inward or outward, but a great deal weaker.

It is a most admirable remedy for such whose livers are annoyed either by heat or cold. The liver is the former of blood, and blood the nourisher of the body, and Agrimony a strengthener of the liver.

I cannot stand to give you a reason in every herb why it cures such diseases; but if you please to pursue my judgment in the herb Wormwood, you shall find them there, and it will be well worth your while to consider it in every herb, you shall find them true throughout the book.

WATER AGRIMONY

It is called in some countries, Water Hemp, Bastard Hemp, and Bastard Agrimony, Eupatorium, and Hepatorium, because it strengthens the liver.

Descript.] The root continues a long time, having many long slender strings. The stalk grows up about two feet high, sometimes higher. They are of a dark purple colour. The branches are many, growing at distances the one from the other, the one from the one side of the stalk, the other from the opposite point. The leaves are fringed, and much indented at the edges. The flowers grow at the top of the branches, of a brown yellow colour, spotted with black spots, having a substance within the midst of them like that of a Daisy. If you rub them between your fingers, they smell like rosin or cedar when it is burnt. The seeds are long, and easily stick to any woollen thing they touch.

Place.] They delight not in heat, and therefore they are not so frequently found in the Southern parts of England as in the northern, where they grow frequently. You may look for them in cold grounds, by ponds and ditches' sides, and also by running waters; sometimes you shall find them grow in the midst of waters.

Time.] They all flower in July or August, and the seed is ripe presently after.

Government and virtues.] It is a plant of Jupiter, as well as the other Agrimony, only this belongs to the celestial sign Cancer. It heals and dries, cuts and cleanses thick and tough humours of the breast, and for this I hold it inferior to but few herbs that grow. It helps the cachexia or evil disposition of the body, the dropsy and yellow-jaundice. It opens obstructions of the liver, mollifies the hardness of the spleen, being applied outwardly. It breaks imposthumes away inwardly. It is an excellent remedy for the third day ague. It provokes urine and the terms; it kills worms, and cleanses the body of sharp humours, which are the cause of itch and scabs; the herb being burnt, the smoke thereof drives away flies, wasps, &c. It strengthens the lungs exceedingly. Country people give it to their cattle when they are troubled with the cough, or broken-winded.

ALEHOOF, OR GROUND-IVY

Several counties give it different names, so that there is scarcely any herb growing of that bigness that has got so many. It is called Cat's-foot, Ground-ivy, Gill-go-by-ground, and Gill-creep-by-ground, Turnhoof, Haymaids, and Alehoof.

Descript.] This well known herb lies, spreads and creeps upon the ground, shoots forth roots, at the corners of tender jointed stalks, set with two round leaves at every joint somewhat hairy, crumpled and unevenly dented about the edges with round dents; at the joints likewise, with the leaves towards the end of the branches, come forth hollow, long flowers of a blueish purple colour, with small white spots upon the lips that hang down. The root is small with strings.

Place.] It is commonly found under hedges, and on the sides of ditches, under houses, or in shadowed lanes, and other waste grounds, in almost every part of this land.

Time.] They flower somewhat early, and abide a great while; the leaves continue green until Winter, and sometimes abide, except the Winter be very sharp and cold.

Government and virtues.] It is an herb of Venus, and therefore cures the diseases she causes by sympathy, and those of Mars by antipathy; you may usually find it all the year long except the year be extremely frosty; it is quick, sharp, and bitter in taste, and is thereby found to be hot and dry; a singular herb for all inward wounds, exulcerated lungs, or other parts, either by itself, or boiled with other the like herbs; and being drank, in a short time it eases all griping pains, windy and choleric humours in the stomach, spleen or belly; helps the yellow jaundice, by opening the stoppings of the gall and liver, and melancholy, by opening the stoppings of the spleen; expels venom or poison, and also the plague; it provokes urine and women's courses; the decoction of it in wine drank for some time together, procures ease to them that are troubled with the sciatica, or hip-gout: as also the gout in hands, knees or feet; if you put to the decoction some honey and a little burnt alum, it is excellently good to gargle any sore mouth or throat, and to wash the sores and ulcers in the privy parts of man or woman; it speedily helps green wounds, being bruised and bound thereto. The juice of it boiled with a little honey and verdigrease, doth wonderfully cleanse fistulas, ulcers, and stays the spreading or eating of cancers and ulcers; it helps the itch, scabs, wheals, and other breakings out in any part of the body. The juice of Celandine, Field-daisies, and Ground-ivy clarified, and a little fine sugar dissolved therein, and dropped into the eyes, is a sovereign remedy for all pains, redness, and watering of them; as also for the pin and web, skins and films growing over the sight, it helps beasts as well as men. The juice dropped into the ears, wonderfully helps the noise and singing of them, and helps the hearing which is decayed. It is good to tun up with new drink, for it will clarify it in a night, that it will be the fitter to be drank the next morning; or if any drink be thick with removing, or any other accident, it will do the like in a few hours.

ALEXANDER

It is called Alisander, Horse-parsley, and Wild-parsley, and the Black Pot-herb; the seed of it is that which is usually sold in apothecaries' shops for Macedonian Parsley-seed.

Descript.] It is usually sown in all the gardens in Europe, and so well known, that it needs no farther description.

Time.] It flowers in June and July; the seed is ripe in August.

Government and virtues.] It is an herb of Jupiter, and therefore friendly to nature, for it warms a cold stomach, and opens a stoppage of the liver and spleen; it is good to move women's courses, to expel the afterbirth, to break wind, to provoke urine, and helps the stranguary; and these things the seeds will do likewise. If either of

them be boiled in wine, or being bruised and taken in wine, is also
effectual against the biting of serpents. And you know what
Alexander pottage is good for, that you may no longer eat it out of
ignorance but out of knowledge.

THE BLACK ALDER-TREE

Descript.] This tree seldom grows to any great bigness but for
the most part abideth like a hedge-bush, or a tree spreading its
branches, the woods of the body being white, and a dark red colet
or heart; the outward bark is of a blackish colour, with many
whitish spots therein; but the inner bark next the wood is yellow,
which being chewed, will turn the spittle into a saffron colour. The
leaves are somewhat like those of an ordinary Alder-tree, or the
Female Cornet, or Dogberry-tree, called in Sussex Dog-wood, but
blacker, and not so long. The flowers are white, coming forth
with the leaves at the joints, which turn into small round berries,
first green, afterwards red, but blackish when they are thorough
ripe, divided, as it were, into two parts, wherein is contained two
small round and flat seeds. The root runneth not deep into the
ground, but spreads rather under the upper crust of the earth.

Place.] This tree or shrub may be found plentifully in St. John's
Wood by Hornsey, and the woods upon Hampstead Heath; as also
a wood called the Old Park, in Barcomb, in Essex, near the brook's
sides.

Time.] It flowers in May, and the berries are ripe in September.

Government and virtues.] It is a tree of Venus, and perhaps under
the celestial sign Cancer. The inner yellow bark hereof purges
downwards both choler and phlegm, and the watery humours of
such that have the dropsy, and strengthens the inward parts again
by binding. If the bark hereof be boiled with Agrimony, Wormwood, Dodder, Hops, and some Fennel, with Smallage, Endive,
and Succory-roots, and a reasonable draught taken every morning
for some time together, it is very effectual against the jaundice,
dropsy, and the evil disposition of the body, especially if some
suitable purging medicines have been taken before, to void the
grosser excrements. It purges and strengthens the liver and spleen,
cleansing them from such evil humours and hardness as they are
afflicted with. It is to be understood that these things are per-
formed by the dried bark; for the fresh green bark taken inwardly
provokes strong vomitings, pains in the stomach, and gripings in
the belly; yet if the decoction may stand and settle two or three days,
until the yellow colour be changed black, it will not work so strongly
as before, but will strengthen the stomach, and procure an appetite

to meat. The outward bark contrariwise doth bind the body, and is helpful for all lasks and fluxes thereof, but this also must be dried first, whereby it will work the better. The inner bark thereof boiled in vinegar is an approved remedy to kill lice, to cure the itch, and take away scabs, by drying them up in a short time. It is singularly good to wash the teeth, to take away the pains, to fasten those that are loose, to cleanse them, and to keep them sound. The leaves are good fodder for kine, to make them give more milk.

If in the Spring-time you use the herbs before mentioned, and will take but a handful of each of them, and to them add an handful of Elder buds, and having bruised them all, boil them in a gallon of ordinary beer, when it is new; and having boiled them half an hour, add to this three gallons more, and let them work together, and drink a draught of it every morning, half a pint or thereabouts; it is an excellent purge for the Spring, to consume the phlegmatic quality the Winter hath left behind it, and withal to keep your body in health, and consume those evil humours which the heat of Summer will readily stir up. Esteem it as a jewel.

THE COMMON ALDER-TREE

Descript.] This grows to a reasonable height, and spreads much if it like the place. It is so generally known to country people, that I conceive it needless to tell that which is no news.

Place and Time.] It delights to grow in moist woods, and watery places; flowering in April or May, and yielding ripe seed in September.

Government and virtues.] It is a tree under the dominion of Venus, and of some watery sign or others, I suppose Pisces; and therefore the decoction, or distilled water of the leaves, is excellent against burnings and inflammations, either with wounds or without, to bathe the place grieved with, and especially for that inflammation in the breast, which the vulgar call an ague.

If you cannot get the leaves (as in Winter it is impossible) make use of the bark in the same manner.

The leaves and bark of the Alder-tree are cooling, drying, and binding. The fresh leaves, laid upon swellings, dissolve them, and stay the inflammation. The leaves put under the bare feet galled with travelling, are a great refreshing to them. The said leaves, gathered while the morning dew is on them, and brought into a chamber troubled with fleas, will gather them thereunto, which being suddenly cast out, will rid the chamber of those troublesome bedfellows.

ANGELICA

To write a description of that which is so well known to be growing almost in every garden, I suppose is altogether needless; yet for its virtue it is of admirable use.

In time of Heathenism, when men had found out any excellent herb, they dedicated it to their gods; as the bay-tree to Apollo, the Oak to Jupiter, the Vine to Bacchus, the Poplar to Hercules. These the idolators following as the Patriarchs they dedicate to their Saints; as our Lady's Thistle to the Blessed Virgin, St. John's Wort to St. John and another Wort to St. Peter, &c. Our physicians must imitate like apes (though they cannot come off half so cleverly) for they blasphemously call Phansies or Heartsease, *an herb of the Trinity*, because it is of three colours; and a certain ointment, *an ointment of the Apostles*, because it consists of twelve ingredients. Alas I am sorry for their folly, and grieved at their blasphemy. God send them wisdom the rest of their age, for they have their share of ignorance already. Oh! Why must ours be blasphemous, because the Heathens and infidels were idolatrous? Certainly they have read so much in old rusty authors, that they have lost all their divinity; for unless it were amongst the Ranters, I never read or heard of such blasphemy. The Heathens and infidels were bad, and ours worse; the idolators give idolatrous names to herbs for their virtues sake, not for their fair looks; and therefore some called this an herb of the *Holy Ghost*; others, more moderate, called it Angelica, because of its angelical virtues, and that name it retains still, and all nations follow it so near as their dialect will permit.

Government and virtues.] It is an herb of the Sun in Leo; let it be gathered when he is there, the Moon applying to his good aspect; let it be gathered either in his hour, or in the hour of Jupiter, let Sol be angular; observe the like in gathering the herbs of other planets, and you may happen to do wonders. In all epidemical diseases caused by Saturn, that is as good a preservative as grows: It resists poison, by defending and comforting the heart, blood, and spirits; it doth the like against the plague and all epidemical diseases, if the root be taken in powder to the weight of half a dram at a time, with some good treacle in Carduus water, and the party thereupon laid to sweat in his bed; if treacle be not to be had take it alone in Carduus or Angelica-water. The stalks or roots candied and eaten fasting, are good preservatives in time of infection; and at other times to warm and comfort a cold stomach. The root also steeped in vinegar, and a little of that vinegar taken sometimes fasting, and the root smelled unto, is good for the same purpose. A water distilled from the root simply, as steeped in wine, and distilled in a glass, is much more effectual than the water of the leaves; and this water, drank two or three spoonfuls at a time, easeth all pains and torments coming of cold and wind, so that the body be not bound; and taken with some of the root in powder at the beginning, helpeth the pleurisy, as also all other diseases of the lungs and breast, as coughs, phthysic, and shortness of breath; and a syrup of the stalks do the like. It helps pains of the cholic, the stranguary and stoppage of the urine, procureth womens' courses, and expelleth the after-birth, openeth the stoppings of the liver and spleen, and briefly easeth and discusseth all windiness and inward swellings. The decoction drank before the fit of an ague, that they may sweat (if possible) before the fit comes, will, in two or three times taking, rid it quite away; it helps digestion and is a remedy for a surfeit. The juice or the water, being dropped into the eyes or ears, helps dimness of sight and deafness; the juice put into the hollow teeth, easeth their pains. The root in powder, made up into a plaster with a little pitch, and laid on the biting of mad dogs, or any other venomous creature, doth wonderfully help. The juice or the waters dropped, or tent wet therein, and put into filthy dead ulcers, or the powder of the root (in want of either) doth cleanse and cause them to heal quickly, by covering the naked bones with flesh; the distilled water applied to places pained with the gout, or sciatica, doth give a great deal of ease.

The wild Angelica is not so effectual as the garden; although it may be safely used to all the purposes aforesaid.

AMARANTHUS

BESIDES its common name, by which it is best known by the florists of our days, it is called Flower Gentle, Flower Velure Floramor, and Velvet Flower.

Descript.] It being a garden flower, and well known to every one that keeps it, I might forbear the description; yet, notwithstanding, because some desire it, I shall give it. It runs up with a stalk a cubit high, streaked, and somewhat reddish towards the root, but very smooth, divided towards the top with small branches, among which stand long broad leaves of a reddish green colour, slippery; the flowers are not properly flowers, but tuffs, very beautiful to behold, but of no smell, of reddish colour; if you bruise them, they yield juice of the same colour, being gathered, they keep their beauty a long time; the seed is of a shining black colour.

Time.] They continue in flower from August till the time the frost nips them.

Government and virtues.] It is under the dominion of Saturn, and is an excellent qualifier of the unruly actions and passions of Venus, though Mars also should join with her. The flowers, dried and beaten into powder, stop the terms in women, and so do almost all other red things. And by the icon, or image of every herb, the ancients at first found out their virtues. Modern writers laugh at them for it; but I wonder in my heart, how the virtues of herbs came at first to be known, if not by their signatures; the moderns have them from the writings of the ancients; the ancients had no writings to have them from: but to proceed. The flowers stop all fluxes of blood; whether in man or woman, bleeding either at the nose or wound. There is also a sort of Amaranthus that bears a white flower, which stops the whites in women, and the running of the reins in men, and is a most gallant antivenereal, and a singular remedy for the French pox.

ANEMONE

CALLED also Wind flower, because they say the flowers never open but when the wind blows. Pliny is my author; if it be not so, blame him. The seed also (if it bears any at all) flies away with the wind.

Place and Time.] They are sown usually in the gardens of the curious, and flower in the Spring-time. As for description I shall pass it, being well known to all those that sow them.

Government and virtues.] It is under the dominion of Mars, being supposed to be a kind of Crow-foot. The leaves provoke the terms mightily, being boiled, and the decoction drank. The body being bathed with the decoction of them, cures the leprosy. The leaves being stamped and the juice snuffed up in the nose, purges the head mightily; so does the root, being chewed in the mouth, for it procures much spitting, and brings away many watery and phlegmatic humours, and is therefore excellent for the lethargy. And when all is done, let physicians prate what they please, all the pills in the dispensatory purge not the head like to hot things held in the mouth. Being made into an ointment, and the eye-lids anointed with it, it helps inflammations of the eyes, whereby it is palpable, that every stronger draws its weaker like. The same ointment is excellently good to cleanse malignant and corroding ulcers.

GARDEN ARRACH

CALLED also Orach, and Arage; it is cultivated for domestic uses.

Descript.] It is so commonly known to every housewife, it were labour lost to describe it.

Time.] It flowers and seeds from June to the end of August.

Government and virtues.] It is under the government of the Moon; in quality cold and moist like unto her. It softens and loosens the body of man being eaten, and fortifies the expulsive faculty in him. The herb, whether it be bruised and applied to the throat, or boiled, and in like manner applied, it matters not much, it is excellently good for swellings in the throat: the best way, I suppose, is to boil it, apply the herb outwardly: the decoction of it, besides, is an excellent remedy for the yellow jaundice.

ARRACH, WILD AND STINKING

CALLED also Vulvaria, from that part of the body upon which the operation is most; also Dog's Arrach, Goat's Arrach, and Stinking Motherwort.

Descript.] This has small and almost round leaves, yet a little pointed and without dent or cut, of a dusky mealy colour, growing on the slender stalks and branches that spread on the ground, with small flowers set with the leaves, and small seeds succeeding like the rest, perishing yearly, and rising again with its own sowing. It smells like rotten fish, or something worse.

Place.] It grows usually upon dunghills.

Time.] They flower in June and July, and their seed is ripe quickly after.

Government and virtues.] Stinking Arrach is used as a remedy to women pained, and almost strangled with the mother, by smelling to it; but inwardly taken there is no better remedy under the moon for that disease. I would be large in commendation of this herb, were I but eloquent. It is an herb under the dominion of Venus, and under the sign Scorpio; it is common almost upon every dung-hill. The works of God are freely given to man, his medicines are common and cheap, and easily to be found. I commend it for an universal medicine for the womb, and such a medicine as will easily, safely, and speedily cure any disease thereof, as the fits of the mother, dislocation, or falling out thereof; cools the womb being over-heated. And let me tell you this, and I will tell you the truth, heat of the womb is one of the greatest causes of hard labour in child-birth. It makes barren women fruitful. It cleanseth the womb if it be foul, and strengthens it exceedingly; it provokes the terms if they be stopped, and stops them if they flow immoderately; you can desire no good to your womb, but this herb will affect it; therefore if you love children, if you love health, if you love ease, keep a syrup always by you, made of the juice of this herb, and sugar (or honey, if it be to cleanse the womb), and let such as be rich keep it for their poor neighbours; and bestow it as freely as I bestow my studies upon them, or else let them look to answer it another day, when the Lord shall come to make inquisition for blood.

ARCHANGEL

To put a gloss upon their practice, the physicians call a herb (which country people vulgarly know by the name of Dead Nettle) Archangel; whether they favour more of superstition or folly, I leave to the judicious reader. There is more curiosity than courtesy to my countrymen used by others in the explanation as well of the names, as description of this so well known herb; which that I may not also be guilty of, take this short description: first, of the Red Archangel. This is likewise called Bee Nettle.

Descript.] This has divers square stalks, somewhat hairy, at the joints whereof grow two sad green leaves dented about the edges, opposite to one another to the lowermost, upon long foot stalks, but without any toward the tops, which are somewhat round, yet pointed, and a little crumpled and hairy; round about the upper joints, where the leaves grow thick, are sundry gaping flowers of a pale reddish colour; after which come the seeds three or four in a husk. The root is small and thready, perishing every year; the whole plant hath a strong smell but not stinking.

White Archangel hath divers square stalks, none standing straight upward, but bending downward, whereon stand two leaves at a joint, larger and more pointed than the other, dented about the edges, and greener also, more like unto Nettle leaves, but not stinking, yet hairy. At the joints, with the leaves, stand larger and more open gaping white flowers, husks round about the stalks, but not with such a bush of leaves as flowers set in the top, as is on the other, wherein stand small roundish black seeds; the root is white, with many strings at it, not growing downward but lying under the upper crust of the earth, and abides many years increasing; this has not so strong a scent as the former.

Yellow Archangel is like the White in the stalks and leaves; but that the stalks are more straight and upright, and the joints with leaves are farther asunder, having longer leaves than the former, and the flowers a little larger and more gaping, of a fair yellow colour in most, in some paler. The roots are like the white, only they creep not so much under the ground.

Place.] They grow almost everywhere (unless it be in the middle of the street), the yellow most usually in the wet grounds of woods, and sometimes in the dryer, in divers counties of this nation.

Time.] They flower from the beginning of the Spring all the Summer long.

Government and virtues.] The Archangels are somewhat hot and drier than the stinging Nettles, and used with better success for the stopping and hardness of the spleen, than they, by using the decoction of the herb in wine, and afterwards applying the herb hot into the region of the spleen as a plaister, or the decoction with spunges. Flowers of the White Archangel are preserved or conserved to be used to stay the whites, and the flowers of the red to stay the reds in women. It makes the head merry, drives away melancholy, quickens the spirits, is good against quartan agues, stancheth bleeding at mouth and nose, if it be stamped and applied to the nape of the neck; the herb also bruised, and with some salt and vinegar and hog's-grease, laid upon a hard tumour or swelling, or that vulgarly called the king's evil, do help to dissolve or discuss them; and being in like manner applied, doth much allay the pains, and give ease to the gout, sciatica, and other pains of the joints and sinews. It is also very effectual to heal green wounds, and old ulcers; also to stay their fretting, gnawing, and spreading. It draws forth splinters, and such like things gotten into the flesh, and is very good against bruises and burnings. But the Yellow Archangel is most commended for old, filthy, corrupt sores and ulcers, yea although they grow to be hollow, and to dissolve tumours. The chief use of them is for women, it being a herb of Venus.

ARSSMART

THE hot Arssmart is called also Waterpepper, or Culrage. The mild Arssmart is called dead Arssmart Persicaria, or Peachwort, because the leaves are so like the leaves of a peach-tree; it is also called Plumbago.

Description of the mild.] This has broad leaves set at the great red joint of the stalks; with semicircular blackish marks on them, usually either bluish or whitish, with such like seed following. The root is long, with many strings thereat, perishing yearly; this has no sharp taste (as another sort has, which is quick and biting) but rather sour like sorrel, or else a little drying, or without taste.

Place.] It grows in watery places, ditches, and the like, which for the most part are dry in summer.

Time.] It flowers in June, and the seed is ripe in August.

Government and virtues.] As the virtue of both these is various, so is also their government; for that which is hot and biting, is under the dominion of Mars, but Saturn, challenges the other, as appears by that leaden coloured spot he hath placed upon the leaf.

It is of a cooling and drying quality, and very effectual for putrefied ulcers in man or beast, to kill worms, and cleanse the putrefied places. The juice thereof dropped in, or otherwise applied, consumes all colds, swellings, and dissolveth the congealed blood of bruises by strokes, falls, &c. A piece of the root, or some of the seeds bruised, and held to an aching tooth, takes away the pain. The leaves bruised and laid to the joint that has a felon thereon, takes it away. The juice destroys worms in the ears, being dropped into them; if the hot Arssmart be strewed in a chamber, it will soon kill all the fleas; and the herb or juice of the cold Arssmart, put to a horse or other cattle's sores, will drive away the fly in the hottest time of Summer; a good handful of the hot biting Arssmart put under a horse's saddle, will make him travel the better, although he were half tired before. The mild Arssmart is good against all imposthumes and inflammations at the beginning, and to heal green wounds.

All authors chop the virtues of both sorts of Arssmart together, as men chop herbs for the pot, when both of them are of contrary qualities. The hot Arssmart grows not so high or tall as the mild doth, but has many leaves of the colour of peach leaves, very seldom or never spotted; in other particulars it is like the former, but may easily be known from it, if you will but be pleased to break a leaf of it cross your tongue, for the hot will make your tongue to smart, but the cold will not. If you see them both together, you may easily distinguish them, because the mild hath far broader leaves.

ASARABACCA

Descript.] Asarabacca appears like an evergreen, keeping its leaves all the Winter, but putting forth new ones in the time of Spring. It has many heads rising from the roots, from whence come many smooth leaves, every one upon his foot stalks, which are rounder and bigger than Violet leaves, thicker also, and of a dark green shining colour on the upper side, and of a pale yellow green underneath, little or nothing dented about the edges, from among which rise small, round, hollow, brown green husks, upon short stalks, about an inch long, divided at the brims into five divisions, very like the cups or heads of the Henbane seed, but that they are smaller; and these be all the flower it carries, which are somewhat sweet, being smelled to, and wherein, when they are ripe, is contained small cornered rough seeds, very like the kernels or stones of grapes, or raisins. The roots are small and whitish, spreading divers ways in the ground, increasing into divers heads; but not running or creeping under the ground as some other creeping herbs do. They are somewhat sweet in smell, resembling Nardus, but more when they are dry than green; and of a sharp and not unpleasant taste.

Place.] It grows frequently in gardens.

Time.] They keep their leaves green all Winter; but shoot forth new in the Spring, and with them come forth those heads or flowers which give ripe seed about Mid-summer, or somewhat after.

Government and virtues.] It is a plant under the dominion of Mars, and therefore inimical to nature. This herb being drank, not only provokes vomiting, but purges downwards, and by urine also, purges both choler and phlegm: If you add to it some spikenard, with the whey of goat's milk, or honeyed water, it is made more strong, but it purges phlegm more manifestly than choler, and therefore does much help pains in the hips, and other parts; being boiled in whey, it wonderfully helps the obstructions of the liver and spleen, and therefore profitable for the dropsy and jaundice; being steeped in wine and drank, it helps those continual agues that come by the plenty of stubborn humours; an oil made thereof by setting in the sun, with some laudanum added to it, provokes sweating (the ridge of the back being anointed therewith), and thereby drives away the shaking fits of the ague. It will not abide any long boiling, for it loseth its chief strength thereby; nor much beating, for the finer powder provokes vomits and urine, and the coarser purgeth downwards.

The common use hereof is, to take the juice of five or seven leaves in a little drink to cause vomiting; the roots have also the same virtue, though they do not operate so forcibly; they are very effectual against the biting of serpents, and therefore are put as an ingredient both into Mithridite and Venice treacle. The leaves and roots being boiled in lye, and the head often washed therewith while it is warm, comforts the head and brain that is ill affected by taking cold, and helps the memory.

I shall desire ignorant people to forbear the use of the leaves; the roots purge more gently, and may prove beneficial to such as have cancers, or old putrefied ulcers, or fistulas upon their bodies, to take a dram of them in powder in a quarter of a pint of white wine in the morning. The truth is, I fancy purging and vomiting medicines as little as any man breathing doth, for they weaken nature, nor shall ever advise them to be used, unless upon urgent necessity. If a physician be nature's servant, it is his duty to strengthen his mistress as much as he can, and weaken her as little as may be.

ASPARAGUS, SPARAGUS, OR SPERAGE

Descript.] It rises up at first with divers white and green scaly heads, very brittle or easy to break while they are young, which afterwards rise up in very long and slender green stalks of the bigness of an ordinary riding wand, at the bottom of most, or bigger, or lesser, as the roots are of growth; on which are set divers branches of green leaves shorter and smaller than fennel to the top; at the joints whereof come forth small yellowish flowers, which turn into round berries, green at first and of an excellent red colour when they are ripe, showing like bead or coral, wherein are contained exceeding hard black seeds; the roots are dispersed from a spongeous head into many long, thick, and round strings, wherein is sucked much nourishment out of the ground, and increaseth plentifully thereby.

PRICKLY ASPARAGUS, OR SPERAGE

Descript.] This grows usually in gardens, and some of it grows wild in Appleton meadows in Gloucestershire, where the poor people gather the buds of young shoots, and sell them cheaper than our garden Asparagus is sold in London.

Time.] For the most part they flower, and bear their berries late in the year, or not at all, although they are housed in Winter.

Government and virtues.] They are both under the dominion of Jupiter. The young buds or branches boiled in ordinary broth, make the belly soluble and open, and boiled in white wine, provoke urine, being stopped, and is good against the stranguary or difficulty of making water; it expelleth the gravel and stone out of the kidneys, and helpeth pains in the reins. And boiled in white wine or vinegar, it is prevalent for them that have their arteries loosened, or are troubled with the hip-gout or sciatica. The decoction of the roots boiled in wine and taken, is good to clear the sight, and being held in the mouth easeth the toothache. The garden asparagus nourisheth more than the wild, yet hath it the same effects in all the aforementioned diseases. The decoction of the root in white wine, and the back and belly bathed therewith, or kneeling or lying down in the same, or sitting therein as a bath, has been found effectual against pains of the reins and bladder, pains of the mother and cholic, and generally against all pains that happen to the lower parts of the body, and no less effectual against stiff and benumbed sinews, or those that are shrunk by cramp and convulsions, and helps the sciatica.

ASH TREE

This is so well known, that time would be misspent in writing a description of it; therefore I shall only insist upon the virtues of it.

Government and virtues.] It is governed by the Sun: and the young tender tops, with the leaves, taken inwardly, and some of them outwardly applied, are singularly good against the bitings of viper, adder, or any other venomous beast; and the water distilled therefrom being taken, a small quantity every morning fasting, is a singular medicine for those that are subject to dropsy, or to abate the greatness of those that are too gross or fat. The decoction of the leaves in white wine helps to break the stone, and expel it, and cures the jaundice. The ashes of the bark of the Ash made into lye, and those heads bathed therewith which are leprous, scabby, or scald, they are thereby cured. The kernels within the husks, commonly called Ashen Keys, prevail against stitches and pains in the sides, proceeding of wind, and voideth away the stone by provoking urine.

I can justly except against none of all this, save only the first, *viz.* That Ash-tree tops and leaves are good against the bitings of serpents and vipers. I suppose this had its rise from Gerrard or Pliny, both which hold that there is such an antipathy between an adder and an Ash-tree, that if an adder be encompassed round with Ash-tree leaves, she will sooner run through the fire than through the leaves. The contrary to which is the truth, as both my eyes are witnesses. The rest are virtues something likely, only if it be in Winter when you cannot get the leaves, you may safely use the bark instead of them. The keys you may easily keep all the year, gathering them when they are ripe.

AVENS, CALLED ALSO COLEWORT, AND HERB BONET

Descript.] The ordinary Avens hath many long, rough, dark green, winged leaves, rising from the root, every one made of many leaves set on each side of the middle rib, the largest three whereof grow at the end, and are snipped or dented round about the edges; the other being small pieces, sometimes two and sometimes four, standing on each side of the middle rib underneath them. Among which do rise up divers rough or hairy stalks about two feet high, branching forth with leaves at every joint not so long as those below, but almost as much cut in on the edges, some into three parts, some into more. On the tops of the branches stand small, pale, yellow flowers consisting of five leaves, like the flowers of Cinquefoil, but large, in the middle whereof stand a small green herb, which when the flower is fallen, grows to be round, being made of many long greenish purple seeds, (like grains) which will stick upon your clothes. The root consists of many brownish strings or fibres, smelling somewhat like unto cloves, especially those which grow in the higher, hotter, and drier grounds, and in free and clear air.

Place.] They grow wild in many places under hedge's sides, and by the pathways in fields; yet they rather delight to grow in shadowy than sunny places.

Time.] They flower in May or June for the most part, and their seed is ripe in July at the farthest.

Government and virtues.] It is governed by Jupiter, and that gives hopes of a wholesome healthful herb. It is good for the diseases of the chest or breast, for pains, and stiches in the side, and to expel crude and raw humours from the belly and stomach, by the sweet savour and warming quality. It dissolves the inward congealed blood happening by falls or bruises, and the spitting of blood, if the roots, either green or dry, be boiled in wine and drank; as also all manner of inward wounds or outward, if washed or bathed therewith. The decoction also being drank, comforts the heart, and strengthens the stomach and a cold brain, and therefore is good in the spring time to open obstructions of the liver, and helps the wind cholic; it also helps those that have fluxes, or are bursten, or have a rupture; it takes away spots or marks in the face, being washed therewith. The juice of the fresh root, or powder of the dried root, has the same effect with the decoction. The root in the Spring-time steeped in wine, gives it a delicate savour and taste, and being drank fasting every morning, comforts the heart, and is a good preservative against the plague, or any other poison. It helps indigestion, and warms a cold stomach, and opens obstructions of the liver and spleen.

It is very safe: you need have no dose prescribed; and is very fit to be kept in every body's house.

BALM

THIS herb is so well known to be an inhabitant almost in every garden, that I shall not need to write any discription thereof, although its virtues, which are many, may not be omitted.

Government and virtues.] It is an herb of Jupiter, and under Cancer, and strengthens nature much in all its actions. Let a syrup made with the juice of it and sugar (as you shall be taught at the latter end of this book) be kept in every gentlewoman's house to relieve the weak stomachs and sick bodies of their poor sickly neighbours; as also the herb kept dry in the house, that so with other convenient simples, you may make it into an electuary with

honey, according as the disease is you shall be taught at the latter
end of my book. The Arabian physicians have extolled the virtues
thereof to the skies; although the Greeks thought it not worth
mentioning. Seraphio says, it causes the mind and heart to become
merry, and revives the heart, faintings and swoonings, especially
of such who are overtaken in sleep, and drives away all troublesome
cares and thoughts out of the mind, arising from melancholy or
black choler; which Avicen also confirms. It is very good to help
digestion, and open obstructions of the brain, and hath so much
purging quality in it (saith Avicen) as to expel those melancholy
vapours from the spirits and blood which are in the heart and
arteries, although it cannot do so in other parts of the body. Dioscorides says, that the leaves steeped in wine, and the wine drank,
and the leaves externally applied, is a remedy against the stings of a
scorpion, and the bitings of mad dogs; and commends the decoction
thereof for women to bathe or sit in to procure their courses; it is
good to wash aching teeth therewith, and profitable for those that
have the bloody flux. The leaves also, with a little nitre taken in
drink, are good against the surfeit of mushrooms, helps the griping
pains of the belly; and being made into an electuary, it is good for
them that cannot fetch their breath. Used with salt, it takes away
wens, kernels, or hard swelling in the flesh or throat; it cleanses foul
sores, and eases pains of the gout. It is good for the liver and spleen.
A tansy or caudle made with eggs, and juice thereof while it is
young, putting to it some sugar and rosewater, is good for a woman
in child-birth, when the after-birth is not thoroughly voided, and
for their faintings upon or in their sore travail. The herb bruised
and boiled in a little wine and oil, and laid warm on a boil, will ripen
it, and break it.

BARBERRY

The shrub is so well known by every boy or girl that has but
attained to the age of seven years, that it needs no description.

Government and virtues.] Mars owns the shrub, and presents it
to the use of my countrymen to purge their bodies of choler. The
inner rind of the Barberry-tree boiled in white wine, and a quarter
of a pint drank each morning, is an excellent remedy to cleanse the
body of choleric humours, and free it from such diseases as choler
causes, such as scabs, itch, tetters, ringworms, yellow jaundice,
boils, &c. It is excellent for hot agues, burnings, scaldings, heat
of the blood, heat of the liver, bloody-flux; for the berries are as
good as the bark, and more pleasing: they get a man a good stomach
to his victuals, by strengthening the attractive faculty which is

under Mars. The hair washed with the lye made of the tree and water, will make it turn yellow, *viz.* of Mars' own colour. The fruit and rind of the shrub, the flowers of broom and of heath, or furz, cleanse the body of choler by sympathy, as the flowers, leaves, and bark of the peach tree do by antipathy, because these are under Mars, that under Venus.

BARLEY

THE continual usefulness hereof hath made all in general so acquainted herewith that it is altogether needless to describe it, several kinds hereof plentifully growing, being yearly sown in this land. The virtues thereof take as follow.

Government and virtues.] It is a notable plant of Saturn: if you view diligently its effects by sympathy and antipathy, you may easily perceive a reason of them, as also why barley bread is so unwholesome for melancholy people. Barley in all the parts and compositions thereof (except malt) is more cooling than wheat, and a little cleansing. And all the preparations thereof, as barley-water and other things made thereof, give great nourishment to persons troubled with fevers, agues, and heats in the stomach. A poultice made of barley meal or flour boiled in vinegar and honey, and a few dry figs put into them, dissolves all imposthumes, and assuages inflammations, being thereto applied. And being boiled with melilot and camomile-flowers, and some linseed, fenugreek, and rue in powder, and applied warm, it eases pains in side and stomach, and windiness of the spleen. The meal of barley and fleawort boiled in water, and made a poultice with honey and oil of lilies applied warm, cures swellings under the ears, throat, neck, and such like; and a plaister made thereof with tar, with sharp vinegar into a poultice, and laid on hot, helps the leprosy; being boiled in red wine with pomegranate rinds and myrtles, stays the lask or other flux of the belly; boiled with vinegar and quince, it eases the pains of the gout; barley-flour, white salt, honey, and vinegar mingled together, takes away the itch speedily and certainly. The water distilled from the green barley in the end of May, is very good for those that have defluctions of humours fallen into their eyes, and eases the pain, being dropped into them; or white bread steeped therein, and bound on the eyes, does the same.

GARDEN BAZIL, OR SWEET BAZIL

Descript.] The greater of Ordinary Bazil rises up usually with one upright stalk, diversive branching forth on all sides, with two leaves at every joint, which are somewhat broad and round, yet pointed, of a pale green colour, but fresh; a little snipped about the edges, and of a strong healthy scent. The flowers are small and white, and standing at the tops of the branches, with two small leaves at the joints, in some places green, in others brown, after which come black seed. The root perishes at the approach of Winter, and therefore must be new sown every year.

Place.] It grows in gardens.

Time.] It must be sowed late, and flowers in the heart of Summer, being a very tender plant.

Government and virtues.] This is the herb which all authors are together by the ears about, and rail at one another (like lawyers). Galen and Dioscorides hold it not fit to be taken inwardly; and Chrysippus rails at it with downright Billingsgate rhetoric; Pliny, and the Arabian physicians defend it.

For my own part, I presently found that speech true:

Non nostrium inter nos tantas componere lites

And away to Dr. Reason went I, who told me it was an herb of Mars, and under the Scorpion, and perhaps therefore called Basilicon; and it is no marvel if it carry a kind of virulent quality with it. Being applied to the place bitten by venomous beasts, or stung by a wasp or hornet, it speedily draws the poison to it, *Every like draws his like*. Mizaldus affirms, that, being laid to rot in horse-dung, it will breed venomous beasts. Hilarius, a French physician, affirms upon his own knowledge, that an acquaintance of his, by common smelling to it, had a scorpion bred in his brain. Something is the matter; this herb and rue will not grow together, no, nor near one another: and we know rue is as great an enemy to poison as any that grows.

To conclude; It expels both birth and after-birth; and as it helps the deficiency of Venus in one kind, so it spoils all her actions in another. I dare write no more of it.

THE BAY TREE

THIS is so well known that it needs no description: I shall therefore only write the virtues thereof, which are many.

Government and virtues.] I shall but only add a word or two to what my friend has written, *viz.*, that it is a tree of the sun, and under the celestial sign Leo, and resists witchcraft very potently, as also all the evils old Saturn can do to the body of man, and they are not a few; for it is the speech of one, and I am mistaken if it were not Mizaldus, that neither witch nor devil, thunder nor lightning, will hurt a man in the place where a Bay-tree is. Galen said, that the leaves or bark do dry and heal very much, and the berries more than the leaves; the bark of the root is less sharp and hot, but more bitter, and hath some astriction withal whereby it is effectual to break the stone, and good to open obstructions of the liver, spleen, and other inward parts, which bring the jaundice, dropsy, &c. The berries are very effectual against all poison of venomous creatures, and the sting of wasps and bees; as also against the pestilence, or other infectious diseases, and therefore put into sundry treacles for that purpose; they likwise procure women's courses, and seven of them given to women in sore travail of child-birth, do cause a speedy delivery, and expel the after-birth, and therefore not to be taken by such as have not gone out their time, lest they procure abortion, or cause labour too soon. They wonder-fully help all cold and rheumatic distillations from the brain to the eyes, lungs or other parts; and being made into an electuary with honey, do help the consumption, old coughs, shortness of breath, and thin rheums; as also the megrim. They mightily expel the wind, and provoke urine; helps the mother, and kill the worms. The leaves also work the like effect. A bath of the decoction of leaves and berries, is singularly good for women to sit in, that are troubled with the mother, or the diseases thereof, or the stoppings of their courses, or for the diseases of the bladder, pains in the bowels by wind and stoppage of the urine. A decoction likewise of equal parts of Bay-berries, cummin seed, hyssop, origanum, and euphorbium, with some honey, and the head bathed therewith, wonderfully helps distillations and rheums, and settles the pallate of the mouth into its place. The oil made of the berries is very comfortable in all cold griefs of the joints, nerves, arteries, stomach, belly, or womb, and helps palsies, convulsions, cramp, aches, tremblings, and numbness in any part, weariness also, and pains that come by sore travelling. All griefs and pains proceeding from wind, either in the head, stomach, back, belly, or womb, by anointing the parts affected there-with. And pains in the ears are also cured by dropping in some of the oil, or by receiving into the ears the fume of the decoction of the berries through a funnel. The oil takes away the marks of the skin and flesh by bruises, falls, &c. and dissolves the congealed blood in them. It helps also the itch, scabs, and weals in the skin.

BEANS

Both the garden and field beans are so well known, that it saves me the labour of writing any description of them. The virtues follow.

Government and virtues.] They are plants of Venus, and the distilled water of the flower of garden beans is good to clean the face and skin from spots and wrinkles, and the meal or flour of them, or the small beans doth the same. The water distilled from the green husk, is held to be very effectual against the stone, and to provoke urine. Bean flour is used in poultices to assuage inflammations arising from wounds, and the swelling of women's breasts caused by the curdling of their milk, and represses their milk. Flour of beans and Fenugreek mixed with honey, and applied to felons, boils, bruises, or blue marks by blows, or the imposthumes in the kernels of the ears, helps them all, and with Rose leaves, Frankincense and the white of an egg, being applied to the eyes, helps them that are swollen or do water, or have received any blow upon them, if used with wine. If a bean be parted in two, the skin being taken away, and laid on the place where the leech hath been set that bleeds too much, stays the bleeding. Bean flour boiled to a poultice with wine and vinegar, and some oil put thereto, eases both pains and swelling of the privities. The husk boiled in water to the consumption of a third part thereof, stays a lask; and the ashes of the husks, made up with old hog's grease, helps the old pains, contusions, and wounds of the sinews, the sciatica and gout. The field beans have all the aforementioned virtues as the garden beans.

Beans eaten are extremely windy meat; but if after the Dutch fashion, when they are half boiled you husk them and then stew them (I cannot tell you how, for I never was a cook in all my life), they are wholesome food.

FRENCH BEANS

Descript.] This French or kidney Bean arises at first but with one stalk, which afterwards divides itself into many arms or branches, but all so weak that if they be not sustained with sticks or poles, they will be fruitless upon the ground. At several places of these branches grow foot stalks, each with three broad round and pointed green leaves at the end of them; towards the top comes forth divers flowers made like to pease blossoms, of the same colour for the most part that the fruit will be of, that is to say, white, yellow, red, blackish, or of a deep purple, but white is the most usual; after which come long and slender flat pods, some crooked, some straight, with a string running down the back thereof, wherein is flattish round fruit made like a kidney; the root long, spreads with many strings annexed to it, and perishes every year.

There is another sort of French bean commonly growing with us in this land, which is called the Scarlet flower Bean.

This rises with sundry branches as the other, but runs higher, to the length of hop-poles, about which they grow twining, but turning contrary to the sun, having footstalks with three leaves on each, as on the others; the flowers also are like the other, and of a most orient scarlet colour. The Beans are larger than the ordinary kind, of a dead purple colour turning black when ripe and dry; the root perishes in Winter.

Government and virtues.] These also belong to Dame Venus, and being dried and beat to powder, are as great strengtheners of the kidneys as any are; neither is there a better remedy than it; a dram at a time taken in white wine to prevent the stone, or to cleanse the kidneys of gravel or stoppage. The ordinary French Beans are of an easy digestion; they move the belly, provoke urine, enlarge the breast that is straightened with shortness of breath, engender sperm, and incite to venery. And the scarlet coloured Beans, in regard of the glorious beauty of their colour, being set near a quick-set hedge, will much adorn the same, by climbing up thereon, so that they may be discerned a great way, not without admiration of the beholders at a distance. But they will go near to kill the quick-sets by cloathing them in scarlet.

LADIES BED-STRAW

BESIDES the common name above written, it is called Cheese-Rennet, because it performs the same office, as also Gailion, Petti-mugget, and Maiden-hair; and by some Wild Rosemary.

Descript.] This rises up with divers small brown, and square upright stalks, a yard high or more; sometimes branches forth into divers parts, full of joints and with divers very fine small leaves at every one of them, little or nothing rough at all; at the tops of the branches grow many long tufts or branches of yellow flowers very thick set together, from the several joints which consist of four leaves apiece, which smell somewhat strong, but not unpleasant. The seed is small and black like poppy seed, two for the most part joined together. The root is reddish, with many small threads fastened to it, which take strong hold of the ground, and creep a little: and the branches leaning a little down to the ground, take root at the joints thereof, whereby it is easily increased.

There is another sort of Ladies Bedstraw growing frequently in England, which bears white flowers as the other doth yellow; but the branches of this are so weak, that unless it be sustained by the hedges, or other things near which it grows, it will lie down on the ground; the leaves a little bigger than the former, and the flowers not so plentiful as these; and the root hereof is also thready and abiding.

Place.] They grow in meadow and pastures both wet and dry, and by the hedges.

Time.] They flower in May for the most part, and the seed is ripe in July and August.

Government and virtues.] They are both herbs of Venus, and therefore strengthening the parts both internal and external, which she rules. The decoction of the former of those being drank, is good to fret and break the stone, provoke the urine, stays inward bleeding and heals inward wounds. The herb or flower bruised and put into the nostrils, stays their bleeding likewise. The flowers and herbs being made into an oil, by being set in the sun, and changed after it has stood ten or twelve days; or into an ointment being boiled in *Axunga*, or sallad oil, with some wax melted therein, after it is strained; either the oil made thereof, or the ointment, do help burnings with fire, or scalding with water. The same also, or the decoction of the herb and flower, is good to bathe the feet of travellers and lacquies, whose long running causes weariness and stiffness in the sinews and joints. If the decoction be used warm, and the joints afterwards anointed with ointment, it helps the dry scab, and the itch in children; and the herb with the white flower is also very good for the sinews, arteries, and joints, to comfort and strengthen them after travel, cold, and pains.

BEETS

OF Beets there are two sorts, which are best known generally, and whereof I shall principally treat at this time, *viz.* the white and red Beets and their virtues.

Descript.] The common white beet has many great leaves next the ground, somewhat large and of a whitish green colour. The stalk is great, strong, and ribbed, bearing great store of leaves upon it, almost to the very top of it. The flowers grow in very long tufts, small at the end, and turning down their heads, which are small, pale greenish-yellow buds, giving cornered prickly seed. The root is great, long, and hard, and when it has given seed is of no use at all.

The common red Beet differs not from the white, but only it is less, and the leaves and the roots are somewhat red; the leaves are differently red, some only with red stalks or veins; some of a fresh red, and others of a dark red. The root thereof is red, spungy, and not used to be eaten.

Government and virtues.] The government of these two sorts of Beets are far different; the red Beet being under Saturn and the white under Jupiter; therefore take the virtues of them apart, each by itself. The white Beet much loosens the belly, and is of a cleansing, digesting quality, and provokes urine. The juice of it opens obstructions both of the liver and spleen, and is good for the headache and swimmings therein, and turnings of the brain; and is effectual also against all venomous creatures; and applied to the temples, stays inflammations of the eyes; it helps burnings, being used with oil, and with a little alum put to it, is good for St. Anthony's fire. It is good for all wheals, pushes, blisters, and blains in the skin: the herb boiled, and laid upon chilblains or kibes, helps them. The decoction thereof in water and some vinegar, heals the itch, if bathed therewith; and cleanses the head of dandruff, scurf and dry scabs, and does much good for fretting and running sores, ulcers, and cankers in the head, legs, or other parts, and is much commended against baldness and shedding the hair.

The red Beet is good to stay the bloody-flux, women's courses, and the whites, and to help the yellow jaundice; the juice of the root put into the nostrils, purges the head, helps the noise in the ears, and the tooth-ache; the juice snuffed up the nose, helps a stinking breath, if the cause lie in the nose, as many times it does, if any bruise has been there: as also want of smell coming that way.

WATER BETONY

CALLED also Brown-wort, and in Yorkshire, Bishop's-leaves.

Descript.] First, of the Water Betony, which rises up with square, hard, greenish stalks, sometimes brown, set with broad dark green leaves dented about the edges with notches somewhat resembling the leaves of the Wood Betony, but much larger too, for the most part set at a joint. The flowers are many, set at the tops of the stalks and branches, being round bellied and open at the brims, and divided into two parts, the uppermost being like a hood, and the lowermost like a hip hanging down, of a dark red colour, which passing, there comes in their places small round heads with small points at the ends, wherein lie small and brownish seeds; the root is a thick bush of strings and shreds, growing from the head.

Place.] It grows by the ditch side, brooks and other watercourses, generally through this land, and is seldom found far from the water-side.

Time.] It flowers about July, and the seed is ripe in August.

Government and virtues.] Water Betony is an herb of Jupiter in Cancer, and is appropriated more to wounds and hurts in the breast than Wood Betony, which follows. It is an excellent remedy for sick hogs. It is of a cleansing quality. The leaves bruised and applied are effectual for all old and filthy ulcers; and especially if the juice of the leaves be boiled with a little honey, and dipped therein, and the sores dressed therewith; as also for bruises and hurts, whether inward or outward. The distilled water of the leaves is used for the same purpose; as also to bathe the face and hands spotted or blemished, or discoloured by sun burning.

I confess I do not much fancy distilled waters, I mean such waters as are distilled cold; some virtues of the herb they may haply have (it were a strange thing else;) but this I am confident of, that being distilled in a pewter still, as the vulgar and apish fashion is, both chemical oil and salt is left behind unless you burn them, and then all is spoiled, water and all, which was good for as little as can be, by such a distillation.

WOOD BETONY

Descript.] Common or Wood Betony has many leaves rising from the root, which are somewhat broad and round at the end, roundly dented about the edges, standing upon long foot stalks, from among which rise up small, square, slender, but upright hairy stalks, with some leaves thereon to a piece at the joints, smaller than the lower, whereon are set several spiked heads of flowers like Lavender, but thicker and shorter for the most part, and of a reddish or purple colour, spotted with white spots both in the upper and lower part. The seeds being contained within the husks that hold the flowers, are blackish, somewhat long and uneven. The roots are many white thready strings: the stalk perishes, but the roots with some leaves thereon, abide all the Winter. The whole plant is somewhat small.

Place.] It grows frequently in woods, and delights in shady places.

Time.] And it flowers in July; after which the seed is quickly ripe, yet in its prime in May.

Government and virtues.] The herb is appropriated to the planet Jupiter, and the sign Aries. Antonius Musa, physician to the Emperor Augustus Cæsar, wrote a peculiar book of the virtues of this herb; and among other virtues saith of it, that it preserves the liver and bodies of men from the danger of epidemical diseases, and from witchcraft also; it helps those that loath and cannot digest their meat, those that have weak stomachs and sour belchings, or continual rising in their stomachs, using it familiarly either green or dry; either the herb, or root, or the flowers, in broth, drink, or meat, or made into conserve, syrup, water, electuary, or powder, as every one may best frame themselves unto, or as the time and season requires; taken any of the aforesaid ways, it helps the jaundice, falling sickness, the palsy, convulsions, or shrinking of the sinews, the gout and those that are inclined to dropsy, those that have continual pains in their heads, although it turn to phrensy. The powder mixed with pure honey is no less available for all sorts of coughs or colds, wheesing, or shortness of breath, distillations of thin rheum upon the lungs, which causes consumptions. The decoction made with Mead, and a little Pennyroyal, is good for those that are troubled with putrid agues, whether quotidian, tertian, or quartan, and to draw down and evacuate the blood and humours, that by falling into the eyes, do hinder the sight; the decoction thereof made in wine and taken, kills the worms in the belly, opens obstructions both of the spleen and liver; cures stitches, and pains in the back and sides, the torments and griping pains in the bowels, and the wind cholic; and mixed with honey purges the belly, helps to bring down women's courses, and is of special use for those that are troubled with the falling down of the mother, and pains thereof, and causes an easy and speedy delivery of women in child-birth. It helps also to break and expel the stone, either in the bladder or kidneys. The decoction with wine gargled in the mouth, eases the tooth-ache. It is commended against the stinging and biting of venomous serpents, or mad dogs, being used inwardly and applied outwardly to the place. A dram of the powder of Betony taken with a little honey in some vinegar, does wonderfully refresh those that are over wearied by travelling. It stays bleeding at the mouth or nose, and helps those that void or spit blood, and those that are bursten or have a rupture, and is good for such as are bruised by any fall or otherwise. The green herb bruised, or the juice applied to any inward hurt, or outward green wound in the head or body, will quickly heal and close it up; as also any vein or sinews that are cut, and will draw forth any broken bone or splinter, thorn or other things got into the flesh. It is no less profitable for old sores or filthy ulcers, yea, tho' they be fistulous and hollow. But some do advise to put a little salt for this purpose, being applied with a little hog's lard, it helps a plague sore, and other boils and pushes. The fumes of the decoction while it is warm, received by a funnel into the ears, eases the pains of them, destroys the worms and cures the running sores in them. The juice dropped into them does the same. The root of Betony is displeasing both to the taste and stomach, whereas the leaves and flowers, by their sweet and spicy taste, are comfortable both to meat and medicine.

These are some of the many virtues Anthony Muse, an expert physician (for it was not the practice of Octavius Cesar to keep fools about him), appropriates to Betony; it is a very precious herb, that is certain, and most fitting to be kept in a man's house, both in syrup, conserve, oil, ointment and plaister. The flowers are usually conserved.

THE BEECH TREE

In treating of this tree, you must understand, that I mean the green mast Beech, which is by way of distinction from that other small rough sort, called in Sussex the smaller Beech, but in Essex Hornbeam.

I suppose it is needless to describe it, being already too well known to my countrymen.

Place.] It grows in woods amongst oaks and other trees, and in parks, forests, and chases, to feed deer; and in other places to fatten swine.

Time.] It blooms in the end of April, or beginning of May, for the most part, and the fruit is ripe in September.

Government and virtues.] It is a plant of Saturn, and therefore performs his qualities and proportion in these operations. The leaves of the Beech tree are cooling and binding, and therefore good to be applied to hot swellings to discuss them; the nuts do much nourish such beasts as feed thereon. The water that is found in the hollow places of decaying Beeches will cure both man and beast of any scurf, or running tetters, if they be washed therewith; you may boil the leaves into a poultice, or make an ointment of them when time of year serves.

BILBERRIES, CALLED BY SOME WHORTS, AND WHORTLE-BERRIES

Descript.] Of these I shall only speak of two sorts which are common in England, viz. the black and red berries. And first of the black.

The small bush creeps along upon the ground, scarcely rising half a yard high, with divers small green leaves set in the green branches, not always one against the other, and a little dented about the edges. At the foot of the leaves come forth small, hollow, pale, bluish coloured flowers, the brims ending at five points, with a reddish thread in the middle, which pass into small round berries of the bigness and colour of juniper berries, but of a purple, sweetish sharp taste; the juice of them gives a purplish colour in their hands and lips that eat and handle them, especially if they break them.

The root grows aslope under ground, shooting forth in sundry places as it creeps. This loses its leaves in Winter.

The Red Bilberry, or Whortle-Bush, rises up like the former, having sundry hard leaves, like the Box-tree leaves, green and round pointed, standing on the several branches, at the top whereof only, and not from the sides, as in the former, come forth divers round, reddish, sappy berries, when they are ripe, of a sharp taste. The root runs in the ground, as in the former, but the leaves of this abide all Winter.

Place.] The first grows in forests, on the heaths, and such like barren places: the red grows in the north parts of this land, as Lancashire, Yorkshire, &c.

Time.] They flower in March and April, and the fruit of the black is ripe in July and August.

Government and virtues.] They are under the dominion of Jupiter. It is a pity they are used no more in physic than they are.

The black Bilberries are good in hot agues and to cool the heat of the liver and stomach; they do somewhat bind the belly, and stay vomiting and loathings; the juice of the berries made in a syrup, or the pulp made into a conserve with sugar, is good for the purposes aforesaid, as also for an old cough, or an ulcer in the lungs, or other diseases therein. The Red Worts are more binding, and stops women's courses, spitting of blood, or any other flux of blood or humours, being used as well outwardly as inwardly.

BIFOIL OR TWOBLADE

Descript.] This small herb, from a root somewhat sweet, shooting downwards many long strings, rises up a round green stalk, bare or naked next the ground for an inch, two or three to the middle thereof as it is in age or growth; as also from the middle upwards to the flowers, having only two broad Plaintain-like leaves (but whiter) set at the middle of the stalk one against another, compassing it round at the bottom of them.

Place.] It is an usual inhabitant in woods, copses, and in many places in this land.

There is another sort, grows in wet grounds and marshes, which is somewhat different from the former. It is a smaller plant, and greener, having sometimes three leaves; the spike of the flowers is less than the former, and the roots of this do run or creep in the ground.

They are often used by many to good purpose for wounds, both green and old, to consolidate or knit ruptures; and well it may, being a plant of Saturn.

THE BIRCH TREE

Descript.] This grows a goodly tall straight tree, fraught with many boughs, and slender branches bending downward: the old being covered with discoloured chapped bark, and the younger being browner by much. The leaves at the first breaking out are crumpled, and afterwards like the beech leaves, but smaller and greener, and dented about the edges. It bears small short catkins, somewhat like those of the hazelnut-tree, which abide on the branches a long time, until growing ripe, they fall on the ground and their seed with them.

Place.] It usually grows in woods.

Government and virtues.] It is a tree of Venus; the juice of the leaves, while they are young, or the distilled water of them, or the water that comes from the tree being bored with an auger, and distilled afterwards; any of these being drank for some days together, is available to break the stone in the kidneys and bladder, and is good also to wash sore mouths.

BIRD'S FOOT

THIS small herb grows not above a span high with many branches spread upon the ground, set with many wings of small leaves. The flowers grow upon the branches, many small ones of a pale yellow colour being set a-head together, which afterwards turn into small jointed pods, well resembling the claw of small birds, whence it took its name.

There is another sort of Bird's Foot in all things like the former, but a little larger; the flowers of a pale whitish and red colour, and the pods distinct by joints like the other, but little more crooked; and the roots do carry many small white knots or kernels amongst the strings.

Place.] These grow on heaths, and many open untilled places of this land.

Time.] They flower and seed in the end of Summer.

Government and virtues.] They belong to Saturn and are of a drying, binding quality, and thereby very good to be used in wound drinks, as also to apply outwardly for the same purpose. But the latter Bird's Foot is found by experience to break the stone in the back or kidneys, and drives them forth, if the decoction thereof be taken; and it wonderfully helps the ruptures, being taken inwardly, and outwardly applied to the place.

All sorts have best operations upon the stone, as ointments and plaisters have upon wounds: and therefore you may make a salt of this for the stone; the way how to do so may be found in my translation of the London Dispensatory; and it may be I may give you it again in plainer terms at the latter end of this book.

BISHOP'S-WEED

BESIDES the common name Bishop's-weed, it is usually known by the Greek name *Ammi* and *Ammois*; some call it Aethiopian Cummin-seed, and others Cummin-royal, as also Herb William, and Bull-wort.

Descript.] Common Bishop's-weed rises up with a round straight stalk, sometimes as high as a man, but usually three or four feet high, beset with divers small, long and somewhat broad leaves, cut in some places, and dented about the edges, growing one against another, of a dark green colour, having sundry branches on them, and at the top small umbels of white flowers, which turn into small round seeds little bigger than Parsley seeds, of a quick hot scent and taste; the root is white and stringy; perishing yearly, and usually rises again on its own sowing.

Place.] It grows wild in many places in England and Wales, as between Greenhithe and Gravesend.

Government and virtues.] It is hot and dry in the third degree, of a bitter taste, and somewhat sharp withal; it provokes lust to purpose; I suppose Venus owns it. It digests humours, provokes urine and women's courses, dissolves wind, and being taken in wine it eases pains and griping in the bowels, and is good against the biting of serpents; it is used to good effect in those medicines which are given to hinder the poisonous operation of Cantharides, upon the passage of the urine: being mixed with honey and applied to black and blue marks, coming of blows or bruises, it takes them away; and being drank or outwardly applied, it abates a high colour, and makes it pale; and the fumes thereof taken with rosin or raisins, cleanses the mother.

BISTORT, OR SNAKEWEED

IT is called Snakeweed, English Serpentary, Dragon-wort, Osterick, and Passions.

Descript.] This has a thick short knobbed root, blackish without, and somewhat reddish within, a little crooked or turned together, of a hard astringent taste, with divers black threads hanging there-from, whence springs up every year divers leaves, standing upon long footstalks, being somewhat broad and long like a dock leaf, and a little pointed at the ends, but that it is of a bluish green colour on the upper side, and of an ash-colour grey, and a little purplish underneath, with divers veins therein, from among which rise up divers small and slender stalks, two feet high, and almost naked and without leaves, or with a very few, and narrow, bearing a spiky bush of pale-coloured flowers; which being past, there abides small seed, like unto Sorrel seed, but greater.

There are other sorts of Bistort growing in this land, but smaller, both in height, root, and stalks, and especially in the leaves. The root blackish without, and somewhat whitish within; of an austere binding taste, as the former.

Place.] They grow in shadowy moist woods, and at the foot of hills, but are chiefly nourished up in gardens. The narrow leafed Bistort grows in the north, in Lancashire, Yorkshire, and Cumberland.

Time.] They flower about the end of May, and the seed is ripe about the beginning of July.

Government and virtues.] It belongs to Saturn, and is in operation cold and dry; both the leaves and roots have a powerful faculty to resist all poison. The root, in powder, taken in drink expels the venom of the plague, the small-pox, measels, purples, or any other infectious disease, driving it out by sweating. The root in powder, the decoction thereof in wine being drank, stays all manner of inward bleeding, or spitting of blood, and any fluxes in the body of either man or woman, or vomiting. It is also very available against ruptures, or burstings, or all bruises from falls, dissolving the congealed blood, and easing the pains that happen thereupon; it also helps the jaundice.

The water, distilled from both leaves and roots, is a singular remedy to wash any place bitten or stung by any venomous creature; as also for any of the purposes before spoken of, and is very good to wash any running sores or ulcers. The decoction of the root in wine being drank, hinders abortion or miscarriage in child-bearing. The leaves also kill the worms in children, and is a great help to them that cannot keep their water; if the juice of Plaintain be added thereto, and outwardly applied, much helps the ghonorrhea, or running of the reins. A dram of the powder of the root, taken in water thereof, wherein some red hot iron or steel hath been quenched, is also an admirable help thereto, so as the body be first prepared and purged from the offensive humours. The leaves, seed, or roots, are all very good in decoction, drinks, or lotions, for inward or outward wounds, or other sores. And the powder, strewed upon any cut or wound in a vein, stays the immoderate bleeding thereof. The decoction of the root in water, where unto some pomegranate peels and flowers are added, injected into the matrix, stays the immoderate flux of the courses. The root thereof, with pelitory of Spain and burnt alum, of each a little quantity, beaten small and into paste with some honey, and a little piece thereof put into a hollow tooth, or held between the teeth, if there be no hollowness in them, stays the defluction of rheum upon them which causes pains, and helps to cleanse the head, and void much offensive water. The distilled water is very effectual to wash sores or cankers in the nose, or any other part; if the powder of the root be applied thereunto afterwards. It is good also to fasten the gums, and to take away the heat and inflammations that happen in the jaws, almonds of the throat, or mouth, if the decoction of the leaves, roots, or seeds bruised, or the juice of them, be applied; but the roots are most effectual to the purposes aforesaid.

ONE-BLADE

Descript.] This small plant never bears more than one leaf, but only when it rises up with its stalk, which thereon bears another, and seldom more, which are of a bluish green colour, broad at the bottom, and pointed with many ribs or veins like Plaintain; at the top of the stalk grows many small flowers star-fashion, smelling somewhat sweet; after which comes small reddish berries when they are ripe. The root small, of the bigness of a rush, lying and creeping under the upper crust of the earth, shooting forth in divers places.

Place.] It grows in moist, shadowy grassy places of woods, in many places of this realm.

Time.] It flowers about May, and the berries are ripe in June, and then quickly perishes, until the next year it springs from the same again.

Government and virtues.] It is a herb of the Sun, and therefore cordial; half a dram, or a dram at most, of the root hereof in powder taken in wine and vinegar, of each a little quantity, and the party presently laid to sweat, is held to be a sovereign remedy for those that are infected with the plague, and have a sore upon them, by expelling the poison, and defending the heart and spirit from danger. It is also accounted a singular good wound herb, and therefore used with other herbs in making such balms as are necessary for curing of wounds, either green or old, and especially if the nerves be hurt.

THE BRAMBLE, OR BLACKBERRY BUSH

It is so well known that it needs no description. The virtues thereof are as follows:

Government and virtues.] It is a plant of Venus in Aries. If any ask the reason why Venus is so prickly ? Tell them it is because she is in the house of Mars. The buds, leaves, and branches, while they are green, are of a good use in the ulcers and putrid sores of the mouth and throat, and of the quinsey, and likewise to heal other fresh wounds and sores; but the flowers and fruit unripe are very binding, and so profitable for the bloody flux, lasks, and are a fit remedy for spitting of blood. Either the decoction of the powder or of the root taken, is good to break or drive forth gravel and the stone in the reins and kidneys. The leaves and brambles, as well green as dry, are exceeding good lotions for sores in the mouth, or secret parts. The decoction of them, and of the dried branches, do much bind the belly and are good for too much flowing of women's courses; the berries of the flowers are a powerful remedy against the poison of the most venomous serpents; as well drank as outwardly applied, helps the sores of the fundament and the piles; the juice of the berries mixed with the juice of mulberries, do bind more effectually, and helps all fretting and eating sores and ulcers wheresoever. The distilled water of the branches, leaves, and flowers, or of the fruit, is very pleasant in taste, and very effectual in fevers and hot distempers of the body, head, eyes, and other parts, and for the purposes aforesaid. The leaves boiled in lye, and the head washed therewith, heals the itch and running sores thereof, and makes the hair black. The powder of the leaves strewed on cankers and running ulcers, wonderfully helps to heal them. Some use to condensate the juice of the leaves, and some the juice of the berries, to keep for their use all the year, for the purposes aforesaid.

BLITES

Descript.] Of these there are two sorts commonly known, viz. white and red. The white has leaves somewhat like to Beets, but smaller, rounder and of a whitish green colour, every one standing upon a small long footstalk: the stalk rises up two or three feet high, with such like leaves thereon; the flowers grow at the top in long round tufts or clusters, wherein are contained small and round seeds; the root is very full of threads or strings.

The red Blite is in all things like the white but that its leaves and tufted heads are exceeding red at first, and after turn more purple.

There are other kinds of Blites which grow different from the two former sorts but little, but only the wild are smaller in every part.

Place.] They grow in gardens, and wild in many places in this land.

Time.] They seed in August and September.

Government and virtues.] They are all of them cooling, drying, and binding, serving to restrain the fluxes of blood in either man or woman, especially the red; which also stays the overflowing of the women's reds, as the white Blites stays the whites in women. It is an excellent secret; you cannot well fail in the use. They are all under the dominion of Venus.

There is another sort of wild Blites like the other wild kinds, but have long and spiky heads of greenish seeds, seeming by the thick setting together to be all seed.

This sort the fishers are delighted with, and it is good and usual bait; for fishes will bite fast enough at them, if you have wit enough to catch them when they bite.

BORAGE AND BUGLOSS

THESE are so well known to the inhabitants in every garden that I hold it needless to describe them.

To these I may add a third sort, which is not so common, nor yet so well known, and therefore I shall give you its name and description.

It is called *Langue de Bœuf*; but why then should they call one herb by the name of Bugloss, and another by the name *Langue de Bœuf*? it is some question to me, seeing one signifies Ox-tongue in Greek, and the other signifies the same in French.

Descript.] The leaves whereof are smaller than those of Bugloss but much rougher; the stalks rising up about a foot and a half high, and is most commonly of a red colour; the flowers stand in scaly round heads, being composed of many small yellow flowers not much unlike to those of Dandelion, and the seed flieth away in down as that doth; you may easily know the flowers by their taste, for they are very bitter.

Place.] It grows wild in many places of this land, and may be plentifully found near London, as between Rotherhithe and Deptford, by the ditch side. Its virtues are held to be the same with Borage and Bugloss, only this is somewhat hotter.

Time.] They flower in June and July, and the seed is ripe shortly after.

Government and virtues.] They are all three herbs of Jupiter and under Leo, all great cordials, and great strengtheners of nature. The leaves and roots are to very good purpose used in putrid and pestilential fevers, to defend the heart, and help to resist and expel the poison, or the venom of other creatures: the seed is of the like effect; and the seed and leaves are good to increase milk in women's breasts; the leaves, flowers, and seed, all or any of them, are good to expel pensiveness and melancholy; it helps to clarify the blood, and mitigate heat in fevers. The juice made into a syrup prevails much to all the purposes aforesaid, and is put, with other cooling, opening and cleansing herbs to open obstructions, and help the yellow jaundice, and mixed with Fumitory, to cool, cleanse, and temper the blood thereby; it helps the itch, ringworms and tetters, or other spreading scabs or sores. The flowers candied or made into a conserve, are helpful in the former cases, but are chiefly used as a cordial, and are good for those that are weak in long sickness, and to comfort the heart and spirits of those that are in a consumption, or troubled with often swoonings, or passions of the heart. The distilled water is no less effectual to all the purposes aforesaid, and helps the redness and inflammations of the eyes, being washed therewith; the herb dried is never used, but the green; yet the ashes thereof boiled in mead, or honied water, is available against the inflammations and ulcers in the mouth or throat, to gargle it therewith; the roots of Bugloss are effectual, being made into a licking electuary for the cough, and to condensate thick phlegm, and the rheumatic distillations upon the lungs.

BLUE-BOTTLE

It is called Syanus, I suppose from the colour of it; Hurt-sickle, because it turns the edge of the sickles that reap the corn; Blueblow, Corn-flower, and Blue-bottle.

Descript.] I shall only describe that which is commonest, and in my opinion most useful; its leaves spread upon the ground, being of a whitish green colour, somewhat on the edges like those of Corn-Scabions, amongst which rises up a stalk divided into divers branches, beset with long leaves of a greenish colour, either but very little indented, or not at all; the flowers are of a bluish colour, from whence it took its name, consisting of an innumerable company of flowers set in a scaly head, not much unlike those of Knap-weed; the seed is smooth, bright, and shining, wrapped up in a woolly mantle; the root perishes every year.

Place.] They grow in corn fields, amongst all sorts of corn (pease, beans, and tares excepted.) If you please to take them up from thence, and transplant them in your garden, especially towards the full of the moon, they will grow more double than they are, and many times change colour.

Time.] They flower from the beginning of May, to the end of the harvest.

Government and virtues.] As they are naturally cold, dry, and binding, so they are under the dominion of Saturn. The powder or dried leaves of the Blue-bottle, or Corn-flower, is given with good success to those that are bruised by a fall, or have broken a vein inwardly, and void much blood at the mouth; being taken in the water of Plaintain, Horsetail, or the greater Confrey, it is a remedy against the poison of the Scorpion, and resists all venoms and poisons. The seed or leaves taken in wine, is very good against the plague, and all infectious diseases, and is very good in pestilential fevers. The juice put into fresh or green wounds, doth quickly solder up the lips of them together, and is very effectual to heal all ulcers and sores in the mouth. The juice dropped into the eyes takes away the heat and inflammation of them. The distilled water of this herb, has the same properties, and may be used for the effects aforesaid.

BRANK URSINE

BESIDES the common name Brank-Ursine, it is also called Bear's-breach, and Acanthus, though I think our English names to be more proper; for the Greek word *Acanthus*, signifies any thistle whatsoever.

Descript.] This thistle shoots forth very many large, thick, sad green smooth leaves on the ground, with a very thick and juicy middle rib; the leaves are parted with sundry deep gashes on the edges; the leaves remain a long time, before any stalk appears, afterwards rising up a reasonable big stalk, three or four feet high, and bravely decked with flowers from the middle of the stalk upwards; for on the lower part of the stalk, there is neither branches nor leaf. The flowers are hooded and gaping, being white in colour, and standing in brownish husk, with a long small undivided leaf under each leaf; they seldom seed in our country. Its roots are many, great and thick, blackish without and whitish within, full of a clammy sap; a piece of them if you set it in the garden, and defend it from the first Winter cold will grow and flourish.

Place.] They are only nursed in the gardens in England, where they will grow very well.

Time.] It flowers in June and July.

Government and virtues.] It is an excellent plant under the dominion of the Moon; I could wish such as are studious would labour to keep it in their gardens. The leaves being boiled and used in clysters, is excellent good to mollify the belly, and make the passage slippery. The decoction drank inwardly, is excellent and good for the bloody-flux. The leaves being bruised, or rather boiled and applied like a poultice are excellent good to unite broken bones and strengthen joints that have been put out. The decoction of either leaves or roots being drank, and the decoction of leaves applied to the place, is excellent good for the king's evil that is broken and runs; for by the influence of the moon, it revives the ends of the veins which are relaxed. There is scarce a better remedy to be applied to such places as are burnt with fire than this is, for it fetches out the fire, and heals it without a scar. This is an excellent remedy for such as are bursten, being either taken inwardly, or applied to the place. In like manner used, it helps the cramp and the gout. It is excellently good in hectic fevers, and restores radical moisture to such as are in consumptions.

BRIONY, OR WILD VINE

IT is called Wild, and Wood Vine, Tamus, or Ladies' Seal. The white is called White Vine by some; and the black, Black Vine.

Descript.] The common White Briony grows ramping upon the hedges, sending forth many long, rough, very tender branches at the beginning, with many very rough, and broad leaves thereon, cut (for the most part) into five partitions, in form very like a vine leaf, but smaller, rough, and of a whitish hoary green colour, spreading very far, spreading and twining with his small claspers (that come forth at the joints with the leaves) very far on whatsoever stands next to it. At the several joints also (especially towards the top of the branches) comes forth a long stalk bearing many whitish flowers together on a long tuft, consisting of five small leaves a-piece, laid open like a star, after which come the berries separated one from another, more than a cluster of grapes, green at the first, and very red when they are thorough ripe, of no good scent, but of a most loathsome taste provokes vomit. The root grows to be exceeding great, with many long twines or branches going from it, of a pale whitish colour on the outside, and more white within, and of a sharp, bitter, loathsome taste.

Place.] It grows on banks, or under hedges, through this land; the roots lie very deep.

Time.] It flowers in July and August, some earlier, and some later than the other.

Government and virtues.] They are furious martial plants. The root of Briony purges the belly with great violence, troubling the stomach and burning the liver, and therefore not rashly to be taken; but being corrected, is very profitable for the diseases of the head, as falling sickness, giddiness, and swimmings, by drawing away much phlegm and rheumatic humours that oppress the head, as also the joints and sinews; and is therefore good for palsies, convulsions, cramps, and stitches in the sides, and the dropsy, and for provoking urine; it cleanses the reins and kidneys from gravel and stone, by opening the obstructions of the spleen, and consume, the hardness and swelling thereof. The decoction of the root in wine, drank once a week at going to bed, cleanses the mother, and helps the rising thereof, expels the dead child; a dram of the root in powder taken in white wine, brings down their courses. An electuary made of the roots and honey, doth mightily cleanse the chest of rotten phlegm, and wonderfully help any old strong cough, to those that are troubled with shortness of breath, and is good for them that are bruised inwardly, to help to expel the clotted or congealed blood. The leaves, fruit, and root do cleanse old and filthy sores, are good against all fretting and running cankers, gangrenes, and tetters and therefore the berries are by some country people called tetter-berries. The root cleanses the skin wonderfully from all black and blue spots, freckles, morphew, leprosy, foul scars, or other deformity whatsoever; also all running scabs and manginess are healed by the powder of the dried root, or the juice thereof, but especially by the fine white hardened juice. The distilled water of the root works the same effects, but more weakly; the root bruised and applied of itself to any place where the bones are broken, helps to draw them forth, as also splinters and thorns in the flesh; and being applied with a little wine mixed therewith, it breaks boils, and helps whitlows on the joints.—For all these latter, beginning at sores, cancers, &c. apply it outwardly, mixing it with a little hog's grease, or other convenient ointment.

As for the former diseases where it must be taken inwardly, it purges very violently, and needs an abler hand to correct it than most country people have.

BROOK LIME, OR WATER-PIMPERNEL

Descript.] This sends forth from a creeping root that shoots forth strings at every joint, as it runs, divers and sundry green stalks, round and sappy with some branches on them, somewhat broad, round, deep green, and thick leaves set by couples thereon; from the bottom whereof shoot forth long foot stalks, with sundry small blue flowers on them, that consist of five small round pointed leaves a piece.

There is another sort nothing different from the former, but that it is greater, and the flowers of a paler green colour.

Place.] They grow in small standing waters, and usually near Water-Cresses.

Time.] And flower in June and July, giving seed the next month after.

Government and virtues.] It is a hot and biting martial plant. Brook-lime and Water-Cresses are generally used together in diet-drink, with other things serving to purge the blood and body from all ill humours that would destroy health, and are helpful to the scurvy. They do all provoke urine, and help to break the stone, and pass it away; they procure women's courses, and expel the dead child. Being fried with butter and vinegar, and applied warm, it helps all manner of tumours, swellings, and inflammations.

Such drinks ought to be made of sundry herbs, according to the malady. I shall give a plain and easy rule at the latter end of this book.

BUTCHER'S BROOM

IT is called Ruscus, and Bruscus, Kneeholm, Kneeholly, Knee-hulver, and Pettigree.

Descript.] The first shoots that sprout from the root of Butcher's Broom, are thick, whitish, and short, somewhat like those of Asparagus, but greater, they rise up to be a foot and half high, are spread into divers branches, green, and somewhat creased with the roundness, tough and flexible, whereon are set somewhat broad and almost round hard leaves and prickly, pointed at the end, of a dark green colour, two at the most part set at a place, very close and near together; about the middle of the leaf, on the back and lower side from the middle rib, breaks forth a small whitish green flower, consisting of four small round pointed leaves, standing upon little or no footstalk, and in the place whereof comes a small round berry, green at the first, and red when it is ripe, wherein are two or three white, hard, round seeds contained. The root is thick, white and great at the head, and from thence sends forth divers thick, white, long, tough strings.

Place.] It grows in copses, and upon heaths and waste grounds, and oftentimes under or near the holly bushes.

Time.] It shoots forth its young buds in the Spring, and the berries are ripe about September, the branches of leaves abiding green all the Winter.

Government and virtues.] It is a plant of Mars, being of a gallant cleansing and opening quality. The decoction of the root made with wine opens obstructions, provokes urine, helps to expel gravel and the stone, the stranguary and women's courses, also the yellow jaundice and the head-ache; and with some honey or sugar put thereunto, cleanses the breast of phlegm, and the chest of such clammy humours gathered therein. The decoction of the root drank, and a poultice made of the berries and leaves applied, are effectual in knitting and consolidating broken bones or parts out of joint. The common way of using it, is to boil the root of it, and Parsley and Fennel and Smallage in white wine, and drink the decoction, adding the like quantity of Grass-root to them: The more of the root you boil, the stronger will the decoction be; it works no ill effects, yet I hope you have wit enough to give the strongest decoction to the strongest bodies.

BROOM, AND BROOM-RAPE

To spend time in writing a description hereof is altogether needless, it being so generally used by all the good housewives almost through this land to sweep their houses with, and therefore very well known to all sorts of people.

The Broom-rape springs up in many places from the roots of the broom (but more often in fields, as by hedge-sides and on heaths). The stalk whereof is of the bigness of a finger or thumb, above two feet high, having a shew of leaves on them, and many flowers at the top, of a reddish yellow colour, as also the stalks and leaves are.

Place.] They grow in many places of this land commonly, and as commonly spoil all the land they grow in.

Time.] They flower in the Summer months, and give their seed before Winter.

Government and virtues.] The juice or decoction of the young branches or seed, or the powder of the seed taken in drink purges downwards, and draws phlegmatic and watery humours from the joints; whereby it helps the dropsy, gout, sciatica, and pains of the hips and joints; it also provokes strong vomits, and helps the pains of the sides, and swelling of the spleen, cleanses also the reins or kidneys and bladder of the stone, provokes urine abundantly, and hinders the growing again of the stone in the body. The continual use of the powder of the leaves and seed doth cure the black jaundice. The distilled water of the flowers is profitable for all the same purposes: it also helps surfeit, and alters the fit of agues, if three or four ounces thereof, with as much of the water of the lesser Centaury, and a little sugar put therein, be taken a little before the fit comes, and the party be laid down to sweat in his bed. The oil or water that is drawn from the end of the green sticks heated in the fire, helps the tooth-ache. The juice of young branches made into an ointment of old hog's grease, and anointed, or the young branches bruised and heated in oil or hog's grease, and laid to the sides pained by wind, as in stitches, or the spleen, ease them in once or twice using it. The same boiled in oil is the safest and surest medicine to kill lice in the head or body of any; and is an especial remedy for joint aches, and swollen knees, that come by the falling down of humours.

The BROOM RAPE *also is not without its virtues.*

The decoction thereof in wine, is thought to be as effectual to void the stone in the kidney or bladder, and to provoke urine, as the Broom itself. The juice thereof is a singular good help to cure as well green wounds, as old and filthy sores and malignant ulcers. The insolate oil, wherein there has been three or four repetitions of infusion of the top stalks, with flowers strained and cleared, cleanses the skin from all manner of spots, marks, and freckles that rise either by the heat of the sun, or the malignity of humours. As for the Broom and Broom-rape, Mars owns them, and is exceeding prejudicial to the liver, I suppose by reason of the antipathy between Jupiter and Mars; therefore if the liver be disaffected, minister none of it.

BUCK'S-HORN PLANTAIN

Descript.] This being sown of seed, rises up at first with small, long, narrow, hairy, dark green leaves like grass, without any division or gash in them, but those that follow are gashed in on both sides the leaves into three or four gashes, and pointed at the ends, resembling the knags of a buck's horn (whereof it took its name), and being well wound round about the root upon the ground, in order one by another, thereby resembling the form of a star, from among which rise up divers hairy stalks, about a hand's breadth high, bearing every one a small, long spiky head, like to those of the common Plantain having such like bloomings and seed after them. The root is single, long and small, with divers strings at it.

Place.] They grow in sandy grounds, as in Tothill-fields by Westminster, and divers other places of this land.

Time.] They flower and seed in May, June, and July, and their green leaves do in a manner abide fresh all the Winter.

Government and virtues.] It is under the dominion of Saturn, and is of a gallant, drying, and binding quality. This boiled in wine and drank, and some of the leaves put to the hurt place, is an excellent remedy for the biting of the viper or adder, which I take to be one and the same. The same being also drank, helps those that are troubled with the stone in the reins or kidneys, by cooling the heat of the part affected, and strengthens them; also weak stomachs that cannot retain, but cast up their meat. It stays all bleeding both at mouth or nose; bloody urine or the bloody-flux, and stops the lask of the belly and bowels. The leaves hereof bruised and laid to their sides that have an ague, suddenly ease the fits; and the leaves and roots applied to the wrists, works the same effect. The herb boiled in ale and wine, and given for some mornings and evenings together, stays the distillation of hot and sharp rheums falling into the eyes from the head, and helps all sorts of sore eyes.

BUCK'S HORN

It is called Hart's-horn, Herba-stella and Herba-stellaria, Sanguinaria, Herb-Eve, Herb-Ivy, Wort-Tresses, and Swine-Cresses.

Descript.] They have many small and weak straggled branches trailing here and there upon the ground. The leaves are many, small and jagged, not much unlike to those of Buck's-horn Plantain, but much smaller, and not so hairy. The flowers grow among the leaves in small, rough, whitish clusters; the seeds are smaller and brownish, of a bitter taste.

Place.] They grow in dry, barren, sandy grounds.

Time.] They flower and seed when the rest of the Plantains do.

Government and virtues.] This is also under the dominion of Saturn; the virtues are held to be the same as Buck's-horn Plaintain, and therefore by all authors it is joined with it. The leaves bruised and applied to the place, stop bleeding. The herbs bruised and applied to warts, will make them consume and waste in a short time.

BUGLE

Besides the name Bugle, it is called Middle Confound and Middle Comfrey, Brown Bugle, and by some Sicklewort, and Herb-Carpenter; though in Essex we call another herb by that name.

Descript.] This has larger leaves than those of the Self-heal, but else of the same fashion, or rather longer; in some green on the upper side, and in others more brownish, dented about the edges, somewhat hairy, as the square stalk is also which rises up to be half a yard high sometimes, with the leaves set by couples, from the middle almost, whereof upwards stand the flowers, together with many smaller and browner leaves than the rest, on the stalk below set at distance, and the stalk bare between them; among which flowers, are also small ones of a bluish and sometimes of an ash colour, fashioned like the flowers of Ground-ivy, after which come small, round blackish seeds. The root is composed of many strings, and spreads upon the ground.

The white flowered Bugle differs not in form or greatness from the former, saving that the leaves and stalks are always green, and never brown, like the other, and the flowers thereof are white.

Place.] They grow in woods, copses, and fields, generally throughout England, but the white flowered Bugle is not so plentiful as the former.

Time.] They flower from May until July, and in the meantime perfect their seed. The roots and leaves next thereunto upon the ground abiding all the Winter.

Government and virtues.] This herb belongs to Dame Venus. If the virtues of it make you fall in love with it (as they will if you be wise) keep a syrup of it to take inwardly, an ointment and plaister of it to use outwardly, always by you.

The decoction of the leaves and flowers made in wine, and taken, dissolves the congealed blood in those that are bruised inwardly by a fall, or otherwise is very effectual for any inward wounds, thrusts, or stabs in the body or bowels; and it is an especial help in all wound-drinks, and for those that are liver-grown (as they call it.) It is wonderful in curing all manner of ulcers and sores, whether new and fresh or old and inveterate; yea, gangrenes and fistulas also, if the leaves bruised and applied, or their juice be used to wash and bathe the place; and the same made into a lotion, and some honey and alum, cures all sores in the mouth and gums, be they ever so foul, or of long continuance; and works no less powerfully and effectually for such ulcers and sores as happen in the secret parts of men and women. Being also taken inwardly, or outwardly applied, it helps those that have broken any bone, or have any member out of joint. An ointment made with the leaves of Bugle, Scabious and Sanicle, bruised and boiled in hog's grease, until the herbs be dry, and then strained forth into a pot for such occasions as shall require; it is so singularly good for all sorts of hurts in the body, that none that know its usefulness will be without it.

The truth is, I have known this herb cure some diseases of Saturn, of which I thought good to quote one. Many times such as give themselves much to drinking are troubled with strange fancies, strange sights in the night time, and some with voices, as also with the disease Ephialtes, or the Mare. I take the reason of this to be (according to Fernelius) a melancholy vapour made thin by excessive drinking strong liquor, and, so flies up and disturbs the fancy, and breeds imaginations like itself, viz. fearful and troublesome. Those I have known cured by taking only two spoonfuls, of the syrup of this herb after supper two hours, when you go to bed. But whether this does it by sympathy, or antipathy, is some doubt in astrology. I know there is great antipathy between Saturn and Venus in matter of procreation, yea, such a one, that the barrenness of Saturn can be removed by none but Venus! nor the lust of Venus be repelled by none but Saturn; but I am not of opinion this is done this way, and my reason is, because these vapours though in quality melancholy, yet by their flying upward, seem to be something aerial; therefore I rather think it is done by antipathy; Saturn being exalted in Libra, in the house of Venus.

BURNET

IT is called Sanguisorbia, Pimpinella, Bipulo, Solbegrella, &c. The common garden Burnet is so well known, that it needs no description. There is another sort which is wild, the description whereof take as follows:

Descript.] The great wild Burnet has winged leaves arising from the roots like the garden Burnet, but not so many; yet each of these leaves are at the least twice as large as the other, and nicked in the same manner about the edges, of a greyish colour on the under side; the stalks are greater, and rise higher, with many such leaves set thereon, and greater heads at the top, of a brownish colour, and out of them come small dark purple flowers, like the former, but greater. The root is black and long like the other, but greater also: it has almost neither scent nor taste therein, like the garden kind.

Place.] It first grows frequently in gardens. The wild kind grows in divers counties of this land, especially in Huntingdon, in Northamptonshire, in the meadows there: as also near London, by Pancras church, and by a causeway-side in the middle of a field by Paddington.

Time.] They flower about the end of June and beginning of July, and their seed is ripe in August.

Government and virtues.] This is an herb the Sun challenges dominion over, and is a most precious herb, little inferior to Betony; the continual use of it preserves the body in health, and the spirits in vigour; for if the Sun be the preserver of life under God, his herbs are the best in the world to do it by. They are accounted to be both of one property, but the lesser is more effectual because quicker and more aromatic. It is a friend to the heart, liver, and other principal parts of a man's body. Two or three of the stalks, with leaves put into a cup of wine, especially claret, are known to quicken the spirits, refresh and cheer the heart, and drive away melancholy. It is a special help to defend the heart from noisome vapours, and from infection of the pestilence, the juice thereof being taken in some drink, and the party laid to sweat thereupon. They have also a drying and an astringent quality, whereby they are available in all manner of fluxes of blood or humours, to staunch bleedings inward or outward, lasks, scourings, the bloody flux, women's too abundant flux of courses, the whites, and the choleric belchings and castings of the stomach, and is a singular wound-herb for all sorts of wounds, both of the head and body, either inward or outward, for all old ulcers, running cankers, and most sores, to be used either by the juice or decoction of the herb, or by the powder of the herb or root, or the water of the distilled herb, or ointment by itself, or with other things to be kept. The seed is also no less effectual both to stop fluxes, and dry up moist sores, being taken in powder inwardly in wine, or steeled water, that is, wherein hot rods of steel have been quenched; or the powder, or the seed mixed with the ointments.

THE BUTTER-BUR, OR PETASITIS

Descript.] This rises up in February, with a thick stalk about a foot high, whereon are set a few small leaves, or rather pieces, and at the top a long spiked head; flowers of a blue or deep red colour, according to the soil where it grows, and before the stalk with the flowers have abiden a month above ground, it will be withered and gone, and blow away with the wind, and the leaves will begin to spring, which being full grown, are very large and broad, being somewhat thin and almost round, whose thick red foot stalks above a foot long, stand towards the middle of the leaves. The lower part being divided into two round parts, close almost one to another, and are of a pale green colour; and hairy underneath. The root is long, and spreads underground, being in some places no bigger than one's finger, in others much bigger, blackish on the outside, and whitish within, of a bitter and unpleasant taste.

Place and Time.] They grow in low and wet grounds by rivers and water sides. Their flower (as is said) rising and decaying in February and March, before their leaves, which appear in April.

Government and virtues.] It is under the dominion of the Sun, and therefore is a great strengthener of the heart, and clearer of the vital spirit. The roots thereof are by long experience found to be very available against the plague and pestilential fevers by provoking sweat; if the powder thereof be taken in wine, it also resists the force of any other poison. The root hereof taken with Zedoary and Angelica, or without them, helps the rising of the mother. The decoction of the root in wine, is singularly good for those that wheese much, or are short-winded. It provokes urine also, and women's courses, and kills the flat and broad worms in the belly. The powder of the root doth wonderfully help to dry up the moisture of the sores that are hard to be cured, and takes away all spots and blemishes of the skin. It were well if gentlewomen would keep this root preserved, to help their poor neighbours. *It is fit the rich should help the poor, for the poor cannot help themselves.*

THE BURDOCK

They are also called Personata, and Loppy-major, great Burdock and Clod-bur. It is so well known, even by the little boys, who pull off the burs to throw and stick upon each other, that I shall spare to write any description of it.

Place.] They grow plentifully by ditches and water-sides, and by the highways almost everywhere through this land.

Government and virtues.] Venus challenges this herb for her own, and by its leaf or seed you may draw the womb which way you please, either upwards by applying it to the crown of the head, in case it falls out; or downwards in fits of the mother, by applying it to the soles of the feet; or if you would stay it in its place, apply it to the navel, and that is one good way to stay the child in it. The Burdock leaves are cooling, moderately drying, and discussing withal, whereby it is good for old ulcers and sores. A dram of the roots taken with Pine kernels, helps them that spit foul, mattery, and bloody phlegm. The leaves applied to the places troubled with the shrinking of the sinews or arteries, gives much ease. The juice of the leaves, or rather the roots themselves, given to drink with old wine, doth wonderfully help the biting of any serpents. And the root beaten with a little salt, and laid on the place, suddenly eases the pain thereof, and helps those that are bit by a mad dog. The juice of the leaves being drank with honey, provokes urine, and remedies the pain of the bladder. The seed being drank in wine forty days together, doth wonderfully help the sciatica. The leaves bruised with the white of an egg, and applied to any place burnt with fire, takes out the fire, gives sudden ease, and heals it up afterwards. The decoction of them fomented on any fretting sore, or canker, stays the corroding quality, which must be afterwards anointed with an ointment made of the same liquor, hog's-grease, nitre, and vinegar boiled together. The roots may be preserved with sugar, and taken fasting, or at other times, for the same purposes, and for consumptions, the stone, and the lask. The seed is much commended to break the stone, and cause it to be expelled by urine, and is often used with other seeds and things to that purpose.

CABBAGES AND COLEWORTS

I SHALL spare labour in writing a description of these, since almost everyone that can but write at all, may describe them from his own knowledge, they being generally so well known, that descriptions are altogether needless.

Place.] They are generally planted in gardens.

Time.] Their flower time is towards the middle or end of July, and the seed is ripe in August.

Government and virtues.] The Cabbages or Coleworts boiled gently in broth, and eaten, do open the body, but the second decoction doth bind the body. The juice thereof drank in wine, helps those that are bitten by an adder, and the decoction of the flowers brings down women's courses. Being taken with honey, it recovers hoarseness, or loss of the voice. The often eating of them well boiled, helps those that are entering into a consumption. The pulp of the middle ribs of Coleworts boiled in almond milk, and made up into an electuary with honey, being taken often, is very profitable for those that are puffy and short winded. Being boiled twice, an old cock boiled in the broth and drank, it helps the pains and the obstructions of the liver and spleen, and the stone in the kidneys. The juice boiled with honey, and dropped into the corner of the eyes, clears the sight, by consuming any film or clouds beginning to dim it; it also consumes the cankers growing therein. They are much commended, being eaten before meat to keep one from surfeiting, as also from being drunk with too much wine, or quickly to make a man sober again that was drunk before. For (as they say) there is such an antipathy or enmity between the Vine and the Coleworts, that the one will die where the other grows. The decoction of Coleworts takes away the pain and ache, and allays the swelling of sores and gouty legs and knees, wherein many gross and watery humours are fallen, the place being bathed therewith warm. It helps also old and filthy sores, being bathed therewith, and heals all small scabs, pushes, and wheals, that break out in the skin. The ashes of Colewort stalks mixed with old hog's-grease, are very effectual to anoint the sides of those that have had long pains therein, or any other place pained with melancholy and windy humours. This was surely Chrysippus's God, and therefore he wrote a whole volume on them and their virtues, and that none of the least neither, for he would be no small fool. He appropriates them to every part of the body, and to every disease in every part; and honest old Cato (they say) used no other physic. I know not what metal their bodies were made of; this I am sure, Cabbages are extremely windy, whether you take them as meat or as medicine: yea, as windy meat as can be eaten, unless you eat bag-pipes or bellows, and they are but seldom eaten in our days; and Colewort flowers are something more tolerable, and the wholesomer food of the two. The Moon challenges the dominion of this herb.

THE SEA COLEWORTS

Descript.] This has divers somewhat long and broad large and thick wrinkled leaves, somewhat crumpled about the edges, and growing each upon a thick footstalk very brittle, of a greyish green colour, from among which rises up a strong thick stalk, two feet high and better, with some leaves thereon to the top, where it branches forth much; and on every branch stands a large bush of pale whitish flowers, consisting of four leaves apiece. The root is somewhat great, shoots forth many branches under ground, keeping the leaves green all the Winter.

Place.] They grow in many places upon the sea-coasts, as well on the Kentish as Essex shores; as at Lid in Kent, Colchester in Essex, and divers other places, and in other counties of this land.

Time.] They flower and seed about the time that other kinds do.

Government and virtues.] The Moon claims the dominion of these also. The broth, or first decoction of the Sea Colewort, doth by the sharp, nitrous, and bitter qualities therein, open the belly, and purge the body; it cleanses and digests more powerfully than the other kind. The seed hereof, bruised and drank, kills worms. The leaves or the juice of them applied to sores or ulcers, cleanses and heals them, and dissolves swellings, and takes away inflammations.

CALAMINT, OR MOUNTAIN-MINT

Descript.] This is a small herb, seldom rising above a foot high, with square, hairy and woody stalks, and two small hoary leaves set at a joint, about the height of Marjoram, or not much bigger, a little dented about the edges, and of a very fierce or quick scent, as the whole herb is. The flowers stand at several spaces of the stalk, from the middle almost upwards, which are small and gaping like to those of the Mints, of a pale bluish colour. After which follow small, round blackish seed. The root is small and woody, with divers small strings spreading within the ground, and dies not, but abides many years.

Place.] It grows on heaths, and uplands, and dry grounds, in many places of this land.

Time.] They flower in July and their seed is ripe quickly after.

Government and virtues.] It is an herb of Mercury, and a strong one too, therefore excellent good in all afflictions of the brain. The decoction of the herb being drank, brings down women's courses, and provokes urine. It is profitable for those that are bursten, or troubled with convulsions or cramps, with shortness of breath, or choleric torments and pains in their bellies or stomach; it also helps the yellow-jaundice, and stays vomiting, being taken in wine. Taken with salt and honey, it kills all manner of worms in the body. It helps such as have the leprosy, either taken inwardly, drinking whey after it, or the green herb outwardly applied. It hinders conception in women, but either burned or strewed in the chamber, it drives away venomous serpents. It takes away black and blue marks in the face, and makes black scars become well coloured, if the green herb (not the dry) be boiled in wine, and laid to the place, or the place washed therewith. Being applied to the hucklebone, by continuance of time, it spends the humours, which cause the pain of the sciatica. The juice being dropped into the ears, kills the worms in them. The leaves boiled in wine, and drank, provoke sweat, and open obstructions of the liver and spleen. It helps them that have a tertian ague (the body being first purged) by taking away the cold fits. The decoction hereof, with some sugar put thereto afterwards, is very profitable for those that be troubled with the over-flowing of the gall, and that have an old cough, and that are scarce able to breathe by shortness of their wind; that have any cold distemper in their bowels, and are troubled with the hardness of the spleen, for all which purposes, both the powder, called Diacaluminthes, and the compound Syrup of Calamint are the most effectual. Let no woman be too busy with it, for it works very violent upon the feminine part.

CAMOMILE

It is so well known everywhere, that it is but lost time and labour to describe it. The virtues thereof are as follow.

A decoction made of Camomile, and drank, takes away all pains and stitches in the side. The flowers of Camomile beaten, and made up into balls with Gill, drive away all sorts of agues, if the part grieved be anointed with that oil, taken from the flowers, from the crown of the head to the sole of the foot, and afterwards laid to sweat in his bed, and that he sweats well. This is Nechessor, an Egyptian's, medicine. It is profitable for all sorts of agues that come either from phlegm, or melancholy, or from an inflammation of the bowels, being applied when the humours causing them shall be concocted; and there is nothing more profitable to the sides and region of the liver and spleen than it. The bathing with a decoction of Camomile takes away weariness, eases pains, to what part of the body soever they be applied. It comforts the sinews that are over-strained, mollifies all swellings. It moderately comforts all parts that have need of warmth, digests and dissolves whatsoever has need thereof, by a wonderful speedy property. It eases all pains of the cholic and stone, and all pains and torments of the belly, and gently provokes urine. The flowers boiled in posset-drink provokes sweat, and helps to expel all colds, aches, and pains whatsoever, and is an excellent help to bring down women's courses. Syrup made of the juice of Camomile, with the flowers, in white wine, is a remedy against the jaundice and dropsy. The flowers boiled in lye, are good to wash the head, and comfort both it and the brain. The oil made of the flowers of Camomile, is much used against all hard swellings, pains or aches, shrinking of the sinews, or cramps, or pains in the joints, or any other part of the body. Being used in clysters, it helps to dissolve the wind and pains in the belly; anointed also, it helps stitches and pains in the sides.

Nechessor saith, the Egyptians dedicated it to the Sun, because it cured agues, and they were like enough to do it, for they were the arrantest apes in their religion that I ever read of. Bachinus, Bena, and Lobel, commend the syrup made of the juice of it and sugar, taken inwardly, to be excellent for the spleen. Also this is certain, that it most wonderfully breaks the stone. Some take it in syrup or decoction, others inject the juice of it into the bladder with a syringe. My opinion is, that the salt of it, taken half a dram in the morning in a little white or Rhenish wine, is better than either; that it is excellent for the stone, appears in this which I have seen tried, *viz.*, that a stone that has been taken out of the body of a man being wrapped in Camomile, will in time dissolve, and in a little time too.

WATER-CALTROPS

THEY are called also Tribulus Aquaticus, Tribulus Lacusoris, Tribulus Marinus, Caltrops, Saligos, Water Nuts, and Water Chesnuts.

Descript.] As for the greater sort of Water Caltrop it is not found here, or very rarely. Two other sorts there are which I shall here describe. The first has a long creeping and jointed root, sending forth tufts at each joint, from which joints rise long, flat, slender, knotted, stalks, even to the top of the water, divided towards the top into many branches, each carrying two leaves on both sides, being about two inches long, and half an inch broad, thin and almost transparent; they look as though they were torn; the flowers are long, thick, and whitish, set together almost like a bunch of grapes, which being gone, there succeed, for the most part, sharp pointed grains all together, containing a small white kernel in them.

The second differs not much from this, save that it delights in more clean water; its stalks are not flat, but round; its leaves are not so long, but more pointed. As for the place we need not determine, for their name shews they grow in water.

Government and virtues.] They are under the dominion of the Moon, and being made into a poultice, are excellently good for hot inflammations, swellings, cankers, sore mouths and throats, being washed with the decoction; it cleanses and strengthens the neck and throat, and helps those swellings which, when people have, they say the almonds of the ears are fallen down. It is excellently good for the rankness of the gums, a safe and present remedy for the king's evil. They are excellent for the stone and gravel, especially the nuts, being dried. They also resist poison, and bitings of venomous beasts.

CAMPION, WILD

Descript.] The wild White Campion has many long and somewhat broad dark green leaves lying upon the ground, and divers ribs therein, somewhat like plantain, but somewhat hairy, broader, but not so long. The hairy stalks rise up in the middle of them three or four feet high, and sometimes more, with divers great white joints at several places thereon, and two such like leaves thereat up to the top, sending forth branches at several joints also; all which bear on several foot-stalks white flowers at the tops of them, consisting of five broad pointed leaves, every one cut in on the end unto the middle, making them seem to be two a-piece, smelling somewhat sweet, and each of them standing in a large green striped hairy husk, large and round below next to the stalk. The seed is small and greyish in the hard heads that come up afterwards. The root is white and long, spreading divers fangs in the ground.

The Red Wild Campion grows in the same manner as the White; but its leaves are not so plainly ribbed, somewhat shorter, rounder, and more woolly in handling. The flowers are of the same form and bigness; but in some of a pale, in others of a bright red colour, cut in at the ends more finely, which makes the leaves look more in number than the other. The seeds and the roots are alike, the roots of both sorts abiding many years.

There are forty-five kinds of Campion more, those of them which are of a physical use, having the like virtues with those above described, which I take to be the two chief kinds.

Place.] They grow commonly through this land by fields and hedge-sides, and ditches.

Time.] They flower in Summer, some earlier than others, and some abiding longer than others.

Government and virtues.] They belong to Saturn, and it is found by experience, that the decoction of the herb, either in white or red wine being drank, doth stay inward bleedings, and applied outwardly it does the like; and being drank, helps to expel urine, being stopped, and gravel and stone in the reins and kidneys. Two drams of the seed drank in wine, purges the body of choleric humours, and helps those that are stung by scorpions, or other venomous beasts, and may be as effectual for the plague. It is of very good use in old sores, ulcers, cankers, fistulas, and the like, to cleanse and heat them, by consuming the moist humours falling into them, and correcting the putrefaction of humours offending them.

CARDUUS BENEDICTUS

It is called Carduus Benedictus, or Blessed Thistle, or Holy Thistle. I suppose the name was put upon it by some that had little holiness themselves.

I shall spare a labour in writing a description of this as almost every one that can but write at all, may describe them from his own knowledge.

Time.] They flower in August, and seed not long after.

Government and virtues.] It is an herb of Mars, and under the sign of Aries. Now, in handling this herb, I shall give you a rational pattern of all the rest; and if you please to view them throughout the book, you shall, to your content, find it true. It helps swimming and giddiness of the head, or the disease called vertigo, because Aries is in the house of Mars. It is an excellent remedy against the yellow jaundice and other infirmities of the gall, because Mars governs choler. It strengthens the attractive faculty in man, and clarifies the blood, because the one is ruled by Mars. The continual drinking the decoction of it, helps red faces, tetters, and ringworms, because Mars causes them. It helps the plague, sores, boils, and itch, the bitings of mad dogs and venomous beasts, all which infirmities are under Mars; thus you see what it doth by sympathy.

By antipathy to other planets it cures the French pox. By antipathy to Venus, who governs it, it strengthens the memory, and cures deafness by antipathy to Saturn, who has his fall in Aries, which rules the head. It cures quartan agues, and other diseases of melancholy, and adust choler, by sympathy to Saturn, Mars being exalted in Capricorn. Also provokes urine, the stopping of which is usually caused by Mars or the Moon.

CARROTS

GARDEN Carrots are so well known, that they need no description; but because they are of less physical use than the wild kind (as indeed almost in all herbs the wild are the most effectual in physic, as being more powerful in operation than the garden kinds,) I shall therefore briefly describe the Wild Carrot.

Descript.] It grows in a manner altogether like the tame, but that the leaves and stalks are somewhat whiter and rougher. The stalks bear large tufts of white flowers, with a deep purple spot in the middle, which are contracted together when the seed begins to ripen, that the middle part being hollow and low, and the outward stalk rising high, makes the whole umbel to show like a bird's nest. The root small, long, and hard, and unfit for meat, being somewhat sharp and strong.

Place.] The wild kind grows in divers parts of this land plenti-fully by the field-sides, and untilled places.

Time.] They flower and seed in the end of Summer.

Government and virtues.] Wild Carrots belong to Mercury, and therefore break wind, and remove stitches in the sides, provoke urine and women's courses, and helps to break and expel the stone; the seed also of the same works the like effect, and is good for the dropsy, and those whose bellies are swelling with wind; helps the cholic, the stone in the kidneys, and rising of the mother; being taken in wine, or boiled in wine and taken, it helps conception. The leaves being applied with honey to running sores or ulcers, do cleanse them.

I suppose the seeds of them perform this better than the roots; and though Galen commended garden Carrots highly to break wind, yet experience teaches they breed it first, and we may thank nature for expelling it, not they; the seeds of them expel wind indeed, and so mend what the root mars.

CARRAWAY

IT is on account of the seeds principally that the Carraway is cultivated.

Descript.] It bears divers stalks of fine cut leaves, lying upon the ground, somewhat like to the leaves of carrots, but not bushing so thick, of a little quick taste in them, from among which rises up a square stalk, not so high as the Carrot, at whose joints are set the like leaves, but smaller and finer, and at the top small open tufts, or umbels of white flowers, which turn into small blackish seed, smaller than the Aniseed, and of a quicker and hotter taste. The root is whitish, small and long, somewhat like unto a parsnip, but with more wrinkled bark, and much less, of a little hot and quick taste, and stronger than the parsnip and abides after seed-time.

Place.] It is usually sown with us in gardens.

Time.] They flower in June and July, and seed quickly after.

Government and virtues.] This is also a Mercurial plant. Carraway seed has a moderate sharp quality, whereby it breaks wind and provokes urine, which also the herb doth. The root is better food than the parsnip; it is pleasant and comfortable to the stomach, and helps digestion. The seed is conducing to all cold griefs of the head and stomach, bowels, or mother, as also the wind in them, and helps to sharpen the eye-sight. The powder of the seed put into a poultice, takes away black and blue spots of blows and bruises. The herb itself, or with some of the seed bruised and fried, laid hot in a bag or double cloth, to the lower parts of the belly, eases the pains of the wind cholic.

The roots of Carraway eaten as men do parsnips, strengthen the stomach of ancient people exceedingly, and they need not to make a whole meal of them neither, and are fit to be planted in every garden.

Carraway comfits, once only dipped in sugar, and half a spoonful of them eaten in the morning fasting, and as many after each meal, is a most admirable remedy, for those that are troubled with wind.

CELANDINE

Descript.] This hath divers tender, round, whitish green stalks, with greater joints than ordinary in other herbs as it were knees, very brittle and easy to break, from whence grow branches with large tender broad leaves, divided into many parts, each of them cut in on the edges, set at the joint on both sides of the branches, of a dark bluish green colour, on the upper side like Columbines, and of a more pale bluish green underneath, full of yellow sap, when any is broken, of a bitter taste, and strong scent. At the flowers, of four leaves a-piece, after which come small long pods, with blackish seed therein. The root is somewhat great at the head, shooting forth divers long roots and small strings, reddish on the outside, and yellow within, full of yellow sap therein.

Place.] They grow in many places by old walls, hedges and waysides in untilled places; and being once planted in a garden, especially some shady places, it will remain there.

Time.] They flower all the Summer, and the seed ripens in the mean time.

Government and virtues.] This is an herb of the Sun, and under the Celestial Lion, and is one of the best cures for the eyes; for, all that know any thing in astrology, know that the eyes are subject to the luminaries; let it then be gathered when the Sun is in Leo, and the Moon in Aries, applying to this time; let Leo arise, then may you make into an oil or ointment, which you please, to anoint your sore eyes with. I can prove it doth both my own experience, and the experience of those to whom I have taught it, that most desperate sore eyes have been cured by this only medicine; and then, I pray, is not this far better than endangering the eyes by the art of the needle? For if this does not absolutely take away the film, it will so facilitate the work, that it might be done without danger. The herb or root boiled in white wine and drank, a few Aniseeds being boiled therewith, opens obstructions of the liver and gall, helps the yellow jaundice; and often using it, helps the dropsy and the itch, and those who have old sores in their legs, or other parts of the body. The juice thereof taken fasting, is held to be of singularly good use against the pestilence. The distilled water, with a little sugar and a little good treacle mixed therewith (the party upon the taking being laid down to sweat a little) has the same effect. The juice dropped into the eyes, cleanses them from films and cloudiness which darken the sight, but it is best to allay the sharpness of the juice with a little breast milk. It is good in all old filthy corroding creeping ulcers wheresoever, to stay their malignity of fretting and running, and to cause them to heal more speedily. The juice often applied to tetters, ring-worms, or other such like spreading cankers, will quickly heal them, and rubbed often upon warts, will take them away. The herb with the roots bruised and bathed with oil of camomile, and applied to the navel, takes away the griping pains of the belly and bowels, and all the pains of the mother; and applied to women's breasts stays the overmuch flowing of the courses. The juice or decoction of the herb gargled between the teeth that ache, eases the pain, and the powder of the dried root laid upon any aching, hollow or loose tooth, will cause it to fall out. The juice mixed with some powder of brimstone is not only good against the itch, but takes away all discolourings of the skin whatsoever: and if it chance that in a tender body it causes any itchings or inflammations, by bathing the place with a little vinegar it is helped.

Another ill-favoured trick have physicians got to use to the eye, and that is worse than the needle; which is to take away the films by corroding or gnawing medicine. That I absolutely protest against.

1. Because the tunicles of the eyes are very thin, and therefore soon eaten asunder.

2. The callus or film that they would eat away, is seldom of an equal thickness in every place, and then the tunicle may be eaten asunder in one place, before the film be consumed in another, and so be a readier way to extinguish the sight than to restore it.

It is called Chelidonium, from the Greek word *Chelidon*, which signifies a swallow; because they say, that if you put out the eyes of young swallows when they are in the nest, the old ones will recover their eyes again with this herb. This I am confident, for I have tried it, that if we mar the very apple of their eyes with a needle, she will recover them again; but whether with this herb or not, I know not.

Also I have read (and it seems to be somewhat probable) that the herb, being gathered as I showed before, and the elements draw apart from it by art of the alchymist, and after they are drawn apart rectified, the earthly quality, still in rectifying them, added to the *Terra damnata* (as Alchymists call it) or *Terra Sacratisima* (as some philosophers call it) the elements so rectified are sufficient for the cure of all diseases, the humours offending being known and the contrary element given. It is an experiment worth the trying, and can do no harm.

THE LESSER CELANDINE, USUALLY KNOWN BY THE NAME OF PILEWORT AND FOGWORT

I WONDER what ailed the ancients to give this the name Celandine, which resembles it neither in nature nor form; it acquired the name of Pilewort from its virtues, and it being no great matter where I set it down, so I set it down at all, I humoured Dr. Tradition so much, as to set him down here.

Descript.] This Celandine or Pilewort (which you please) doth spread many round pale green leaves, set on weak and trailing branches which lie upon the ground, and are flat, smooth, and somewhat shining, and in some places (though seldom) marked with black spots, each standing on a long foot-stalk, among which rise small yellow flowers, consisting of nine or ten small narrow leaves, upon slender foot-stalks, very like unto Crowsfoot, where-unto the seed also is not unlike being many small kernels like a grain of corn sometimes twice as long as others, of a whitish colour, with fibres at the end of them.

Place.] It grows for the most part in moist corners of fields and places that are near water sides, yet will abide in drier ground if they be a little shady.

Time.] It flowers betimes, about March or April, is quite gone by May; so it cannot be found till it spring again.

Government and virtues.] It is under the dominion of Mars, and behold here another verification of the learning of the ancients, *viz.* that the virtue of an herb may be known by its signature, as plainly appears in this; for if you dig up the root of it, you shall perceive the perfect image of the disease which they commonly call the piles. It is certain by good experience, that the decoction of the leaves and roots wonderfully helps piles and hæmorrhoids, also kernels by the ears and throat, called the king's evil, or any other hard wens or tumours.

Here's another secret for my countrymen and women, a couple of them together; Pilewort made into an oil, ointment, or plaister, readily cures both the piles, or hæmorrhoids, and the king's evil. The very herb borne about one's body next the skin helps in such diseases, though it never touch the place grieved; let poor people make use of it for those uses; with this I cured my own daughter of the king's evil, broke the sore, drew out a quarter of a pint of corruption, cured without any scar at all in one week's time.

THE ORDINARY SMALL CENTAURY

Descript.] This grows up most usually but with one round and somewhat crusted stalk, about a foot high or better, branching forth at the top into many sprigs, and some also from the joints of the stalks below; the flowers thus stand at the tops as it were in one umbel or tuft, are of a pale red, tending to carnation colour, consisting of five, sometimes six small leaves, very like those of St. John's Wort, opening themselves in the day time and closing at night, after which come seeds in little short husk, in forms like unto wheat corn. The leaves are small and somewhat round; the root small and hard, perishing every year. The whole plant is of an exceeding bitter taste.

There is another sort in all things like the former, save only it bears white flowers.

Place.] They grow ordinarily in fields, pastures, and woods, but that with the white flowers not so frequently as the other.

Time.] They flower in July or thereabouts, and seeds within a month after.

Government and virtues.] They are under the dominion of the Sun, as appears in that their flowers open and shut as the Sun, either shows or hides his face. This herb, boiled and drank, purges choleric and gross humours, and helps the sciatica; it opens obstructions of the liver, gall, and spleen, helps the jaundice, and eases the pains in the sides and hardness of the spleen, used outwardly, and is given with very good effect in agues. It helps those that have the dropsy, or the green-sickness, being much used by the Italians in powder for that purpose. It kills the worms in the belly, as is found by experience. The decoction thereof, *viz.* the tops of the stalks, with the leaves and flowers, is good against the cholic, and to bring down women's courses, helps to avoid the dead birth, and eases pains of the mother, and is very effectual in all pains of the joints, as the gout, cramps, or convulsions. A dram of the powder taken in wine, is a wonderful good help against the biting and poison of an adder. The juice of the herb with a little honey put to it, is good to clear the eyes from dimness, mists and clouds that offend or hinder sight. It is singularly good both for green and fresh wounds, as also for old ulcers and sores, to close up the one and cleanse the other, and perfectly to cure them both, although they are hollow or fistulous; the green herb especially, being bruised and laid thereto. The decoction thereof dropped into the ears, cleanses them from worms, cleanses the foul ulcers and spreading scabs of the head, and takes away all freckles, spots, and marks in the skin, being washed with it; the herb is so safe you cannot fail in the using of it, only giving it inwardly for inward diseases. It is very wholesome, but not very toothsome.

There is beside these, another small Centaury, which bears a yellow flower; in all other respects it is like the former, save that the leaves are larger, and of a darker green, and the stalks pass through the midst of them, as it does in the herb Thorowan. They are all of them, as I told you, under the government of the Sun; yet this, if you observe it, you shall find an excellent truth; in diseases of the blood, use the red Centaury; if of choler, use the yellow; but if phlegm or water, you will find the white best.

THE CHERRY-TREE

I suppose there are few but know this tree, for its fruit's sake; and therefore I shall spare writing a description thereof.

Place.] For the place of its growth, it is afforded room in every orchard.

Government and virtues.] It is a tree of *Venus.* Cherries, as they are of different tastes, so they are of different qualities. The sweet pass through the stomach and the belly more speedily, but are of little nourishment; the tart or sour are more pleasing to an hot stomach, procure appetite to meat, to help and cut tough phlegm, and gross humours; but when these are dried, they are more binding to the belly than when they are fresh, being cooling in hot diseases, and welcome to the stomach, and provokes urine. The gum of the Cherry-tree, desolved in wine is good for a cold, cough, and hoarseness of the throat; mends the colour in the face, sharpens the eyesight, provokes appetite, and helps to break and expel the stone, and dissolved, the water thereof is much used to break the stone, and to expel gravel and wind.

WINTER-CHERRIES

Descript.] The Winter Cherry has a running or creeping root in the ground, of the bigness many times one's little finger, shooting forth at several joints in several places, whereby it quickly spreads a great compass of ground. The stalk rises not above a yard high, whereon are set many broad and long green leaves, somewhat like nightshades, but larger; at the joints, whereof come forth whitish flowers made of five leaves a piece, which afterwards turn into green berries inclosed with thin skins, which change to be reddish when they grow ripe, the berry likewise being reddish, and as large as a cherry; wherein are contained many flat and yellowish seeds lying within the pulp, which being gathered and strung up, will keep all the year to be used upon occasions.

Place.] They grow not naturally in this land, but are cherished in gardens for their virtues.

Time.] They flower not until the middle or latter end of July; and the fruit is ripe about August, or the beginning of September.

Government and virtues.] This also is a plant of Venus. They are of great use in physic. The leaves being cooling, may be used in inflammations, but not opening as the berries and fruit are; which by drawing down the urine provoke it to be voided plentifully when it is stopped or grown hot, sharp, and painful in the passage; it is good also to expel the stone and gravel out of the reins, kidneys and bladder, helping to dissolve the stone, and voiding it by grit or gravel sent forth in the urine; it also helps much to cleanse inward imposthumes or ulcers in the reins of bladder, or in those that void a bloody or foul urine. The distilled water of the fruit, or the leaves together with them, or the berries, green or dry, distilled with a little milk and drank morning and evening with a little sugar, is effectual to all the purposes before specified, and especially against the heat and sharpness of the urine. I shall only mention one way, amongst many others, which might be used for ordering the berries, to be helpful for the urine and the stone; which is this: Take three or four good handfuls of the berries, either green or fresh, or dried, and having bruised them, put them into so many gallons of beer or ale when it is new tunned up. This drink taken daily, has been found to do much good to many, both to ease the pains, and expel urine and the stone, and to cause the stone not to engender. The decoction of the berries in wine and water is the most usual way; but the powder of them taken in drink is more effectual.

CHERVIL

It is called Cerefolium, Mirrhis, and Mirrha, Chervil, Sweet Chervil, and Sweet Cicely.

Descript.] The garden Chervil doth at first somewhat resemble Parsley, but after it is better grown, the leaves are much cut in and jagged, resembling hemlock, being a little hairy and of a whitish green colour, sometimes turning reddish in the Summer, with the stalks also; it rises a little above half a foot high, bearing white flowers in spiked tufts, which turn into long and round seeds pointed at the ends, and blackish when they are ripe; of a sweet taste, but no smell, though the herb itself smells reasonably well. The root is small and long, and perishes every year, and must be sown a-new in spring, for seed after July for Autumn fails.

The wild Chervil grows two or three feet high with yellow stalks and joints, set with broader and more hairy leaves, divided into sundry parts, nicked about the edges, and of a dark green colour, which likewise grow reddish with the stalks; at the tops whereof stands small white tufts of flowers, afterwards smaller and longer seed. The root is white, hard, and enduring long. This has little or no scent.

Place.] The first is sown in gardens for a sallad herb; the second grows wild in many of the meadows of this land, and by the hedge sides, and on heaths.

Time.] They flower and seed early, and thereupon are sown again in the end of Summer.

Government and virtues.] The garden Chervil being eaten, doth moderately warm the stomach, and is a certain remedy (saith Tragus) to dissolve congealed or clotted blood in the body, or that which is clotted by bruises, falls, &c. The juice or distilled water thereof being drank, and the bruised leaves laid to the place, being taken either in meat or drink, it is good to help to provoke urine, or expel the stone in the kidneys, to send down women's courses, and to help the pleurisy and pricking of the sides.

The wild Chervil bruised and applied, dissolves swellings in any part, or the marks of congealed blood by bruises or blows, in a little space.

SWEET CHERVIL, OR SWEET CICELY

Descript.] This grows very like the great hemlock, having large spread leaves cut into divers parts, but of a fresher green colour than the Hemlock, tasting as sweet as the Anniseed. The stalks rise up a yard high, or better, being creased or hollow, having leaves at the joints, but lesser; and at the tops of the branched stalks, umbels or tufts of white flowers; after which comes long crested black shining seed, pointed at both ends, tasting quick, yet sweet and pleasant. The root is great and white, growing deep in the ground, and spreading sundry long branches therein, in taste and smell stronger than the leaves or seeds, and continuing many years.

Place.] This grows in gardens.

Government and virtues.] These are all three of them of the nature of Jupiter, and under his dominion. This whole plant, besides its pleasantness in sallads, has its physical virtue. The root boiled, and eaten with oil and vinegar, (or without oil) do much please and warm old and cold stomachs oppressed with wind or phlegm, or those that have the phthisic or consumption of the lungs. The same drank with wine is a preservation from the plague. It provokes women's courses, and expels the after-birth, procures an appetite to meat, and expels wind. The juice is good to heal the ulcers of the head and face; the candied roots hereof are held as effectual as Angelica, to preserve from infection in the time of a plague, and to warm and comfort a cold weak stomach. It is so harmless, you cannot use it amiss.

CHESNUT TREE

It were as needless to describe a tree so commonly known as to tell a man he had gotten a mouth; therefore take the government and virtues of them thus:

The tree is abundantly under the dominion of Jupiter, and therefore the fruit must needs breed good blood, and yield commendable nourishment to the body; yet if eaten over-much, they make the blood thick, procure head ache, and bind the body; the inner skin, that covers the nut, is of so binding a quality, that a scruple of it being taken by a man, or ten grains by a child, soon stops any flux whatsoever. The whole nut being dried and beaten into powder, and a dram taken at a time, is a good remedy to stop the terms in women. If you dry Chesnuts, (only the kernels I mean) both the barks being taken away, beat them into powder, and make the powder up into an electuary with honey, so have you an admirable remedy for the cough and spitting of blood.

EARTH CHESNUTS

They are called Earth-nuts, Earth Chesnuts, Ground Nuts, Ciper-nuts, and in Sussex Pig-nuts. A description of them were needless, for every child knows them.

Government and virtues.] They are something hot and dry in quality, under the dominion of Venus, they provoke lust exceedingly, and stir up to those sports she is mistress of; the seed is excellent good to provoke urine; and so also is the root, but it doth not perform it so forcibly as the seed both. The root being dried and beaten into powder, and the powder made into an electuary, is as singular a remedy for spitting and pissing of blood, as the former Chesnut was for coughs.

CHICKWEED

It is so generally known to most people, that I shall not trouble you with the description thereof, nor myself with setting forth the several kinds, since but only two or three are considerable for their usefulness.

Place.] They are usually found in moist and watery places, by wood sides, and elsewhere.

Time.] They flower about June, and their seed is ripe in July.

Government and virtues.] It is a fine soft pleasing herb under the dominion of the Moon. It is found to be effectual as Purslain to all the purposes whereunto it serves, except for meat only. The herb bruised, or the juice applied (with cloths or sponges dipped therein) to the region of the liver, and as they dry, to have it fresh applied, doth wonderfully temperate the heat of the liver, and is effectual for all imposthumes and swellings whatsoever, for all redness in the face, wheals, pushes, itch, scabs; the juice either simply used, or boiled with hog's grease and applied, helps cramps, convulsions, and palsy. The juice, or distilled water, is of much good use for all heats and redness in the eyes, to drop some thereof into them; as also into the ears, to ease pains in them; and is of good effect to ease pains from the heat and sharpness of the blood in the piles, and generally all pains in the body that arise of heat. It is used also in hot and virulent ulcers and sores in the privy parts of men and women, or on the legs, or elsewhere. The leaves boiled with marsh-mallows, and made into a poultice with fenugreek and linseed, applied to swellings or imposthumes, ripen and break them, or assuage the swellings and ease the pains. It helps the sinews when they are shrunk by cramps, or otherwise, and to extend and make them pliable again by this medicine. Boil a handful of Chickweed, and a handful of red rose leaves dried, in a quart of muscadine, until a fourth part be consumed; then put to them a pint of oil of trotters or sheep's feet; let them boil a good while, still stirring them well; which being strained, anoint the grieved place therewith, warm against the fire, rubbing it well with one hand: and bind also some of the herb (if you will) to the place, and, with God's blessing, it will help it in three times dressing.

CHICK-PEASE, OR CICERS

Descript.] The garden sorts whether red, black, or white, bring forth stalks a yard long, whereon do grow many small and almost round leaves, dented about the edges, set on both sides of a middle rib. At the joints come forth one or two flowers, upon sharp foot stalks, pease-fashion, either white or whitish, or purplish red, lighter or deeper, according as the pease that follow will be, that are contained in small, thick, and short pods, wherein lie one or two pease, more usually pointed at the lower end, and almost round at the head, yet a little cornered or sharp; the root is small, and perishes yearly.

Place and Time.] They are sown in gardens, or fields as pease, being sown later than pease, and gathered at the same time with them, or presently after.

Government and virtues.] They are both under the dominion of Venus. They are less windy than beans, but nourish more; they provoke urine, and are thought to increase sperm; they have a cleansing faculty, whereby they break the stone in the kidneys. To drink the cream of them, being boiled in water, is the best way. It moves the belly downwards, provokes women's courses and urine, increases both milk and seed. One ounce of Cicers, two ounces of French barley, and a small handful of Marsh-mallow roots, clean washed and cut, being boiled in the broth of a chicken, and four ounces taken in the morning, and fasting two hours after, is a good medicine for a pain in the sides. The white Cicers are used more for meat than medicine, yet have the same effect, and are thought more powerful to increase milk and seed. The wild Cicers are so much more powerful than the garden kinds, by how much they exceed them in heat and dryness; whereby they do more open obstructions, break the stone, and have all the properties of cutting, opening, digesting, and dissolving; and this more speedily and certainly than the former.

CINQUEFOIL, OR FIVE-LEAVED GRASS; CALLED IN SOME COUNTIES, FIVE-FINGERED GRASS

Descript.] It spreads and creeps far upon the ground, with long slender strings like straw-berries, which take root again, and shoot forth many leaves, made of five parts, and sometimes of seven, dented about the edges, and somewhat hard. The stalks are slender, leaning downwards and bear many small yellow flowers thereon, with some yellow threads in the middle, standing about a smooth green head, which, when it is ripe, is a little rough, and contains small brownish seeds. The root is of a blackish brown colour, as big as one's little finger, but growing long, with some threads thereat; and by the small string it quickly spreads over the ground.

Place.] It grows by wood sides, hedge sides, the path-way in fields, and in the borders and corners of them almost through all this land.

Time.] It flowers in summer, some sooner, some later.

Government and virtues.] This is an herb of Jupiter, and therefore strengthens the part of the body it rules; let Jupiter be angular and strong when it is gathered; and if you give but a scruple (which is but twenty grains,) of it at a time, either in white wine, or in white wine vinegar, you shall very seldom miss the cure of an ague, be it what ague soever, in three fits, as I have often proved to the admiration both of myself and others; let no man despise it because it is plain and easy, the ways of God are all such. It is an especial herb used in all inflammations and fevers, whether infectious or pestilential; or among other herbs to cool and temper the blood and humours in the body. As also for all lotions, gargles, infections, and the like, for sore mouths, ulcers, cancers, fistulas, and other corrupt, foul, or running sores. The juice hereof drank, about four ounces at a time, for certain days together, cures the quinsey and yellow jaundice; and taken for thirty days together, cures the falling sickness. The roots boiled in milk, and drank, is a most effectual remedy for all fluxes in man or woman, whether the white or red, as also the bloody flux. The roots boiled in vinegar, and the decoction thereof held in the mouth, eases the pains of the toothache. The juice or decoction taken with a little honey, helps the hoarseness of the throat, and is very good for the cough of the lungs. The distilled water of both roots and leaves, is also effectual to all the purposes aforesaid; and if the hands be often washed therein, and suffered at every time to dry in of itself without wiping, it will in a short time help the palsy, or shaking in them. The root boiled in vinegar, helps all knots, kernels, hard swellings, and lumps growing in any part of the flesh, being thereto applied, as also inflammations, and St. Anthony's fire, all imposthumes, and painful sores with heat and putrefaction, the shingles also, and all other sorts of running and foul scabs, sores and itch. The same also boiled in wine, and applied to any joint full of pain, ache, or the gout in the hands or feet, or the hip gout, called the Sciatica, and the decoction thereof drank the while, doth cure them, and eases much pain in the bowels. The roots are likewise effectual to help ruptures or bursting, being used with other things available to that purpose, taken either inwardly or outwardly, or both; as also bruises or hurts by blows, falls, or the like, and to stay the bleeding of wounds in any parts inward or outward.

Some hold that one leaf cures a quotidian, three a tertian, and four a quartan ague, and a hundred to one if it be not Dioscorides; for he is full of whimsies. The truth is, I never stood so much upon the number of the leaves, nor whether I give it in powder or decoction. If Jupiter were strong, and the Moon applying to him, or his good aspect at the gathering, I never knew it miss the desired effect.

CIVES

CALLED also Rush Leeks, Chives, Civet, and Sweth.

Government and virtues.] I confess I had not added these, had it not been for a country gentleman, who by a letter certified me, that amongst other herbs, I had left these out; they are indeed a kind of leek, hot and dry in the fourth degree as they are, and so under the dominion of Mars; if they be eaten raw, (I do not mean raw, opposite to roasted or boiled, but raw, opposite to chymical preparation) they send up very hurtful vapours to the brain, causing troublesome sleep, and spoiling the eye-sight, yet of them prepared by the art of the alchymist, may be made an excellent remedy for the stoppage of the urine.

CLARY, OR MORE PROPERLY CLEAR-EYE

Descript.] Our ordinary garden Clary has four square stalks, with broad, rough, wrinkled, whitish, or hoary green leaves somewhat evenly cut in on the edges, and of a strong sweet scent, growing some near the ground, and some by couples upon stalks. The flowers grow at certain distances, with two small leaves at the joints under them, somewhat like unto the flowers of Sage, but smaller, and of a whitish blue colour. The seed is brownish, and somewhat flat, or not so round as the wild. The roots are blackish, and spread not far, and perish after the seed time. It is usually sown, for it seldom rises of its own sowing.

Place.] This grows in gardens.

Time.] It flowers in June and July, some a little later than others, and their seed is ripe in August, or thereabouts.

Government and virtues.] It is under the dominion of the Moon. The seed put into the eyes clears them from motes, and such like things gotten within the lids to offend them, as also clears them from white and red spots on them. The mucilage of the seed made with water, and applied to tumours, or swellings, disperses and takes them away; as also draws forth splinters, thorns, or other things gotten into the flesh. The leaves used with vinegar, either by itself, or with a little honey, doth help boils, felons, and the hot inflammation that are gathered by their pains, if applied before it be grown too great. The powder of the dried root put into the nose, provokes sneezing, and thereby purges the head and brain of much rheum and corruption. The seed or leaves taken in wine, provokes to venery. It is of much use both for men and women that have weak backs, and helps to strengthen the reins: used either by itself, or with other herbs conducing to the same effect, and in tansies often. The fresh leaves dipped in a batter of flour, eggs, and a little milk, and fried in butter, and served to the table, is not unpleasant to any, but exceedingly profitable for those that are troubled with weak backs, and the effects thereof. The juice of the herb put into ale or beer, and drank, brings down women's courses, and expels the after-birth.

WILD CLARY

WILD Clary is most blasphemously called Christ's Eye, because it cures diseases of the eye. I could wish for my soul, blasphemy, ignorance, and tyranny, were ceased among physicians, that they may be happy, and I joyful.

Descript.] It is like the other Clary, but lesser, with many stalks about a foot and a half high. The stalks are square, and somewhat hairy; the flowers of a bluish colour. He that knows the common Clary cannot be ignorant of this.

Place.] It grows commonly in this nation in barren places; you may find it plentifully, if you look in the fields near Gray's Inn, and near Chelsea.

Time.] They flower from the beginning of June to the latter end of August.

Government and virtues.] It is something hotter and drier than the garden Clary is, yet nevertheless under the dominion of the Moon, as well as that; the seeds of it being beat to powder, and drank with wine, is an admirable help to provoke lust. A decoction of the leaves being drank, warms the stomach, and it is a wonder if it should not, the stomach being under Cancer, the house of the Moon. Also it helps digestion, scatters congealed blood in any part of the body. The distilled water hereof cleanses the eyes of redness, waterishness and heat. It is a gallant remedy for dimness of sight, to take one of the seeds of it, and put into the eyes, and there let it remain till it drops out of itself, (the pain will be nothing to speak of,) it will cleanse the eyes of all filthy and putrefied matter; and in often repeating it, will take off a film which covers the sight: a handsomer, safer, and easier remedy by a great deal, than to tear it off with a needle.

CLEAVERS

IT is also called Aperine, Goose-shade, Goose-grass, and Cleavers.

Descript.] The common Cleavers have divers very rough square stalks, not so big as the top of a point, but rising up to be two or three yards high sometimes, if it meet with any tall bushes or trees whereon it may climb, yet without any claspers, or else much lower, and lying on the ground, full of joints, and at every one of them shoots forth a branch, besides the leaves thereat, which are usually six, set in a round compass like a star, or a rowel of a spur. From between the leaves or the joints towards the tops of the branches, come forth very small white flowers, at every end, upon small thready foot-stalks, which after they have fallen, there do shew two small round and rough seeds joined together which, when they are ripe, grow hard and whitish, having a little hole on the side, something like unto a navel. Both stalks, leaves, and seeds are so rough, that they will cleave to any thing that will touch them. The root is small and thready, spreading much to the ground, but dies every year.

Place.] It grows by the hedge and ditchsides in many places of this land, and is so troublesome an inhabitant in gardens, that it ramps upon, and is ready to choak whatever grows near it.

Time.] It flowers in June or July, and the seed is ripe and falls again in the end of July or August, from whence it springs up again, and not from the old roots.

Government and virtues.] It is under the dominion of the Moon. The juice of the herb and the seed together taken in wine, helps those bitten with an adder, by preserving the heart from the venom. It is familiarly taken in broth to keep them lean and lank, that are apt to grow fat. The distilled water drank twice a day, helps the yellow jaundice, and the decoction of the herb, in experience, is found to do the same, and stays lasks and bloody-fluxes. The juice of the leaves, or they a little bruised, and applied to any bleeding wounds, stays the bleeding. The juice also is very good to close up the lips of green wounds, and the powder of the dried herb strewed thereupon doth the same, and likewise helps old ulcers. Being boiled in hog's grease, it helps all sorts of hard swellings or kernels in the throat, being anointed therewith. The juice dropped into the ears, takes away the pain of them.

It is a good remedy in the Spring, eaten (being first chopped small, and boiled well) in water-gruel, to cleanse the blood, and strengthen the liver, thereby to keep the body in health, and fitting it for that change of season that is coming.

CLOWN'S WOODS

Descript.] It grows up sometimes to two or three feet high, but usually about two feet, with square green rough stalks, but slender, joined somewhat far asunder, and two very long, somewhat narrow, dark green leaves, bluntly dented about the edges thereof, ending in a long point. The flowers stand towards the tops, compassing the stalks at the joints with the leaves, and end likewise in a spiked top, having long and much gaping hoods of a purplish red colour, with whitish spots in them, standing in somewhat round husks, wherein afterwards stand blackish round seeds. The root is composed of many long strings, with some tuberous long knobs growing among them, of a pale yellowish or whitish colour, yet some times of the year these knobby roots in many places are not seen in this plant. This plant smells somewhat strong.

Place.] It grows in sundry counties of this land, both north and west, and frequently by path-sides in the fields near about London, and within three or four miles distant about it, yet it usually grows in or near ditches.

Time.] It flowers in June or July, and the seed is ripe soon after.

Government and virtues.] It is under the dominion of the planet Saturn. It is singularly effectual in all fresh and green wounds, and therefore bears not this name for nought. And it is very available in staunching of blood and to dry up the fluxes of humours in old fretting ulcers, cankers, &c. that hinder the healing of them.

A syrup made of the juice of it, is inferior to none for inward wounds, ruptures of veins, bloody flux, vessels broken, spitting, urining, or vomiting blood. Ruptures are excellent and speedily, ever to admiration, cured by taking now and then a little of the syrup, and applying an ointment or plaister of this herb to the place. Also, if any vain be swelled or muscle, apply a plaister of this herb to it, and if you add a little Comfrey to it, it will not be amiss. I assure thee the herb deserves commendation, though it has gotten such a clownish name; and whosoever reads this, (if he try it, as I have done,) will commend it; only take notice that it is of a dry earthy quality.

COCK'S HEAD, RED FITCHING, OR MEDICK FETCH

Descript.] This has divers weak but rough stalks, half a yard long, leaning downward, but set with winged leaves, longer and more pointed than those of Lintels, and whitish underneath; from the tops of these stalks arise up other slender stalks, naked without leaves unto the tops, where there grow many small flowers in manner of a spike, of a pale reddish colour with some blueness among them; after which rise up in their places, round rough, and somewhat flat heads. The root is tough, and somewhat woody, yet lives and shoots a-new every year.

Place.] It grows upon hedges, and sometimes in the open fields, in divers places of this land.

Time.] They flower all the months of July and August, and the seed ripen in the meanwhile.

Government and virtues.] It is under the dominion of Venus. It has power to rarify and digest, and therefore the green leaves bruised and laid as a plaister, disperse knots, nodes, or kernels in the flesh; and if, when dry, it be taken in wine, it helps the stranguary; and being anointed with oil, it provokes sweat. It is a singular food for cattle, to cause them to give store of milk; and why then may it not do the like, being boiled in ordinary drink, for nurses.

COLUMBINES

THESE are so well known, growing almost in every garden, that I think I may save the expense of time in writing a description of them.

Time.] They flower in May, and abide not for the most part when June is past, perfecting their seed in the meantime.

Government and virtues.] It is also an herb of Venus. The leaves of Columbines are commonly used in lotions with good success for sore mouths and throats. Tragus saith, that a dram of the seed taken in wine with a little saffron, opens obstructions of the liver, and is good for the yellow jaundice, if the party after the taking thereof be laid to sweat well in bed. The seed also taken in wine causes a speedy delivery of women in childbirth: if one draught suffice not, let her drink the second, and it will be effectual. The Spaniards used to eat a piece of the root thereof in the morning fasting, many days together, to help them when troubled with the stone in the reins or kidneys.

COLTSFOOT

CALLED also Coughwort, Foals's-foot, Horse-hoof, and Bull's-foot.

Descript.] This shoots up a slender stalk, with small yellowish flowers somewhat earlier, which fall away quickly, and after they are past, come up somewhat round leaves, sometimes dented about the edges, much lesser, thicker, and greener than those of butter-bur, with a little down or frieze over the green leaf on the upper side, which may be rubbed away, and whitish or meally underneath. The root is small and white, spreading much under ground, so that where it takes it will hardly be driven away again, if any little piece be abiding therein; and from thence spring fresh leaves.

Place.] It grows as well in wet grounds as in drier places.

Time.] And flowers in the end of February, the leaves begin to appear in March.

Government and virtues.] The plant is under Venus, the fresh leaves or juice, or a syrup thereof is good for a hot dry cough, or wheezing, and shortness of breath. The dry leaves are best for those that have thin rheums and distillations upon their lungs, causing a cough, for which also the dried leaves taken as tobacco, or the root is very good. The distilled water hereof simply, or with Elder flowers and Nightshade, is a singularly good remedy against all hot agues, to drink two ounces at a time, and apply cloths wet therein to the head and stomach, which also does much good, being applied to any hot swellings and inflammations. It helps St. Anthony's fire, and burnings, and is singularly good to take away wheals and small pushes that arise through heat; as also the burning heat of the piles, or privy parts, cloths wet therein being thereunto applied.

COMFREY

THIS is a very common but a very neglected plant. It contains very great virtues.

Descript.] The common Great Comfrey has divers very large hairy green leaves lying on the ground, so hairy or prickly, that if they touch any tender parts of the hands, face, or body, it will cause it to itch; the stalks that rise from among them, being two or three feet high, hollow and cornered, is very hairy also, having many such like leaves as grow below, but less and less up to the top. At the joints of the stalks it is divided into many branches, with some leaves thereon, and at the ends stand many flowers in order one above another, which are somewhat long and hollow like the finger of a glove, of a pale whitish colour, after which come small black seeds. The roots are great and long, spreading great thick branches under ground, black on the outside, and whitish within, short and easy to break, and full of glutinous or clammy juice, of little or no taste at all.

There is another sort in all things like this, only somewhat less, and bears flowers of a pale purple colour.

Place.] They grow by ditches and water-sides, and in divers fields that are moist, for therein they chiefly delight to grow. The first generally through all the land, and the other but in some places. By the leave of my authors, I know the first grows in dry places.

Time.] They flower in June or July, and give their seed in August.

Government and virtues.] This is an herb of Saturn, and I suppose under the sign Capricorn, cold, dry, and earthy in quality. What was spoken of Clown's Woundwort may be said of this. The Great Comfrey helps those that spit blood or make a bloody urine. The root boiled in water or wine, and the decoction drank, helps all inward hurts, bruises, wounds, and ulcer of the lungs, and causes the phlegm that oppresses them to be easily spit forth. It helps the defluction of rheum from the head upon the lungs, the fluxes of blood or humours by the belly, women's immoderate courses, as well the reds as the whites, and the running of the reins happening by what cause soever. A syrup made thereof is very effectual for all those inward griefs and hurts, and the distilled water for the same purpose also, and for outward wounds and sores in the fleshy or sinewy part of the body whatsoever, as also to take away the fits of agues, and to allay the sharpness of humours. A decoction of the leaves hereof is available to all the purposes, though not so effectual as the roots. The roots being outwardly applied, help fresh wounds or cuts immediately, being bruised and laid thereto; and is special good for ruptures and broken bones; yea, it is said to be so powerful to consolidate and knit together, that if they be boiled with dissevered pieces of flesh in a pot, it will join them together again. It is good to be applied to women's breasts that grow sore by the abundance of milk coming into them; also to repress the over much bleeding of the hæmorrhoids, to cool the inflammation of the parts thereabouts, and to give ease of pains. The roots of Comfrey taken fresh, beaten small, and spread upon leather, and laid upon any place troubled with the gout, doth presently give ease of the pains; and applied in the same manner, gives ease to pained joints, and profits very much for running and moist ulcers, gangrenes, mortifications, and the like, for which it hath by often experience been found helpful.

CORALWORT

It is also called by some Toothwort, Tooth Violet, Dog-Teeth Violet, and Dentaria.

Descript.] Of the many sorts of this herb two of them may be found growing in this nation; the first of which shoots forth one or two winged leaves, upon long brownish foot-stalks, which are doubled down at their first coming out of the ground; when they are fully opened they consist of seven leaves, most commonly of a sad green colour, dented about the edges, set on both sides the middle rib one against another, as the leaves of the ash tree; the stalk bears no leaves on the lower half of it; the upper half bears sometimes three or four, each consisting of five leaves, sometimes of three; on the top stand four or five flowers upon short foot-stalks, with long husks; the flowers are very like the flowers of Stockgilli-flowers, of a pale purplish colour, consisting of four leaves apiece, after which come small pods, which contain the seed; the root is very smooth, white and shining; it does not grow downwards, but creeps along under the upper crust of the ground, and consists of divers small round knobs set together; towards the top of the stalk there grows some single leaves, by each of which comes a small cloven bulb, which when it is ripe, if it be set in the ground, it will grow to be a root.

As for the other Coralwort, which grows in this nation, it is more scarce than this, being a very small plant, much like Crowfoot, therefore some think it to be one of the sorts of Crowfoot. I know not where to direct you to it, therefore I shall forbear the description.

Place.] The first grows in Mayfield in Sussex, in a wood called Highread, and in another wood there also, called Fox-holes.

Time.] They flower from the latter end of April to the middle of May, and before the middle of July they are gone, and not to be found.

Government and virtues.] It is under the dominion of the Moon. It cleanses the bladder, and provokes urine, expels gravel, and the stone; it eases pains in the sides and bowels, is excellently good for inward wounds, especially such as are made in the breast or lungs, by taking a dram of the powder of the root every morning in wine; the same is excellently good for ruptures, as also to stop fluxes; an ointment made of it is exceedingly good for wounds and ulcers, for it soon dries up the watery humours which hinder the cure.

COSTMARY, OR ALCOST, OR BALSAM HERB

THIS is so frequently known to be an inhabitant in almost every garden, that I suppose it needless to write a description thereof.

Time.] It flowers in June and July.

Government and virtues.] It is under the dominion of Jupiter. The ordinary Costmary, as well as Maudlin, provokes urine abundantly, and moistens the hardness of the mother; it gently purges choler and phlegm, extenuating that which is gross, and cutting that which is tough and glutinous, cleanses that which is foul, and hinders putrefaction and corruption; it dissolves without attraction, opens obstructions, and helps their evil effects, and it is a wonderful help to all sorts of dry agues. It is astringent to the stomach, and strengthens the liver, and all the other inward parts; and taken in whey works more effectually. Taken fasting in the morning, it is very profitable for pains in the head that are continual, and to stay, dry up, and consume all thin rheums or distillations from the head into the stomach, and helps much to digest raw humours that are gathered therein. It is very profitable for those that are fallen into a continual evil disposition of the whole body, called Cachexia, but especially in the beginning of the disease. It is an especial friend and helps to evil, weak and cold livers. The seed is familiarly given to children for the worms, and so is the infusion of the flowers in white wine given them to the quantity of two ounces at a time; it makes an excellent salve to cleanse and heal old ulcers, being boiled with oil of olive, and Adder's tongue with it, and after it is strained, put a little wax, rosin, and turpentine, to bring it to a convenient body.

CUDWEED, OR COTTONWEED

BESIDES Cudweed and Cottonweed, it is also Called Chaffweed, Dwarf Cotton, and Petty Cotton.

Descript.] The common Cudweed rises up with one stalk sometimes, and sometimes with two or three, thick set on all sides with small, long and narrow whitish or woody leaves, from the middle of the stalk almost up to the top, with every leaf stands small flowers of a dun or brownish yellow colour, or not so yellow as others; in which herbs, after the flowers are fallen, come small seed wrapped up, with the down therein, and is carried away with the wind; the root is small and thready.

There are other sorts hereof, which are somewhat less than the former, not much different, save only that the stalks and leaves are shorter, so that the flowers are paler and more open.

Place.] They grow in dry, barren, sandy, and gravelly grounds, in most places of this land.

Time.] They flower about July, some earlier, some later, and their seed is ripe in August.

Government and virtues.] Venus is Lady of it. The plants are all astringent, binding, or drying, and therefore profitable for de-fluctions of rheum from the head, and to stays fluxes of blood where-soever, the decoction being made into red wine and drank, or the powder taken therein. It also helps the bloody-flux, and eases the torments that come thereby, stays the immoderate courses of women, and is also good for inward or outward wounds, hurts, and bruises, and helps children both of bursting and the worms, and being either drank or injected, for the disease called Tenesmus, which is an often provocation to the stool without doing any think. The green leaves bruised, and laid to any green wound, stays the bleeding, and heals it up quickly. The juice of the herb taken in wine and milk, is, as Pliny saith, a sovereign remedy against the mumps and quinsey; and further saith, That whosoever shall so take it, shall never be troubled with that disease again.

COWSLIPS, OR PEAGLES

Both the wild and garden Cowslips are so well known, that I neither trouble myself nor the reader with a description of them.

Time.] They flower in April and May.

Government and virtues.] Venus lays claim to this herb as her own, and it is under the sign Aries, and our city dames know well enough the ointment or distilled water of it adds beauty, or at least restores it when it is lost. The flowers are held to be more effectual than the leaves, and the roots of little use. An ointment being made with them, takes away spots and wrinkles of the skin, sun-burning, and freckles, and adds beauty exceedingly; they remedy all in-firmities of the head coming of heat and wind, as vertigo, ephialtes, false apparitions, phrensies, falling-sickness, palsies, convulsions, cramps, pains in the nerves; the roots ease pains in the back and bladder, and open the passages of urine. The leaves are good in wounds, and the flowers take away trembling. If the flowers be not well dried, and kept in a warm place, they will soon putrefy and look green. Have a special eye over them. If you let them see the Sun ounce a month, it will do neither the Sun nor them harm.

Because they strengthen the brain and nerves, and remedy palsies, and Greeks gave them the name Paralysis. The flowers preserved or conserved, and the quantity of a nutmeg eaten every morning, is a sufficient dose for inward diseases; but for wounds, spots, wrinkles, and sunburnings, an ointment is made of the leaves, and hog's grease.

CRAB'S CLAWS

CALLED also Water Sengreen, Knight's Pond Water, Water House-leek, Pond Weed, and Fresh-water Soldier.

Descript.] It has sundry long narrow leaves, with sharp prickles on the edges of them, also very sharp pointed; the stalks which bear flowers, seldom grow so high as the leaves, bearing a forked head, like a Crab's Claw, out of which comes a white flower, consisting of three leaves, with divers yellowish hairy threads in the middle; it takes root in the mud at the bottom of the water.

Place.] It grows plentifully in the fens in Lincolnshire.

Time.] It flowers in June, and usually from thence till August.

Government and virtues.] It is a plant under the dominion of Venus, and therefore a great strengthener of the reins; it is excellently good for inflammation which is commonly called St. Anthony's Fire; it assuages inflammations, and swellings in wounds: and an ointment made of it is excellently good to heal them; there is scarcely a better remedy growing than this is, for such as have bruised their kidneys, and upon that account discharge blood; a dram of the powder of the herb taken every morning, is a very good remedy to stop the terms.

BLACK CRESSES

Descript.] It has long leaves, deeply cut and jagged on both sides, not much unlike wild mustard; the stalk small, very limber, though very tough: you may twist them round as you may a willow before they break. The flowers are very small and yellow, after which comes small pods, which contains the seed.

Place.] It is a common herb, grows usually by the way-side, and sometimes upon mud walls about London, but it delights to grow most among stones and rubbish.

Time.] It flowers in June and July, and the seed is ripe in August and September.

Government and virtues.] It is a plant of a hot and biting nature, under the dominion of Mars. The seed of Black Cresses strengthens the brain exceedingly, being, in performing that office, little inferior to mustard seed, if at all; they are excellently good to stay those rheums which may fall down from the head upon the lungs; you may beat the seed into powder, if you please, and make it up into an electuary with honey; so you have an excellent remedy by you, not only for the premises, but also for the cough, yellow jaundice and sciatica. This herb boiled into a poultice, is an excellent remedy for inflammations; both in women's breasts, and men's testicles.

SCIATICA CRESSES

Descript.] These are of two kinds. The first rises up with a round stalk about two feet high, spreads into divers branches, whose lower leaves are somewhat larger than the upper, yet all of them cut or torn on the edges, somewhat like the garden Cresses, but smaller, the flowers are small and white, growing at the tops of branches, where afterwards grow husks with small brownish seeds therein very strong and sharp in taste, more than the Cresses of the garden; the root is long, white, and woody.

The other has the lower leaves whole somewhat long and broad, not torn at all, but only somewhat deeply dented about the edges towards the ends; but those that grow up higher are smaller. The flowers and seeds are like the former, and so is the root likewise, and both root and seeds as sharp as it.

Place.] They grow in the way-sides in untilled places, and by the sides of old walls.

Time.] They flower in the end of June, and their seed is ripe in July.

Government and virtues.] It is a Saturnine plant. The leaves, but especially the root, taken fresh in Summer-time, beaten or made into a poultice or salve with old hog's grease, and applied to the places pained with the sciatica, to continue thereon four hours if it be on a man, and two hours on a woman; the place afterwards bathed with wine and oil mixed together, and then wrapped with wool or skins, after they have sweat a little, will assuredly cure not only the same disease in hips, knuckle-bone, or other of the joints, as gout in the hands or feet, but all other old griefs of the head, (as inveterate rheums,) and other parts of the body that are hard to be cured. And if of the former griefs any parts remain, the same medicine after twenty days, is to be applied again. The same is also effectual in the diseases of the spleen; and applied to the skin, takes away the blemish thereof, whether they be scars, leprosy, scabs, or scurf, which although it ulcerate the part, yet that is to be helped afterwards with a salve made of oil and wax. Esteem this as another secret.

WATER CRESSES

Descript.] Our ordinary Water Cresses spread forth with many weak, hollow, sappy stalks, shooting out fibres at the joints and upwards long winged leaves made of sundry broad sappy almost round leaves, of a brownish colour. The flowers are many and white standing on long foot-stalks after which come small yellow seed, contained in small long pods like horns. The whole plant abides green in the winter, and tastes somewhat hot and sharp.

Place.] They grow, for the most part, in small standing waters, yet sometimes in small rivulets of running water.

Time.] They flower and seed in the beginning of Summer.

Government and virtues.] It is an herb under the dominion of the Moon. They are more powerful against the scurvy, and to cleanse the blood and humours, than Brooklime is, and serve in all the other uses in which Brooklime is available, as to break the stone, and provoke urine and woman's courses. The decoction thereof cleanses ulcers, by washing them therewith. The leaves bruised, or the juice, is good, to be applied to the face or other parts troubled with freckles, pimples, spots, or the like, at night, and washed away in the morning. The juice mixed with vinegar, and the fore part of the head bathed therewith, is very good for those that are dull and drowsy, or have the lethargy.

Water-cress pottage is a good remedy to cleanse the blood in the spring, and help headaches, and consume the gross humours winter has left behind; those that would live in health, may use it if they please; if they will not, I cannot help it. If any fancy not pottage, they may eat the herb as a sallad.

CROSSWORT

THIS herb receives its name from the situation of its leaves.

Descript.] Common Crosswort grows up with square hairy brown stalks a little above a foot high, having four small broad and pointed, hairy yet smooth thin leaves, growing at every joint, each against other one way, which has caused the name. Towards the tops of the stalks at the joints, with the leaves in three or four rows downwards, stand small, pale yellow flowers, after which come small blackish round seeds, four for the most part, set in every husk. The root is very small, and full of fibres, or threads, taking good hold of the ground, and spreading with the branches over a great deal of ground, which perish not in winter, although the leaves die every year and spring again anew.

Place.] It grows in many moist grounds, well in meadows as untilled places, about London, in Hampstead church-yard, at Wye in Kent, and sundry other places.

Time.] It flowers from May all the Summer long, in one place or other, as they are more open to the sun; the seed ripens soon after.

Government and virtues.] It is under the dominion of Saturn. This is a singularly good wound herb, and is used inwardly, not only to stay bleeding of wounds, but to consolidate them, as it doth outwardly any green wound, which it quickly solders up, and heals. The decoction of the herb in wine, helps to expectorate the phlegm out of the chest, and is good for obstructions in the breast, stomach, or bowels, and helps a decayed appetite. It is also good to wash any wound or sore with, to cleanse and heal it. The herb bruised, and then boiled applied outwardly for certain days together, renewing it often: and in the mean time the decoction of the herb in wine, taken inwardly every day, doth certainly cure the rupture in any, so as it be not too inveterate; but very speedily, if it be fresh and lately taken.

CROWFOOT

MANY are the names this furious biting herb has obtained, almost enough to make up a Welchman's pedigree, if he fetch no farther than John of Gaunt, or William the Conqueror; for it is called Frog's-foot, from the Greek name Barrakion: Crowfoot, Gold Knobs, Gold Cups, King's Knob, Baffiners, Troilflowers, Polts, Locket Goulons, and Butterflowers.

Abundance are the sorts of this herb, that to describe them all, would tire the patience of Socrates himself, but because I have not yet attained to the spirit of Socrates, I shall but describe the most usual.

Descript.] The most common Crowfoot has many thin great leaves, cut into divers parts, in taste biting and sharp, biting and blistering the tongue. It bears many flowers, and those of a bright, resplendent, yellow colour. I do not remember, that I ever saw any thing yellower. Virgins, in ancient time, used to make powder of them to furrow bride beds; after which flowers come small heads, some spiked and rugged like a Pine-Apple.

Place.] They grow very common everywhere; unless you turn your head into a hedge you cannot but see them as you walk.

Time.] They flower in May and June, even till September.

Government and virtues.] This fiery and hot-spirited herb of Mars is no way fit to be given inwardly, but an ointment of the leaves or flowers will draw a blister, and may be so fitly applied to the nape of the neck to draw back rheum from the eyes. The herb being bruised and mixed with a little mustard, draws a blister as well, and as perfectly as Cantharides, and with far less danger to the vessels of urine, which Cantharides naturally delight to wrong. I knew the herb once applied to a pestilential rising that was fallen down, and it saved life even beyond hope; it were good to keep an ointment and plaister of it, if it were but for that.

CUCKOW-POINT

It is called Aron, Janus, Barba-aron, Calve's-foot, Ramp, Starchwort, Cuckow-point, and Wake Robin.

Descript.] This shoots forth three, four or five leaves at the most, from one root, every one whereof is somewhat large and long, broad at the bottom next the stalk, and forked, but ending in a point, without a cut on the edge, of a full green colour, each standing upon a thick round stalk, of a hand-breadth long, or more, among which, after two or three months that they begin to wither, rises up a bare, round, whitish green stalk, spotted and streaked with purple, somewhat higher than the leaves. At the top whereof stands a long hollow husk close at the bottom, but open from the middle upwards, ending in a point: in the middle whereof stands the small long pestle or clapper, smaller at the bottom than at the top, of a dark purple colour, as the husk is on the inside, though green without; which, after it hath so abided for some time, the husk with the clapper decays, and the foot or bottom thereof grows to be a small long bunch of berries, green at the first, and of a yellowish red colour when they are ripe, of the bigness of a hazel-nut kernel, which abides thereon almost until Winter; the root is round, and somewhat long, for the most part lying along, the leaves shooting forth at the largest end, which, when it bears its berries, are somewhat wrinkled and loose, another growing under it, which is solid and firm, with many small threads hanging thereat. The whole plant is of a very sharp biting taste, pricking the tongue as nettles do the hands, and so abides for a great while without alteration. The root thereof was anciently used instead of starch to starch linen with.

There is another sort of Cuckow-point, with less leaves than the former, and some times harder, having blackish spots upon them, which for the most part abide longer green in Summer than the former, and both leaves and roots are more sharp and fierce than it. In all things else it is like the former.

Place.] These two sorts grow frequently almost under every hedge-side in many places of this land.

Time.] They shoot forth leaves in the Spring, and continue but until the middle of Summer, or somewhat later; their husks appearing before the fall away, and their fruit shewing in April.

Government and virtues.] It is under the dominion of Mars. Tragus reports, that a dram weight, or more, if need be, of the spotted Wake Robin, either fresh and green, or dried, having been eaten and taken, is a present and sure remedy for poison and the plague. The juice of the herb taken to the quantity of a spoonful has the same effect. But if there be a little vinegar added thereto, as well as to the root aforesaid, it somewhat allays the sharp biting taste thereof upon the tongue. The green leaves bruised, and laid upon any boil or plague sore, doth wonderfully help to draw forth the poison. A dram of the powder of the dried root taken with twice so much sugar in the form of a licking electuary, or the green root, doth wonderfully help those that are pursy and short-winded, as also those that have a cough; it breaks, digests, and rids away phlegm from the stomach, chest, and lungs. The milk wherein the root has been boiled is effectual also for the same purpose. The said powder taken in wine or other drink, or the juice of the berries, or the powder of them, or the wine wherein they have been boiled, provokes urine, and brings down women's courses and purges them effectually after child-bearing, to bring away the after-birth. Taken with sheep's milk, it heals the inward ulcers of the bowels. The distilled water thereof is effectual to all the purposes aforesaid. A spoonful taken at a time heals the itch; an ounce or more taken a time for some days together, doth help the rupture. The leaves either green or dry, or the juice of them, doth cleanse all manner of rotten and filthy ulcers, in what part of the body soever; and heals the stinking sores in the nose, called Polypus. The water wherein the root has been boiled, dropped into the eyes, cleanses them from any film or skin, cloud or mists, which begin to hinder the sight, and helps the watering and redness of them, or when, by some chance, they become black and blue. The root mixed with bean-flour, and applied to the throat or jaws that are inflamed, helps them. The juice of the berries boiled in oil of roses, or beaten into powder mixed with the oil, and dropped into the ears, eases pains in them. The berries or the roots beaten with the hot ox-dung, and applied, eases the pains of the gout. The leaves and roots boiled in wine with a little oil, and applied to the piles, or the falling down of the fundament, eases them, and so doth sitting over the hot fumes thereof. The fresh roots bruised and distilled with a little milk, yields a most sovereign water to cleanse the skin from scurf, freckles, spots, or blemishes whatsoever therein.

Authors have left large commendations of this herb you see, but

for my part, I have neither spoken with Dr. Reason nor Dr.
Experience about it.

CUCUMBERS

Government and virtues.] There is no dispute to be made, but
that they are under the dominion of the Moon, though they are
so much cried out against for their coldness, and if they were but
one degree colder they would be poison. The best of Galenists hold
them to be cold and moist in the second degree, and then not so hot
as either lettuce or purslain. They are excellently good for a hot
stomach, and hot liver; the unmeasurable use of them fills the body
full of raw humours, and so indeed the unmeasurable use of any
thing else doth harm. The face being washed with their juice,
cleanses the skin, and is excellently good for hot rheums in the eyes;
the seed is excellently good to provoke urine, and cleanses the
passages thereof when they are stopped: there is not a better
remedy for ulcers in the bladder growing, than Cucumbers are.
The usual course is, to use the seeds in emulsions, as they make
almond milk; but a far better way (in my opinion) is this. When
the season of the year is, take the Cucumbers and bruise them well,
and distil the water from them, and let such as are troubled with
ulcers in the bladder drink no other drink. The face being washed
with the same water, cures the reddest face that is; it is also excellently good for sun-burning, freckles, and morphew.

DAISIES

THESE are so well known almost to every child, that I suppose it
needless to write any description of them. Take therefore the virtues
of them as follows.

Government and virtues.] The herb is under the sign Cancer,
and under the dominion of Venus, and therefore excellently good
for wounds in the breast, and very fitting to be kept both in oils,
ointments, and plaisters, as also in syrup. The greater wild Daisy
is a wound herb of good respect, often used in those drinks or salves
that are for wounds, either inward or outward. The juice or distilled water of these, or the small Daisy, doth much temper the heat
of choler, and refresh the liver, and the other inward parts. A
decoction made of them and drank, helps to cure the wounds made
in the hollowness of the breast. The same also cures all ulcers and
pustules in the mouth or tongue, or in the secret parts. The leaves
bruised and applied to the privities, or to any other parts that are

swollen and hot, doth dissolve it, and temper the heat. A decoction made thereof, of Wallwort and Agrimony, and the places fomented and bathed therewith warm, gives great ease to them that are troubled with the palsy, sciatica, or the gout. The same also disperses and dissolves the knots or kernels that grow in the flesh of any part of the body, and bruises and hurts that come of falls and blows; they are also used for ruptures, and other inward burnings, with very good success. An ointment made thereof doth wonderfully help all wounds that have inflammations about them, or by reason of moist humours having access unto them, are kept long from healing, and such are those, for the most part, that happen to joints of the arms or legs. The juice of them dropped into the running eyes of any, doth much help them.

DANDELION, VULGARLY CALLED PISS-A-BEDS

Descript.] It is well known to have many long and deep gashed leaves, lying on the ground round about the head of the roots; the ends of each gash or jag, on both sides looking downwards towards the roots; the middle rib being white, which being broken, yields abundance of bitter milk, but the root much more; from among the leaves, which always abide green, arise many slender, weak, naked, foot-stalks, every one of them bearing at the top one large yellow flower, consisting of many rows of yellow leaves, broad at the points, and nicked in with deep spots of yellow in the middle, which growing ripe, the green husk wherein the flowers stood turns itself down to the stalk, and the head of down becomes as round as a ball: with long seed underneath, bearing a part of the down on the head of every one, which together is blown away with the wind, or may be at once blown away with one's mouth. The root growing downwards exceedingly deep, which being broken off within the ground, will yet shoot forth again, and will hardly be destroyed where it hath once taken deep root in the ground.

Place.] It grows frequently in all meadows and pasture-grounds.

Time.] It flowers in one place or other almost all the year long.

Government and virtues.] It is under the dominion of Jupiter. It is of an opening and cleansing quality, and therefore very effectual for the obstructions of the liver, gall and spleen, and the diseases that arise from them, as the jaundice and hypocondriac; it opens the passages of the urine both in young and old; powerfully cleanses imposthumes and inward ulcers in the urinary passage, and by its drying and temperate quality doth afterwards heal them; for which purpose the decoction of the roots or leaves in white wine, or the leaves chopped as pot-herbs, with a few Alisanders, and boiled in their broth, are very effectual. And whoever is drawing towards a consumption or an evil disposition of the whole body, called Cachexia, by the use hereof for some time together, shall find a wonderful help. It helps also to procure rest and sleep to bodies distempered by the heat of ague fits, or other wise. The distilled water is effectual to drink in pestilential fevers, and to wash the sores.

You see here what virtues this common herb hath, and that is the reason the French and Dutch so often eat them in the Spring; and now if you look a little farther, you may see plainly without a pair of spectacles, that foreign physicians are not so selfish as ours are, but more communicative of the virtues of plants to people.

DARNEL

It is called Jam and Wray: in Sussex they call it Crop, it being a pestilent enemy among corn.

Descript.] This has all the winter long, sundry long, flat, and rough leaves, which, when the stalk rises, which is slender and jointed, are narrower, but rough still; on the top grows a long spike, composed of many heads set one above another, containing two or three husks, with a sharp but short beard of awns at the end; the seed is easily shaken out of the ear, the husk itself being somewhat rough.

Place.] The country husbandmen do know this too well to grow among their corn, or in the borders and pathways of the other fields that are fallow.

Government and virtues.] It is a malicious part of sullen Saturn. As it is not without some vices, so hath it also many virtues. The meal of Darnel is very good to stay gangrenes, and other such like fretting and eating cankers, and putrid sores. It also cleanses the skin of all leprosies, morphews, ringworms, and the like, if it be used with salt and raddish roots. And being used with quick brimstone and vinegar, it dissolves knots and kernels, and breaks those that are hard to be dissolved, being boiled in wine with pigeon's dung and Linseed. A decoction thereof made with water and honey, and the places bathed therewith, is profitable for the sciatica. Darnel meal applied in a poultice draws forth splinters and broken bones in the flesh. The red Darnel, boiled in red wine and taken, stays the lask and all other fluxes, and women's bloody issues; and restrains urine that passes away too suddenly.

DILL

Descript.] The common Dill grows up with seldom more than one stalk, neither so high, nor so great usually as Fennel, being round and fewer joints thereon, whose leaves are sadder, and somewhat long, and so like Fennel that it deceives many, but harder in handling, and somewhat thicker, and of a strong unpleasant scent. The tops of the stalks have four branches and smaller umbels of yellow flowers, which turn into small seed, somewhat flatter and thinner than Fennel seed. The root is somewhat small and woody, perishes every year after it hath borne seed: and is also unprofitable, being never put to any use.

Place.] It is most usually sown in gardens and grounds for the purpose, and is also found wild in many places.

Government and virtues.] Mercury has the dominion of this plant, and therefore to be sure it strengthens the brain. The Dill being boiled and drank, is good to ease swellings and pains; it also stays the belly and stomach from casting. The decoction therefore helps women that are troubled with the pains and windiness of the mother, if they sit therein. It stays the hiccough, being boiled in wine, and but smelled unto being tied in a cloth. The seed is of more use than the leaves, and more effectual to digest raw and vicious humours, and is used in medicines that serve to expel wind, and the pains proceeding therefrom. The seed, being roasted or fried, and used in oils or plasters, dissolves the imposthumes in the fundament; and dries up all moist ulcers, especially in the fundament; an oil made of Dill is effectual to warm or dissolve humours and imposthumes, and the pains, and to procure rest. The decoction of Dill, be it herb or seed (only if you boil the seed you must bruise it) in white wine, being drank, it is a gallant expeller of wind, and provoker of the terms.

DEVIL'S-BIT

Descript.] This rises up with a round green smooth stalk, about two feet high, set with divers long and somewhat narrow, smooth, dark green leaves, somewhat nipped about the edges, for the most part, being else all whole, and not divided at all, or but very seldom, even to the tops of the branches, which yet are smaller than those below, with one rib only in the middle. At the end of each branch stands a round head of many flowers set together in the same manner, or more neatly than Scabious, and of a bluish purple colour, which being past, there follows seed which falls away. The root is somewhat thick, but short and blackish, with many strings, abiding after seed time many years. This root was longer, until the devil (as the friars say) bit away the rest of it for spite, envying its usefulness to mankind; for sure he was not troubled with any disease for which it is proper.

There are two other sorts hereof, in nothing unlike the former, save that the one bears white, and the other bluish-coloured flowers.

Place.] The first grows as well in dry meadows and fields as moist, in many places of this land. But the other two are more rare, and hard to be met with, yet they are both found growing wild about Appledore, near Rye in Kent.

Time.] They flower not usually until August.

Government and virtues.] The plant is venereal, pleasing, and harmless. The herb or the root (all that the devil hath left of it) being boiled in wine, and drank, is very powerful against the plague, and all pestilential diseases or fevers, poisons also, and the bitings of venemous beasts. It helps also those that are inwardly bruised by any casuality, or outwardly by falls or blows, dissolving the clotted blood; and the herb or root beaten and outwardly applied, takes away the black and blue marks that remain in the skin. The decoction of the herb, with honey of roses put therein, is very effectual to help the inveterate tumours and swellings of the almonds and throat, by often gargling the mouth therewith. It helps also to procure women's courses, and eases all pains of the mother and to break and discuss wind therein, and in the bowels. The powder of the root taken in drink, drives forth the worms in the body. The juice or distilled water of the herb, is effectual for green wounds, or old sores, and cleanses the body inwardly, and the seed outwardly, from sores, scurf, itch, pimples, freckles, morphew, or other deformities thereof, especially if a little vitriol be dissolved therein.

DOCK

MANY kinds of these are so well known, that I shall not trouble you with a description of them. My book grows big too fast.

Government and virtues.] All Docks are under Jupiter, of which the Red Dock, which is commonly called Bloodwort, cleanses the blood, and strengthens the liver; but the yellow Dock-root is best to be taken when either the blood or liver is affected by choler. All of them have a kind of cooling (but not all alike) drying quality, the sorrel being most cold, and the Blood-worts most drying. Of the Burdock, I have spoken already by itself. The seed of most of the other kinds, whether the gardens or fields, do stay lasks and fluxes of all sorts, the loathing of the stomach through choler, and is helpful for those that spit blood. The roots boiled in vinegar help the itch, scabs, and breaking out of the skin, if it be bathed therewith. The distilled water of the herb and roots have the same virtue, and cleanses the skin from freckles, morphews, and all other spots and discolourings therein.

All Docks being boiled with meat, make it boil the sooner. Besides Blood-wort is exceeding strengthening to the liver, and procures good blood, being as wholesome a pot herb as any growing in a garden; yet such is the nicety of our times, forsooth, that women will not put it into a pot, because it makes the pottage black; pride and ignorance (a couple of monsters in the creation) preferring nicety before health.

DODDER OF THYME, EPITHYMUM, AND OTHER DODDERS

Descript.] This first from seed gives roots in the ground, which shoot forth threads or strings, grosser or finer as the property of the plant wherein it grows, and the climate doth suffer, creeping and spreading on that plant whereon it fastens, be it high or low. The strings have no leaves at all on them, but wind and interlace themselves, so thick upon a small plant, that it takes away all comfort of the sun from it; and is ready to choak or strangle it. After these strings are risen to that height, that they may draw nourishment from that plant, they seem to be broken off from the ground, either by the strength of their rising, or withered by the heat of the Sun. Upon these strings are found clusters of small heads or husks, out of which shoot forth whitish flowers, which afterwards give small pale white coloured seed, somewhat flat, and twice as big as Poppy-seed. It generally participates of the nature of the plant which it climbs upon; but the Dodder of Thyme is accounted the best, and is the only true Epithymum.

Government and virtues.] All Dodders are under Saturn. Tell not me of physicians crying up Epithymum, or that Dodder which grows upon Thyme, (most of which comes from Hemetius in Greece, or Hybla in Sicily, because those mountains abound with Thyme,) he is a physician indeed, that hath wit enough to choose the Dodder according to the nature of the disease and humour peccant. We confess, Thyme is the hottest herb it usually grows upon; and therefore that which grows upon Thyme is hotter than that which grows upon cold herbs; for it draws nourishment from what it grows upon, as well as from the earth where its root is, and thus you see old Saturn is wise enough to have two strings to his bow. This is accounted the most effectual for melancholy diseases, and to purge black or burnt choler, which is the cause of many diseases of the head and brain, as also for the trembling of the heart, faintings and swoonings. It is helpful in all diseases and griefs of the spleen, and melancholy that arises from the windiness of the hypochondria. It purges also the reins or kidneys by urine; it opens obstructions of the gall, whereby it profits them that have the jaundice; as also the leaves, the spleen. Purging the veins of the choleric and phlegmatic humours, and helps children in agues, a little worm seed being put thereto.

The other Dodders do, as I said before, participate of the nature of those plants whereon they grow. As that which hath been found growing upon nettles in the west-country, hath by experience been found very effectual to procure plenty of urine where it hath been stopped or hindered. And so of the rest.

Sympathy and antipathy are two hinges upon which the whole mode of physic turns; and that physician who minds them not, is like a door off from the hooks, more like to do a man mischief, than to secure him. Then all the diseases Saturn causes, this helps by sympathy, and strengthens all the parts of the body he rules; such as be caused by Sol, it helps by antipathy. What those diseases are, see my judgment of diseases by astrology; and if you be pleased to look at the herb Wormwood, you shall find a rational way for it.

DOG'S-GRASS, OR COUCH GRASS

Descript.] It is well known, that the grass creeps far about under ground, with long white joined roots, and small fibres almost at every joint, very sweet in taste, as the rest of the herb is, and interlacing one another, from whence shoot forth many fair grassy leaves, small at the ends, and cutting or sharp on the edges. The stalks are jointed like corn, with the like leaves on them, and a large spiked head, with a long husk in them, and hard rough seed in them. If you know it not by this description, watch the dogs when they are sick, and they will quickly lead you to it.

Place.] It grows commonly through this land in divers ploughed grounds to the no small trouble of the husbandmen, as also of the gardeners, in gardens, to weed it out, if they can; for it is a constant customer to the place it get footing in.

Government and virtues.] 'Tis under the dominion of Jupiter, and is the most medicinal of all the Quick-grasses. Being boiled and drank, it opens obstructions of the liver and gall, and the stopping of urine, and eases the griping pains of the belly and inflammations; wastes the matter of the stone in the bladder, and the ulcers thereof also. The roots bruised and applied, do consolidate wounds. The seed doth more powerfully expel urine, and stays the lask and vomiting. The distilled water alone, or with a little wormseed, kills the worms in children.

The way of use is to bruise the roots, and having well boiled them in white wine, drink the decoction: 'Tis opening but not purging, very safe: 'Tis a remedy against all diseases coming of stopping, and such are half those that are incident to the body of man; and although a gardener be of another opinion, yet a physician holds half an acre of them to be worth five acres of Carrots twice told over.

DOVE'S-FOOT, OR CRANE'S-BILL

Descript.] This has divers small, round, pale-green leaves, cut in about the edges, much like mallow, standing upon long, reddish, hairy stalks lying in a round compass upon the ground; among which rise up two or three, or more, reddish, jointed, slender, weak, hairy stalks, with some like leaves thereon, but smaller, and more cut in up to the tops, where grow many very small bright red flowers of five leaves a-piece; after which follow small heads, with small short beaks pointed forth, as all other sorts of those herbs do.

Place.] It grows in pasture grounds, and by the path-sides in many places, and will also be in gardens.

Time.] It flowers in June, July, and August, some earlier and some later; and the seed is ripe quickly after.

Government and virtues.] It is a very gentle, though martial plant. It is found by experience to be singularly good for wind cholic, as also to expel the stone and gravel in the kidneys. The decoction thereof in wine, is an excellent good cure for those that have inward wounds, hurts, or bruises, both to stay the bleeding, to dissolve and expel the congealed blood, and to heal the parts, as also to cleanse and heal outward sores, ulcers and fistulas; and for green wounds, many do only bruise the herb, and apply it to the places, and it heals them quickly. The same decoction in wine fomented to any place pained with the gout, or to joint-aches, or pains of the sinews, gives much ease. The powder or decoction of the herb taken for some time together, is found by experience to be singularly good for ruptures and burstings in people, either young or old.

DUCK'S MEAT

THIS is so well known to swim on the tops of standing waters, as ponds, pools, and ditches, that it is needless further to describe it.

Government and virtues.] Cancer claims the herb, and the Moon will be Lady of it; a word is enough to a wise man. It is effectual to help inflammations, and St. Anthony's Fire, as also the gout, either applied by itself, or in a poultice with Barley meal. The distilled water by some is highly esteemed against all inward inflammations and pestilent fevers; as also to help the redness of the eyes, and swellings of privities, and of the breasts before they be grown too much. The fresh herb applied to the forehead, eases the pains of the headache coming of heat.

DOWN, OR COTTON-THISTLE

Descript.] This has large leaves lying on the ground, somewhat cut in, and as it were crumpled on the edges, of a green colour on the upper side, but covered with long hairy wool, or Cotton Down, set with most sharp and cruel pricks, from the middle of whose head of flowers, thrust forth many purplish crimson threads, and sometimes (although very seldom) white ones. The seed that follows in the heads, lying in a great deal of white down, is somewhat large, long, and round, like the seed of ladies thistle, but paler. The root is great and thick, spreading much, yet it usually dies after seed-time.

Place.] It grows in divers ditches, banks, and in cornfields, and highways, generally everywhere throughout the land.

Time.] It flowers and bears seed about the end of Summer, when other thistles do flower and seed.

Government and virtues.] Mars owns the plant, and manifest to the world, that though it may hurt your finger, it will help your body; for I fancy it much for the ensuing virtues. Pliny and Dioscorides write, That the leaves and roots thereof taken in drink, help those that have a crick in their neck; whereby they cannot turn their neck but their whole body must turn also (sure they do not mean those that have got a crick in their neck by being under the hangman's hand.) Galen saith, that the root and leaves hereof are of a healing quality, and good for such persons as have their bodies drawn together by some spasm or convulsion, as it is with children that have the rickets.

DRAGONS

THEY are so well known to everyone that plants them in their gardens, they need no description; if not, let them look down to the lower end of the stalks, and see how like a snake they look.

Government and virtues.] The plant is under the dominion of Mars, and therefore it would be a wonder if it should want some obnoxious quality or other. In all herbs of that quality, the safest way is either to distil the herb in an alembick, in what vehicle you please, or else to press out the juice, and distil that in a glass still, in sand. It scours and cleanses the internal parts of the body mightily, and it clears the external parts also, being externally applied, from freckles, morphew, and sun-burning. Your best way to use it externally, is to mix it with vinegar; an ointment of it is held to be good in wounds and ulcers; it consumes cankers, and that flesh growing in the nostrils, which they call Polypus. Also the distilled water being dropped into the eyes, takes away spots there, or the pin and web, and mends the dimness of sight; it is excellently good against pestilence and poison. Pliny and Dioscorides affirm, that no serpent will meddle with him that carries this herb about him.

THE ELDER TREE

I HOLD it needless to write any description of this, since every boy that plays with a pop-gun will not mistake another tree instead of Elder. I shall therefore in this place only describe the Dwarf-Elder, called also Dead-wort, and Wall-wort.

THE DWARF-ELDER

Descript.] This is but an herb every year, dying with his stalks to the ground, and rising afresh every Spring, and is like unto the Elder both in form and quality, rising up with a square, rough, hairy stalks, four feet high, or more sometimes. The winged leaves are somewhat narrower than the Elder, but else like them. The flowers are white with a dash of purple, standing in umbels, very like the Elder also, but more sweet in scent, after which come small blackish berries, full of juice while they are fresh, wherein is small hard kernels, or seed. The root doth creep under the upper crust of the ground, springing in divers places, being of the bigness of one's finger or thumb sometimes.

Place.] The Elder-tree grows in hedges, being planted there to strengthen the fences and partitions of ground, and to hold the banks by ditches and water-courses.

The Dwarf Elder grows wild in many places of England, where being once gotten into a ground, it is not easily gotten forth again.

Time.] Most of the Elder Trees, flower in June, and their fruit is ripe for the most part in August. But the Dwarf Elder, or Wall-wort, flowers somewhat later, and his fruit is not ripe until September.

Government and virtues.] Both Elder and Dwarf Tree are under the dominion of Venus. The first shoots of the common Elder boiled like Asparagus, and the young leaves and stalks boiled in fat broth, doth mightily carry forth phlegm and choler. The middle or inward bark boiled in water, and given in drink, works much more violently; and the berries, either green or dry, expel the same humour, and are often given with good success to help the dropsy; the bark of the root boiled in wine, or the juice thereof drank, works the same effects, but more powerfully than either the leaves or fruit. The juice of the root taken, doth mightily procure vomitings, and purges the watery humours of the dropsy. The decoction of the root taken, cures the biting of an adder, and biting of mad dogs. It mollifies the hardness of the mother, if women sit thereon, and opens their veins, and brings down their courses. The berries boiled in wine perform the same effect; and the hair of the head washed therewith is made black. The juice of the green leaves applied to the hot inflammations of the eyes, assuages them; the juice of the leaves snuffed up into the nostrils, purges the tunicles of the brain; the juice of the berries boiled with honey and dropped into the ears, helps the pains of them; the decoction of the berries in wine, being drank, provokes urine; the distilled water of the flowers is of much use to clean the skin from sun-burning, freckles, morphew, or the like; and takes away the head-ache, coming of a cold cause, the head being bathed therewith. The leaves or flowers distilled in the month of May, and the legs often washed with the said distilled water, it takes away the ulcers and sores of them. The eyes washed therewith, it takes away the redness and bloodshot; and the hands washed morning and evening therewith, helps the palsy, and shaking of them.

The Dwarf Elder is more powerful than the common Elder in opening and purging choler, phlegm, and water; in helping the gout, piles, and women's diseases, colours the hair black, helps the inflammations of the eyes, and pains in the ears, the biting of serpents, or mad dogs, burnings and scaldings, the wind cholic, cholic, and stone, the difficulty of urine, the cure of old sores and fistulous ulcers. Either leaves or bark of Elder, stripped upwards as you gather it, causes vomiting. Also, Dr. Butler, in a manuscript of his, commends Dwarf Elder to the sky of dropsies, *viz.* to drink it, being boiled in white wine; to drink the decoction I mean, not the Elder.

THE ELM TREE

This tree is so well known, growing generally in all counties of this land, that it is needless to describe it.

Government and virtues.] It is a cold and saturnine plant. The leaves thereof bruised and applied, heal green wounds, being bound thereon with its own bark. The leaves or the bark used with vinegar, cures scurf and leprosy very effectually. The decoction of the leaves, bark, or root, being bathed, heals broken bones. The water that is found in the bladders on the leaves, while it is fresh, is very effectual to cleanse the skin, and make it fair; and if cloaths be often wet therein, and applied to the ruptures of children, it heals them, if they be well bound up with a truss. The said water put into a glass, and set into the ground, or else in dung for twenty-five days, the mouth thereof being close stopped, and the bottom set upon a layer of ordinary salt, that the fœces may settle and water become clear, is a singular and sovereign balm for green wounds, being used with soft tents. The decoction of the bark of the root, fomented, mollifies hard tumours, and the shrinking of the sinews. The roots of the Elm, boiled for a long time in water, and the fat arising on the top thereof, being clean skimmed off, and the place anointed therewith that is grown bald, and the hair fallen away, will quickly restore them again. The said bark ground with brine or pickle, until it come to the form of a poultice and laid on the place pained with the gout, gives great ease. The decoction of the bark in water, is excellent to bathe such places as have been burnt with fire.

ENDIVE

Descript.] Common garden Endive bears a longer and larger leaf than Succory, and abides but one year, quickly running up to a stalk and seed, and then perishes; it has blue flowers, and the seed of the ordinary Endive is so like Succory seed, that it is hard to distinguish them.

Government and virtues.] It is a fine cooling, cleansing, jovial plant. The decoction of the leaves, or the juice, or the distilled water of Endive, serve well to cool the excessive heat of the liver and stomach, and in the hot fits of agues, and all other inflammations in any part of the body; it cools the heat and sharpness of the urine, and excoriation in the urinary parts. The seeds are of the same property, or rather more powerful, and besides are available for fainting, swoonings, and passions of the heart. Outwardly applied, they serve to temper the sharp humours of fretting ulcers, hot tumours, swellings, and pestilential sores; and wonderfully help not only the redness and inflammations of the eyes, but the dimness of the sight also; they are also used to allay the pains of the gout. You cannot use it amiss; a syrup of it is a fine cooling medicine for fevers.

ELECAMPANE

Descript.] It shoots forth many large leaves, long and broad, lying near the ground, small at both ends, somewhat soft in handling of a whitish green on the upper side, and grey underneath, each set upon a short footstalk, from among which arise up divers great and strong hairy stalks, three or four feet high, with some leaves thereupon, compassing them about at the lower end, and are branched towards the tops, bearing divers great and large flowers, like those of the corn marigold, both the border of leaves, and the middle thrum being yellow, which turn into down, with long, small, brownish seeds amongst it, and is carried away with the wind. The root is great and thick, branched forth divers ways, blackish on the outside and whitish within, of a very bitter taste, and strong, but good scent, especially when they are dried, no part else of the plant having any smell.

Place.] It grows on moist grounds, and shadowy places oftener than in the dry and open borders of the fields and lanes, and in other waste places, almost in every county of this land.

Time.] It flowers in the end of June and July, and the seed is ripe in August. The roots are gathered for use, as well in the Spring before the leaves come forth, as in Autumn or Winter.

Government and virtues.] It is a plant under the dominion of Mercury. The fresh roots of Elecampane preserved with sugar, or made into a syrup or conserve, are very effectual to warm a cold windy stomach, or the pricking therein, and stitches in the sides caused by the spleen; and to help the cough, shortness of breath, and wheezing in the lungs. The dried root made into powder, and mixed with sugar, and taken, serves to the same purpose, and is also profitable for those who have their urine stopped, or the stopping of women's courses, the pains of the mother and the stone in the reins, kidneys, or bladder; it resists poison, and stays the spreading of the venom of serpents, as also putrid and pestilential fevers, and the plague itself. The roots and herbs beaten and put into new ale or beer, and daily drank, clears, strengthens, and quickens the sight of the eyes wonderfully. The decoction of the roots in wine, or the juice taken therein, kills and drives forth all manner of worms in the belly, stomach, and maw; and gargled in the mouth, or the root chewed, fastens loose teeth, and helps to keep them from putrefaction; and being drank is good for those that spit blood, helps to remove cramps or convulsions, gout, sciatica, pains in the joints, applied outwardly or inwardly, and is also good for those that are bursten, or have any inward bruise. The root boiled well in vinegar beaten afterwards, and made into an ointment with hog's suet, or oil of trotters is an excellent remedy for scabs or itch in young or old; the places also bathed or washed with the decoction doth the same; it also helps all sorts of filthy old putrid sores or cankers whatsoever. In the roots of this herb lieth the chief effect for the remedies aforesaid. The distilled water of the leaves and roots together, is very profitable to cleanse the skin of the face, or other parts, from any morphew, spots, or blemishes therein, and make it clear.

ERINGO, OR SEA-HOLLY

Descript.] The first leaves of our ordinary Sea-holly, are nothing so hard and prickly as when they grow old, being almost round, and deeply dented about the edges, hard and sharp pointed, and a little crumpled, of a bluish green colour, every one upon a long foot stalk; but those that grow up higher with the stalk, do as it were compass it about. The stalk itself is round and strong, yet somewhat crested, with joints and leaves set thereat, but more divided, sharp and prickly; and branches rising from thence, which have likewise other small branches, each of them having several bluish round prickly heads, with many small jagged prickly leaves under them, standing like a star, and sometimes found greenish or whitish. The root grows wonderfully long, even to eight or ten feet in length, set with rings and circles towards the upper part, cut smooth and without joints down lower, brownish on the outside, and very white within, with a pith in the middle; of a pleasant taste, but much more, being artificially preserved, and candied with sugar.

Place.] It is found about the sea coast in almost every county of this land which borders upon the sea.

Time.] It flowers in the end of Summer, and gives ripe seed within a month after.

Government and virtues.] The plant is venereal, and breeds seed exceedingly, and strengthens the spirit procreative; it is hot and moist, and under the celestial Balance. The decoction of the root hereof in wine, is very effectual to open obstructions of the spleen and liver, and helps yellow jaundice, dropsy, pains of the loins, and wind cholic, provokes urine, and expels the stone, procures women's courses. The continued use of the decoction for fifteen days, taken fasting, and next to bedward, doth help the stranguary, the difficulty and stoppage of urine, and the stone, as well as all defects of the reins and kidneys; and if the said drink be continued longer, it is said that it cures the stone; it is found good against the French pox. The roots bruised and applied outwardly, help the kernels of the throat, commonly called the king's evil; or taking inwardly, and applied to the place stung or bitten by any serpent, heal it speedily. If the roots be bruised, and boiled in old hog's grease, or salted lard, and broken bones, thorns &c. remaining in the flesh, they do not only draw them forth, but heal up the place again, gathering new flesh where it was consumed. The juice of the leaves dropped into the ear, helps imposthumes therein. The distilled water of the whole herb, when the leaves and stalks are young, is profitable drank for all the purposes aforesaid; and helps the melancholy of the heart, and is available in quartan and quotidian agues; as also for them that have their necks drawn awry, and cannot turn them without turning their whole body.

EYEBRIGHT

Descript.] Common Eyebright is a small low herb, rising up usually but with one blackish green stalk a span high, or not much more, spread from the bottom into sundry branches, whereon are small and almost round yet pointed dark green leaves, finely snipped about the edges, two always set together, and very thick. At the joints with the leaves, from the middle upward, come forth small white flowers, marked with purple and yellow spots, or stripes; after which follow small round heads, with very small seed therein. The root is long, small and thready at the end.

Place.] It grows in meadows, and grassy places in this land.

Government and virtues.] It is under the sign of the Lion, and Sol claims dominion over it. If the herb was but as much used as it is neglected, it would half spoil the spectacle maker's trade; and a man would think, that reason should teach people to prefer the preservation of their natural before artificial spectacles; which that they may be instructed how to do, take the virtues of Eyebright as follows.

The juice or distilled water of Eyebright, taken inwardly in white wine or broth, or dropped into the eyes for divers days together, helps all infirmities of the eyes that cause dimness of sight. Some make conserve of the flowers to the same effect. Being used any of the ways, it also helps a weak brain, or memory. This tunned up with strong beer, that it may work together, and drank, or the powder of the dried herb mixed with sugar, a little Mace, and Fennel seed, and drank, or eaten in broth; or the said powder made into an electuary with sugar, and taken, has the same powerful effect to help and restore the sight, decayed through age; and Arnoldus de Ville Nova saith, it hath restored sight to them that have been blind a long time before.

FERN

Descript.] Of this there are two kinds principally to be treated of, *viz.* the Male and Female. The Female grows higher than the Male, but the leaves thereof are smaller, and more divided and dented, and of as strong a smell as the male; the virtue of them are both alike, and therefore I shall not trouble you with any description or distinction of them.

Place.] They grow both in heaths and in shady places near the hedge-sides in all counties of this land.

Time.] They flower and give their seed at Midsummer.

The Female Fern is that plant which is in Sussex, called Brakes, the seed of which some authors hold to be so rare. Such a thing there is I know, and may be easily had upon Midsummer Eve, and for ought I know, two or three days after it, if not more.

Government and virtues.] It is under the dominion of Mercury, both Male and Female. The roots of both these sorts of Fern being bruised and boiled in Mead, or honeyed water, and drank, kills both the broad and long worms in the body, and abates the swelling and hardness of the spleen. The green leaves eaten, purge the belly of choleric and waterish humours that trouble the stomach. They are dangerous for women with child to meddle with, by reason they cause abortions. The roots bruised and boiled in oil, or hog's grease, make a very profitable ointment to heal wounds, or pricks gotten in the flesh. The powder of them used in foul ulcers, dries up their malignant moisture, and causes their speedier healing. Fern being burned, the smoke thereof drives away serpents, gnats, and other noisome creatures, which in fenny countries do in the night time, trouble and molest people lying in their beds with their faces uncovered; it causes barrenness.

OSMOND ROYAL, OR WATER FERN

Descript.] This shoots forth in Spring time (for in the Winter the leaves perish) divers rough hard stalks, half round, and yellowish, or flat on the other side, two feet high, having divers branches of winged yellowish green leaves on all sides, set one against another, longer, narrower, and not nicked on the edges as the former. From the top of some of these stalks grow forth a long bush of small and more yellow, green, scaly aglets, set in the same manner on the stalks as the leaves are, which are accounted the flowers and seeds. The root is rough, thick and scabby: with a white pith in the middle, which is called the heart thereof.

Place.] It grows on moors, bogs, and watery places, in many parts of this land.

Time.] It is green all the summer, and the root only abides in winter.

Government and virtues.] Saturn owns the plant. This has all the virtues mentioned in the former Ferns, and is much more effectual than they, both for inward and outward griefs, and is accounted singularly good in wounds, bruises, or the like. The decoction to be drank, or boiled into an ointment of oil, as a balsam or balm, and so it is singularly good against bruises, and bones broken, or out of joint, and gives much ease to the cholic and splenetic diseases: as also for ruptures or burstings. The decoction of the root in white wine, provokes urine exceedingly, and cleanses the bladder and passages of urine.

FEVERFEW OR FEATHERFEW

Descript.] Common Featherfew has large, fresh, green leaves, much torn or cut on the edges. The stalks are hard and round, set with many such like leaves, but smaller, and at the tops stand many single flowers, upon small foot stalks, consisting of many small white leaves standing round about a yellow thrum in the middle. The root is somewhat hard and short, with many strong fibres about it. The scent of the whole plant is very strong, and the taste is very bitter.

Place.] This grows wild in many places of the land, but is for the most part nourished in gardens.

Time.] It flowers in the months of June and July.

Government and virtues.] Venus commands this herb, and has commended it to succour her sisters (women) and to be a general strengthener of their wombs, and remedy such infirmities as a careless midwife hath there caused; if they will but be pleased to make use of her herb boiled in white wine, and drink the decoction; it cleanses the womb, expels the after-birth, and doth a woman all the good she can desire of an herb. And if any grumble because they cannot get the herb in winter, tell them, if they please, they may make a syrup of it in summer; it is chiefly used for the disease of the mother, whether it be the strangling or rising of the mother, or hardness, or inflammation of the same, applied outwardly thereunto. Or a decoction of the flowers in wine, with a little Nutmeg or Mace put therein, and drank often in a day, is an approved remedy to bring down women's courses speedily, and helps to expel the dead birth and after-birth. For a woman to sit over the hot fumes of the decoction of the herb made in water or wine, is effectual for the same; and in some cases to apply the boiled herb warm to the privy parts. The decoction thereof made with some sugar, or honey put thereto, is used by many with good success to help the cough and stuffing of the chest, by colds, as also to cleanse the reins and bladder, and helps to expel the stone in them. The powder of the herb taken in wine, with some Oxymel, purges both choler and phlegm, and is available for those that are short winded, and are troubled with melancholy and heaviness, or sadness of spirits. It is very effectual for all pains in the head coming of a cold cause, the herb being bruised and applied to the crown of the head. As also for the vertigo, that is a running or swimming in the head. The decoction thereof drank warm, and the herb bruised with a few corns of Bay salt, and applied to the wrists before the coming of the ague fits, doth take them away. The distilled water takes away freckles, and other spots and deformities in the face. The herb bruised and heated on a tile, with some wine to moisten it, or fried with a little wine and oil in a frying-pan, and applied warm outwardly to the places, helps the wind and cholic in the lower part of the belly. It is an especial remedy against opium taken too liberally.

FENNEL

EVERY garden affords this so plentifully, that it needs no description.

Government and virtues.] One good old fashion is not yet left off, *viz.* to boil Fennel with fish; for it consumes that phlegmatic humour, which fish most plentifully afford and annoy the body with, though few that use it know wherefore they do it. I suppose the reason of its benefit this way is because it is an herb of Mercury, and under Virgo, and therefore bears antipathy to Pisces. Fennel is good to break wind, to provoke urine, and ease the pains of the stone, and helps to break it. The leaves or seed, boiled in barley water and drank are good for nurses, to increase their milk, and make it more wholesome for the child. The leaves, or rather the seeds, boiled in water, stays the hiccough, and takes away the loathings which oftentimes happen to the stomachs of sick and feverish persons, and allays the heat thereof. The seed boiled in wine and drank, is good for those that are bitten with serpents, or have eaten poisonous herbs, or mushrooms. The seed and the roots much more, help to open obstructions of the liver, spleen, and gall, and thereby help the painful and windy swellings of the spleen, and the yellow jaundice; as also the gout and cramps. The seed is of good use in medicines to help shortness of breath and wheezing by stopping of the lungs. It helps also to bring down the courses, and to

cleanse the parts after delivery. The roots are of most use in physic
drinks, and broth that are taken to cleanse the blood, to open
obstructions of the liver, so provoke urine, and amend the ill colour
in the face after sickness, and to cause a good habit through the
body. Both leaves, seeds, and roots thereof are much used in drink
or broth, to make people more lean that are too fat. The distilled
water of the whole herb, or the condensate juice dissolved, but
especially the natural juice, that in some counties issues out hereof
of its own accord, dropped into the eyes, cleanses them from mists
and films that hinder the sight. The sweet Fennel is much weaker
in physical uses than the common Fennel. The wild Fennel is
stronger and hotter than the tame, and therefore most powerful
against the stone, but not so effectual to encrease milk, because of
its dryness.

SOW-FENNEL, OR HOG'S-FENNEL

Besides the common name in English, Hog's Fennel, and the
Latin name Peucidanum, is called Hoar-strange, and Hoar-strong,
Sulphur-wort, and Brimstone-wort.

Descript.] The common Sow-Fennel has divers branched stalks
of thick and somewhat long leaves, three for the most part joined
together at a place, among which arises a crested straight stalk, less
than Fennel, with some joints thereon, and leaves growing thereat,
and towards the tops some branches issuing from thence; likewise
on the tops of the stalks and branches stand divers tufts of yellow
flowers, whereafter grows somewhat flat, thin, and yellowish seed,
bigger than Fennel seed. The roots grow great and deep, with many
other parts and fibres about them of a strong scent like hot brimstone, and yield forth a yellowish milk, or clammy juice, almost
like a gum.

Place.] It grows plentifully in the salt low marshes near Faver-
sham in Kent.

Time.] It flowers plentifully in July and August.

Government and virtues.] This is also an herb of Mercury. The
juice of Sow-Fennel (saith Dioscorides, and Galen,) used with
vinegar and rose water, or the juice with a little Euphorbium put
to the nose, helps those that are troubled with the lethargy, frenzy,
giddiness of the head, the falling sickness, long and inveterate
head-aches, the palsy, sciatica, and the cramp, and generally all the
diseases of the sinews, used with oil and vinegar. The juice dissolved in wine, or put into an egg, is good for a cough, or shortness
of breath, and for those that are troubled with wind in the body.
It purges the belly gently, expels the hardness of the spleen, gives

ease to women that have sore travail in child-birth, and eases the pains of the reins and bladder, and also the womb. A little of the juice dissolved in wine, and dropped into the ears, eases much of the pains in them, and put into a hollow tooth, eases the pain thereof. The root is less effectual to all the aforesaid disorders; yet the powder of the root cleanses foul ulcers, being put into them, and takes out splinters of broken bones, or other things in the flesh, and heals them up perfectly: as also, dries up old and inveterate running sores, and is of admirable virtue in all green wounds.

FIG-WORT, OR THROAT-WORT

Descript.] Common great Fig-wort sends divers great, strong, hard, square brown stalks, three or four feet high, whereon grow large, hard, and dark green leaves, two at a joint, harder and larger than Nettle leaves, but not stinking; at the tops of the stalks stand many purple flowers set in husks, which are sometimes gaping and open, somewhat like those of Water Betony; after which come hard round heads, with a small point in the middle, wherein lie small brownish seed. The root is great, white, and thick, with many branches at it, growing aslope under the upper crust of the ground, which abides many years, but keeps not his green leaves in Winter.

Place.] It grows frequently in moist and shadowy woods, and in the lower parts of the fields and meadows.

Time.] It flowers about July, and the seed will be ripe about a month after the flowers are fallen.

Government and virtues.] Some Latin authors call it Cervicaria, because it is appropriated to the neck; and we Throat-wort, because it is appropriated to the throat. Venus owns the herb, and the Celestial Bull will not deny it; therefore a better remedy cannot be for the king's evil, because the Moon that rules the disease, is exalted there. The decoction of the herb taken inwardly, and the bruised herb applied outwardly, dissolves clotted and congealed blood within the body, coming by any wounds, bruise or fall; and is no less effectual for the king's evil, or any other knobs, kernel, bunches, or wens growing in the flesh wheresoever; and for the hæmorrhoids, or piles. An ointment made hereof may be used at all times when the fresh herb is not to be had. The distilled water of the whole plant, roots and all, is used for the same purposes, and dries up the superfluous, virulent moisture of hollow and corroding ulcers; it takes away all redness, spots, and freckles in the face, as also the scurf, and any foul deformity therein, and the leprosy likewise.

FILIPENDULA, OR DROP-WORT

Descript.] This sends forth many leaves, some larger, some smaller, set on each side of a middle rib, and each of them dented about the edges, somewhat resembling wild Tansy, or rather Agrimony, but harder in handling; among which rise up one or more stalks, two or three feet high, with the leaves growing thereon, and sometimes also divided into other branches spreading at the top into many white, sweet-smelling flowers, consisting of five leaves a-piece, with some threads in the middle of them, standing together in a pith or umble, each upon a small foot stalk, which after they have been blown upon a good while, do fall away, and in their places appear small, round, chaffy heads like buttons, wherein are the chaffy seeds set and placed. The root consists of many small, black, tuberous pieces, fastened together by many small, long, blackish strings, which run from one to another.

Place.] It grows in many places of this land, in the corners of dry fields and meadows, and the hedge sides.

Time.] They flower in June and July, and their seed is ripe in August.

Government and virtues.] It is under the dominion of Venus. It effectually opens the passages of the urine, helps the stranguary; the stone in the kidneys or bladder, the gravel, and all other pains of the bladder and reins, by taking the roots in powder, or a decoction of them in white wine, with a little honey. The roots made into powder, and mixed with honey in the form of an electuary, doth much help them whose stomachs are swollen, dissolving and breaking the wind which was the cause thereof; and is also very effectual for all the diseases of the lungs, as shortness of breath, wheezing, hoarseness of the throat, and the cough; and to expectorate tough phlegm, or any other parts thereabout.

THE FIG-TREE

To give a description of a tree so well known to every body that keep it in his garden, were needless. They prosper very well in our English gardens, yet are fitter for medicine than for any other profit which is gotten by the fruit of them.

Government and virtues.] The tree is under the dominion of Jupiter. The milk that issues out from the leaves or branches where they are broken off, being dropped upon warts, takes them away. The decoction of the leaves is excellently good to wash sore heads with: and there is scarcely a better remedy for the leprosy than it is. It clears the face also of morphew, and the body of white scurf, scabs, and running sores. If it be dropped into old fretting ulcers, it cleanses out the moisture, and brings up the flesh; because you cannot have the leaves green all the year, you may make an ointment of them whilst you can. A decoction of the leaves being drank inwardly, or rather a syrup made of them, dissolves congealed blood caused by bruises or falls, and helps the bloody flux. The ashes of the wood made into an ointment with hog's grease, helps kibes and chilblains. The juice being put into an hollow tooth, eases pain: as also pain and noise in the ears, being dropped into them; and deafness. An ointment made of the juice and hog's grease, is an excellent remedy for the bitten of mad dogs, or other venomous beasts as most are. A syrup made of the leaves, or green fruit, is excellently good for coughs, hoarseness, or shortness of breath, and all diseases of the breast and lungs; it is also extremely good for the dropsy and falling sickness. They say that the Fig Tree, as well as the Bay Tree, is never hurt by lightning; as also, if you tie a bull, be he ever so mad, to a Fig Tree, he will quickly become tame and gentle. As for such figs as come from beyond sea, I have little to say, because I write not of exoticks.

THE YELLOW WATER-FLAG, OR FLOWER-DE-LUCE

Descript.] This grows like the Flower-de-luce, but it has much longer and narrower sad green leaves, joined together in that fashion; the stalk also growing oftentimes as high, bearing small yellow flowers shaped like the Flower-de-luce, with three falling leaves, and other three arched that cover their bottoms; but instead of the three upright leaves, as the Flower-de-luce has, this has only three short pieces standing in their places, after which succeed thick and long three square heads, containing in each part somewhat big and flat seed, like those of the Flower-de-luce. The root is long and slender, of a pale brownish colour on the outside, and of a horse-flesh colour on the inside, with many hard fibres thereat, and very harsh in taste.

Place.] It usually grows in watery ditches, ponds, lakes, and moor sides, which are always overflowed with water.

Time.] It flowers in July, and the seed is ripe in August.

Government and virtues.] It is under the dominion of the Moon. The root of this Water-flag is very astringent, cooling, and drying; and thereby helps all lasks and fluxes, whether of blood or humours, as bleeding at the mouth, nose, or other parts, bloody flux, and the immoderate flux of women's courses. The distilled water of the whole herb, flowers and roots, is a sovereign good remedy for watering eyes, both to be dropped into them, and to have cloths or sponges wetted therein, and applied to the forehead. It also helps the spots and blemishes that happen in and about the eyes, or in any other parts. The said water fomented on swellings and hot inflammations of women's breasts, upon cancers also, and those spreading ulcers called *Noli me tangere*, do much good. It helps also foul ulcers in the privities of man or woman; but an ointment made of the flowers is better for those external applications.

FLAX-WEED, OR TOAD-FLAX

Descript.] Our common Flax-weed has divers stalks full fraught with long and narrow ash-coloured leaves, and from the middle of them almost upward, stored with a number of pale yellow flowers, of a strong unpleasant scent, with deeper yellow mouths, and black-ish flat seed in round heads. The root is somewhat woody and white, especially the main downright one, with many fibres, abiding many years, shooting forth roots every way round about, and new branches every year.

Place.] This grows throughout this land, both by the way sides and in meadows, as also by hedge-sides, and upon the sides of banks, and borders of fields.

Time.] It flowers in Summer, and the seed is ripe usually before the end of August.

Government and virtues.] Mars owns the herb. In Sussex we call it Gallwort, and lay it in our chicken's water to cure them of the gall; it relieves them when they are drooping. This is fre-quently used to spend the abundance of those watery humours by urine which cause the dropsy. The decoction of the herb, both leaves and flowers, in wine, taken and drank, doth somewhat move the belly downwards, opens obstructions of the liver, and helps the yellow jaundice; expels poison, provokes women's courses, drives forth the dead child, and after-birth. The distilled water of the herb and flowers is effectual for all the same purposes; being drank with a dram of the powder of the seeds of bark or the roots of Wall-wort, and a little Cinnamon, for certain days together, it is held a singular remedy for the dropsy. The juice of the herb, or the distilled water, dropped into the eyes, is a certain remedy for all heat, in-flammation, and redness in them. The juice or water put into foul ulcers, whether they be cancerous or fistulous, with tents rolled therein, or parts washed and injected therewith, cleanses them thoroughly from the bottom, and heals them up safely. The same juice or water also cleanses the skin wonderfully of all sorts of de-formity, as leprosy, morphew, scurf, wheals, pimples, or spots, applied of itself, or used with some powder of Lupines.

FLEA-WORT

Descript.] Ordinary Flea-wort rises up with a stalk two feet high or more, full of joints and branches on every side up to the top, and at every joint two small, long and narrow whitish green leaves somewhat hairy. At the top of every branch stand divers small, short scaly, or chaffy heads out of which come forth small whitish yellow threads, like to those of the Plantain herbs, which are the bloomings of flowers. The seed enclosed in these heads is small and shining while it is fresh, very like unto fleas both for colour and bigness, but turning black when it grows old. The root is not long, but white, hard and woody, perishing every year, and rising again of its own seed for divers years, if it be suffered to shed. The whole plant is somewhat whitish and hairy, smelling somewhat like rosin.

There is another sort hereof, differing not from the former in the manner of growing, but only that the stalk and branches being somewhat greater, do a little more bow down to the ground. The leaves are somewhat greater, the heads somewhat less, the seed alike; and the root and leaves abide all winter, and perish not as the former.

Place.] The first grows only in gardens, the second plentifully in fields that are near the sea.

Time.] They flower in July or thereabouts.

Government and virtues.] The herb is cold, and dry, and saturnine. I suppose it obtained the name of Flea-wort, because the seeds are so like Fleas. The seeds fried, and taken, stays the flux or lask of the belly, and the corrosions that come by reason of hot choleric, or sharp and malignant humours, or by too much purging of any violent medicine, as Scammony, or the like. The mucilage of the seed made with Rose-water, and a little sugar-candy put thereto, is very good in all hot agues and burning fevers, and other inflammations, to cool the thirst, and lenify the dryness and roughness of the tongue and throat. It helps also hoarseness of the voice, and diseases of the breast and lungs, caused by heat, or sharp salt humours, and the pleurisy also. The mucilage of the seed made with Plantain water, whereunto the yoke of an egg or two, and a little Populeon are put, is a most safe and sure remedy to ease the sharpness, pricking, and pains of the hæmorrhoids or piles, if it be laid on a cloth, and bound thereto. It helps all inflammations in any part of the body, and the pains that come thereby, as the headache and megrims, and all hot imposthumes, swellings, or breaking out of the skin, as blains, wheals, pushes, purples, and the like, as also the joints of those that are out of joint, the pains of the gout and sciatica, the burstings of young children, and the swellings of the

navel, applied with oil of roses and vinegar. It is also good to heal
the nipples and sore breasts of women, being often applied thereunto. The juice of the herb with a little honey put into the ears
helps the running of them, and the worms breeding in them. The
same also mixed with hog's grease, and applied to corrupt and filthy
ulcers, cleanses them and heals them.

FLUX-WEED

Descript.] It rises up with a round upright hard stalk, four or
five feet high, spread into sundry branches, whereon grow many
greyish green leaves, very finely cut and severed into a number of
short and almost round parts. The flowers are very small and
yellow, growing spike fashion, after which come small long pods,
with small yellowish seed in them. The root is long and woody,
perishing every year.

There is another sort, differing in nothing, save only it has somewhat broad leaves; they have a strong evil savour, being smelled
unto, and are of a drying taste.

Place.] They flower wild in the fields by hedge-sides and highways, and among rubbish and other places.

Time.] They flower and seed quickly after, namely in June and July.

Government and virtues.] This herb is saturnine also. Both the
herb and seed of Flux-weed is of excellent use to stay the flux or
lask of the belly, being drank in water wherein gads of steel heated
have been often quenched; and is no less effectual for the same
purpose than Plantain or Comfrey, and to restrain any other flux
of blood in man or woman, as also to consolidate bones broken or
out of joint. The juice thereof drank in wine, or the decoction of
the herb drank, doth kill the worms in the stomach or belly, or the
worms that grow in putrid and filthy ulcers, and made into a salve
doth quickly heal all old sores, how foul or malignant soever they be.
The distilled water of the herb works the same effect, although
somewhat weaker, yet it is a fair medicine, and more acceptable to
be taken. It is called Flux-weed because it cures the flux, and for its
uniting broken bones, &c. Paracelsus extol it to the skies. It is
fitting that syrup, ointment, and plaisters of it were kept in your house.

FLOWER-DE-LUCE

I⊤ is so well known, being nourished up in most gardens, that I
shall not need to spend time in writing a description thereof.

Time.] The flaggy kinds thereof have the most physical uses;
the dwarf kinds thereof flowers in April, the greater sorts in May.

Government and virtues.] The herb is Luner. The juice or decoction of the green root of the flaggy kind of Flower-de-luce, with a little honey drank, doth purge and cleanse the stomach of gross and tough phlegm, and choler therein; it helps the jaundice and the dropsy, evacuating those humours both upwards and downwards; and because it somewhat hurts the stomach, is not to be taken without honey and spikenard. The same being drank, doth ease the pains and torments of the belly and sides, the shaking of agues, the diseases of the liver and spleen, the worms of the belly, the stone in the reins, convulsions and cramps that come of old humours; it also helps those whose seed passes from them unawares. It is a remedy against the bitings and stingings of venomous creatures, being boiled in water and vinegar and drank. Boiled in water and drank, it provokes urine, helps the cholic, brings down women's courses; and made up into a pessary with honey, and put up into the body, draws forth the dead child. It is much commended against the cough, to expectorate rough phlegm. It much eases pains in the head, and procures sleep; being put into the nostrils it procures sneezing, and thereby purges the head of phlegm. The juice of the root applied to the piles or hæmorrhoids, gives much ease. The decoction of the roots gargled in the mouth, eases the tooth-ache, and helps the stinking breath. Oil called Oleum Irinum, if it be rightly made of the great broad flag Flower-de-luce and not of the great bulbous blue Flower-de-luce, (as is used by some apothecaries) and roots of the same, of the flaggy kinds, is very effectual to warm and comfort all cold joints and sinews, as also the gout and sciatica, and mollifies, dissolves and consumes tumours and swellings in any part of the body, as also of the matrix; it helps the cramp, or convulsions of the sinews. The head and temples anointed therewith, helps the catarrh or thin rheum distilled from thence; and used upon the breast or stomach, helps to extenuate the cold tough phlegm; it helps also the pains and noise in the ears, and the stench of the nostrils. The root itself, either green or in powder, helps to cleanse, heal, and incarnate wounds, and to cover the naked bones with flesh again, that ulcers have made bare; and is also very good to cleanse and heal up fistulas and cankers that are hard to be cured.

FLUELLIN, OR LLUELLIN

Descript.] It shoots forth many long branches partly lying upon the ground, and partly standing upright, set with almost red leaves, yet a little pointed, and sometimes more long than round, without order thereon, somewhat hairy, and of an evil greenish white colour;

at the joints all along the stalks, and with the leaves come forth small flowers, one at a place, upon a very small short foot-stalk, gaping somewhat like Snapdragons, or rather like Toad-flax, with the upper jaw of a yellow colour, and the lower of a purplish, with a small heel or spur behind; after which come forth small round heads, containing small black seed. The root is small and thready, dying every year, and rises itself again of its own sowing.

There is another sort of Lluellin which has longer branches wholly trailing upon the ground, two or three feet long, and somewhat more thin, set with leaves thereon, upon small foot-stalks. The leaves are a little larger, and somewhat round, and cornered sometimes in some places on the edges; but the lower part of them being the broadest, hath on each side a small point, making it seem as if they were ears, sometimes hairy, but not hoary, and of a better green colour than the former. The flowers come forth like the former, but the colours therein are more white than yellow, and the purple not so far. It is a large flower, and so are the seed and seed-vessels. The root is like the other, and perishes every year.

Place.] They grow in divers corn fields, and in borders about them, and in other fertile grounds about Southfleet in Kent abundantly; at Buchrite, Hamerton, and Rickmanworth in Huntingdonshire, and in divers other places.

Time.] They are in flower about June and July, and the whole plant is dry and withered before August be done.

Government and virtues.] It is a Lunar herb. The leaves bruised and applied with barley meal to watering eyes that are hot and inflamed by defluxions from the head, do very much help them, as also the fluxes of blood or humours, as the lask, bloody flux, women's courses, and stays all manner of bleeding at the nose, mouth, or any other place, or that comes by any bruise or hurt, or bursting a vein; it wonderfully helps all those inward parts that need consolidating or strengthening, and is no less effectual both to heal and close green wounds, than to cleanse and heal all foul or old ulcers, fretting or spreading cankers or the like. This herb is of a fine cooling, drying quality, and an ointment or plaister of it might do a man a courtesy that hath any hot virulent sores. 'Tis admirable for the ulcers of the French pox; if taken inwardly, may cure the desease.

FOX-GLOVE

Descript.] It has many long and broad leaves lying upon the ground dented upon the edges, a little soft or woolly, and of a hoary green colour, among which rise up sometimes sundry stalks,

but one very often, bearing such leaves thereon from the bottom
to the middle, from whence to the top it is stored with large and
long hollow reddish purple flowers, a little more long and eminent
at the lower edge, with some white spots within them, one above
another with small green leaves at every one, but all of them turning
their heads one way, and hanging downwards, having some threads
also in the middle, from whence rise round heads, pointed sharp at
the ends, wherein small brown seed lies. The roots are so many
small fibres, and some greater strings among them; the flowers
have no scent, but the leaves have a bitter hot taste.

Place.] It grows on dry sandy ground for the most part, and as
well on the higher as the lower places under hedge-sides in almost
every county of this land.

Time.] It seldom flowers before July, and the seed is ripe in
August.

Government and virtues.] The plant is under the dominion of
Venus, being of a gentle cleansing nature, and withal very friendly
to nature. The herb is familiarly and frequently used by the
Italians to heal any fresh or green wound, the leaves being but
bruised and bound thereon; and the juice thereof is also used in old
sores, to cleanse, dry, and heal them. The decoction hereof made
up with some sugar or honey, is available to cleanse and purge the
body both upwards and downwards, sometimes of tough phlegm
and clammy humours, and to open obstructions of the liver and
spleen. It has been found by experience to be available for the king's
evil, the herb bruised and applied, or an ointment made with the
juice thereof, and so used; and a decoction of two handfuls thereof,
with four ounces of Polipody in ale, has been found by late experience to cure divers of the falling sickness, that have been troubled
with it above twenty years. I am confident that an ointment of it is
one of the best remedies for scabby head that is.

FUMITORY

Descript.] Our common Fumitory is a tender sappy herb, sends
forth from one square, a slender weak stalk, and leaning downwards
on all sides, many branches two or three feet long, with finely cut
and jagged leaves of a whitish or rather bluish sea green colour.
At the tops of the branches stand many small flowers, as it were in
a long spike one above another, made like little birds, of a reddish
purple colour, with whitish bellies, after which come small round
husks, containing small black seeds. The root is yellow, small, and
not very long, full of juice while it is green, but quickly perishes with

the ripe seed. In the corn fields in Cornwall, it bears white flowers.

Place.] It grows in corn fields almost every where, as well as in gardens.

Time.] It flowers in May, for the most part, and the seed ripens shortly after.

Government and virtues.] Saturn owns the herb, and presents it to the world as a cure for his own disease, and a strengthener of the parts of the body he rules. If by my astrological judgment of diseases, from the decumbiture, you find Saturn author of the disease, or if by direction from a nativity you fear a saturnine disease approaching, you may by this herb prevent it in the one, and cure it in the other, and therefore it is fit you keep a syrup of it always by you. The juice or syrup made thereof, or the decoction made in whey by itself, with some other purging or opening herbs and roots to cause it to work the better (itself being but weak) is very effectual for the liver and spleen, opening the obstructions thereof, and clarifying the blood from saltish, choleric, and adust humours, which cause leprosy, scabs, tetters, and itches, and such like breakings-out of the skin, and after the purgings doth strengthen all the inward parts. It is also good against the yellow-jaundice, and spends it by urine, which it procures in abundance. The powder of the dried herb given for some time together, cures melancholy, but the seed is strongest in operation for all the former diseases. The distilled water of the herb is also of good effect in the former diseases, and conduces much against the plague and pestilence, being taken with good treacle. The distilled water also, with a little water and honey of roses, helps all sores of the mouth or throat, being gargled often therewith. The juice dropped into the eyes, clears the sight and takes away redness and other defects in them, although it procure some pain for the present, and cause tears. Dioscorides saith it hinders any fresh springing of hairs on the eye-lids (after they are pulled away) if the eye-lids be anointed with the juice hereof, with Gum Arabic dissolved therein. The juice of the Fumitory and Docks mingled with vinegar, and the places gently washed therewith, cures all sorts of scabs, pimples, blotches, wheals, and pushes which arise on the face or hands or any other parts of the body.

THE FURZE BUSH

It is as well known by this name, as it is in some counties by the name of Gorz or Whins, that I shall not need to write any description thereof, my intent being to teach my countrymen what they know not, rather than to tell them again of that which is general known before.

Place.] They are known to grow on dry barren heaths, and other waste, gravelly or sandy grounds, in all counties of this land.

Time.] They also flower in the Summer months.

Government and virtues.] Mars owns the herb. They are hot and dry, and open obstructions of the liver and spleen. A decoction made with the flowers thereof hath been found effectual against the jaundice, as also to provoke urine, and cleanse the kidneys from gravel or stone ingendered in them. Mars doth also this by sympathy.

GARLICK

THE offensiveness of the breath of him that hath eaten Garlick, will lead you by the nose to the knowledge hereof, and (instead of a description) direct you to the place where it grows in gardens, which kinds are the best, and most physical.

Government and virtues.] Mars owns this herb. This was anciently accounted the poor man's treacle, it being a remedy for all diseases and hurts (except those which itself breed.) It provokes urine, and women's courses, helps the biting of mad dogs and other venomous creatures, kills worms in children, cuts and voids tough phlegm, purges the head, helps the lethargy, is a good preservative against, and a remedy for any plague, sore, or foul ulcers; takes away spots and blemishes in the skin, eases pains in the ears, ripens and breaks imposthumes, or other swellings. And for all those diseases the onions are as effectual. But the Garlick hath some more peculiar virtues besides the former, *viz.* it hath a special quality to discuss inconveniences coming by corrupt agues or mineral vapours; or by drinking corrupt and stinking waters; as also by taking wolf-bane, henbane, hemlock, or other poisonous and dangerous herbs. It is also held good in hydropick diseases, the jaundice, falling sickness, cramps, convulsions, the piles or hæmorrhoids, or other cold diseases. Many authors quote many diseases this is good for; but conceal its vices. Its heat is very vehement, and all vehement hot things send up but ill-favoured vapours to the brain. In coleric men it will add fuel to the fire; in men oppressed by melancholy, it will attenuate the humour, and send up strong fancies, and as many strange visions to the head; therefore let it be taken inwardly with great moderation; outwardly you may make more bold with it.

GENTIAN, FELWORT, OR BALDMONY

IT is confessed that Gentian, which is most used amongst us, is brought over from beyond sea, yet we have two sorts of it growing frequently in our nation, which, besides the reasons so frequently alledged why English herbs should be fittest for English bodies, has been proved by the experience of divers physicians, to be not a wit inferior in virtue to that which comes from beyond sea, therefore be pleased to take the description of them as follows.

Descript.] The greater of the two hath many small long roots thrust down deep into the ground, and abiding all the Winter. The stalks are sometimes more, sometimes fewer, of a brownish green colour, which is sometimes two feet high, if the ground be fruitful, having many long, narrow, dark green leaves, set by couples up to the top; the flowers are long and hollow, of a purple colour, ending in fine corners. The smaller sort which is to be found in our land, grows up with sundry stalks, not a foot high, parted into several small branches, whereon grow divers small leaves together, very like those of the lesser Centaury, of a whitish green colour; on the tops of these stalks grow divers perfect blue flowers, standing in long husks, but not so big as the other; the root is very small, and full of threads.

Place.] The first grows in divers places of both the East and West counties, and as well in wet as in dry grounds; as near Longfield, by Gravesend, near Cobham in Kent, near Lillinstone in Kent, also in a chalk pit hard by a paper-mill not far from Dartford in Kent. The second grows also in divers places in Kent, as about Southfleet, and Longfield; upon Barton's hills in Bedfordshire; also not far from St. Albans, upon a piece of waste chalky ground, as you go out by Dunstable way towards Gorhambury.

Time.] They flower in August.

Government and virtues.] They are under the dominion of Mars, and one of the principal herbs he is ruler of. They resist putrefactions, poison, and a more sure remedy cannot be found to prevent the pestilence than it is; it strengthens the stomach exceedingly, helps digestion, comforts the heart, and preserves it against faintings and swoonings. The powder of the dry roots helps the biting of mad dogs and venomous beasts, open obstructions of the liver, and restores an appetite for their meat to such as have lost it. The herb steeped in wine, and the wine drank, refreshes such as be overweary with traveling, and grow lame in their joints, either by cold or evil lodgings; it helps stitches, and griping pains in the sides; is an excellent remedy for such as are bruised by falls; it provokes urine and the terms exceedingly, therefore let it not be given to women with child. The same is very profitable for such as are troubled with cramps and convulsions, to drink the decoction. Also they say it breaks the stone, and helps ruptures most certainly: it is excellent in all cold diseases, and such as are troubled with tough phlegm, scabs, itch, or any fretting sores and ulcers; it is an admirable remedy to kill the worms, by taking half a dram of the powder in a morning in any convenient liquor; the same is excellently good to be taken inwardly for the king's evil. It helps agues of all sorts, and the yellow jaundice, as also the bots in cattle; when kine are bitten on the udder by any venomous beast, do but stroke the place with the decoction of any of these, and it will instantly heal them.

CLOVE GILLIFLOWERS

It is vain to describe an herb so well known.

Government and virtues.] They are gallant, fine, temperate flowers, of the nature and under the dominion of Jupiter; yea, so temperate, that no excess, neither in heat, cold, dryness, nor moisture, can be perceived in them; they are great strengtheners both of the brain and heart, and will therefore serve either for cordials or cephalics, as your occasion will serve. There is both a syrup and a conserve made of them alone, commonly to be had at every apothecary's. To take now and then a little of either, strengthens nature much, in such as are in consumptions. They are also excellently good in hot pestilent fevers, and expel poison.

GERMANDER

Descript.] Common Germander shoots forth sundry stalks, with small and somewhat round leaves, dented about the edges. The flowers stand at the tops of a deep purple colour. The root is composed of divers sprigs, which shoots forth a great way round about, quickly overspreading a garden.

Place.] It grows usually with us in gardens.

Time.] And flowers in June and July.

Government and virtues.] It is a most prevalent herb of Mercury, and strengthens the brain and apprehension exceedingly when weak, and relieves them when drooping. This taken with honey (saith Dioscorides) is a remedy for coughs, hardness of the spleen and difficulty of urine, and helps those that are fallen into a dropsy, especially at the beginning of the disease, a decoction being made thereof when it is green, and drank. It also brings down women's courses, and expels the dead child. It is most effectual against the poison of all serpents, being drank in wine, and the bruised herb outwardly applied; used with honey, it cleanses old and foul ulcers; and made into an oil, and the eyes anointed therewith, takes away the dimness and moistness. It is likewise good for the pains in the sides and cramps. The decoction thereof taken for four days together, drives away and cures both tertain and quartan agues. It is also good against all diseases of the brain, as continual head-ache, falling-sickness, melancholy, drowsiness and dullness of the spirits, convulsions and palsies. A dram of the seed taken in powder purges by urine, and is good against the yellow jaundice. The juice of the leaves dropped into the ears kills the worms in them. The tops thereof, when they are in flowers, steeped twenty-four hours in a drought of white wine, and drank, kills the worms in the belly.

STINKING GLADWIN

Descript.] This is one of the kinds of Flower-de-luce, having divers leaves arising from the roots, very like a Flower-de-luce, but that they are sharp-edged on both sides, and thicker in the middle, of a deeper green colour narrower and sharper pointed, and a strong ill-scent, if they be bruised between the fingers. In the middle rises up a reasonably strong stalk, a yard high at least, bearing three or four flowers at the top, made somewhat like the flowers of the Flower-de-luce, with three upright leaves, of a dead purplish ash-colour, with some veins discoloured in them; the other three do not fall down, nor are the three other small ones so arched, nor cover the lower leaves as the Flower-de-luce doth, but stand loose or asunder from them. After they are past, there come up three square hard husks, opening wide into three parts when they are ripe, wherein lie reddish seed, turns black when it hath abiden long. The root is like that of the Flower-de-luce, but reddish on the outside, and whitish within, very sharp and hot in the taste, of as evil a scent as the leaves.

Place.] This grows as well in upland grounds, as in moist places, woods, and shadowy places by the sea-side in many places of this land, and is usually nursed up in gardens.

Time.] It flowers not until July, and the seed is ripe in August or September, yet the husks after they are ripe, opening themselves, will hold their seed with them for two or three months, and not shed them.

Government and virtues.] It is supposed to be under the dominion of Saturn. It is used by many country people to purge corrupt phlegm and choler, which they do by drinking the decoction of the roots; and some to make it more gentle, do but infuse the sliced roots in ale; and some take the leaves, which serve well for the weaker stomach. The juice hereof put up, or snuffed up the nose, causes sneezing, and draws from the head much corruption; and the powder thereof doth the same. The powder thereof drank in wine, helps those that are troubled with the cramps and convulsions, or with the gout and sciatica, and gives ease to those that have griping pains in their body and belly, and helps those that have the stranguary. It is given with much profit to those that have had long fluxes by the sharp and evil quality of humours, which it stays, having first cleansed and purged them by the drying and binding property therein. The root boiled in wine and drank, doth effectually procure women's courses, and used as a pessary, works the same effect, but causes abortion in women with child. Half a dram of the seed beaten to powder, and taken in wine, doth speedily cause one to make water abundantly. The same taken with vinegar, dissolves the hardness and swellings of the spleen. The root is very effectual in all wounds, especially of the head; as also to draw forth any splinters, thorns, or broken bones, or any other thing sticking in the flesh, without causing pains, being used with a little verdigrease and honey, and the great Centaury root. The same boiled in vinegar, and laid upon an eruption or swelling, doth very effectually dissolve and consume them; yea, even the swellings of the throat called the king's evil; the juice of the leaves or roots heals the itch, and all running or spreading scabs, sores, blemishes, or scars in the skin, wheresoever they be.

GOLDEN ROD

Descript.] This rises up with brownish small round stalks, two feet high, and sometimes more, having thereon many narrow and long dark green leaves, very seldom with any dents about the edges, or any stalks or white spots therein, yet they are sometimes so found divided at the tops into many small branches, with divers small yellow flowers on every one of them, all which are turned one way, and being ripe, do turn into down, and are carried away by the wind. The root consists of many small fibres, which grows not deep in the ground, but abides all the winter therein, shooting forth new branches every year, the old one lying down to the ground.

Place.] It grows in the open places of woods and copses, on both moist and dry grounds, in many places of this land.

Time.] It flowers about the month of July.

Government and virtues.] Venus claims the herb, and therefore to be sure it respects beauty lost. Arnoldus de Villa Nova commends it much against the stone in the reins and kidneys, and to provoke urine in abundance, whereby also the gravel and stone may be voided. The decoction of the herb, green or dry, or the

distilled water thereof, is very effectual for inward bruises, as also
to be outwardly applied, it stays bleeding in any part of the body,
and of wounds; also the fluxes of humours, the bloody-flux, and
women's courses; and is no less prevalent in all ruptures or burstings, being drank inwardly, and outwardly applied. It is a sovereign
wound herb, inferior to none, both for the inward and outward
hurts; green wounds, old sores and ulcers, are quickly cured therewith. It also is of especial use in all lotions for sores or ulcers in
the mouth, throat, or privy parts of man or woman. The decoction
also helps to fasten the teeth that are loose in the gums.

GOUT-WORT, OR HERB GERRARD

Descript.] It is a low herb, seldom rising half a yard high, having
sundry leaves standing on brownish green stalks by three, snipped
about, and of a strong unpleasant savour. The umbels of the
flowers are white, and the seed blackish, the root runs in the ground,
quickly taking a great deal of room.

Place.] It grows by hedge and wallsides, and often in the border
and corner of fields, and in gardens also.

Time.] It flowers and seeds about the end of July.

Government and virtues.] Saturn rules it. Neither is it to be supposed Gout-wort hath its name for nothing but upon experiment
to heal the gout and sciatica; as also joint-aches, and other cold
griefs. The very bearing of it about one eases the pains of the gout,
and defends him that bears it from the disease.

GROMEL

OF this I shall briefly describe their kinds, which are principally
used in physic, the virtues whereof are alike, though somewhat
different in their manner and form of growing.

Descript.] The greater Gromel grows up with slender hard and
hairy stalks, trailing and taking root in the ground, as it lies thereon,
and parted into many other small branches with hairy dark green
leaves thereon. At the joints, with the leaves, come forth very small
blue flowers, and after them hard stony roundish seed. The root is
long and woody, abiding the Winter, and shoots forth fresh stalks
in the spring.

The smaller wild Gromel sends forth divers upright hard
branched stalks, two or three feet high full of joints, at every one of
which grow small, long, hard, and rough leaves like the former, but

less; among which leaves come forth small white flowers, and after them greyish round seed like the former; the root is not very big, but with many strings thereat.

The garden Gromel has divers upright, slender, woody, hairy stalks, blown and cressed very little branched, with leaves like the former, and white flowers; after which, in rough brown husks, is contained a white, hard, round seed, shining like pearls, and greater than either the former; the root is like the first described, with divers branches and sprigs thereat, which continues (as the first doth) all the Winter.

Place.] The two first grow wild in barren or untilled places, and by the way side in many places of this land. The last is a nursling in the gardens of the curious.

Time.] They all flower from Midsummer until September sometimes, and in the mean time the seed ripens.

Government and virtues.] The herb belongs to Dame Venus; and therefore if Mars cause the cholic or stone, as usually he doth, if in Virgo, this is your cure. These are accounted to be of as singular force as any herb or seed whatsoever, to break the stone and to void it, and the gravel either in the reins or bladder, as also to provoke urine being stopped, and to help stranguary. The seed is of greatest use, being bruised and boiled in white wine or in broth, or the like, or the powder of the seed taken therein. Two drams of the seed in powder taken with women's breast milk, is very effectual to procure a very speedy delivery to such women as have sore pains in their travail, and cannot be delivered. The herb itself, (when the seed is not to be had) either boiled, or the juice thereof drank, is effectual to all the purposes aforesaid, but not so powerful or speedy in operation.

GOOSEBERRY BUSH

CALLED also Feapberry, and in Sussex Dewberry-Bush, and in some Counties Wineberry.

Government and virtues.] They are under the dominion of Venus. The berries, while they are unripe, being scalded or baked, are good to stir up a fainting or decayed appetite, especially such whose stomachs are afflicted by choleric humours. They are excellently good to stay longings of women with child. You may keep them preserved with sugar all the year long. The decoction of the leaves of the tree cools hot swellings and inflammations; as also St. Anthony's fire. The ripe Gooseberries being eaten, are an excellent remedy to allay the violent heat both of the stomach and liver. The young and tender leaves break the stone, and expel gravel both from the kidneys and bladder. All the evil they do to the body of man is, they are supposed to breed crudities, and by crudities, worms.

WINTER-GREEN

Descript.] This sends forth seven, eight, or nine leaves from a small brown creeping root, every one standing upon a long foot stalk, which are almost as broad as long, round pointed, of a sad green colour, and hard in handling, and like the leaf of a Pear-tree; from whence arises a slender weak stalk, yet standing upright, bearing at the top many small white sweet-smelling flowers, laid open like a star, consisting of five round pointed leaves, with many yellow threads standing in the middle about a green head, and a long stalk with them, which in time grows to be the seed-vessel, which being ripe is found five square, with a small point at it, wherein is contained seed as small as dust.

Place.] It grows seldom in fields, but frequent in the woods northwards, *viz.* in Yorkshire, Lancashire, and Scotland.

Time.] It flowers about June and July.

Government and virtues.] Winter-green is under the dominion of Saturn, and is a singularly good wound herb, and an especial remedy for healing green wounds speedily, the green leaves being bruised and applied, or the juice of them. A salve made of the green herb stamped, or the juice boiled with hog's lard, or with salad oil and wax, and some turpentine added to it, is a sovereign salve, and highly extolled by the Germans, who use it to heal all manner of wounds and sores. The herb boiled in wine and water, and given to drink to them that have any inward ulcers in their kidneys, or neck of the bladder, doth wonderfully help them. It stays all fluxes, as the lask, bloody fluxes, women's courses, and bleeding of wounds, and takes away any inflammations rising upon pains of the heart; it is no less helpful for foul ulcers hard to be cured; as also for cankers or fistulas. The distilled water of the herb effectually performs the same things.

GROUNDSEL

Descript.] Our common Groundsel has a round green and somewhat brownish stalk, spreading toward the top into branches, set with long and somewhat narrow green leaves, cut in on the edges, somewhat like the oak-leaves, but less, and round at the end. At the tops of the branches stand many small green heads, out of which grow several small, yellow threads or thumbs, which are the flowers, and continue many days blown in that manner, before it pass away into down, and with the seed is carried away in the wind. The root is small and thready, and soon perishes, and as soon rises again of its own sowing, so that it may be seen many months in the year both green and in flower, and seed; for it will spring and seed twice in a year at least, if it be suffered in a garden.

Place.] They grow almost every where, as well on tops of walls, as at the foot amongst rubbish and untilled grounds, but especially in gardens.

Time.] It flowers, as was said before, almost every month throughout the year.

Government and virtues.] This herb is Venus's mistress-piece, and is as gallant and universal a medicine for all diseases coming of heat, in what part of the body soever they be, as the sun shines upon; it is very safe and friendly to the body of man: yet causes vomiting if the stomach be afflicted; if not, purging: and it doth it with more gentleness than can be expected; it is moist, and something cold withal, thereby causing expulsion, and repressing the heat caused by the motion of the internal parts in purges and vomits. Lay by our learned receipts; take so much Sena, so much Scammony, so much Colocynthis, so much infusion of Crocus Metallorum, &c. this herb alone preserved in a syrup, in a distilled water, or in an ointment, shall do the deed for you in all hot diseases, and, shall do it, 1, Safely; 2, Speedily.

The decoction of this herb (saith Dioscorides) made with wine, and drank, helps the pains of the stomach, proceeding of choler, (which it may well do by a vomit) as daily experience shews. The juice thereof taken in drink, or the decoction of it in ale, gently performs the same. It is good against the jaundice and falling sickness, being taken in wine; as also against difficulty of making water. It provokes urine, expels gravel in the reins or kidneys; a dram thereof given in oxymel, after some walking or stirring of the body. It helps also the sciatica, griping of the belly, the cholic, defects of the liver, and provokes women's courses. The fresh herb boiled, and made into a poultice, applied to the breasts of women that are swollen with pain and heat, as also the privy parts of man or woman, the seat or fundament, or the arteries, joints, and sinews, when they are inflamed and swollen, doth much ease them; and used with some salt, helps to dissolve knots or kernels in any part of the body. The juice of the herb, or as (Dioscorides saith) the leaves and flowers, with some fine Frankincense in powder, used in wounds of the body, nerves or sinews, doth singularly help to heal them. The distilled water of the herb performs well all the aforesaid cures, but especially for inflammations or watering of the eyes, by reason of the defluxion of rheum unto them.

HEART'S-EASE

THIS is that herb which such physicians as are licensed to blaspheme by authority, without danger of having their tongues burned through with an hot iron, called an herb of the Trinity. It is also called by those that are more moderate, Three Faces in a Hood, Live in Idleness, Cull me to you; and in Sussex we call them Pancies.

Place.] Besides those which are brought up in gardens, they grow commonly wild in the fields, especially in such as are very barren: sometimes you may find it on the tops of the high hills.

Time.] They flower all the Spring and Summer long.

Government and virtues.] The herb is really saturnine, something cold, viscous, and slimy. A strong decoction of the herbs and flowers (if you will, you may make it into syrup) is an excellent cure for the French pox, the herb being a gallant antivenereal: and that antivenereals are the best cure for that disease, far better and safer than to torment them with the flux, divers foreign physicians have confessed. The spirit of it is excellently good for the convulsions in children, as also for the falling sickness, and a gallant remedy for the inflammation of the lungs and breasts, pleurisy, scabs, itch, &c. It is under the celestial sign Cancer.

ARTICHOKES

THE Latins call them Cinera, only our college calls them Artichocus.

Government and virtues.] They are under the dominion of Venus, and therefore it is no marvel if they provoke lust, as indeed they do, being somewhat windy meat; and yet they stay the involuntary course of natural seed in man, which is commonly called nocturnal pollutions. And here I care not greatly if I quote a little of Galen's nonsense in his treatise of the faculties of nourishment. He saith, they contain plenty of choleric juice, (which notwithstanding I can scarcely believe,) of which he saith is engendered melancholy juice, and of that melancholy juice thin choleric blood. But, to proceed; this is certain, that the decoction of the root boiled in wine, or the root bruised and distilled in wine in an alembic, and being drank, purges by urine exceedingly.

HART'S-TONGUE

Descript.] This has divers leaves arising from the root, every one severally, which fold themselves in their first springing and spreading: when they are full grown, are about a foot long, smooth and green above but hard and with little sap in them, and streaked on the back, athwart on both sides of the middle rib, with small and somewhat long and brownish marks; the bottoms of the leaves are a little bowed on each side of the middle rib, somewhat small at the end. The root is of many black threads, folded or interlaced together.

Time.] It is green all the Winter; but new leaves spring every year.

Government and virtues.] Jupiter claims dominion over this herb, therefore it is a singular remedy for the liver, both to strengthen it when weak, and ease it when afflicted, you shall do well to keep it in a syrup all the year. For though authors say it is green all the year, I scarcely believe it. Hart's Tongue is much commended against the hardness and stoppings of the spleen and liver, and against the heat of the liver and stomach, and against lasks, and the bloody-flux. The distilled water thereof is also very good against the passions of the heart, and to stay the hiccough, to help the falling of the palate, and to stay the bleeding of the gums, being gargled in the mouth. Dioscorides saith, it is good against the stinging or biting of serpents. As for the use of it, my direction at the latter end will be sufficient, and enough for those that are studious in physic, to whet their brains upon for one year or two.

HAZEL-NUT

Hazel Nuts are so well known to every body, that they need no description.

Government and virtues.] They are under the dominion of Mercury. The parted kernels made into an electuary, or the milk drawn from the kernels with mead or honeyed water, is very good to help an old cough; and being parched, and a little pepper put to them and drank, digests the distillations of rheum from the head. The dried husks and shells, to the weight of two drams, taken in red wine, stays lasks and women's courses, and so doth the red skin that covers the kernels, which is more effectual to stay women's courses.

And if this be true, as it is, then why should the vulgar so familiarly affirm, that eating nuts causes shortness of breath, than which nothing is falser? For, how can that which strengthens the lungs, cause shortness of breath? I confess, the opinion is far older than I am; I knew tradition was a friend to error before, but never that he was the father of slander. Or are men's tongues so given to slander one another, that they must slander Nuts too, to keep their tongues in use? If any part of the Hazel Nut be stopping, it is the husks and shells, and no one is so mad as to eat them unless physically; and the red skin which covers the kernel, you may easily pull off. And so thus have I made an apology for Nuts, which cannot speak for themselves.

HAWK-WEED

THERE are several sorts of Hawk-weed, but they are similar in virtues.

Descript.] It has many large leaves lying upon the ground, much rent or torn on the sides into gashes like Dandelion, but with greater parts, more like the smooth Sow Thistle, from among which rises a hollow, rough stalk, two or three feet high, branched from the middle upward, whereon are set at every joint longer leaves, little or nothing rent or cut, bearing on them sundry pale, yellow flowers, consisting of many small, narrow leaves, broad pointed, and nicked in at the ends, set in a double row or more, the outermost being larger than the inner, which form most of the Hawk-weeds (for there are many kinds of them) do hold, which turn into down, and with the small brownish seed is blown away with the wind. The root is long and somewhat great, with many small fibres thereat. The whole plant is full of bitter-milk.

Place.] It grows in divers places about the field sides, and the path-ways in dry grounds.

Time.] It flowers and flies away in the Summer months.

Government and virtues.] Saturn owns it. Hawk-weed (saith Dioscorides) is cooling, somewhat drying and binding, and therefore good for the heat of the stomach, and gnawings therein; for inflammations and the hot fits of agues. The juice thereof in wine, helps digestion, discusses wind, hinders crudities abiding in the stomach, and helps the difficulty of making water, the biting of venomous serpents, and stinging of the scorpion, if the herb be also outwardly applied to the place, and is very good against all other poisons. A scruple of the dried root given in wine and vinegar, is profitable for those that have the dropsy. The decoction of the herb taken in honey, digests the phlegm in the chest or lungs, and with Hyssop helps the cough. The decoction thereof, and of wild Succory, made with wine, and taken, helps the wind cholic and hardness of the spleen; it procures rest and sleep, hinders venery and venerous dreams, cooling heats, purges the stomach, increases blood, and helps the diseases of the reins and bladder. Outwardly applied, it is singularly good for all the defects and diseases of the eyes, used with some women's milk; and used with good success in fretting or creeping ulcers, especially in the beginning. The

green leaves bruised, and with a little salt applied to any place
burnt with fire, before blisters do rise, helps them; as also inflammations, St. Anthony's fire, and all pushes and eruptions, hot and salt
phlegm. The same applied with meal and fair water in manner of
a poultice, to any place affected with convulsions, the cramp, and
such as are out of joint, doth give help and ease. The distilled
water cleanses the skin, and takes away freckles, spots, morphew,
or wrinkles in the face.

HAWTHORN

IT is not my intention to trouble you with a description of this tree,
which is so well known that it needs none. It is ordinarily but a
hedge bush, although being pruned and dressed, it grows to a tree
of a reasonable height.

As for the Hawthorn Tree at Glastonbury, which is said to flower
yearly on Christmas-day, it rather shews the superstition of those
that observe it for the time of its flowering, than any great wonder,
since the like may be found in divers other places of this land; as
in Whey-street in Romney Marsh, and near unto Nantwich in
Cheshire, by a place called White Green, where it flowers about
Christmas and May. If the weather be frosty, it flowers not until
January, or that the hard weather be over.

Government and virtues.] It is a tree of Mars. The seeds in the
berries beaten to powder being drank in wine, are held singularly
good against the stone, and are good for the dropsy. The distilled
water of the flowers stay the lask. The seed cleared from the down,
bruised and boiled in wine, and drank, is good for inward tormenting pains. If cloths or sponges be wet in the distilled water, and
applied to any place wherein thorns and splinters, or the like, do
abide in the flesh, it will notably draw them forth.

And thus you see the thorn gives a medicine for its own pricking,
and so doth almost every thing else.

HEMLOCK

Descript.] The common great Hemlock grows up with a green
stalk, four or five feet high, or more, full of red spots sometimes,
and at the joints very large winged leaves set at them, which are
divided into many other winged leaves, one set against the other,
dented about the edges, of a sad green colour, branched towards the
top, where it is full of umbels of white flowers, and afterwards with
whitish flat seed. The root is long, white, and sometimes crooked,

and hollow within. The whole plant, and every part, has a strong, heady, and ill-savoured scent, much offending the senses.

Place.] It grows in all counties of this land, by walls and hedge-sides, in waste grounds and untilled places.

Time.] It flowers and seeds in July, or thereabouts.

Government and virtues.] Saturn claims dominion over this herb, yet I wonder why it may not be applied to the privities in a Priapism, or continual standing of the yard, it being very beneficial to that disease. I suppose, my author's judgment was first upon the opposite disposition of Saturn to Venus in those faculties, and therefore he forbade the applying of it to those parts, that it might not cause barrenness, or spoil the spirit procreative; which if it do, yet applied to the privities, it stops its lustful thoughts. Hemlock is exceedingly cold, and very dangerous, especially to be taken inwardly. It may safely be applied to inflammations, tumours, and swellings in any part of the body (save the privy parts) as also to St. Anthony's fire, wheals, pushes, and creeping ulcers that arise of hot sharp humours, by cooling and repelling the heat; the leaves bruised and laid to the brow or forehead are good for their eyes that are red and swollen; as also to take away a pin and web growing in the eye; this is a tried medicine: Take a small handful of this herb, and half so much bay salt, beaten together, and applied to the contrary wrist of the hand, for 24 hours, doth remove it in thrice dressing. If the root thereof be roasted under the embers, wrapped in double wet paper, until it be soft and tender, and then applied to the gout in the hands or fingers, it will quickly help this evil. If any through mistake eat the herb Hemlock instead of Parsley, or the roots instead of a Parsnip (both of which it is very like) whereby happens a kind of frenzy, or perturbation of the senses, as if they were stupid and drunk, the remedy is (as Pliny saith) to drink of the best and strongest pure wine, before it strikes to the heart, or Gentian put in wine, or a draught of vinegar, wherewith Tragus doth affirm, that he cured a woman that had eaten the root.

HEMP

This is so well known to every good housewife in the country, that I shall not need to write any description of it.

Time.] It is sown in the very end of March, or beginning of April, and is ripe in August or September.

Government and virtues.] It is a plant of Saturn, and good for something else, you see, than to make halters only. The seed of Hemp consumes wind, and by too much use thereof disperses it so much that it dries up the natural seed for procreation; yet, being boiled in milk and taken, helps such as have a hot dry cough. The Dutch make an emulsion out of the seed, and give it with good success to those that have the jaundice, especially in the beginning of the disease, if there be no ague accompanying it, for it opens obstructions of the gall, and causes digestion of choler. The emulsion or decoction of the seed stays lasks and continual fluxes, eases the cholic, and allays the troublesome humours in the bowels, and stays bleeding at the mouth, nose, or other places, some of the leaves, being fried with the blood of them that bleed, and so given them to eat. It is held very good to kill the worms in men or beasts; and the juice dropped into the ears kills worms in them; and draws forth earwigs, or other living creatures gotten into them. The decoction of the root allays inflammations of the head, or any other parts: the herb itself, or the distilled water thereof doth the like. The decoction of the root eases the pains of the gout, the hard humours of knots in the joints, the pains and shrinking of the sinews, and the pains of the hips. The fresh juice mixed with a little oil and butter, is good for any place that hath been burnt with fire, being thereto applied.

HENBANE

Descript.] Our common Henbane has very large, thick, soft, woolly leaves, lying on the ground, much cut in, or torn on the edges, of a dark, ill greyish green colour; among which arise up divers thick and short stalks, two or three feet high, spread into divers small branches, with lesser leaves on them, and many hollow flowers, scarce appearing above the husk, and usually torn on one side, ending in five round points, growing one above another, of a deadish yellowish colour, somewhat paler towards the edges, with many purplish veins therein, and of a dark, yellowish purple in the bottom of the flower, with a small point of the same colour in the middle, each of them standing in a hard close husk, which after the flowers are past, grow very like the husk of Asarabacca, and somewhat sharp at the top points, wherein is contained much small seed, very like Poppy seed, but of a dusky, greyish colour. The root is great, white, and thick, branching forth divers ways under ground, so like a Parsnip root (but that it is not so white) that it has deceived others. The whole plant more than the root, has a very heavy, ill, soporiferous smell, somewhat offensive.

Place.] It commonly grows by the waysides, and under hedge-sides and walls.

Time.] It flowers in July, and springs again yearly of its own seed. I doubt my authors mistook July for June, if not for May.

Government and virtues.] I wonder how astrologers could take on them to make this an herb of Jupiter; and yet Mizaldus, a man of a penetrating brain, was of that opinion as well as the rest; the herb is indeed under the dominion of Saturn, and I prove it by this argument: All the herbs which delight most to grow in saturnine places, are saturnine herbs. But Henbane delights most to grow in saturnine places, and whole cart loads of it may be found near the places where they empty the common Jakes, and scarce a ditch to be found without it growing by it. Ergo, it is an herb of Saturn. The leaves of Henbane do cool all hot inflammations in the eyes, or any other part of the body; and are good to assuage all manner of swellings of the privities, or women's breasts, or elsewhere, if they be boiled in wine, and either applied themselves, or the fomentation warm; it also assuages the pain of the gout, the sciatica, and other pains in the joints which arise from a hot cause. And applied with vinegar to the forehead and temples, helps the head-ache and want of sleep in hot fevers. The juice of the herb or seed, or the oil drawn from the seed, does the like. The oil of the seed is helpful for deafness, noise, and worms in the ears, being dropped therein; the juice of the herb or root doth the same. The decoction of the herb or seed, or both, kills lice in man or beast. The fume of the dried herb, stalks and seed, burned, quickly heals swellings, chilblains or kibes in the hands or feet, by holding them in the fume thereof. The remedy to help those that have taken Henbane is to drink goat's milk, honeyed water, or pine kernels, with sweet wine; or, in the absence of these, Fennel seed, Nettle seed, the seed of Cresses, Mustard, or Radish; as also Onions or Garlic taken in wine, do all help to free them from danger, and restore them to their due temper again.

Take notice, that this herb must never be taken inwardly; outwardly, an oil ointment, or plaister of it, is most admirable for the gout, to cool the veneral heat of the reins in the French pox; to stop the tooth-ache, being applied to the aching side: to allay all inflammations, and to help the diseases before premised.

HEDGE HYSSOP

DIVERS sorts there are of this plant; the first of which is an Italian by birth, and only nursed up here in the gardens of the curious. Two or three sorts are found commonly growing wild here, the description of two of which I shall give you.

Descript.] The first is a smooth, low plant, not a foot high, very bitter in taste, with many square stalks, diversly branched from the bottom to the top, with divers joints, and two small leaves at each joint, broader at the bottom than they are at the end, a little dented about the edges, of a sad green colour, and full of veins. The flowers stand at the joints, being of a fair purple colour, with some white spots in them, in fashion like those of dead nettles. The seed is small and yellow, and the roots spread much under ground.

The second seldom grows half a foot high, sending up many small branches, whereon grow many small leaves, set one against the other, somewhat broad, but very short. The flowers are like the flowers of the other fashion, but of a pale reddish colour. The seeds are small and yellowish. The root spreads like the other, neither will it yield to its fellow one ace of bitterness.

Place.] They grow in wet low grounds, and by the water-sides; the last may be found among the bogs on Hampstead Heath.

Time.] They flower in June or July, and the seed is ripe presently after.

Government and virtues.] They are herbs of Mars, and as choleric and churlish as he is, being most violent purges, especially of choler and phlegm. It is not safe taking them inwardly, unless they be well rectified by the art of the alchymist, and only the purity of them given; so used they may be very helpful both for the dropsy, gout, and sciatica; outwardly used in ointments they kill worms, the belly anointed with it, and are excellently good to cleanse old and filthy ulcers.

BLACK HELLEBORE

It is also called Setter-wort, Setter-grass, Bear's-foot, Christmas-herb, and Christmas-flowers.

Descript.] It hath sundry fair green leaves rising from the root, each of them standing about an handful high from the earth; each leaf is divided into seven, eight, or nine parts, dented from the middle of the leaf to the point on both sides, abiding green all the Winter; about Christmas-time, if the weather be any thing temperate, the flowers appear upon foot stalks, also consisting of five large, round, white leaves a-piece, which sometimes are purple towards the edges, with many pale yellow thumbs in the middle; the seeds are divided into several cells, like those of Columbines, save only that they are greater; the seeds are in colour black, and in form long and round. The root consists of numberless blackish strings all united into one head. There is another Black Hellebore, which grows up and down in the woods very like this, but only that the leaves are smaller and narrower, and perish in the Winter, which this doth not.

Place.] The first is maintained in gardens. The second is commonly found in the woods in Northamptonshire.

Time.] The first flowers in December or January; the second in February or March.

Government and virtues.] It is an herb of Saturn, and therefore no marvel if it has some sullen conditions with it, and would be far safer, being purified by the art of the alchymist than given raw. If any have taken any harm by taking it, the common cure is to take goat's milk. If you cannot get goat's milk, you must make a shift with such as you can get. The roots are very effectual against all melancholy diseases, especially such as are of long standing, as quartan agues and madness; it helps the falling sickness, the leprosy, both the yellow and black jaundice, the gout, sciatica, and convulsions; and this was found out by experience, that the root of that which grows wild in our country, works not so churlishly as those do which are brought from beyond sea, as being maintained by a more temperate air. The root used as a pessary, provokes the terms exceedingly; also being beaten into powder, and strewed upon foul ulcers, it consumes the dead flesh, and instantly heals them; nay, it will help gangrenes in the beginning. Twenty grains taken inwardly is a sufficient dose for one time, and let that be corrected with half so much cinnamon; country people used to rowel their cattle with it. If a beast be troubled with a cough, or have taken any poison, they bore a hole through the ear, and put a piece of the root in it, this will help him in 24 hours time. Many other uses farriers put it to which I shall forbear.

HERB ROBERT

The Herb Robert is held in great estimation by farmers, who use it in diseases of their cattle.

Descript.] It rises up with a reddish stalk two feet high, having divers leaves thereon, upon very long and reddish foot-stalks, divided at the ends into three or five divisions, each of them cut in on the edges, which sometimes turn reddish. At the tops of the stalks come forth divers flowers made of five leaves, much larger than the Dove's-foot, and of a more reddish colour; after which come black heads, as in others. The root is small and thready, and smells, as the whole plant, very strong, almost stinking.

Place.] This grows frequently every where by the way-sides, upon ditch banks and waste grounds wheresoever one goes.

Time.] It flowers in June and July chiefly, and the seed is ripe shortly after.

Government and virtues.] It is under the dominion of Venus. Herb Robert is commended not only against the stone, but to stay blood, where or howsoever flowing; it speedily heals all green wounds, and is effectual in old ulcers in the privy parts, or elsewhere. You may persuade yourself this is true, and also conceive a good reason for it, do but consider it is an herb of Venus, for all it hath a man's name.

HERB TRUE-LOVE, OR ONE-BERRY

Descript.] Ordinary Herb True-love has a small creeping root running under the uppermost crust of the ground, somewhat like couch grass root, but not so white, shooting forth stalks with leaves, some whereof carry no berries, the others do; every stalk smooth without joints, and blackish green, rising about half a foot high, if it bear berries, otherwise seldom so high, bearing at the top four leaves set directly one against another, in manner of a cross or ribband tied (as it is called in a true-loves knot,) which are each of them apart somewhat like unto a night-shade leaf, but somewhat broader, having sometimes three leaves, sometimes five, sometimes six, and those sometimes greater than in others, in the middle of the four leaves rise up one small slender stalk, about an inch high, bearing at the tops thereof one flower spread open like a star, consisting of four small and long narrow pointed leaves of a yellowish green colour, and four others lying between them lesser than they; in the middle whereof stands a round dark purplish button or head, compassed about with eight small yellow mealy threads with three colours, making it the more conspicuous, and lovely to behold. This button or head in the middle, when the other leaves are withered, becomes a blackish purple berry, full of juice, of the bigness of a reasonable grape, having within it many white seeds. The whole plant is without any manifest taste.

Place.] It grows in woods and copses, and sometimes in the corners or borders of fields, and waste grounds in very many places of this land, and abundantly in the woods, copses, and other places about Chislehurst and Maidstone in Kent.

Time.] They spring up in the middle of April or May, and are in flower soon after. The berries are ripe in the end of May, and in some places in June.

Government and virtues.] Venus owns it; the leaves or berries hereof are effectual to expel poison of all sorts, especially that of the aconites; as also, the plague, and other pestilential disorders; Matthiolus saith, that some that have lain long in a lingering sickness, and others that by witchcraft (as it was thought) were become half foolish, by taking a dram of the seeds or berries hereof in powder every day for 20 days together, were restored to their former health. The roots in powder taken in wine eases the pains of the cholic speedily. The leaves are very effectual as well for green wounds, as to cleanse and heal up filthy old sores and ulcers; and is very powerful to discuss all tumours and swellings in the privy parts, the groin, or in any part of the body, and speedily to allay all inflammations. The juice of the leaves applied to felons, or those nails of the hands or toes that have imposthumes or sores gathered together at the roots of them, heals them in a short space. The herb is not to be described for the premises, but is fit to be nourished in every good woman's garden.

HYSSOP

HYSSOP is so well known to be an inhabitant in every garden, that it will save me labour in writing a description thereof. The virtues are as follow.

Government and virtues.] The herb is Jupiter's, and the sign Cancer. It strengthens all the parts of the body under Cancer and Jupiter; which what they may be, is found amply described in my astrological judgment of diseases. Dioscorides saith, that Hyssop boiled with rue and honey, and drank, helps those that are troubled with coughs, shortness of breath, wheezing and rheumatic distillation upon the lungs; taken also with oxymel, it purges gross humours by stool; and with honey, kills worms in the belly; and with fresh and new figs bruised, helps to loosen the belly, and more forcibly if the root of Flower-de-luce and cresses be added thereto. It amends and cherishes the native colour of the body, spoiled by the yellow jaundice; and being taken with figs and nitre, helps the dropsy and spleen; being boiled with wine, it is good to wash inflammations, and takes away the black and blue spots and marks that come by strokes, bruises, or falls, being applied with warm water. It is an excellent medicine for the quinsy, or swellings in the throat, to wash and gargle it, being boiled in figs; it helps the toothache, being boiled in vinegar and gargled therewith. The hot vapours of the decoction taken by a funnel in at the ears, eases the inflammations and singing noise of them. Being bruised, and salt, honey, and cummin seed put to it, helps those that are stung by serpents. The oil thereof (the head being anointed) kills lice, and takes away itching of the head. It helps those that have the falling sickness, which way soever it be applied. It helps to expectorate tough phlegm, and is effectual in all cold griefs or diseases of the chests or lungs, being taken either in syrup or licking medicine.

The green herb bruised and a little sugar put thereto, doth quickly heal any cut or green wounds, being thereunto applied.

HOPS

THESE are so well known that they need no description; I mean the manured kind, which every good husband or housewife is acquainted with.

Descript.] The wild hop grows up as the other doth, ramping upon trees or hedges, that stand next to them, with rough branches and leaves like the former, but it gives smaller heads, and in far less plenty than it, so that there is scarcely a head or two seen in a year on divers of this wild kind, wherein consists the chief difference.

Place.] They delight to grow in low moist grounds, and are found in all parts of this land.

Time.] They spring not until April, and flower not until the latter end of June; the heads are not gathered until the middle or latter end of September.

Government and virtues.] It is under the dominion of Mars. This, in physical operations, is to open obstructions of the liver and spleen, to cleanse the blood, to loosen the belly, to cleanse the reins from gravel, and provoke urine. The decoction of the tops of Hops, as well of the tame as the wild, works the same effects. In cleansing the blood they help to cure the French diseases, and all manner of scabs, itch, and other breakings-out of the body; as also all tetters, ringworms, and spreading sores, the morphew and all discolouring of the skin. The decoction of the flowers and hops, do help to expel poison that any one hath drank. Half a dram of the seed in powder taken in drink, kills worms in the body, brings down women's courses, and expels urine. A syrup made of the juice and sugar, cures the yellow jaundice, eases the head-ache that comes of heat, and tempers the heat of the liver and stomach, and is profitably given in long and hot agues that rise in choler and blood. Both the wild and the manured are of one property, and alike effectual in all the aforesaid diseases. By all these testimonies beer appears to be better than ale.

Mars owns the plant, and then Dr. Reason will tell you how it performs these actions.

HOREHOUND

THERE are two kinds of Horehound, the white and the black. The black sort is likewise called Hen-bit; but the white one is here spoken of.

Descript.] Common Horehound grows up with square hairy stalks, half a yard or two feet high, set at the joints with two round crumpled rough leaves of a sullen hoary green colour, of a reasonable good scent, but a very bitter taste. The flowers are small, white, and gaping, set in a rough, hard prickly husk round about the joints, with the leaves from the middle of the stalk upward, wherein afterward is found small round blackish seed. The root is blackish, hard and woody, with many strings, and abides many years.

Place.] It is found in many parts of this land, in dry grounds, and waste green places.

Time.] It flowers in July, and the seed is ripe in August.

Government and virtues.] It is an herb of Mercury. A decoction of the dried herb, with the seed, or the juice of the green herb taken with honey, is a remedy for those that are short-winded, have a cough, or are fallen into a consumption, either through long sickness, or thin distillations of rheum upon the lungs. It helps to expectorate tough phlegm from the chest, being taken from the roots of Iris or Orris. It is given to women to bring down their courses, to expel the after-birth, and to them that have taken poison, or are stung or bitten by venomous serpents. The leaves used with honey, purge foul ulcers, stay running or creeping sores, and the growing of the flesh over the nails. It also helps pains of the sides. The juice thereof with wine and honey, helps to clear the eyesight, and snuffed up into the nostrils purges away the yellow-jaundice, and with a little oil of roses dropped into the ears, eases the pains of them. Galen saith, it opens obstructions both of the liver and spleen, and purges the breast and lungs of phlegm: and used outwardly it both cleanses and digests. A decoction of Horehound (saith Matthiolus) is available for those that have hard livers, and for such as have itches and running tetters. The powder hereof taken, or the decoction, kills worms. The green leaves bruised, and boiled in old hog's grease into an ointment, heals the biting of dogs, abates the swellings and pains that come by any pricking of thorns, or such like means; and used with vinegar, cleanses and heals tetters. There is a syrup made of Horehound to be had at the apothecaries, very good for old coughs, to rid the tough phlegm; as also to void cold rheums from the lungs of old folks, and for those that are asthmatic or short-winded.

HORSETAIL

OF that there are many kinds, but I shall not trouble you nor myself with any large description of them, which to do, were but, as the proverb is, To find a knot in a rush, all the kinds thereof being nothing else but knotted rushes, some with leaves, and some with-out. Take the description of the most eminent sort as follows.

Descript.] The great Horsetail at the first springing has heads somewhat like those of asparagus, and afterwards grow to be hard, rough, hollow stalks, jointed at sundry places up to the top, a foot high, so made as if the lower parts were put into the upper, where grow on each side, a bush of small long rush-like hard leaves, each part resembling a horsetail, from whence it is so called. At the tops of the stalks come forth small catkins, like those of trees. The root creeps under ground, having joints at sundry places.

Place.] This (as most of the other sorts hereof) grows in wet grounds.

Time.] They spring up in April, and their blooming catkins in July, seeding for the most part in August, and then perish down to the ground, rising afresh in the Spring.

Government and virtues.] The herb belongs to Saturn, yet is very harmless, and excellently good for the things following: Horsetail, the smoother rather than the rough, and the leaves rather than the bark is most physical. It is very powerful to staunch bleeding either inward or outward, the juice or the decoction thereof being drank, or the juice, decoction, or distilled water applied outwardly. It also stays all sorts of lasks and fluxes in man or woman and bloody urine; and heals also not only the inward ulcers, and the excoriation of the entrails, bladder, &c. but all other sorts of foul, moist and running ulcers, and soon solders together the tops of green wounds. It cures all ruptures in children. The decoction thereof in wine being drank, provokes urine, and helps the stone and stranguary; and the distilled water thereof drank two or three times in a day, and a small quantity at a time, also eases the bowels, and is effectual against a cough that comes by distillations from the head. The juice or distilled water being warmed, and hot inflammations, pustules or red wheals, and other breakings-out in the skin, being bathed therewith, doth help them, and doth no less the swelling heat and inflammation of the lower parts in men and women.

HOUSELEEK OR SENGREEN

BOTH these are so well known to my countrymen, that I shall not need to write any description of them.

Place.] It grows commonly upon walls and house-sides, and flowers in July.

Government and virtues.] It is an herb of Jupiter, and it is reported by Mezaldus, to preserve what it grows upon from fire and lightning. Our ordinary Houseleek is good for all inward heats as well as outward, and in the eyes or other parts of the body; a posset made with the juice of Houseleek, is singularly good in all hot agues, for it cools and tempers the blood and spirits, and quenches the thirst; and also good to stay all hot defluctions or sharp and salt rheums in the eyes, the juice being dropped into them, or into the ears. It helps also other fluxes of humours in the bowels, and the immoderate courses of women. It cools and restrains all other hot inflammations, St. Anthony's fire, scaldings and burnings, the shingles, fretting ulcers, cankers, tetters, ring-worms, and the like; and much eases the pains of the gout proceeding from any hot cause. The juice also takes away warts and corns in the hands or feet, being often bathed therewith, and the skin and leaves being laid on them afterwards. It eases also the head-ache, and distempered heat of the brain in frenzies, or through want of sleep, being applied to the temples and forehead. The leaves bruised and laid upon the crown or seam of the head stays bleeding at the nose very quickly. The distilled water of the herb is profitable for all the purposes aforesaid. The leaves being gently rubbed on any place stung with nettles or bees, doth quickly take away the pain.

HOUND'S TONGUE

Descript.] The great ordinary Hound's Tongue has many long and somewhat narrow, soft, hairy, darkish green leaves, lying on the ground, somewhat like unto Bugloss leaves, from among which rises up a rough hairy stalk about two feet high, with some smaller leaves thereon, and branched at the tops into divers parts, with a small leaf at the foot of every branch, which is somewhat long, with many flowers set along the same, which branch is crooked or turned inwards before it flowers, and opens by degrees as the flowers blow, which consist of small purplish red leaves of a dead colour, rising out of the husks wherein they stand with some threads in the middle. It has sometimes a white flower. After the flowers are past, there comes rough flat seed, with a small pointle in the middle, easily cleaving to any garment that it touches, and not so easily pulled off again. The root is black, thick, and long, hard to break, and full of clammy juice, smelling somewhat strong, of an evil scent, as the leaves also do.

Place.] It grows in moist places of this land, in waste grounds, and untilled places, by highway sides, lanes, and hedge-sides.

Time.] It flowers about May or June, and the seed is ripe shortly after.

Government and virtues.] It is a plant under the dominion of Mercury. The root is very effectually used in pills, as well as the decoction, or otherwise, to stay all sharp and thin defluxions of rheum from the head into the eyes or nose, or upon the stomach or lungs, as also for coughs and shortness of breath. The leaves boiled in wine (saith Dioscorides, but others do rather appoint it to be made with water, and add thereto oil and salt) molifies or opens the belly downwards. It also helps to cure the biting of a mad dog, some of the leaves being also applied to the wound. The leaves bruised, or the juice of them boiled in hog's lard, and applied, helps falling away of the hair, which comes of hot and sharp humours; as also for any place that is scalded or burnt; the leaves bruised and laid to any green wound doth heal it up quickly: the root baked under the embers, wrapped in paste or wet paper, or in a wet double cloth, and thereof a suppository made, and put up into or applied to the fundament, doth very effectually help the painful piles or hæmorrhoids. The distilled water of the herbs and roots is very good to all the purposes aforesaid, to be used as well inwardly to drink, as outwardly to wash any sore place, for it heals all manner of wounds and punctures, and those foul ulcers that arise by the French pox. Mizaldus adds that the leaves laid under the feet, will keep the dogs from barking at you. It is called Hound's-tongue, because it ties the tongues of hounds; whether true, or not, I never tried, yet I cured the biting of a mad dog with this only medicine.

HOLLY, HOLM, OR HULVER BUSH

For to describe a tree so well known is needless.

Government and virtues.] The tree is Saturnine. The berries expel wind, and therefore are held to be profitable in the cholic. The berries have a strong faculty with them; for if you eat a dozen of them in the morning fasting when they are ripe and not dried, they purge the body of gross and clammy phlegm: but if you dry the berries, and beat them into powder, they bind the body, and stop fluxes, bloody-fluxes, and the terms in women. The bark of the tree, and also the leaves, are excellently good, being used in fomentations for broken bones, and such members as are out of joint. Pliny saith, the branches of the tree defend houses from lightning, and men from witchcraft.

ST. JOHN'S WORT

This is a very beautiful shrub, and is a great ornament to our meadows.

Descript.] Common St. John's Wort shoots forth brownish, up-right, hard, round stalks, two feet high, spreading many branches from the sides up to the tops of them, with two small leaves set one against another at every place, which are of a deep green colour, somewhat like the leaves of the lesser Centaury, but narrow, and full of small holes in every leaf, which cannot be so well perceived, as when they are held up to the light; at the tops of the stalks and branches stand yellow flowers of five leaves a-piece, with many yellow threads in the middle, which being bruised do yield a reddish juice like blood; after which come small round heads, wherein is contained small blackish seed smelling like rosin. The root is hard and woody, with divers strings and fibres at it, of a brownish colour, which abides in the ground many years, shooting anew every Spring.

Place.] This grows in woods and copses, as well those that are shady, as open to the sun.

Time.] They flower about Midsummer and July, and their seed is ripe in the latter end of July or August.

Government and virtues.] It is under the celestial sign Leo, and the dominion of the Sun. It may be, if you meet a Papist, he will tell you, especially if he be a lawyer, that St. John made it over to him by a letter of attorney. It is a singular wound herb; boiled in wine and drank, it heals inward hurts or bruises; made into an ointment, it open obstructions, dissolves swellings, and closes up the lips of wounds. The decoction of the herb and flowers, espe-cially of the seed, being drank in wine, with the juice of knot-grass, helps all manner of vomiting and spitting of blood, is good for those that are bitten or stung by any venomous creature, and for those that cannot make water. Two drams of the seed of St. John's Wort made into powder, and drank in a little broth, doth gently expel choler or congealed blood in the stomach. The decoction of the leaves and seeds drank somewhat warm before the fits of agues, whether they be tertains or quartans, alters the fits, and, by often using, doth take them quite away. The seed is much commended, being drank for forty days together, to help the sciatica, the falling sickness, and the palsy.

IVY

It is so well known to every child almost, to grow in woods upon the trees, and upon the stone walls of churches, houses, &c. and sometimes to grow alone of itself, though but seldom.

Time.] It flowers not until July, and the berries are not ripe till Christmas, when they have felt Winter frosts.

Government and virtues.] It is under the dominion of Saturn. A pugil of the flowers, which may be about a dram, (saith Dioscorides) drank twice a day in red wine, helps the lask, and bloody flux. It is an enemy to the nerves and sinews, being much taken inwardly, but very helpful to them, being outwardly applied. Pliny saith, the yellow berries are good against the jaundice; and taken before one be set to drink hard, preserves from drunkenness, and helps those that spit blood; and that the white berries being taken inwardly, or applied outwardly, kills the worms in the belly. The berries are a singular remedy to prevent the plague, as also to free them from it that have got it, by drinking the berries thereof made into a powder, for two or three days together. They being taken in wine, do certainly help to break the stone, provoke urine, and women's courses. The fresh leaves of Ivy, boiled in vinegar, and applied warm to the sides of those that are troubled with the spleen, ache, or stitch in the sides, do give much ease. The same applied with some Rosewater, and oil of Roses, to the temples and forehead, eases the head-ache, though it be of long continuance. The fresh leaves boiled in wine, and old filthy ulcers hard to be cured washed therewith, do wonderfully help to cleanse them. It also quickly heals green wounds, and is effectual to heal all burnings and scaldings, and all kinds of exulcerations coming thereby, or by salt phlegm or humours in other parts of the body. The juice of the berries or leaves snuffed up into the nose, purges the head and brain of thin rheum that makes defluxions into the eyes and nose, and curing the ulcers and stench therein; the same dropped into the ears helps the old and running sores of them; those that are troubled with the spleen shall find much ease by continual drinking out of a cup made of Ivy, so as the drink may stand some small time therein before it be drank. Cato saith, That wine put into such a cup, will soak through it, by reason of the antipathy that is between them.

There seems to be a very great antipathy between wine and Ivy; for if one hath got a surfeit by drinking of wine, his speediest cure is to drink a draught of the same wine wherein a handful of Ivy leaves, being first bruised, have been boiled.

JUNIPER BUSH

FOR to give a description of a bush so commonly known is needless.

Place.] They grow plentifully in divers woods in Kent, Warney common near Brentwood in Essex, upon Finchley Common without Highgate; hard by the New-found Wells near Dulwich, upon a Common between Mitcham and Croydon, in the Highgate near Amersham in Buckinghamshire, and many other places.

Time.] The berries are not ripe the first year, but continue green two Summers and one Winter before they are ripe; at which time they are all of a black colour, and therefore you shall always find upon the bush green berries; the berries are ripe about the fall of the leaf.

Government and virtues.] This admirable solar shrub is scarce to be paralleled for its virtues. The berries are hot in the third degree, and dry but in the first, being a most admirable counter-poison, and as great a resister of the pestilence, as any growing: they are excellent good against the bitings of venomous beasts, they provoke urine exceedingly, and therefore are very available to dysuries and stranguaries. It is so powerful a remedy against the dropsy, that the very lye made of the ashes of the herb being drank, cures the disease. It provokes the terms, helps the fits of the mother, strengthens the stomach exceedingly, and expels the wind. Indeed there is scarce a better remedy for wind in any part of the body, or the cholic, than the chymical oil drawn from the berries; such country people as know not how to draw the chymical oil, may content themselves by eating ten or a dozen of the ripe berries every morning fasting. They are admirably good for a cough, shortness of breath, and consumption, pains in the belly, ruptures, cramps, and convulsions. They give safe and speedy delivery to women with child, they strengthen the brain exceedingly, help the memory, and fortify the sight by strengthening the optic nerves; are excellently good in all sorts of agues; help the gout and sciatica, and strengthen the limbs of the body. The ashes of the wood is a speedy remedy to such as have the scurvy, to rub their gums with. The berries stay all fluxes, help the hæmorrhoids or piles, and kill worms in children. A lye made of the ashes of the wood, and the body bathed with it, cures the itch, scabs and leprosy. The berries break the stone, procure appetite when it is lost, and are excellently good for all palsies, and falling-sickness.

KIDNEYWORT, OR WALL PENNYROYAL, OR WALL PENNYWORT

Descript.] It has many thick, flat, and round leaves growing from the root, every one having a long footstalk, fastened underneath, about the middle of it, and a little unevenly weaved sometimes about the edges, of a pale green colour, and somewhat yellow on the upper side like a saucer; from among which arise one or more tender, smooth, hollow stalks half a foot high, with two or three small leaves thereon, usually not round as those below, but somewhat long, and divided at the edges: the tops are somewhat divided into long branches, bearing a number of flowers, set round about a long spike one above another, which are hollow and like a little bell of a whitish green colour, after which come small heads, containing very small brownish seed, which falling on the ground, will plentifully spring up before Winter, if it have moisture. The root is round and most usually smooth, greyish without, and white within, having small fibres at the head of the root, and bottom of the stalk.

Place.] It grows very plentifully in many places of this land, but especially in all the west parts thereof, upon stone and mud walls, upon rocks also, and in stony places upon the ground, at the bottom of old trees, and sometimes on the bodies of them that are decayed and rotten.

Time.] It usually flowers in the beginning of May, and the seed ripening quickly after, sheds itself; so that about the end of May, usually the stalks and leaves are withered, dry, and gone until September, then the leaves spring up again, and so abide all winter.

Government and virtues.] Venus challenges the herb under Libra. The juice or the distilled water being drank, is very effectual for all inflammations and unnatural heats, to cool a fainting hot stomach, a hot liver, or the bowels: the herb, juice, or distilled water thereof, outwardly applied, heals pimples, St. Anthony's fire, and other outward heats. The said juice or water helps to heal sore kidneys, torn or fretted by the stone, or exulcerated within; it also provokes urine, is available for the dropsy, and helps to break the stone. Being used as a bath, or made into an ointment, it cools the painful piles or hæmorrhoidal veins. It is no less effectual to give ease to the pains of the gout, the sciatica, and helps the kernels or knots in the neck or throat, called the king's evil: healing kibes and chilblains if they be bathed with the juice, or anointed with ointment made thereof, and some of the skin of the leaf upon them: it is also used in green wounds to stay the blood, and to heal them quickly.

KNAPWEED

Descript.] The common sort hereof has many long and somewhat dark green leaves, rising from the root, dented about the edges, and sometimes a little rent or torn on both sides in two or three places, and somewhat hairy withal; amongst which arises a long round stalk, four or five feet high, divided into many branches, at the tops whereof stand great scaly green heads, and from the middle of them thrust forth a number of dark purplish red thrumbs or threads, which after they are withered and past, there are found divers black seeds, lying in a great deal of down, somewhat like unto Thistle seed, but smaller; the root is white, hard and woody, and divers fibres annexed thereunto, which perishes not, but abides with leaves thereon all the Winter, shooting out fresh every spring.

Place.] It grows in most fields and meadows, and about their borders and hedges, and in many waste grounds also every where.

Time.] It usually flowers in June and July, and the seed is ripe shortly after.

Government and virtues.] Saturn challenges the herb for his own. This Knapweed helps to stay fluxes, both of blood at the mouth or nose, or other outward parts, and those veins that are inwardly broken, or inward wounds, as also the fluxes of the belly; it stays distillation of thin and sharp humours from the head upon the stomach and lungs; it is good for those that are bruised by any fall, blows or otherwise, and is profitable for those that are bursten, and have ruptures, by drinking the decoction of the herb and roots in wine, and applying the same outwardly to the place. It is singularly good in all running sores, cancerous and fistulous, drying up of the moisture, and healing them up so gently, without sharpness; it doth the like to running sores or scabs of the head or other parts. It is of special use for the soreness of the throat, swelling of the uvula and jaws, and excellently good to stay bleeding, and heal up all green wounds.

KNOTGRASS

It is generally known so well that it needs no description.

Place.] It grows in every county of this land by the highway sides, and by foot-paths in fields; as also by the sides of old walls.

Time.] It springs up late in the Spring, and abides until the Winter, when all the branches perish.

Government and virtues.] Saturn seems to me to own the herb, and yet some hold the Sun; out of doubt 'tis Saturn. The juice of the common kind of Knotgrass is most effectual to stay bleeding of the mouth, being drank in steeled or red wine; and the bleeding at the nose, to be applied to the forehead or temples, or to be squirted up into the nostrils. It is no less effectual to cool and temper the heat of the blood and stomach, and to stay any flux of the blood and humours, as lasks, bloody-flux, women's courses, and running of the reins. It is singularly good to provoke urine, help the stranguary, and allays the heat that comes thereby; and is powerful by urine to expel the gravel or stone in the kidneys and bladder, a dram of the powder of the herb being taken in wine for many days together. Being boiled in wine and drank, it is profitable to those that are stung or bitten by venomous creatures, and very effectual to stay all defluxions of rheumatic humours upon the stomach and kills worms in the belly or stomach, quiets inward pains that arise from the heat, sharpness and corruption of blood and choler. The distilled water hereof taken by itself or with the powder of the herb or seed, is very effectual to all the purposes aforesaid, and is accounted one of the most sovereign remedies to cool all manner of inflammations, breaking out through heat, hot swellings and imposthumes, gangrene and fistulous cankers, or foul filthy ulcers, being applied or put into them; but especially for all sorts of ulcers and sores happening in the privy parts of men and women. It helps all fresh and green wounds, and speedily heals them. The juice dropped into the ears, cleanses them being foul, and having running matter in them.

It is very prevalent for the premises; as also for broken joints and ruptures.

LADIES' MANTLE

Descript.] It has many leaves rising from the root standing upon long hairy foot-stalks, being almost round, and a little cut on the edges, into eight or ten parts, making it seem like a star, with so many corners and points, and dented round about, of a light green colour, somewhat hard in handling, and as it were folded or plaited at first, and then crumpled in divers places, and a little hairy, as the stalk is also, which rises up among them to the height of two or three feet; and being weak, is not able to stand upright, but bended to the ground, divided at the top into two or three small branches, with small yellowish green heads, and flowers of a whitish colour breaking out of them; which being past, there comes a small yellowish seed like a poppy seed. The root is somewhat long and black, with many strings and fibres thereat.

Place.] It grows naturally in many pastures and wood sides in Hertfordshire, Wiltshire, and Kent, and other places of this land.

Time.] It flowers in May and June, abides after seedtime green all the Winter.

Government and virtues.] Venus claims the herb as her own. Ladies' Mantle is very proper for those wounds that have inflammations, and is very effectual to stay bleeding, vomitings, fluxes of all sorts, bruises by falls or otherwise, and helps ruptures; and such women as have large breasts, causing them to grow less and hard, being both drank and outwardly applied; the distilled water drank for 20 days together helps conception, and to retain the birth; if the women do sometimes also sit in a bath made of the decoction of the herb. It is one of the most singular wound herbs that is, and therefore highly prized and praised by the Germans, who use it in all wounds inward and outward, to drink a decoction thereof, and wash the wounds therewith, or dip tents therein, and put them into the wounds, which wonderfully dries up all humidity of the sores, and abates inflammations therein. It quickly heals all green wounds, not suffering any corruption to remain behind, and cures all old sores, though fistulous and hollow.

LAVENDER

BEING an inhabitant almost in every garden, it is so well known, that it needs no description.

Time.] It flowers about the end of June, and beginning of July.

Government and virtues.] Mercury owns the herb; and it carries his effects very potently. Lavender is of a special good use for all the griefs and pains of the head and brain that proceed of a cold cause, as the apoplexy, falling-sickness, the dropsy, or sluggish malady, cramps, convulsions, palsies, and often faintings. It strengthens the stomach, and frees the liver and spleen from obstructions, provokes women's courses, and expels the dead child and after-birth. The flowers of Lavender steeped in wine, helps them to make water that are stopped, or are troubled with the wind or cholic, if the place be bathed therewith. A decoction made with the flowers of Lavender, Hore-hound, Fennel and Asparagus root, and a little Cinnamon, is very profitably used to help the falling-sickness, and the giddiness or turning of the brain: to gargle the mouth with the decoction thereof is good against the tooth-ache. Two spoonfuls of the distilled water of the flowers taken, helps them that have lost their voice, as also the tremblings and passions of the heart, and faintings and swooning, not only being drank, but applied to the temples, or nostrils to be smelled unto; but it is not safe to use it where the body is replete with blood and humours, because of the hot and subtile spirits wherewith it is possessed. The chymical oil drawn from Lavender, usually called Oil of Spike, is of so fierce and piercing a quality, that it is cautiously to be used, some few drops being sufficient, to be given with other things, either for inward or outward griefs.

LAVENDER-COTTON

IT being a common garden herb, I shall forbear the description, only take notice, that it flowers in June and July.

Government and virtues.] It is under the dominion of Mercury. It resists poison, putrefaction, and heals the biting of venomous beasts. A dram of the powder of the dried leaves taken every morning fasting, stops the running of the reins in men, and whites in women. The seed beaten into powder, and taken as worm-seed, kills the worms, not only in children, but also in people of riper years; the like doth the herb itself, being steeped in milk, and the milk drank; the body bathed with the decoction of it, helps scabs and itch.

LADIES-SMOCK, OR CUCKOW-FLOWER

This is a very pretty ornament to the sides of most meadows.

Descript.] The root is composed of many small white threads from whence spring up divers long stalks of winged leaves, consisting of round, tender, dark, green leaves, set one against another upon a middle rib, the greatest being at the end, amongst which arise up divers tender, weak, round, green stalks, somewhat streaked, with longer and smaller leaves upon them; on the tops of which stand flowers, almost like the Stock Gilliflowers, but rounder, and not so long, of a blushing white colour; the seed is reddish, and grows to small branches, being of a sharp biting taste, and so has the herb.

Place.] They grow in moist places, and near to brooksides.

Time.] They flower in April and May, and the lower leaves continue green all the Winter.

Government and virtues.] They are under the dominion of the Moon, and very little inferior to Water Cresses in all their operations; they are excellently good for the scurvy, they provoke urine, and break the stone, and excellently warm a cold and weak stomach, restoring lost appetite, and help digestion.

LETTUCE

It is so well known, being generally used as a Sallad-herb, that it is altogether needless to write any description thereof.

Government and virtues.] The Moon owns them, and that is the reason they cool and moisten what heat and dryness Mars causeth, because Mars has his fall in Cancer; and they cool the heat because the Sun rules it, between whom and the Moon is a reception in the generation of men, as you may see in my Guide for Women. The juice of Lettuce mixed or boiled with Oil of Roses, applied to the forehead and temples procures sleep, and eases the headache proceeding of an hot cause. Being eaten boiled, it helps to loosen the belly. It helps digestion, quenches thirst, increases milk in nurses, eases griping pains in the stomach or bowels, that come of choler. Applied outwardly to the region of the heart, liver or reins, or by bathing the said places with the juice of distilled water, wherein some white Sanders, or red Roses are put; not only represses the heat and inflammations therein, but comforts and strengthens those parts, and also tempers the heat of urine. Galen advises old men to use it with spice; and where spices are wanting, to add Mints, Rocket, and such like hot herbs, or else Citron Lemon, or Orange seeds, to abate the cold of one and heat of the other. The seed and distilled water of the Lettuce work the same effects in all things; but the use of Lettuce is chiefly forbidden to those that are short-winded, or have any imperfection in the lungs, or spit blood.

WATER LILY

Of these there are two principally noted kinds, *viz*. the White and the Yellow.

Descript.] The White Lily has very large and thick dark green leaves lying on the water, sustained by long and thick foot-stalks, that arise from a great, thick, round, and long tuberous black root spongy or loose, with many knobs thereon, green on the outside, but as white as snow within, consisting of divers rows of long and somewhat thick and narrow leaves, smaller and thinner the more inward they be, encompassing a head with many yellow threads or thrums in the middle; where, after they are past, stand round Poppy-like heads, full of broad oily and bitter seed.

The yellow kind is little different from the former, save only that it has fewer leaves on the flowers, greater and more shining seed, and a whitish root, both within and without. The root of both is somewhat sweet in taste.

Place.] They are found growing in great pools, and standing waters, and sometimes in slow running rivers, and lesser ditches of water, in sundry places of this land.

Time.] They flower most commonly about the end of May, and their seed is ripe in August.

Government and virtues.] The herb is under the dominion of the Moon, and therefore cools and moistens like the former. The leaves and flowers of the Water Lilies are cold and moist, but the roots and seeds are cold and dry; the leaves do cool all inflammations, both outward and inward heat of agues; and so doth the flowers also, either by the syrup or conserve; the syrup helps much to procure rest, and to settle the brain of frantic persons, by cooling the hot distemperature of the head. The seed as well as the root is effectual to stay fluxes of blood or humours, either of wounds or of the belly; but the roots are most used, and more effectual to cool, bind, and restrain all fluxes in man or woman. The root is likewise very good for those whose urine is hot and sharp, to be boiled in wine and water, and the decoction drank. The distilled water of the flowers is very effectual for all the diseases aforesaid, both inwardly taken, and outwardly applied; and is much commended to take away freckles, spots, sunburn, and morphew from the face, or other parts of the body. The oil made of the flowers, as oil of Roses is made, is profitably used to cool hot tumours, and to ease the pains, and help the sores.

LILY OF THE VALLEY

CALLED also Conval Lily, Male Lily, and Lily Confancy.

Descript.] The root is small, and creeps far in the ground, as grass roots do. The leaves are many, against which rises up a stalk half a foot high, with many white flowers, like little bells with turned edges of a strong, though pleasing smell; the berries are red, not much unlike those of Asparagus.

Place.] They grow plentifully upon Hampstead-Heath, and many other places in this nation.

Time.] They flower in May, and the seed is ripe in September.

Government and virtues.] It is under the dominion of Mercury, and therefore it strengthens the brain, recruits a weak memory, and makes it strong again. The distilled water dropped into the eyes, helps inflammations there; as also that infirmity which they call a pin and web. The spirit of the flowers distilled in wine, restores lost speech, helps the palsy, and is excellently good in the apoplexy, comforts the heart and vital spirits. Gerrard saith, that the flowers being close stopped up in a glass, put into an ant-hill, and taken away again a month after, ye shall find a liquor in the glass, which, being outwardly applied, helps the gout.

WHITE LILIES

IT were in vain to describe a plant so commonly known in every one's garden; therefore I shall not tell you what they are, but what they are good for.

Government and virtues.] They are under the dominion of the Moon, and by antipathy to Mars expel poison; they are excellently good in pestilential fevers, the roots being bruised and boiled in wine, and the decoction drank; for it expels the venom to the exterior parts of the body. The juice of it being tempered with barley meal, baked, and so eaten for ordinary bread, is an excellent cure for the dropsy. An ointment made of the root, and hog's grease, is excellently good for scald heads, unites the sinews when they are cut, and cleanses ulcers. The root boiled in any convenient decoction, gives speedy delivery to women in travail, and expels the afterbirth. The root roasted, and mixed with a little hog's grease, makes a gallant poultice to ripen and break plague-sores. The ointment is excellently good for swellings in the privities, and will cure burnings and scaldings without a scar, and trimly deck a blank place with hair.

LIQUORICE

Descript.] Our English Liquorice rises up with divers woody stalks, whereon are set at several distances many narrow, long, green leaves, set together on both sides of the stalk, and an odd one at the end, very well resembling a young ash tree sprung up from the seed. This by many years continuance in a place without removing, and not else, will bring forth flowers, many standing together spike fashion, one above another upon the stalk, of the form of pease blossoms, but of a very pale blue colour, which turn into long, somewhat flat and smooth cods, wherein is contained a small round, hard seed. The roots run down exceeding deep into the ground, with divers other small roots and fibres growing with them, and shoot out suckers from the main roots all about, whereby it is much increased, of a brownish colour on the outside, and yellow within.

Place.] It is planted in fields and gardens, in divers places of this land, and thereof good profit is made.

Government and virtues.] It is under the dominion of Mercury. Liquorice boiled in fair water, with some Maiden-hair and figs, makes a good drink for those that have a dry cough or hoarseness, wheezing or shortness of breath, and for all the griefs of the breast and lungs, phthisic or consumptions caused by the distillation of salt humours on them. It is also good in all pains of the reins, the stranguary, and heat of urine. The fine powder of Liquorice blown through a quill into the eyes that have a pin and web (as they call it) or rheumatic distillations in them, doth cleanse and help them. The juice of Liquorice is as effectual in all the diseases of the breast and lungs, the reins and bladder, as the decoction. The juice distilled in Rose-water, with some Gum Tragacanth, is a fine licking medicine for hoarseness, wheezing, &c.

LIVERWORT

THERE are, according to some botanists, upwards of three hundred different kinds of Liverwort.

Descript.] Common Liverwort grows close, and spreads much upon the ground in moist and shady places, with many small green leaves, or rather (as it were) sticking flat to one another, very unevenly cut in on the edges, and crumpled; from among which arise small slender stalks, an inch or two high at most, bearing small star-like flowers at the top; the roots are very fine and small.

Government and virtues.] It is under the dominion of Jupiter, and under the sign Cancer. It is a singularly good herb for all the diseases of the liver, both to cool and cleanse it, and helps the inflammations in any part, and the yellow jaundice likewise. Being bruised and boiled in small beer, and drank, it cools the heat of the liver and kidneys, and helps the running of the reins in men, and the whites in women; it is a singular remedy to stay the spreading of tetters, ringworms, and other fretting and running sores and scabs, and is an excellent remedy for such whose livers are corrupted by surfeits, which cause their bodies to break out, for it fortifies the liver exceedingly, and makes it impregnable.

LOOSESTRIFE OR WILLOW-HERB

Descript.] Common yellow Loosestrife grows to be four or five feet high, or more, with great round stalks, a little crested, diversly branched from the middle of them to the tops into great and long branches, on all which, at the joints, there grow long and narrow leaves, but broader below, and usually two at a joint, yet sometimes three or four, somewhat like willow leaves, smooth on the edges, and of a fair green colour from the upper joints of the branches, and at the tops of them also stand many yellow flowers of five leaves a-piece, with divers yellow threads in the middle, which turn into small round heads, containing small cornered seeds: the root creeps under ground, almost like couchgrass, but greater, and shoots up every Spring brownish heads which afterwards grow up into stalks. It has no scent or taste, and is only astringent.

Place.] It grows in many places of the land in moist meadows, and by water sides.

Time.] It flowers from June to August.

Government and virtues.] This herb is good for all manner of bleeding at the mouth, nose, or wounds, and all fluxes of the belly, and the bloody-flux, given either to drink or taken by clysters; it stays also the abundance of women's courses; it is a singular good wound-herb for green wounds, to stay the bleeding, and quickly close together the lips of the wound, if the herb be bruised, and the juice only applied. It is often used in gargles for sore mouths, as also for the secret parts. The smoak hereof being bruised, drives away flies and gnats, which in the night time molest people inhabiting near marshes, and in the fenny countries.

LOOSESTRIFE, WITH SPIKED HEADS OF FLOWERS

It is likewise called Grass-polly.

Descript.] This grows with many woody square stalks, full of joints, about three feet high at least; at every one whereof stand two long leaves, shorter, narrower, and a greener colour than the former, and some brownish. The stalks are branched into many long stems of spiked flowers half a foot long, growing in bundles one above another, out of small husks, very like the spiked heads of Lavender, each of which flowers have five round-pointed leaves of a purple violet colour, or somewhat inclining to redness; in which husks stand small round heads after the flowers are fallen, wherein is contained small seed. The root creeps under ground like unto the yellow, but is greater than it, and so are the heads of the leaves when they first appear out of the ground, and more brown than the other.

Place.] It grows usually by rivers, and ditch-sides in wet ground, as about the ditches at and near Lambeth, and in many places of this land.

Time.] It flowers in the months of June and July.

Government and virtues.] It is an herb of the Moon, and under the sign Cancer; neither do I know a better preserver of the sight when it is well, nor a better cure for sore eyes than Eyebright, taken inwardly, and this used outwardly; it is cold in quality. This herb is nothing inferior to the former, it having not only all the virtues which the former hath, but more peculiar virtues of its own, found out by experience; as, namely, The distilled water is a present remedy for hurts and blows on the eyes, and for blindness, so as the Christalline humours be not perished or hurt; and this hath been sufficiently proved true by the experience of a man of judgment, who kept it long to himself as a great secret. It clears the eyes of dust, or any thing gotten into them, and preserves the sight. It is also very available against wounds and thrusts, being made into an ointment in this manner: To every ounce of the water, add two drams of May butter without salt, and of sugar and wax, of each as much also; let them boil gently together. Let tents dipped into the liquor that remains after it is cold, be put into the wounds, and the place covered with a linen cloth doubled and anointed with the ointment; and this is also an approved medicine. It likewise cleanses and heals all foul ulcers, and sores whatsoever, and stays their inflammations by washing them with the water, and laying on them a green leaf or two in the Summer, or dry leaves in the Winter. This water, gargled warm in the mouth, and sometimes drank also, doth cure the quinsy, or king's evil in the throat. The said water applied warm, takes away all spots, marks, and scabs in the skin; and a little of it drank, quenches thirst when it is extreme.

LOVAGE

Descript.] It has many long and green stalks of large winged leaves, divided into many parts, like Smallage, but much larger and greater, every leaf being cut about the edges, broadest forward, and smallest at the stalk, of a sad green colour, smooth and shining; from among which rise up sundry strong, hollow green stalks, five or six, sometimes seven or eight feet high, full of joints, but lesser leaves set on them than grow below; and with them towards the tops come forth large branches, bearing at their tops large umbels of yellow flowers, and after them flat brownish seed. The roots grow thick, great and deep, spreading much, and enduring long, of a brownish colour on the outside, and whitish within. The whole plant and every part of it smelling strong, and aromatically, and is of a hot, sharp, biting taste.

Place.] It is usually planted in gardens, where, if it be suffered, it grows huge and great.

Time.] It flowers in the end of July and seeds in August.

Government and virtues.] It is an herb of the Sun, under the sign Taurus. If Saturn offend the throat (as he always doth if he be occasioner of the malady, and in Taurus is the Genesis) this is your cure. It opens, cures and digests humours, and mightily provokes women's courses and urine. Half a dram at a time of the dried root in powder taken in wine, doth wonderfully warm a cold stomach, helps digestion, and consumes all raw and superfluous moisture therein; eases all inward gripings and pains, dissolves wind, and resists poison and infection. It is a known and much praised remedy to drink the decoction of the herb for any sort of ague, and to help the pains and torments of the body and bowels coming of cold. The seed is effectual to all the purposes aforesaid (except the last) and works more powerfully. The distilled water of the herb helps the quinsy in the throat, if the mouth and throat be gargled and washed therewith, and helps the pleurisy, being drank three or four times. Being dropped into the eyes, it takes away the redness or dimness of them; it likewise takes away spots or freckles in the face. The leaves bruised, and fried with a little hog's lard, and put hot to any blotch or boil, will quickly break it.

LUNGWORT

Descript.] This is a kind of moss, that grows on sundry sorts of trees, especially oaks and beeches, with broad, greyish, tough leaves diversly folded, crumpled, and gashed in on the edges, and some spotted also with many small spots on the upper-side. It was never seen to bear any stalk or flower at any time.

Government and virtues.] Jupiter seems to own this herb. It is of great use to physicians to help the diseases of the lungs, and for coughs, wheezings, and shortness of breath, which it cures both in man and beast. It is very profitable to put into lotions that are taken to stay the moist humours that flow to ulcers, and hinder their healing, as also to wash all other ulcers in the privy parts of a man or woman. It is an excellent remedy boiled in beer for broken-winded horses.

MADDER

Descript.] Garden Madder shoots forth many very long, weak, four-square, reddish stalks, trailing on the ground a great way, very rough or hairy, and full of joints. At every one of these joints come forth divers long and narrow leaves, standing like a star about the stalks, round also and hairy, towards the tops whereof come forth many small pale yellow flowers, after which come small round heads, green at first, and reddish afterwards, but black when they are ripe, wherein is contained the seed. The root is not very great, but exceeding long, running down half a man's length into the ground, red and very clear, while it is fresh, spreading divers ways.

Place.] It is only manured in gardens, or larger fields, for the profit that is made thereof.

Time.] It flowers towards the end of Summer, and the seed is ripe quickly after.

Government and virtues.] It is an herb of Mars. It hath an opening quality, and afterwards to bind and strengthen. It is a sure remedy for the yellow jaundice, by opening the obstructions of the liver and gall, and cleansing those parts; it opens also the obstructions of the spleen, and diminishes the melancholy humour. It is available for the palsy and sciatica, and effectual for bruises inward and outward, and is therefore much used in vulnerary drinks. The root for all those aforesaid purposes, is to be boiled in wine or water, as the cause requires, and some honey and sugar put thereunto afterwards. The seed hereof taken in vinegar and honey, helps the swelling and hardness of the spleen. The decoction of the leaves and branches is a good fomentation for women that have not their courses. The leaves and roots beaten and applied to any part that is discoloured with freckles, morphew, the white scurf, or any such deformity of the skin, cleanses thoroughly, and takes them away.

MAIDEN HAIR

Descript.] Our common Maiden-Hair doth, from a number of hard black fibres, send forth a great many blackish shining brittle stalks, hardly a span long, in many not half so long, on each side set very thick with small, round, dark green leaves, and spotted on the back of them like a fern.

Place.] It grows upon old stone walls in the West parts in Kent, and divers other places of this land; it delights likewise to grow by springs, wells, and rocky moist and shady places, and is always green.

WALL RUE, OR, WHITE MAIDEN-HAIR

Descript.] This has very fine, pale green stalks, almost as fine as hairs, set confusedly with divers pale green leaves on every short foot stalk, somewhat near unto the colour of garden Rue, and not much differing in form but more diversly cut in on the edges, and thicker, smooth on the upper part, and spotted finely underneath.

Place.] It grows in many places of this land, at Dartford, and the bridge at Ashford in Kent, at Beaconsfield in Buckinghamshire, at Wolly in Huntingdonshire, on Framlingham Castle in Suffolk, on the church walls at Mayfield in Sussex, in Somersetshire, and divers other places of this land; and is green in Winter as well as Summer.

Government and virtues.] Both this and the former are under the dominion of Mercury, and so is that also which follows after, and the virtue of both are so near alike, that though I have described them and their places of growing severally, yet I shall in writing the virtues of them, join them both together as follows.

The decoction of the herb Maiden-Hair being drank, helps those that are troubled with the cough, shortness of breath, the yellow jaundice, diseases of the spleen, stopping of urine, and helps exceedingly to break the stone in the kidneys, (in all which diseases the Wall Rue is also very effectual). It provokes women's courses, and stays both bleedings and fluxes of the stomach and belly, especially when the herb is dry; for being green, it loosens the belly, and voids choler and phlegm from the stomach and liver; it cleanses the lungs, and by rectifying the blood, causes a good colour to the whole body. The herb boiled in oil of Camomile, dissolves knots, allays swellings, and dries up moist ulcers. The lye made thereof is singularly good to cleanse the head from scurf, and from dry and running sores, stays the falling or shedding of the hair, and causes it to grow thick, fair, and well coloured; for which purpose some boil it in wine, putting some Smallage seed thereto, and afterwards some oil. The Wall Rue is as effectual as Maiden-Hair, in all diseases of the head, or falling and recovering of the hair again, and generally for all the aforementioned diseases. And besides, the powder of it taken in drink for forty days together, helps the burstings in children.

GOLDEN MAIDEN HAIR

To the former give me leave to add this, and I shall say no more but only describe it to you, and for the virtues refer you to the former, since whatever is said of them, may be also said of this.

Descript.] It has many small, brownish, red hairs, to make up the form of leaves growing about the ground from the root; and in the middle of them, in Summer, rise small stalks of the same colour, set with very fine yellowish green hairs on them, and bearing a small gold, yellow head, less than a wheat corn, standing in a great husk. The root is very small and thready.

Place.] It grows in bogs and moorish places, and also on dry shady places, as Hampstead Heath, and elsewhere.

MALLOWS AND MARSHMALLOWS

COMMON MALLOWS are generally so well known that they need no description.

Our common Marshmallows have divers soft hairy white stalks, rising to be three or four feet high, spreading forth many branches, the leaves whereof are soft and hairy, somewhat less than the other Mallow leaves, but longer pointed, cut (for the most part) into some few divisions, but deep. The flowers are many, but smaller also than the other Mallows, and white, or tending to a bluish colour. After which come such long, round cases and seeds, as in the other Mallows. The roots are many and long, shooting from one head, of the bigness of a thumb or finger, very pliant, tough, and being like liquorice, of a whitish yellow colour on the outside, and more whitish within, full of a slimy juice, which being laid in water, will thicken, as if it were a jelly.

Place.] The common Mallows grow in every county of this land. The common Marsh-mallows in most of the salt marshes, from Woolwich down to the sea, both on the Kentish and Essex shores, and in divers other places of this land.

Time.] They flower all the Summer months, even until the Winter do pull them down.

Government and virtues.] Venus owns them both. The leaves of either of the sorts, both specified, and the roots also boiled in wine or water, or in broth with Parsley or Fennel roots, do help to open the body, and are very convenient in hot agues, or other distempers of the body, to apply the leaves so boiled warm to the belly. It not only voids hot, choleric, and other offensive humours, but eases the pains and torments of the belly coming thereby; and are therefore used in all clysters conducing to those purposes. The same used by nurses procures them store of milk. The decoction of the seed of any of the common Mallows made in milk or wine, doth marvellously help excoriations, the phthisic pleurisy, and other diseases of the chest and lungs, that proceed of hot causes, if it be continued taking for some time together. The leaves and roots work the same effects. They help much also in the excoriations of the bowels, and hardness of the mother, and in all hot and sharp diseases thereof. The juice drank in wine, or the decoction of them therein, do help women to a speedy and easy delivery. Pliny saith, that whosoever takes a spoonful of any of the Mallows, shall that day be free from all diseases that may come unto him; and that it is especially good for the falling-sickness. The syrup also and conserve made of the flowers, are very effectual for the same diseases, and to open the body, being costive. The leaves bruised, and laid to the eyes with a little honey, take away the imposthumations of them. The leaves bruised or rubbed upon any place stung with bees, wasps, or the like, presently take away the pain, redness, and swelling that rise thereupon. And Dioscorides saith, The decoction of the roots and leaves helps all sorts of poison, so as the poison be presently voided by vomit. A poultice made of the leaves boiled and bruised, with some bean or barley flower, and oil of Roses added, is an especial remedy against all hard tumours and inflammations, or imposthumes, or swellings of the privities, and other parts, and eases the pains of them; as also against the hardness of the liver or spleen, being applied to the places. The juice of Mallows boiled in old oil and applied, takes away all roughness of the skin, as also the scurf, dandriff, or dry scabs in the head, or other parts, if they be anointed therewith, or washed with the decoction, and preserves the hair from falling off. It is also effectual against scaldings and burnings, St. Anthony's fire, and all other hot, red, and painful swellings in any part of the body. The flowers boiled in oil or water (as every one is disposed) whereunto a little honey and allum is put, is an excellent gargle to wash, cleanse or heal any sore mouth or throat in a short space. If the feet be bathed or washed with the decoction of the leaves, roots, and flowers, it helps much the defluxions of rheum from the head; if the head be washed therewith, it stays the falling and shedding of the hair. The green leaves (saith Pliny) beaten with nitre, and applied, draw out thorn or prickles in the flesh.

The Marshmallows are more effectual in all the diseases before mentioned. The leaves are likewise used to loosen the belly gently, and in decoctions or clysters to ease all pains of the body, opening the strait passages, and making them slippery, whereby the stone may descend the more easily and without pain, out of the reins, kidneys, and bladder, and to ease the torturing pains thereof. But the roots are of more special use for those purposes, as well for coughs, hoarseness, shortness of breath and wheezings, being boiled in wine, or honeyed water, and drank. The roots and seeds hereof boiled in wine or water, are with good success used by them that have excoriations in the bowels, or the bloody flux, by qualifying the violence of sharp fretting humours, easing the pains, and healing the soreness. It is profitably taken by them that are troubled with ruptures, cramps, or convulsions of the sinews; and boiled in white wine, for the imposthumes by the throat, commonly called the king's evil, and of those kernels that rise behind the ears, and inflammations or swellings in women's breasts. The dried roots boiled in milk and drank, is especially good for the chin-cough. Hippocrates used to give the decoction of the roots, or the juice thereof, to drink, to those that are wounded, and ready to faint through loss of blood, and applied the same, mixed with honey and rosin, to the wounds. As also, the roots boiled in wine to those that have received any hurt by bruises, falls, or blows, or had any bone or member out of joint, or any swelling-pain, or ache in the muscles, sinews or arteries. The muscilage of the roots, and of Linseed and Fenugreek put together, is much used in poultices, ointments, and plaisters, to molify and digest all hard swellings, and the inflammation of them, and to ease pains in any part of the body. The seed

either green or dry, mixed with vinegar, cleanses the skin of
morphew, and all other discolourings, being boiled therewith in
the Sun.

You may remember that not long since there was a raging
disease called the bloody-flux; the college of physicians not knowing
what to make of it, called it the inside plague, for their wits were at
Ne plus ultra about it. My son was taken with the same disease, and
the excoriation of his bowels was exceeding great; myself being in
the country, was sent for up, the only thing I gave him, was Mallows bruised and boiled both in milk and drink, in two days (the
blessing of God being upon it) it cured him. And I here, to shew
my thankfulness to God, in communicating it to his creatures,
leave it to posterity.

MAPLE TREE

Government and virtues.] It is under the dominion of Jupiter.
The decoction either of the leaves or bark, must needs strengthen
the liver much, and so you shall find it to do, if you use it. It is
excellently good to open obstructions both of the liver and spleen,
and eases pains of the sides thence proceeding.

WIND MARJORAM

CALLED also Origanum, Eastward Marjoram, Wild Marjoram, and
Grove Marjoram.

Descript.] Wild or field Marjoram hath a root which creeps much
under ground, which continues a long time, sending up sundry-
brownish, hard, square stalks, with small dark green leaves, very
like those of Sweet Marjoram, but harder, and somewhat broader;
at the top of the stalks stand tufts of flowers, of a deep purplish
red colour. The seed is small and something blacker than that of
Sweet Marjoram.

Place.] It grows plentifully in the borders of corn fields, and in
some copses.

Time.] It flowers towards the latter end of the Summer.

Government and virtues.] This is also under the dominion of
Mercury. It strengthens the stomach and head much, there being
scarce a better remedy growing for such as are troubled with a sour
humour in the stomach; it restores the appetite being lost; helps the
cough, and consumption of the lungs; it cleanses the body of
choler, expels poison, and remedies the infirmities of the spleen;
helps the bitings of venomous beasts, and helps such as have

poisoned themselves by eating Hemlock, Henbane, or Opium. It provokes urine and the terms in women, helps the dropsy, and the scurvy, scabs, itch, and yellow jaundice. The juice being dropped into the ears, helps deafness, pain and noise in the ears. And thus much for this herb, between which and adders, there is a deadly antipathy.

SWEET MARJORAM

SWEET Marjoram is so well known, being an inhabitant in every garden, that it is needless to write any description thereof, neither of the Winter Sweet Marjoram, or Pot Marjoram.

Place.] They grow commonly in gardens; some sorts grow wild in the borders of corn fields and pastures, in sundry places of this land; but it is not my purpose to insist upon them. The garden kinds being most used and useful.

Time.] They flower in the end of Summer.

Government and virtues.] It is an herb of Mercury, and under Aries, and therefore is an excellent remedy for the brain and other parts of the body and mind, under the dominion of the same planet. Our common Sweet Marjoram is warming and comfortable in cold diseases of the head, stomach, sinews, and other parts, taken inwardly, or outwardly applied. The decoction thereof being drank, helps all diseases of the chest which hinder the freeness of breathing, and is also profitable for the obstructions of the liver and spleen. It helps the cold griefs of the womb, and the windiness thereof, and the loss of speech, by resolution of the tongue. The decoction thereof made with some Pellitory of Spain, and long Pepper, or with a little Acorns or Origanum, being drank, is good for those that cannot make water, and against pains and torments in the belly; it provokes women's courses, if it be used as a pessary. Being made into powder, and mixed with honey, it takes away the black marks of blows, and bruises, being thereunto applied; it is good for the inflammations and watering of the eyes, being mixed with fine flour, and laid unto them. The juice dropped into the ears eases the pains and singing noise in them. It is profitably put into those ointments and salves that are warm, and comfort the outward parts, as the joints and sinews, for swellings also, and places out of joint. The powder thereof snuffed up into the nose provokes sneezing, and thereby purges the brain; and chewed in the mouth, draws forth much phlegm. The oil made thereof, is very warm and comfortable to the joints that are stiff, and the sinews that are hard, to molify and supple them. Marjoram is much used in all odoriferous water, powders, &c. that are for ornament or delight.

MARIGOLDS

THESE being so plentiful in every garden, and so well known that they need no description.

Time.] They flower all the Summer long, and sometimes in Winter, if it be mild.

Government and virtues.] It is an herb of the Sun, and under Leo. They strengthen the heart exceedingly, and are very expulsive, and a little less effectual in the smallpox and measles than saffron. The juice of Marigold leaves mixed with vinegar, and any hot swelling bathed with it, instantly gives ease, and assuages it. The flowers, either green or dried, are much used in possets, broths, and drink, as a comforter of the heart and spirits, and to expel any malignant or pestilential quality which might annoy them. A plaister made with the dry flowers in powder, hog's-grease, turpentine, and rosin, applied to the breast, strengthens and succours the heart infinitely in fevers, whether pestilential or not.

MASTERWORT

Descript.] Common Masterwort has divers stalks of winged leaves divided into sundry parts, three for the most part standing together at a small foot-stalk on both sides of the greater, and three likewise at the end of the stalk, somewhat broad, and cut in on the edges into three or more divisions, all of them dented about the brims, of a dark green colour, somewhat resembling the leaves of Angelica, but that these grow lower to the ground, and on lesser stalks; among which rise up two or three short stalks about two feet high, and slender, with such like leaves at the joints which grow below, but with lesser and fewer divisions, bearing umbels of white flowers, and after them thin, flat blackish seeds, bigger than Dill seeds. The root is somewhat greater and growing rather sideways than down deep in the ground, shooting forth sundry heads, which taste sharp, biting on the tongue, and is the hottest and sharpest part of the plant, and the seed next unto it being somewhat blackish on the outside, and smelling well.

Place.] It is usually kept in gardens with us in England.

Time.] It flowers and seeds about the end of August.

Government and virtues.] It is an herb of Mars. The root of Masterwort is hotter than pepper, and very available in cold griefs and diseases both of the stomach and body, dissolving very powerfully upwards and downwards. It is also used in a decoction with wine against all cold rheums, distillations upon the lungs, or shortness of breath, to be taken morning and evening. It also provokes urine, and helps to break the stone, and expel the gravel from the kidneys; provokes women's courses, and expels the dead birth. It is singularly good for strangling of the mother, and other such like feminine diseases. It is effectual also against the dropsy, cramps, and falling sickness; for the decoction in wine being gargled in the mouth, draws down much water and phlegm, from the brain, purging and easing it of what oppresses it. It is of a rare quality against all sorts of cold poison, to be taken as there is cause; it provokes sweat. But lest the taste hereof, or of the seed (which works to the like effect, though not so powerfully) should be too offensive, the best way is to take the water distilled both from the herb and root. The juice hereof dropped, or tents dipped therein, and applied either to green wounds or filthy rotten ulcers, and those that come by envenomed weapons, doth soon cleanse and heal them. The same is also very good to help the gout coming of a cold cause.

SWEET MAUDLIN

Descript.] Common Maudlin hath somewhat long and narrow leaves, snipped about the edges. The stalks are two feet high, bearing at the tops many yellow flowers set round together and all of an equal height, in umbels or tufts like unto tansy; after which follow small whitish seed, almost as big as wormseed.

Place and time.] It grows in gardens, and flowers in June and July.

Government and virtues.] The Virtues hereof being the same with Costmary or Alecost, I shall not make any repetition thereof, lest my book grow too big; but rather refer you to Costmary for satisfaction.

THE MEDLAR

Descript.] The Tree grows near the bigness of the Quince Tree, spreading branches reasonably large, with longer and narrower leaves than either the apple or quince, and not dented about the edges. At the end of the sprigs stand the flowers, made of five white, great, broad-pointed leaves, nicked in the middle with some white threads also; after which comes the fruit, of a brownish green colour, being ripe, bearing a crown as it were on the top, which were the five green leaves; and being rubbed off, or fallen away, the head of the fruit is seen to be somewhat hollow. The fruit is very harsh before it is mellowed, and has usually five hard kernels within it. There is another kind hereof nothing differing from the former, but that it hath some thorns on it in several places, which the other hath not; and usually the fruit is small, and not so pleasant.

Time and place.] They grow in this land, and flower in May for the most part, and bear fruit in September and October.

Government and virtues.] The fruit is old Saturn's, and sure a better medicine he hardly hath to strengthen the retentive faculty; therefore it stays women's longings. The good old man cannot endure women's minds should run a gadding. Also a plaister made of the fruit dried before they are rotten, and other convenient things, and applied to the reins of the back, stops miscarriage in women with child. They are powerful to stay any fluxes of blood or humours in men or women; the leaves also have this quality. The decoction of them is good to gargle and wash the mouth, throat and teeth, when there is any defluxions of blood to stay it, or of humours, which causes the pains and swellings. It is a good bath for women, that have their courses flow too abundant: or for the piles when they bleed too much. If a poultice or plaister be made with dried medlars, beaten and mixed with the juice of red roses, whereunto a few cloves and nutmegs may be added, and a little red coral also, and applied to the stomach that is given to casting or loathing of meat, it effectually helps. The dried leaves in powder strewed on fresh bleeding wounds restrains the blood, and heals up the wound quickly. The medlar-stones made into powder, and drank in wine, wherein some Parsley-roots have lain infused all night, or a little boiled, do break the stone in the kidneys, helping to expel it.

MELLILOT, OR KING'S CLAVER

Descript.] This hath many green stalks, two or three feet high, rising from a tough, long, white root, which dies not every year, set round about at the joints with small and somewhat long, well-smelling leaves, set three together, unevenly dented about the edges. The flowers are yellow, and well-smelling also, made like other trefoil, but small, standing in long spikes one above another, for an hand breath long or better, which afterwards turn into long crooked pods, wherein is contained flat seed, somewhat brown.

Place.] It grows plentifully in many places of this land, as in the edge of Suffolk and in Essex, as also in Huntingdonshire, and in other places, but most usually in corn fields, in corners of meadows.

Time.] It flowers in June and July, and is ripe quickly after.

Government and virtues.] Mellilot, boiled in wine, and applied, mollifies all hard tumours and inflammations that happen in the eyes, or other parts of the body, and sometimes the yolk of a roasted egg, or fine flour, or poppy seed, or endive, is added unto it. It helps the spreading ulcers in the head, it being washed with a lye made thereof. It helps the pains of the stomach, being applied fresh, or boiled with any of the aforenamed things; also, the pains of the ears, being dropped into them; and steeped in vinegar, or rose water, it mitigates the head-ache. The flowers of Mellilot or Camomile are much used to be put together in clysters to expel wind, and ease pains; and also in poultices for the same purpose, and to assuage swelling tumours in the spleen or other parts, and helps inflammations in any part of the body. The juice dropped into the eyes, is a singularly good medicine to take away the film or skin that clouds or dims the eye-sight. The head often washed with the distilled water of the herb and flower, or a lye made therewith, is effectual for those that suddenly lose their senses; as also to strengthen the memory, to comfort the head and brain, and to preserve them from pain, and the apoplexy.

FRENCH AND DOG MERCURY

Descript.] This rises up with a square green stalk full of joints, two feet high, or thereabouts, with two leaves at every joint, and the branches likewise from both sides of the stalk, set with fresh green leaves, somewhat broad and long, about the bigness of the leaves of Bazil, finely dented about the edges; towards the tops of the stalks and branches, come forth at every joint in the male Mercury two small, round green heads, standing together upon a short foot stalk, which growing ripe, are seeds, not having flowers. The female stalk is longer, spike-fashion, set round about with small green husks, which are the flowers, made small like bunches of grapes, which give no seed, but abiding long upon the stalks without shedding. The root is composed of many small fibres, which perishes every year at the first approach of Winter, and rises again of its own sowing; and if once it is suffered to sow itself, the ground will never want afterwards, even both sorts of it.

DOG MERCURY

HAVING described unto you that which is called French Mercury, I come now to shew you a description of this kind also.

Descript.] This is likewise of two kinds, male and Female, having many stalks slender and lower than Mercury, without any branches at all upon them, the root is set with two leaves at every joint, somewhat greater than the female, but more pointed and full of veins, and somewhat harder in handling: of a dark green colour, and less dented or snipped about the edges. At the joints with the leaves come forth longer stalks than the former, with two hairy round seeds upon them, twice as big as those of the former Mercury. The taste hereof is herby, and the smell somewhat strong and virulent. The female has much harder leaves standing upon longer foot-stalks, and the stalks are also longer: from the joints come forth spikes of flowers like the French Female Mercury. The roots of them both are many, and full of small fibres which run under ground, and mat themselves very much, not perishing as the former Mer-curies do, but abide the Winter, and shoot forth new branches every year, for the old lie down to the ground.

Place.] The male and female French Mercury are found wild in divers places of this land, as by a village called Brookland in Rumney Marsh in Kent.

The Dog Mercury in sundry places of Kent also, and elsewhere; but the female more seldom than the male.

Time.] They flower in the Summer months, and therein give their seed.

Government and virtues.] Mercury, they say, owns the herb, but I rather think it is Venus's, and I am partly confident of it too, for I never heard that Mercury ever minded women's business so much: I believe he minds his study more. The decoction of the leaves of Mercury, or the juice thereof in broth, or drank with a little sugar put to it, purges choleric and waterish humours. Hippo-crates commended it wonderfully for women's diseases, and applied to the secret parts, to ease the pains of the mother; and used the decoction of it, both to procure women's courses, and to expel the after-birth; and gave the decoction thereof with myrrh or pepper, or used to apply the leaves outwardly against the stranguary and diseases of the reins and bladder. He used it also for sore and watering eyes, and for the deafness and pains in the ears, by drop-ping the juice thereof into them, and bathing them afterwards in white wine. The decoction thereof made with water and a cock chicken, is a most safe medicine against the hot fits of agues. It also cleanses the breast and lungs of phlegm, but a little offends the stomach. The juice or distilled water snuffed up into the nostrils, purges the head and eyes of catarrhs and rheums. Some use to drink two or three ounces of the distilled water, with a little sugar put to it, in the morning fasting, to open and purge the body of gross, viscous, and melancholy humours. Matthiolus saith, that both the seed of the male and female Mercury boiled with Worm-wood and drank, cures the yellow jaundice in a speedy manner. The leaves or the juice rubbed upon warts, takes them away. The juice mingled with some vinegar, helps all running scabs, tetters, ringworms, and the itch. Galen saith, that being applied in manner of a poultice to any swelling or inflammation, it digests the swelling, and allays the inflammation, and is therefore given in clysters to evacuate from the belly offensive humours. The Dog Mercury, although it be less used, yet may serve in the same manner, to the same purpose, to purge waterish and melancholy humours.

MINT

Of all the kinds of Mint, the Spear Mint, or Heart Mint, being most usual, I shall only describe as follows:

Descript.] Spear Mint has divers round stalks, and long but narrowish leaves set thereon, of a dark green colour. The flowers stand in spiked heads at the tops of the branches, being of a pale blue colour. The smell or scent thereof is somewhat near unto Bazil; it encreases by the root under ground as all the others do.

Place.] It is an usual inhabitant in gardens; and because it seldom gives any good seed, the seed is recompensed by the plentiful increase of the root, which being once planted in a garden, will hardly be rid out again.

Time.] It flowers not until the beginning of August, for the most part.

Government and virtues.] It is an herb of Venus. Dioscorides saith it hath a healing, binding and drying quality, and therefore the juice taken in vinegar, stays bleeding. It stirs up venery, or bodily lust; two or three branches thereof taken in the juice of four pomegranates, stays the hiccough, vomiting, and allays the choler. It dissolves imposthumes being laid to with barley-meal. It is good to repress the milk in women's breasts, and for such as have swollen, flagging, or great breasts. Applied with salt, it helps the biting of a mad dog; with mead and honeyed water, it eases the pains of the ears, and takes away the roughness of the tongue, being rubbed thereupon. It suffers not milk to curdle in the stomach, if the leaves thereof be steeped or boiled in it before you drink it. Briefly it is very profitable to the stomach. The often use hereof is a very powerful medicine to stay women's courses and the whites. Applied to the forehead and temples, it eases the pains in the head, and is good to wash the heads of young children therewith, against all manner of breakings-out, sores or scabs, therein. It is also profitable against the poison of venomous creatures. The distilled water of Mint is available to all the purposes aforesaid, yet more weakly. But if a spirit thereof be rightly and chymically drawn, it is much more powerful than the herb itself. Simeon Sethi saith, it helps a cold liver, strengthens the belly, causes digestion, stays vomits and hiccough; it is good against the gnawing of the heart, provokes appetite, takes away obstructions of the liver, and stirs up bodily lust; but therefore too much must not be taken, because it makes the blood thin and wheyish, and turns it into choler, and therefore choleric persons must abstain from it. It is a safe medicine for the biting of a mad dog, being bruised with salt and laid thereon. The powder of it being dried and taken after meat, helps digestion, and those that are splenetic. Taken with wine, it helps women in their sore travail in child-bearing. It is good against the gravel and stone in the kidneys, and the stranguary. Being smelled unto, it is comfortable for the head and memory. The decoction hereof gargled in the mouth, cures the gums and mouth that are sore, and mends an ill-savoured breath; as also the Rue and Coriander, causes the palate of the mouth to turn to its place, the decoction being gargled and held in the mouth.

The virtues of the Wild or Horse Mint, such as grow in ditches (whose description I purposely omitted, in regard they are well known) are serviceable to dissolve wind in the stomach, to help the cholic, and those that are short-winded, and are an especial remedy for those that have veneral dreams and pollutions in the night, being outwardly applied. The juice dropped into the ears eases the pains of them, and destroys the worms that breed therein. They are good against the venomous biting of serpents. The juice laid on warm, helps the king's evil, or kernels in the throat. The decoction or distilled water helps a stinking breath, proceeding from corruption of the teeth, and snuffed up the nose, purges the head. Pliny saith, that eating of the leaves hath been found by experience to cure the leprosy, applying some of them to the face, and to help the scurf or dandriff of the head used with vinegar. They are extremely bad for wounded people; and they say a wounded man that eats Mint, his wound will never be cured, and that is a long day.

MISSELTO

Descript.] This rises up from the branch or arm of the tree whereon it grows, with a woody stem, putting itself into sundry branches, and they again divided into many other smaller twigs, interlacing themselves one within another, very much covered with a greyish green bark, having two leaves set at every joint, and at the end likewise, which are somewhat long and narrow, small at the bottom, but broader towards the end. At the knots or joints of the boughs and branches grow small yellow flowers, which run into small, round, white, transparent berries, three or four together, full of a glutinous moisture, with a blackish seed in each of them, which was never yet known to spring, being put into the ground, or any where else to grow.

Place.] It grows very rarely on oaks with us; but upon sundry others as well timber as fruit trees, plentifully in woody groves, and the like, through all this land.

Time.] It flowers in the Spring-time, but the berries are not ripe until October, and abides on the branches all the Winter, unless the blackbirds, and other birds, do devour them.

Government and virtues.] This is under the dominion of the Sun, I do not question; and can also take for granted, that which grows upon oaks, participates something of the nature of Jupiter, because an oak is one of his trees; as also that which grows upon pear trees, and apple trees, participates something of his nature, because he rules the tree it grows upon, having no root of its own. But why that should have most virtues that grows upon oaks I know not, unless because it is rarest and hardest to come by; and our college's opinion is in this contrary to scripture, which saith, *God's tender mercies are over all his works*; and so it is, let the college of physicians walk as contrary to him as they please, and that is as contrary as the east to the west. Clusius affirms that which grows upon pear trees to be as prevalent, and gives order, that it should not touch the ground after it is gathered; and also saith, that, being hung about the neck, it remedies witchcraft. Both the leaves and berries of Misselto do heat and dry, and are of subtle parts; the birdlime doth molify hard knots, tumours, and imposthumes; ripens and discusses them, and draws forth thick as well as thin humours from the remote parts of the body, digesting and separating them. And being mixed with equal parts of rozin and wax, doth molify the hardness of the spleen, and helps old ulcers and sores. Being mixed with Sandaric and Orpiment, it helps to draw off foul nails; and if quick-lime and wine lees be added thereunto, it works the stronger. The Misselto itself of the oak (as the best) made into powder, and given in drink to those that have the falling sickness, does assuredly heal them, as Matthiolus saith: but it is fit to use it for forty days together. Some have so highly esteemed it for the virtues thereof, that they have called it *Lignum Sanctiæ Crucis*, Wood of the Holy Cross, believing it helps the falling sickness, apoplexy and palsy very speedily, not only to be inwardly taken, but to be hung at their neck. Tragus saith, that the fresh wood of any Misselto bruised, and the juice drawn forth and dropped in the ears that have imposthumes in them, doth help and ease them within a few days.

MONEYWORT, OR HERB TWOPENCE

Descript.] The common Moneywort sends forth from a small thready root divers long, weak, and slender branches, lying and running upon the ground two or three feet long or more, set with leaves two at a joint one against another at equal distances, which are almost round, but pointed at the ends, smooth, and of a good green colour. At the joints with the leaves from the middle forward come forth at every point sometimes one yellow flower, and sometimes two, standing each on a small foot-stalk, and made of five leaves, narrow-pointed at the end, with some yellow threads in the middle, which being past, there stand in their places small round heads of seed.

Place.] It grows plentifully in almost all places of this land, commonly in moist grounds by hedge-sides, and in the middle of grassy fields.

Time.] They flower in June and July, and their seed is ripe quickly after.

Government and virtues.] Venus owns it. Moneywort is singularly good to stay all fluxes in man or woman, whether they be lasks, bloody-fluxes, bleeding inwardly or outwardly, or the weakness of the stomach that is given to casting. It is very good also for the ulcers or excoriations of the lungs, or other inward parts. It is exceedingly good for all wounds, either fresh or green, to heal them speedily, and for all old ulcers that are of spreading natures. For all which purposes the juice of the herb, or the powder drank in water wherein hot steel hath been often quenched; or the decoction of the green herb in wine or water drank, or used to the outward place, to wash or bathe them, or to have tents dipped therein and put into them, are effectual.

MOONWORT

Descript.] It rises up usually with but one dark green, thick and flat leaf, standing upon a short foot-stalk not above two fingers breadth; but when it flowers it may be said to bear a small slender stalk about four or five inches high, having but one leaf in the middle thereof, which is much divided on both sides into sometimes five or seven parts on a side, sometimes more; each of which parts is small like the middle rib, but broad forwards, pointed and round, resembling therein a half-moon, from whence it took the name; the uppermost parts or divisions being bigger than the lowest. The stalks rise above this leaf two or three inches, bearing many branches of small long tongues, every one like the spiky head of the adder's tongue, of a brownish colour, (which, whether I shall call them flowers, or the seed, I well know not) which, after they have continued awhile, resolve into a mealy dust. The root is small and fibrous. This hath sometimes divers such like leaves as are before described, with so many branches or tops rising from one stalk, each divided from the other.

Place.] It grows on hills and heaths, yet where there is much grass, for therein it delights to grow.

Time.] It is to be found only in April and May; for in June, when any hot weather comes, for the most part it is withered and gone.

Government and virtues.] The Moon owns the herb. Moonwort is cold and drying more than Adder's Tongue, and is therefore held to be more available for all wounds both inward and outward. The leaves boiled in red wine, and drank, stay the immoderate flux of women's courses, and the whites. It also stays bleeding, vomiting, and other fluxes. It helps all blows and bruises, and to consolidate all fractures and dislocations. It is good for ruptures, but is chiefly used, by most with other herbs, to make oils or balsams to heal fresh or green wounds (as I said before) either inward or outward, for which it is excellently good.

Moonwort is an herb which (they say) will open locks, and unshoe such horses as tread upon it. This some laugh to scorn, and those no small fools neither; but country people, that I know, call it Unshoe the Horse. Besides I have heard commanders say, that on White Down in Devonshire, near Tiverton, there were found thirty horse shoes, pulled off from the feet of the Earl of Essex's horses, being there drawn up in a body, many of them being but newly shod, and no reason known, which caused much admiration: the herb described usually grows upon heaths.

MOSSES

I SHALL not trouble the reader with a description of these, since my intent is to speak only of two kinds, as the most principal, viz. Ground Moss and Tree Moss, both which are very well known.

Place.] The Ground Moss grows in our moist woods, and at the bottom of hills, in boggy grounds, and in shadowy ditches, and many other such like places. The Tree Moss grows only on trees.

Government and virtues.] All sorts of Mosses are under the dominion of Saturn. The Ground Moss is held to be singularly good to break the stone, and to expel and drive it forth by urine, being boiled in wine and drank. The herb being bruised and boiled in water, and applied, eases all inflammations and pains coming from an hot cause; and is therefore used to ease the pains of the gout.

The Tree Mosses are cooling and binding, and partake of a digesting and molifying quality withal, as Galen saith. But each

Moss partakes of the nature of the tree from whence it is taken; therefore that of the oak is more binding, and is of good effect to stay fluxes in man or woman; as also vomiting or bleeding, the powder thereof being taken in wine. The decoction thereof in wine is very good for women to be bathed in, that are troubled with the overflowing of their courses. The same being drank, stays the stomach that is troubled with casting, or hiccough; and, as Avicena saith, it comforts the heart. The powder thereof taken in drink for some time together, is thought available for the dropsy. The oil that has had fresh Moss steeped therein for a time, and afterwards boiled and applied to the temples and forehead, marvellously eases the head-ache coming of a hot cause; as also the distillations of hot rheums or humours in the eyes, or other parts. The ancients much used it in their ointments and other medicines against the lassitude, and to strengthen and comfort the sinews. For which, if it was good then, I know no reason but it may be found so still.

MOTHERWORT

Descript.] This hath a hard, square, brownish, rough, strong stalk, rising three or four feet high at least, spreading into many branches, whereon grow leaves on each side, with long foot-stalks, two at every joint, which are somewhat broad and long, as if it were rough or crumpled, with many great veins therein of a sad green colour, and deeply dented about the edges, and almost divided. From the middle of the branches up to the tops of them (which are long and small) grow the flowers round them at distances, in sharp pointed, rough, hard husks, of a more red or purple colour than Balm or Horehound, but in the same manner or form as the Horehound, after which come small, round, blackish seeds in great plenty. The root sends forth a number of long strings and small fibres, taking strong hold in the ground, of a dark yellowish or brownish colour, and abides as the Horehound does: the smell of the one not much differs from the other.

Place.] It grows only in gardens with us in England.

Government and virtues.] Venus owns the herb, and it is under Leo. There is no better herb to take melancholy vapours from the heart, to strengthen it, and make a merry, cheerful, blithe soul than this herb. It may be kept in a syrup or conserve; therefore the Latins called it Cardiaca. Besides, it makes women joyful mothers of children, and settles their wombs as they should be, therefore we call it Motherwort. It is held to be of much use for the trembling of the heart, and faintings and swoonings; from whence it took the name Cardiaca. The powder thereof, to the quantity of a spoonful, drank in wine, is a wonderful help to women in their sore travail, as also for the suffocating or risings of the mother, and for these effects, it is likely it took the name of Motherwort with us. It also provokes urine and women's courses, cleanses the chest of cold phlegm, oppressing it, kills worms in the belly. It is of good use to warm and dry up the cold humours, to digest and disperse them that are settled in the veins, joints, and sinews of the body, and to help cramps and convulsions.

MOUSE-EAR

Descript.] Mouse-ear is a low herb, creeping upon the ground by small strings, like the Strawberry plant, whereby it shoots forth small roots, whereat grow, upon the ground, many small and somewhat short leaves, set in a round form together, and very hairy, which, being broken, do give a whitish milk. From among these leaves spring up two or three small hoary stalks about a span high, with a few smaller leaves thereon; at the tops whereof stands usually but one flower, consisting of many pale yellow leaves, broad at the point, and a little dented in, set in three or four rows (the greater uppermost) very like a Dandelion flower, and a little reddish underneath about the edges, especially if it grow in a dry ground; which after they have stood long in flower do turn into down, which with the seed is carried away with the wind.

Place.] It grows on ditch banks, and sometimes in ditches, if they be dry, and in sandy grounds.

Time.] It flowers about June or July, and abides green all the Winter.

Government and virtues.] The Moon owns this herb also; and though authors cry out upon Alchymists, for attempting to fix quicksilver, by this herb and Moonwort, a Roman would not have judged a thing by the success; if it be to be fixed at all, it is by lunar influence. The juice thereof taken in wine, or the decoction thereof drank, doth help the jaundice, although of long continuance, to drink thereof morning and evening, and abstain from other drink two or three hours after. It is a special remedy against the stone, and the tormenting pains thereof: as also other tortures and griping pains of the bowels. The decoction thereof with Succory and Century is held very effectual to help the dropsy, and them that are inclining thereunto, and the diseases of the spleen. It stays the fluxes of blood, either at the mouth or nose, and inward bleeding also, for it is a singular wound herb for wounds both inward and outward. It helps the bloody flux, and helps the abundance of women's courses. There is a syrup made of the juice hereof and sugar, by the apothecaries of Italy, and other places, which is of much account with them, to be given to those that are troubled with the cough or phthisic. The same also is singularly good for ruptures or burstings. The green herb bruised and presently bound to any cut or wound, doth quickly solder the lips thereof. And the juice, decoction, or powder of the dried herb is most singular to stay the malignity of spreading and fretting cankers and ulcers whatsoever, yea in the mouth and secret parts. The distilled water of the plant is available in all the diseases aforesaid, and to wash outward wounds and sores, by applying tents of cloths wet therein.

MUGWORT

Descript.] Common Mugwort hath divers leaves lying upon the ground, very much divided, or cut deeply in about the brims, somewhat like Wormwood, but much larger, of a dark green colour on the upper side, and very hoary white underneath. The stalks rise to be four or five feet high, having on it such like leaves as those below, but somewhat smaller, branching forth very much towards the top, whereon are set very small, pale, yellowish flowers like buttons, which fall away, and after them come small seeds, inclosed in round heads. The root is long and hard, with many small fibres growing from it, whereby it takes strong hold on the ground; but both stalks and leaves do lie down every year, and the root shoots anew in the Spring. The whole plant is of a reasonable scent, and is more easily propagated by the slips than the seed.

Place.] It grows plentifully in many places of this land, by the water-sides; as also by small water courses, and in divers other places.

Time.] It flowers and seeds in the end of Summer.

Government and virtues.] This is an herb of Venus, therefore maintains the parts of the body she rules, remedies the diseases of the parts that are under her signs, Taurus and Libra. Mugwort is with good success put among other herbs that are boiled for women to apply the hot decoction to draw down their courses, to help the delivery of the birth, and expel the after-birth. As also for the obstructions and inflammations of the mother. It breaks the stone, and opens the urinary passages where they are stopped. The juice thereof made up with Myrrh, and put under as a pessary, works the same effects, and so does the root also. Being made up with hog's grease into an ointment, it takes away wens and hard knots and kernels that grow about the neck and throat, and eases the pains about the neck more effectually, if some Field Daisies be put with it. The herb itself being fresh, or the juice thereof taken, is a special remedy upon the overmuch taking of opium. Three drams of the powder of the dried leaves taken in wine, is a speedy and the best certain help for the sciatica. A decoction thereof made with Camomile and Agrimony, and the place bathed therewith while it is warm, takes away the pains of the sinews, and the cramp.

THE MULBERRY-TREE

THIS is so well known where it grows, that it needs no description.

Time.] It bears fruit in the months of July and August.

Government and virtues.] Mercury rules the tree, therefore are its effects variable as his are. The Mulberry is of different parts; the ripe berries, by reason of their sweetness and slippery moisture, opening the body, and the unripe binding it, especially when they are dried, and then they are good to stay fluxes, lasks, and the abundance of women's courses. The bark of the root kills the broad worms in the body. The juice, or the syrup made of the juice of the berries, helps all inflammations or sores in the mouth, or throat, and palate of the mouth when it is fallen down. The juice of the leaves is a remedy against the biting of serpents, and for those that have taken aconite. The leaves beaten with vinegar, are good to lay on any place that is burnt with fire. A decoction made of the bark and leaves is good to wash the mouth and teeth when they ache. If the root be a little slit or cut, and a small hole made in the ground next thereunto, in the Harvest-time, it will give out a certain juice, which being hardened the next day, is of good use to help the tooth-ache, to dissolve knots, and purge the belly. The leaves of Mulberries are said to stay bleeding at the mouth or nose, or the bleeding of the piles, or of a wound, being bound unto the places. A branch of the tree taken when the moon is at the full, and bound to the wrists of a woman's arm, whose courses come down too much, doth stay them in a short space.

MULLEIN

Descript.] Common White Mullein has many fair, large, woolly white leaves, lying next the ground, somewhat larger than broad, pointed at the end, and as it were dented about the edges. The stalk rises up to be four or five feet high, covered over with such like leaves, but less, so that no stalk can be seen for the multitude of leaves thereon up to the flowers, which come forth on all sides of the stalk, without any branches for the most part, and are many set together in a long spike, in some of a yellow colour, in others more pale, consisting of five round pointed leaves, which afterwards have small round heads, wherein is small brownish seed contained. The root is long, white, and woody, perishing after it hath borne seed.

Place.] It grows by way-sides and lanes, in many places of this land.

Time.] It flowers in July or thereabouts.

Government and virtues.] It is under the dominion of Saturn. A small quantity of the root given in wine, is commended by Dioscorides, against lasks and fluxes of the belly. The decoction hereof drank, is profitable for those that are bursten, and for cramps and convulsions, and for those that are troubled with an old cough. The decoction thereof gargled, eases the pains of the tooth-ache. And the oil made by the often infusion of the flowers, is of very good effect for the piles. The decoction of the root in red wine or in water, (if there be an ague) wherein red hot steel hath been often quenched, doth stay the bloody-flux. The same also opens obstructions of the bladder and reins. A decoction of the leaves hereof, and of Sage, Marjoram, and Camomile flowers, and the places bathed therewith, that have sinews stiff with cold or cramps, doth bring them much ease and comfort. Three ounces of the distilled water of the flowers drank morning and evening for some days together, is said to be the most excellent remedy for the gout. The juice of the leaves and flowers being laid upon rough warts, as also the powder of the dried roots rubbed on, doth easily take them away, but doth no good to smooth warts. The powder of the dried flowers is an especial remedy for those that are troubled with the belly-ache, or the pains of the cholic. The decoction of the root, and so likewise of the leaves, is of great effect to dissolve the tumours, swellings, or inflammations of the throat. The seed and leaves boiled in wine, and applied, draw forth speedily thorns or splinters gotten into the flesh, ease the pains, and heal them also. The leaves bruised and wrapped in double papers, and covered with hot ashes and embers to bake a while, and then taken forth and laid warm on any blotch or boil happening in the groin or share, doth dissolve and heal them. The seed bruised and boiled in wine, and laid on any member that has been out of joint, and newly set again, takes away all swelling and pain thereof.

MUSTARD

Descript.] Our common Mustard hath large and broad rough leaves, very much jagged with uneven and unorderly gashes, somewhat like turnip leaves, but less and rougher. The stalk rises to be more than a foot high, and sometimes two feet high, being round, rough, and branches at the top, bearing such like leaves thereon as grow below, but lesser, and less divided, and divers yellow flowers one above another at the tops, after which come small rough pods, with small, lank, flat ends, wherein is contained round yellowish seed, sharp, hot, and biting upon the tongue. The root is small, long, and woody, when it bears stalks, and perishes every year.

Place.] This grows with us in gardens only, and other manured places.

Time.] It is an annual plant, flowering in July, and the seed is ripe in August.

Government and virtues.] It is an excellent sauce for such whose blood wants clarifying, and for weak stomachs, being an herb of Mars, but naught for choleric people, though as good for such as are aged, or troubled with cold diseases. Aries claims something to do with it, therefore it strengthens the heart, and resists poison. Let such whose stomachs are so weak they cannot digest their meat, or appetite it, take of Mustard-seed a dram, Cinnamon as much, and having beaten them to powder, and half as much Mastich in powder, and with gum Arabic dissolved in rose-water, make it up into troches, of which they may take one of about half a dram weight an hour or two before meals; let old men and women make much of this medicine, and they will either give me thanks, or shew manifest ingratitude. Mustard seed hath the virtue of heat, discussing, ratifying, and drawing out splinters of bones, and other things of the flesh. It is of good effect to bring down women's courses, for the falling-sickness or lethargy, drowsy forgetful evil, to use it both inwardly and outwardly, to rub the nostrils, forehead and temples, to warm and quicken the spirits; for by the fierce sharpness it purges the brain by sneezing, and drawing down rheum and other viscous humours, which by their distillations upon the lungs and chest, procure coughing, and therefore, with some, honey added thereto, doth much good therein. The decoction of the seed made in wine, and drank, provokes urine, resists the force of poison, the malignity of mushrooms, and venom of scorpions, or other venomous creatures, if it be taken in time; and taken before the cold fits of agues, alters, lessens, and cures them. The seed taken either by itself, or with other things, either in an electuary or drink, doth mightily stir up bodily lust, and helps the spleen and pains in the sides, and gnawings in the bowels; and used as a gargle draws up the palate of the mouth, being fallen down; and also it dissolves the swellings about the throat, if it be outwardly applied. Being chewed in the mouth it oftentimes helps the tooth-ache. The outward application hereof upon the pained place of the sciatica, discusses the humours, and eases the pains, as also the gout, and other joint aches; and is much and often used to ease pains in the sides or loins, the shoulder, or other parts of the body, upon the plying thereof to raise blisters, and cures the disease by drawing it to the outward parts of the body. It is also used to help the falling of the hair. The seed bruised mixed with honey, and applied, or made up with wax, takes away the marks and black and blue spots of bruises, or the like, the roughness or scabbiness of the skin, as also the leprosy, and lousy evil. It helps also the crick in the neck. The distilled water of the herb, when it is in the flower, is much used to drink inwardly to help in any of the diseases aforesaid, or to wash the mouth when the palate is down, and for the disease of the throat to gargle, but outwardly also for scabs, itch, or other the like infirmities, and cleanses the face from morphew, spots, freckles, and other deformities.

THE HEDGE-MUSTARD

Descript.] This grows up usually but with one blackish green stalk, tough, easy to bend, but not to break, branched into divers parts, and sometimes with divers stalks set full of branches, whereon grow long, rough, or hard rugged leaves, very much tore or cut on the edges in many parts, some bigger, and some less, of a dirty green colour. The flowers are small and yellow, that grow on the tops of the branches in long spikes, flowering by degrees; so that continuing long in flower, the stalk will have small round cods at the bottom, growing upright and close to the stalk, while the top flowers yet shew themselves, in which are contained small yellow seed, sharp and strong, as the herb is also. The root grows down slender and woody, yet abiding and springing again every year.

Place.] This grows frequently in this land, by the ways and hedge-sides, and sometimes in the open fields.

Time.] It flowers most usually about July.

Government and virtues.] Mars owns this herb also. It is singularly good in all the diseases of the chest and lungs, hoarseness of voice: and by the use of the decoction thereof for a little space, those have been recovered who had utterly lost their voice, and almost their spirits also. The juice thereof made into a syrup, or licking medicine, with honey or sugar, is no less effectual for the same purpose, and for all other coughs, wheezing, and shortness of breath. The same is also profitable for those that have the jaundice, pleurisy, pains in the back and loins, and for torments in the belly, or cholic, being also used in clysters. The seed is held to be a special remedy against poison and venom. It is singularly good for the sciatica, and in joint-aches, ulcers, and cankers in the mouth, throat, or behind the ears, and no less for the hardness and swelling of the testicles, or of women's breasts.

NAILWORT, OR WHITLOW-GRASS

Descript.] This very small and common herb hath no roots, save only a few strings: neither doth it ever grow to be above a hand's breadth high, the leaves are very small, and something long, not much unlike those of Chickweed, among which rise up divers slender stalks, bearing many white flowers one above another, which are exceeding small; after which come small flat pouches containing the seed, which is very small, but of a sharp taste.

Place.] It grows commonly upon old stone and brick walls, and sometimes in gravelly grounds, especially if there be grass or moss near to shadow it.

Time.] They flower very early in the year, sometimes in January, and in February; for before the end of April they are not to be found.

Government and virtues.] It is held to be exceedingly good for those imposthumes in the joints, and under the nails, which they call Whitlows, Felons, Andicorns and Nail-wheals.

NEP, OR CATMINT

Descript.] Common Garden Nep shoots forth hard four-square stalks, with a hoariness on them, a yard high or more, full of branches, bearing at every joint two broad leaves like balm, but longer pointed, softer, white, and more hoary, nicked about the edges, and of a strong sweet scent. The flowers grow in large tufts at the tops of the branches, and underneath them likewise on the stalks many together, of a whitish purple colour. The roots are composed of many long strings or fibres, fastening themselves stronger in the ground, and abide with green leaves thereon all the winter.

Place.] It is only nursed up in our gardens.

Time.] And it flowers in July, or thereabouts.

Government and virtues.] It is an herb of Venus. Nep is generally used for women to procure their courses, being taken inwardly or outwardly, either alone, or with other convenient herbs in a decoction to bathe them, or sit over the hot fumes thereof; and by the frequent use thereof, it takes away barrenness, and the wind, and pains of the mother. It is also used in pains of the head coming of any cold cause, catarrhs, rheums, and for swimming and giddiness thereof, and is of special use for the windiness of the stomach and belly. It is effectual for any cramp, or cold aches, to dissolve cold and wind that afflict the place, and is used for colds, coughs, and shortness of breath. The juice thereof drank in wine, is profitable for those that are bruised by an accident. The green herb bruised and applied to the fundament and lying there two or three hours, eases the pains of the piles; the juice also being made up into an ointment, is effectual for the same purpose. The head washed with a decoction thereof, it takes away scales, and may be effectual for other parts of the body also.

NETTLES

NETTLES are so well known, that they need no description; they may be found by feeling, in the darkest night.

Government and virtues.] This is also an herb Mars claims dominion over. You know Mars is hot and dry, and you know as well that Winter is cold and moist; then you may know as well the reason why Nettle-tops eaten in the Spring consume the phlegmatic superfluities in the body of man, that the coldness and moistness of Winter hath left behind. The roots or leaves boiled, or the juice of either of them, or both made into an electuary with honey and sugar, is a safe and sure medicine to open the pipes and passages of the lungs, which is the cause of wheezing and shortness of breath, and helps to expectorate tough phlegm, as also to raise the imposthumed pleurisy; and spend it by spitting; the same helps the swelling of the almonds of the throat, the mouth and throat being gargled therewith. The juice is also effectual to settle the palate of the mouth in its place, and to heal and temper the inflammations and soreness of the mouth and throat. The decoction of the leaves in wine, being drank, is singularly good to provoke women's courses, and settle the suffocation, strangling of the mother, and all other diseases thereof; it is also applied outwardly with a little myrrh. The same also, or the seed provokes urine, and expels the gravel and stone in the reins or bladder, often proved to be effectual in many that have taken it. The same kills the worms in children, eases pains in the sides, and dissolves the windiness in the spleen, as also in the body, although others think it only powerful to provoke venery. The juice of the leaves taken two or three days together, stays bleeding at the mouth. The seed being drank, is a remedy against the stinging of venomous creatures, the biting of mad dogs, the poisonous qualities of Hemlock, Henbane, Nightshade, Mandrake, or other such like herbs that stupify or dull the senses; as also the lethargy, especially to use it outwardly, to rub the forehead or temples in the lethargy, and the places stung or bitten with beasts, with a little salt. The distilled water of the herb is also effectual (though not so powerful) for the diseases aforesaid; as for outward wounds and sores to wash them, and to cleanse the skin from morphew, leprosy, and other discolourings thereof. The seed or leaves bruised, and put into the nostrils, stays the bleeding of them, and takes away the flesh growing in them called polypus. The juice of the leaves, or the decoction of them, or of the root, is singularly good to wash either old, rotten, or stinking sores or fistulous, and gangrenes, and such as fretting, eating, or corroding scabs, manginess, and itch, in any part of the body, as also green wounds, by washing them therewith, or applying the green herb bruised thereunto, yea, although the flesh were separated from the bones; the same applied to our wearied members, refresh them, or to place those that have been out of joint, being first set up again, strengthens, dries, and comforts them, as also those places troubled with aches and gouts, and the defluxion of humours upon the joints or sinews; it eases the pains, and dries or dissolves the defluctions. An ointment made of the juice, oil, and a little wax, is singularly good to rub cold and benumbed members. An handful of the leaves of green Nettles, and another of Wallwort, or Deanwort, bruised and applied simply themselves to the gout, sciatica, or joint aches in any part, hath been found to be an admirable help thereunto.

NIGHTSHADE

Descript.] Common Nightshade hath an upright, round green, hollow stalk, about a foot or half a yard high, bushing forth in many branches, whereon grow many green leaves, somewhat broad, and pointed at the ends, soft and full of juice, somewhat like unto Bazil, but longer and a little unevenly dented about the edges. At the tops of the stalks and branches come forth three or four more white flowers made of five small pointed leaves a-piece, standing on a stalk together, one above another, with yellow pointels in the middle, composed of four or five yellow threads set together, which afterwards run into so many pendulous green berries, of the bigness of small pease, full of green juice, and small whitish round flat seed lying within it. The root is white, and a little woody when it hath given flower and fruit, with many small fibres at it. The whole plant is of a waterish insipid taste, but the juice within the berries is somewhat viscous, and of a cooling and binding quality.

Place.] It grows wild with us under our walls, and in rubbish, the common paths, and sides of hedges and fields, as also in our gardens here in England, without any planting.

Time.] It lies down every year, and rises up again of its own sowing, but springs not until the latter end of April at the soonest.

Government and virtues.] It is a cold Saturnine plant. The common Nightshade is wholly used to cool hot inflammations either inwardly or outwardly, being no ways dangerous to any that use it, as most of the rest of the Nightshades are; yet it must be used moderately. The distilled water only of the whole herb is fittest and safest to be taken inwardly. The juice also clarified and taken, being mingled with a little vinegar, is good to wash the mouth and throat that is inflamed. But outwardly the juice of the herb or berries, with oil of roses and a little vinegar and ceruse laboured together in a leaden mortar, is very good to anoint all hot inflammations in the eyes. It also doth much good for the shingles, ringworms, and in all running, fretting and corroding ulcers, applied thereunto. The juice dropped into the ears, eases pains thereof that arise of heat of inflammations. And Pliny saith, it is good for hot swellings under the throat. Have a care you mistake not the deadly Nightshade for this; if you know it not, you may let them both alone, and take no harm, having other medicines sufficient in the book.

THE OAK

IT is so well known (the timber thereof being the glory and safety of this nation by sea) that it needs no description.

Government and virtues.] Jupiter owns the tree. The leaves and bark of the Oak, and the acorn cups, do bind and dry very much. The inner bark of the tree, and the thin skin that covers the acorn, are most used to stay the spitting of blood, and the bloody-flux. The decoction of that bark, and the powder of the cups, do stay vomitings, spitting of blood, bleeding at the mouth, or other fluxes of blood, in men or women; lasks also, and the nocturnal involuntary flux of men. The acorn in powder taken in wine, provokes urine, and resists the poison of venomous creatures. The decoction of acorns and the bark made in milk and taken, resists the force of poisonous herbs and medicines, as also the virulency of cantharides, when one by eating them hath his bladder exulcerated, and voids bloody urine. Hippocrates saith, he used the fumes of Oak leaves to women that were troubled with the strangling of the mother; and Galen applied them, being bruised, to cure green wounds. The distilled water of the Oaken bud, before they break out into leaves is good to be used either inwardly or outwardly, to assuage inflammations, and to stop all manner of fluxes in man or woman. The same is singularly good in pestilential and hot burning fevers; for it resists the force of the infection, and allays the heat. It cools the heat of the liver, breaking the stone in the kidneys, and stays women's courses. The decoction of the leaves works the same effects. The water that is found in the hollow places of old Oaks, is very effectual against any foul or spreading scabs. The distilled water (or concoction, which is better) of the leaves, is one of the best remedies that I know of for the whites in women.

OATS

ARE so well known that they need no description.

Government and virtues.] Oats fried with bay salt, and applied to the sides, take away the pains of stitches and wind in the sides or the belly. A poultice made of meal of Oats, and some oil of Bays put thereunto, helps the itch and the leprosy, as also the fistulas of the fundament, and dissolves hard imposthumes. The meal of Oats boiled with vinegar, and applied, takes away freckles and spots in the face, and other parts of the body.

ONE BLADE

Descript.] This small plant never bears more than one leaf, but only when it rises up with his stalk, which thereon bears another, and seldom more, which are of a blueish green colour, pointed, with many ribs or veins therein, like Plantain. At the top of the stalk grow many small white flowers, star fashion, smelling somewhat sweet; after which come small red berries, when they are ripe. The root is small, of the bigness of a rush, lying and creeping under the upper crust of the earth, shooting forth in divers places.

Place.] It grows in moist, shadowy and grassy places of woods, in many parts of this land.

Time.] It flowers about May, and the berries are ripe in June, and then quickly perishes, until the next year it springs from the same root again.

Government and virtues.] It is a precious herb of the Sun. Half a dram, or a dram at most, in powder of the roots hereof taken in wine and vinegar, of each equal parts, and the party laid presently to sweat thereupon, is held to be a sovereign remedy for those that are infected with the plague, and have a sore upon them, by expelling the poison and infection, and defending the heart and spirits from danger. It is a singularly good wound herb, and is thereupon used with other the like effects in many compound balms for curing of wounds, be they fresh and green, or old and malignant, and especially if the sinews be burnt.

ORCHIS

IT has almost as many several names attributed to the several sorts of it, as would almost fill a sheet of paper; as dog-stones, goat-stones, fool-stones, fox-stones, satiricon, cullians, together with many others too tedious to rehearse.

Descript.] To describe all the several sorts of it were an endless piece of work: therefore I shall only describe the roots because they are to be used with some discretion. They have each of them a double root within, some of them are round, in others like a hand; these roots alter every year by course, when the one rises and waxes full, the other waxes lank, and perishes. Now, it is that which is full which is to be used in medicines, the other being either of no use at all, or else, according to the humour of some, it destroys and disannuls the virtues of the other, quite undoing what that doth.

Time.] One or other of them may be found in flower from the beginning of April to the latter end of August.

Government and virtues.] They are hot and moist in operation, under the dominion of Dame Venus, and provoke lust exceedingly, which, they say, the dried and withered roots do restrain. They are held to kill worms in children; as also, being bruised and applied to the place, to heal the king's evil.

ONIONS

THEY are so well known, that I need not spend time about writing a description of them.

Government and virtues.] Mars owns them, and they have gotten this quality, to draw any corruption to them, for if you peel one, and lay it upon a dunghill, you shall find it rotten in half a day, by drawing putrefaction to it; then, being bruised and applied to a plague sore, it is very probable it will do the like. Onions are flatulent, or windy; yet they do somewhat provoke appetite, increase thirst, ease the belly and bowels, provoke women's courses, help the biting of a mad dog, and of other venomous creatures, to be used with honey and rue, increase sperm, especially the seed of them. They also kill worms in children if they drink the water fasting wherein they have been steeped all night. Being roasted under the embers, and eaten with honey or sugar and oil, they much conduce to help an inveterate cough, and expectorate the tough phlegm. The juice being snuffed up into the nostrils, purges the head, and helps the lethargy, (yet the often eating them is said to procure pains in the head). It hath been held by divers country people a great preservative against infection to eat Onions fasting with bread and salt. As also to make a great Onion hollow, filling the place with good treacle, and after to roast it well under the embers, which, after taking away the outermost skin thereof, being beaten together, is a sovereign salve for either plague or sore, or any other putrefied ulcer. The juice of Onions is good for either scalding or burning by fire, water, or gunpowder, and used with vinegar, takes away all blemishes, spots and marks in the skin: and dropped in the ears, eases the pains and noise of them. Applied also with figs beaten together, helps to ripen and break imposthumes, and other sores.

Leeks are as like them in quality, as the pome-water is like an apple. They are a remedy against a surfeit of mushrooms, being baked under the embers and taken, and being boiled and applied very warm, help the piles. In other things they have the same property as the Onions, although not so effectual.

ORPINE

Descript.] Common Orpine rises up with divers rough brittle stalks, thick set with fat and fleshy leaves, without any order, and little or nothing dented about the edges, of a green colour. The flowers are white, or whitish, growing in tufts, after which come small chaffy husks, with seeds like dust in them. The roots are divers thick, round, white tuberous clogs; and the plant grows not so big in some places as in others where it is found.

Place.] It is frequent in almost every county of this land, and is cherished in gardens with us, where it grows greater than that which is wild, and grows in shadowy sides of fields and woods.

Time.] It flowers about July, and the seed is ripe in August.

Government and virtues.] The Moon owns the herb, and he that knows but her exaltatation, knows what I say is true. Orpine is seldom used in inward medicines with us, although Tragus saith from experience in Germany, that the distilled water thereof is profitable for gnawings or excoriations in the stomach or bowels, or for ulcers in the lungs, liver, or other inward parts, as also in the matrix, and helps all those diseases, being drank for certain days together. It stays the sharpness of humours in the bloody-flux, and other fluxes in the body, or in wounds. The root thereof also performs the like effect. It is used outwardly to cool any heat or inflammation upon any hurt or wound, and eases the pains of them; as, also, to heal scaldings or burnings, the juice thereof being beaten with some green sallad oil, and anointed. The leaf bruised, and laid to any green wound in the hand or legs, doth heal them quickly; and being bound to the throat much helps the quinsy; it helps also ruptures and burstenness. If you please to make the juice thereof into a syrup with honey or sugar, you may safely take a spoonful or two at a time, (let my author say what he will) for a quinsy, and you shall find the medicine pleasant, and the cure speedy.

PARSLEY

THIS is so well known, that it needs no description.

Government and virtues.] It is under the dominion of Mercury; is very comfortable to the stomach; helps to provoke urine and women's courses, to break wind both in the stomach and bowels, and doth a little open the body, but the root much more. It opens obstructions both of liver and spleen, and is therefore accounted one of the five opening roots. Galen commended it against the falling sickness, and to provoke urine mightily; especially if the roots be boiled, and eaten like Parsnips. The seed is effectual to provoke urine and women's courses, to break wind, to break the stone, and ease the pains and torments thereof; it is also effectual against the venom of any poisonous creature, and the danger that comes to them that have the lethargy, and is as good against the cough. The distilled water of Parsley is a familiar medicine with nurses to give their children when they are troubled with wind in the stomach or belly which they call the frets; and is also much available to them that are of great years. The leaves of Parsley laid to the eyes that are inflamed with heat, or swollen, doth much help them, if it be used with bread or meal; and being fried with butter, and applied to women's breasts that are hard through the curdling of their milk, it abates the hardness quickly; and also takes away black and blue marks coming of bruises or falls. The juice thereof dropped into the ears with a little wine, eases the pains. Tragus sets down an excellent medicine to help the jaundice and falling sickness, the dropsy, and stone in the kidneys, in this manner: Take of the seed of Parsley, Fennel, Annise and Carraways, of each an ounce; of the roots of Parsley, Burnet, Saxifrage, and Carraways, of each an ounce and an half; let the seeds be bruised, and the roots washed and cut small; let them lie all night to steep in a bottle of white wine, and in the morning be boiled in a close earthen vessel until a third part or more be wasted; which being strained and cleared, take four ounces thereof morning and evening first and last, abstaining from drink after it for three hours. This opens obstructions of the liver and spleen, and expels the dropsy and jaundice by urine.

PARSLEY PIERT, OR PARSLEY BREAKSTONE

Descript.] The root, although it be very small and thready, yet it continues many years, from which arise many leaves lying along on the ground, each standing upon a long small foot-stalk, the leaves as broad as a man's nail, very deeply dented on the edges, somewhat like a parsley-leaf, but of a very dusky green colour. The stalks are very weak and slender, about three or four fingers in length, set so full of leaves that they can hardly be seen, either having no foot-stalk at all, or but very short; the flowers are so small they can hardly be seen, and the seed as small as may be.

Place.] It is a common herb throughout the nation, and rejoices in barren, sandy, moist places. It may be found plentifully about Hampstead Heath, Hyde Park, and in Tothill-fields.

Time.] It may be found all the Summer-time, even from the beginning of April to the end of October.

Government and virtues.] Its operation is very prevalent to provoke urine, and to break the stone. It is a very good sallad herb. It were good the gentry would pickle it up as they pickle up Samphire for their use all the Winter. I cannot teach them how to do it; yet this I can tell them, it is a very wholesome herb. They may also keep the herb dry, or in a syrup, if they please. You may take a dram of the powder of it in white wine; it would bring away gravel from the kidneys insensibly, and without pain. It also helps the stranguary.

PARSNIPS

THE garden kind thereof is so well known (the root being commonly eaten) that I shall not trouble you with any description of it. But the wild kind being of more physical use, I shall in this place describe it unto you.

Descript.] The wild Parsnip differs little from the garden, but grows not so fair and large, nor hath so many leaves, and the root is shorter, more woody, and not so fit to be eaten, and therefore more medicinal.

Place.] The name of the first shews the place of its growth. The other grows wild in divers places, as in the marshes in Rochester, and elsewhere, and flowers in July; the seed being ripe about the beginning of August, the second year after its sowing; for if they do flower the first year, the country people call them Madneps.

Government and virtues.] The garden Parsnips are under Venus. The garden Parsnip nourishes much, and is good and wholesome nourishment, but a little windy, whereby it is thought to procure bodily lust; but it fastens the body much, if much need. It is conducible to the stomach and reins, and provokes urine. But the wild Parsnips hath a cutting, attenuating, cleansing, and opening quality therein. It resists and helps the bitings of serpents, eases the pains and stitches in the sides, and dissolves wind both in the stomach and bowels, which is the cholic, and provokes urine. The root is often used, but the seed much more. The wild being better than the tame, shews Dame Nature to be the best physician.

COW PARSNIPS

Descript.] This grows with three or four large, spread winged, rough leaves, lying often on the ground, or else raised a little from it, with long, round, hairy foot-stalks under them, parted usually into five divisions, the two couples standing each against the other; and one at the end, and each leaf, being almost round, yet somewhat deeply cut in on the edges in some leaves, and not so deep in others, of a whitish green colour, smelling somewhat strongly; among which rises up a round, crusted, hairy stalk, two or three feet high, with a few joints and leaves thereon, and branched at the top, where stand large umbels of white, and sometimes reddish flowers, and after them flat, whitish, thin, winged seed, two always joined together. The root is long and white, with two or three long strings growing down into the ground, smelling likewise strongly and unpleasant.

Place.] It grows in moist meadows, and the borders and corners of fields, and near ditches, through this land.

Time.] It flowers in July, and seeds in August.

Government and virtues.] Mercury hath the dominion over them. The seed thereof, as Galen saith, is of a sharp and cutting quality, and therefore is a fit medicine for a cough and shortness of breath, the falling sickness and jaundice. The root is available to all the purposes aforesaid, and is also of great use to take away the hard skin that grows on a fistula, if it be but scraped upon it. The seed hereof being drank, cleanses the belly from tough phlegmatic matter therein, eases them that are liver-grown, women's passions of the mother, as well being drank as the smoke thereof received, and likewise raises such as are fallen into a deep sleep, or have the lethargy, by burning it under their nose. The seed and root boiled in oil, and the head rubbed therewith, helps not only those that are fallen into a frenzy, but also the lethargy or drowsy evil, and those that have been long troubled with the head-ache, if it be likewise used with Rue. It helps also the running scab and shingles. The juice of the flowers dropped into the ears that run and are full of matter, cleanses and heals them.

THE PEACH TREE

Descript.] A Peach tree grows not so great as the Apricot tree, yet spreads branches reasonable well, from whence spring smaller reddish twigs, whereon are set long and narrow green leaves dented about the edges. The blossoms are greater than the plumb, and of a light purple colour; the fruit round, and sometimes as big as a reasonable Pippin, others smaller, as also differing in colour and taste, as russet, red, or yellow, waterish or firm, with a frize or cotton all over, with a cleft therein like an Apricot, and a rugged, furrowed, great stone within it, and a bitter kernel within the stone. It sooner waxes old, and decays, than the Apricot, by much.

Place.] They are nursed in gardens and orchards through this land.

Time.] They flower in the Spring, and fructify in Autumn.

Government and virtues.] Lady Venus owns this tree, and by it opposes the ill effects of Mars, and indeed for children and young people, nothing is better to purge choler and the jaundice, than the leaves or flowers of this tree being made into a syrup or conserve. Let such as delight to please their lust regard the fruit; but such as have lost their health, and their children's, let them regard what I say, they may safely give two spoonfuls of the syrup at a time; it is as gentle as Venus herself. The leaves of peaches bruised and laid on the belly, kill worms, and so they do also being boiled in ale and drank, and open the belly likewise; and, being dried, is a far safer medicine to discuss humours. The powder of them strewed upon fresh bleeding wounds stays their bleeding, and closes them up. The flowers steeped all night in a little wine standing warm, strained forth in the morning, and drank fasting, doth gently open the belly, and move it downward. A syrup made of them, as the syrup of roses is made, works more forcibly than that of roses, for it provokes vomiting, and spends waterish and hydropic humours by the continuance thereof. The flowers made into a conserve, work the same effect. The liquor that dropped from the tree, being wounded, is given in the decoction of Coltsfoot, to those that are troubled with a cough or shortness of breath, by adding thereunto some sweet wine, and putting some saffron also therein. It is good for those that are hoarse, or have lost their voice; helps all defects of the lungs, and those that vomit and spit blood. Two drams hereof given in the juice of lemons, or of radish, is good for them that are troubled with the stone, the kernels of the stones do wonderfully ease the pains and wringings of the belly through wind or sharp humours, and help to make an excellent medicine for the stone upon all occasions, in this manner: *I take fifty kernels of peach-stones, and one hundred of the kernels of cherry-stones, a handful of elder flowers fresh or dried, and three pints of Muscadel; set them in a close pot into a bed of horse-dung for ten days, after which distil in a glass with a gentle fire,* and keep it for your use. You may drink upon occasion three or four ounces at a time. The milk or cream of these kernels being drawn forth with some Vervain water and applied to the forehead and temples, doth much help to procure rest and sleep to sick persons wanting it. The oil drawn from the kernels, the temples being therewith anointed, doth the like. The said oil put into clysters, eases the pains of the wind cholic: and anointed on the lower part of the belly, doth the like, and dropped into the ears, eases pains in them; the juice of the leaves doth the like. Being also anointed on the forehead and temples, it helps the megrim, and all other pains in the head. If the kernels be bruised and boiled in vinegar, until they become thick, and applied to the head, it marvellously procures the hair to grow again upon bald places, or where it is too thin.

THE PEAR TREE

PEAR Trees are so well known, that they need no description.

Government and virtues.] The Tree belongs to Venus, and so doth the Apple tree. For their physical use they are best discerned by their taste. All the sweet and luscious sorts, whether manured or wild, do help to move the belly downwards, more or less. Those that are hard and sour, do, on the contrary, bind the belly as much, and the leaves do so also. Those that are moist do in some sort cool, but harsh or wild sorts much more, and are very good in repelling medicines; and if the wild sort be boiled with mushrooms, it makes them less dangerous. The said Pears boiled with a little honey, help much the oppressed stomach, as all sorts of them do, some more, some less: but the harsher sorts do more cool and bind, serving well to be bound to green wounds, to cool and stay the blood, and heal up the green wound without farther trouble, or inflammation, as Galen saith he hath found by experience. The wild Pears do sooner close up the lips of green wounds than others.

Schola Selerni advises to drink much wine after Pears, or else (say they) they are as bad as poison; nay, and they curse the tree for it too; but if a poor man find his stomach oppressed by eating Pears, it is but working hard, and it will do as well as drinking wine.

PELLITORY OF SPAIN

COMMON Pellitory of Spain, if it be planted in our gardens, will prosper very well; yet there is one sort growing ordinarily here wild, which I esteem to be little inferior to the other, if at all. I shall not deny you the description of them both.

Descript.] Common Pellitory is a very common plant, and will not be kept in our gardens without diligent looking to. The root goes down right into the ground bearing leaves, being long and finely cut upon the stalk, lying on the ground, much larger than the leaves of the Camomile are. At the top it bears one single large flower at a place, having a border of many leaves, white on the upper side, and reddish underneath, with a yellow thrum in the middle, not standing so close as that of Camomile.

The other common Pellitory which grows here, hath a root of a sharp biting taste, scarcely discernible by the taste from that before described, from whence arise divers brittle stalks, a yard high and more, with narrow leaves finely dented about the edges, standing one above another up to the tops. The flowers are many and white, standing in tufts like those of Yarrow, with a small yellowish thrum in the middle. The seed is very small.

Place.] The last grows in fields by the hedge sides and paths, almost everywhere.

Time.] It flowers at the latter end of June and July.

Government and virtues.] It is under the government of Mercury, and I am persuaded it is one of the best purgers of the brain that grows. An ounce of the juice taken in a draught of Muskadel an hour before the fit of the ague comes, it will assuredly drive away the ague at the second or third time taken at the farthest. Either the herb or root dried and chewed in the mouth, purges the brain of phlegmatic humours; thereby not only easing pains in the head and teeth, but also hinders the distilling of the brain upon the lungs and eyes, thereby preventing coughs, phthisicks and consumption, the apoplexy and falling sickness. It is an excellently approved remedy in the lethargy. The powder of the herb or root being snuffed up the nostrils, procures sneezing, and eases the head-ache; being made into an ointment with hog's grease, it takes away black and blue spots occasioned by blows or falls, and helps both the gout and sciatica.

PELLITORY OF THE WALL

Descript.] It rises with brownish, red, tender, weak, clear, and almost transparent stalks, about two feet high, upon which grow at the joints two leaves somewhat broad and long, of a dark green colour, which afterwards turn brownish, smooth on the edges, but rough and hairy, as the stalks are also. At the joints with the leaves from the middle of the stalk upwards, where it spreads into branches, stand many small, pale, purplish flowers in hairy, rough heads, or husks, after which come small, black, rough seed, which will stick to any cloth or garment that shall touch it. The root is somewhat long, with small fibres thereat, of a dark reddish colour, which abides the Winter, although the stalks and leaves perish and spring every year.

Place.] It grows wild generally through the land, about the borders of fields, and by the sides of walls, and among rubbish. It will endure well being brought up in gardens, and planted on the shady side, where it will spring of its own sowing.

Time.] It flowers in June and July, and the seed is ripe soon after.

Government and virtues.] It is under the dominion of Mercury. The dried herb Pellitory made up into an electuary with honey, or the juices of the herb, or the decoction thereof made up with sugar or honey, is a singular remedy for an old or dry cough, the shortness of breath, and wheezing in the throat. Three ounces of the juice thereof taken at a time, doth wonderfully help stopping of the urine, and to expel the stone or gravel in the kidneys or bladder, and is therefore usually put among other herbs used in clysters to mitigate pains in the back, sides, or bowels, proceeding of wind, stopping of urine, the gravel or stone, as aforesaid. If the bruised herb, sprinkled with some Muskadel, be warmed upon a tile, or in a dish upon a few quick coals in a chafing-dish, and applied to the belly, it works the same effect. The decoction of the herb being drank, eases pains of the mother, and brings down women's courses. It also eases those griefs that arise from obstructions of the liver, spleen, and reins. The same decoction, with a little honey added thereto, is good to gargle a sore throat. The juice held a while in the mouth, eases pains in the teeth. The distilled water of the herb drank with some sugar, works the same effects, and cleanses the skin from spots, freckles, purples, wheals, sun-burn, morphew, &c. The juice dropped into the ears, eases the noise in them, and takes away the pricking and shooting pains therein. The same, or the distilled water, assuages hot and swelling imposthumes, burnings and scaldings by fire or water; as also all other hot tumours and inflammations, or breakings-out, of heat, being bathed often with wet cloths dipped therein. The said juice made into a liniment with ceruss, and oil of roses, and anointed therewith, cleanses foul rotten ulcers, and stays spreading or creeping ulcers, and running scabs or sores in children's heads; and helps to stay the hair from falling off the head. The said ointment, or the herb applied to the fundament, opens the piles, and eases their pains; and being mixed with goats' tallow, helps the gout. The juice is very effectual to cleanse fistulas, and to heal them up safely; or the herb itself bruised and applied with a little salt. It is likewise also effectual to heal any green wound; if it be bruised and bound thereto for three days, you shall need no other medicine to heal it further. A poultice made hereof with Mallows, and boiled in wine and wheat bran and bean flour, and some oil put thereto, and applied warm to any bruised sinews, tendon, or muscle, doth in a very short time restore them to their strength, taking away the pains of the bruises, and dissolves the congealed blood coming of blows, or falls from high places.

The juice of Pellitory of the Wall clarified and boiled in a syrup with honey, and a spoonful of it drank every morning by such as are subject to the dropsy; if continuing that course, though but once a week, they ever have the dropsy, let them but come to me, and I will cure them *gratis*.

PENNYROYAL

PENNYROYAL is so well known unto all, I mean the common kind, that it needs no description.

There is a greater kind than the ordinary sort found wild with us, which so abides, being brought into gardens, and differs not from it, but only in the largeness of the leaves and stalks, in rising higher, and not creeping upon the ground so much. The flowers whereof are purple, growing in rundles about the stalks like the other.

Place.] The first, which is common in gardens, grows also in many moist and watery places of this land.

The second is found wild in effect in divers places by the highways from London to Colchester, and thereabouts, more abundantly than in any other counties, and is also planted in their gardens in Essex.

Time.] They flower in the latter end of Summer, about August.

Government and virtues.] The herb is under Venus. Dioscorides saith, that Pennyroyal makes thin tough phlegm, warms the coldness of any part whereto it is applied, and digests raw or corrupt matter. Being boiled and drank, it provokes women's courses, and expels the dead child and after-birth, and stays the disposition to vomit, being taken in water and vinegar mingled together. And being mingled with honey and salt, it voids phlegm out of the lungs, and purges melancholy by the stool. Drank with wine, it helps such as are bitten and stung with venomous beasts, and applied to the nostrils with vinegar, revives those that are fainting and swooning. Being dried and burnt, it strengthens the gums. It is helpful to those that are troubled with the gout, being applied of itself to the place until it was red; and applied in a plaister, it takes away spots or marks in the face; applied with salt, it profits those that are splenetic, or livergrown. The decoction doth help the itch, if washed therewith. The green herb bruised and put into vinegar, cleanses foul ulcers, and takes away the marks of bruises and blows about the eyes, and all discolourings of the face by fire, yea, and the leprosy, being drank and outwardly applied. Boiled in wine with honey and salt, it helps the tooth-ache. It helps the cold griefs by the joints, taking away the pains, and warms the cold part, being fast bound to the place, after a bathing or sweating in a hot house. Pliny adds, that Pennyroyal and Mints together, help faintings, being put into vinegar, and smelled unto, or put into the nostrils or mouth. It eases head-aches, pains of the breast and belly, and gnawings of the stomach; applied with honey, salt, and vinegar, it helps cramps or convulsions of the sinews. Boiled in milk, and drank, it is effectual for the cough, and for ulcers and sores in the mouth; drank in wine it provokes women's courses, and expels the dead child, and after-birth. Matthiolus saith, The decoction thereof being drank, helps the jaundice and dropsy, all pains of the head and sinews that come of a cold cause, and clears the eye-sight. It helps the lethargy, and applied with barley-meal, helps burnings; and put into the ears, eases the pains of them.

MALE AND FEMALE PEONY

Descript.] Male Peony rises up with brownish stalks, whereon grow green and reddish leaves, upon a stalk without any particular division in the leaf at all. The flowers stand at the top of the stalks, consisting of five or six broad leaves, of a fair purplish red colour, with many yellow threads in the middle standing about the head, which after rises up to be the seed vessels, divided into two, three, or four crooked pods like horns, which being full ripe, open and turn themselves down backwards, shewing with them divers round, black, shining seeds, having also many crimson grains, intermixed with black, whereby it makes a very pretty shew. The roots are great, thick and long, spreading and running down deep in the ground.

The ordinary Female Peony hath as many stalks, and more leaves on them than the Male; the leaves not so large, but nicked on the edges, some with great and deep, others with small cuts and divisions, of a dead green colour. The flowers are of a strong heady scent, usually smaller, and of a more purple colour than the Male, with yellow thrums about the head, as the Male hath. The seed vessels are like horns, as in the Male, but smaller, the seed is black, but less shining. The root consists of many short tuberous clogs, fastened at the end of long strings, and all from the heads of the roots, which is thick and short, and of the like scent with the Male.

Place and Time.] They grow in gardens, and flower usually about May.

Government and virtues.] It is an herb of the Sun, and under the Lion. Physicians say, Male Peony roots are best; but Dr. Reason told me Male Peony was best for men, and Female Peony for women, and he desires to be judged by his brother Dr. Experience. The roots are held to be of more virtue than the seed; next the flowers; and, last of all, the leaves. The roots of the Male Peony, fresh gathered, having been found by experience to cure the falling sickness; but the surest way is, besides hanging it about the neck, by which children have been cured, to take the root of the Male Peony washed clean, and stamped somewhat small, and laid to infuse in sack for 24 hours at the least, afterwards strain it, and take it first and last, morning and evening, a good draught for sundry days together, before and after a full moon: and this will also cure old persons, if the disease be not grown too old, and past cure, especially if there be a due and orderly preparation of the body with posset-drink made of Betony, &c. The root is also effectual for women that are not sufficiently cleansed after child-birth, and such as are troubled with the mother; for which likewise the black seed beaten to powder, and given in wine, is also available. The black seed also taken before bed-time, and in the morning, is very effectual for such as in their sleep are troubled with the disease called Ephialtes, or Incubus, but we do commonly call it the Night-mare: a disease which melancholy persons are subject unto. It is also good against melancholy dreams. The distilled water or syrup made of the flowers, works the same effects that the root and seed do, although more weakly. The Female is often used for the purpose aforesaid, by reason the Male is so scarce a plant, that it is possessed by few, and those great lovers of rarities in this kind.

PEPPERWORT, OR DITTANDER

Descript.] Our common Pepperwort sends forth somewhat long and broad leaves, of a light bluish green colour, finely dented about the edges, and pointed at the ends, standing upon round hard stalks, three or four feet high, spreading many branches on all sides, and having many small white flowers at the tops of them, after which follow small seeds in small heads. The root is slender, running much under ground, and shooting up again in many places, and both leaves and roots are very hot and sharp of taste, like pepper, for which cause it took the name.

Place.] It grows naturally in many places of this land, as at Clare in Essex; also near unto Exeter in Devonshire; upon Rochester common in Kent; in Lancashire, and divers other places; but usually kept in gardens.

Time.] It flowers in the end of June, and in July.

Government and virtues.] Here is another martial herb for you, make much of it. Pliny and Paulus Ægineta say, that Pepperwort is very successful for the sciatica, or any other gout or pain in the joints, or any other inveterate grief. The leaves hereof to be bruised, and mixed with old hog's grease, and applied to the place, and to continue thereon four hours in men, and two hours in women, the place being afterwards bathed with wine and oil mixed together, and then wrapped up with wool or skins, after they have sweat a little. It also amends the deformities or discolourings of the skin, and helps to take away marks, scars, and scabs, or the foul marks of burning with fire or iron. The juice hereof is by some used to be given in ale to drink, to women with child, to procure them a speedy delivery in travail.

PERIWINKLE

Descript.] The common sort hereof hath many branches trailing or running upon the ground, shooting out small fibres at the joints as it runs, taking thereby hold in the ground, and rooteth in divers places. At the joints of these branches stand two small, dark-green, shining leaves, somewhat like bay leaves, but smaller, and with them come forth also the flowers (one at a joint) standing upon a tender foot-stalk, being somewhat long and hollow, parted at the brims, sometimes into four, sometimes into five leaves. The most ordinary sorts are of a pale blue colour; some are pure white, some of a dark reddish purple colour. The root is little bigger than rush, bushing in the ground, and creeping with his branches far about, whereby it quickly possesses a great compass, and is therefore most usually planted under hedges where it may have room to run.

Place.] Those with the pale blue, and those with the white flowers, grow in woods and orchards, by the hedge-sides, in divers places of this land; but those with the purple flowers, in gardens only.

Time.] They flower in March and April.

Government and virtues.] Venus owns this herb, and saith, That the leaves eaten by man and wife together, cause love between them. The Periwinkle is a great binder, stays bleeding both at mouth and nose, if some of the leaves be chewed. The French used it to stay women's courses. Dioscorides, Galen, and Ægineta, commend it against the lasks and fluxes of the belly to be drank in wine.

ST. PETER'S WORT

IF Superstition had not been the father of Tradition, as well as Ignorance the Mother of Devotion, this herb, (as well as St. John's Wort) hath found some other name to be known by; but we may say of our forefathers, as St. Paul of the Athenians, *I perceive in many things you are too superstitious*. Yet seeing it is come to pass, that custom having got in possession, pleads prescription for the name, I shall let it pass, and come to the description of the herb, which take as follows.

Descript.] It rises up with square upright stalks for the most part, some greater and higher than St. John's Wort (and good reason too, St. Peter being the greater apostle, (ask the Pope else;) for though God would have the saints equal, the Pope is of another opinion,) but brown in the same manner, having two leaves at every joint, somewhat like, but larger, than St. John's Wort, and a little rounder pointed, with few or no holes to be seen thereon, and having sometimes some smaller leaves rising from the bosom of the greater, and sometimes a little hairy also. At the tops of two stalks stand many star-like flowers, with yellow threads in the middle, very like those of St. John's Wort, insomuch that this is hardly discerned from it, but only by the largeness and height, the seed being alike also in both. The root abides long, sending forth new shoots every year.

Place.] It grows in many groves, and small low woods, in divers places of this land, as in Kent, Huntingdon, Cambridge, and Northamptonshire; as also near watercourses in other places.

Time.] It flowers in June and July, and the seed is ripe in August.

Government and virtues.] There is not a straw to choose between this and St. John's Wort, only St. Peter must have it lest he should want pot herbs. It is of the same property as St. John's Wort, but somewhat weaker, and therefore more seldom used. Two drams of the seed taken at a time in honied water, purges choleric humours, (as saith Dioscorides, Pliny, and Galen,) and thereby helps those that are troubled with the sciatica. The leaves are used as St. John's Wort, to help those places of the body that have been burnt with fire.

PIMPERNEL

Descript.] Common Pimpernel hath divers weak square stalks lying on the ground, beset all with two small and almost round leaves at every joint, one against another, very like Chickweed, but hath no foot-stalks; for the leaves, as it were, compass the stalk. The flowers stand singly each by themselves at them and the stalk, consisting of five small round-pointed leaves, of a pale red colour, tending to an orange, with so many threads in the middle, in whose places succeed smooth round heads, wherein is contained small seed. The root is small and fibrous, perishing every year.

Place.] It grows almost every where, as well in the meadows and corn-fields, as by the way-sides, and in gardens, arising of itself.

Time.] It flowers from May until April, and the seed ripens in the mean time, and falls.

Government and virtues.] It is a gallant solar herb, of a cleansing attractive quality, whereby it draws forth thorns or splinters, or other such like things gotten into the flesh; and put up into the nostrils, purges the head; and Galen saith also, they have a drying faculty, whereby they are good to solder the lips of wounds, and to cleanse foul ulcers. The distilled water or juice is much esteemed by French dames to cleanse the skin from any roughness and deformity, or discolouring thereof; being boiled in wine and given to drink, it is a good remedy against the plague, and other pestilential fevers, if the party after taking it be warm in his bed, and sweat for two hours after, and use the same for twice at least. It helps also all stingings and bitings of venomous beasts, or mad dogs, being used inwardly, and applied outwardly. The same also opens obstructions of the liver, and is very available against the infirmities of the reins. It provokes urine, and helps to expel the stone and gravel out of the kidneys and bladder, and helps much in all inward pains and ulcers. The decoction, or distilled water, is no less effectual to be applied to all wounds that are fresh and green, or old, filthy, fretting, and running ulcers, which it very effectually cures in a short space. A little mixed with the juice, and dropped into the eyes, cleanses them from cloudy mists, or thick films which grow over them, and hinder the sight. It helps the tooth-ache, being dropped into the ear on a contrary side of the pain. It is also effectual to ease the pains of the hæmorrhoids or piles.

GROUND PINE, OR CHAMEPITYS

Descript.] Our common Ground Pine grows low, seldom rising above a hand's breadth high, shooting forth divers small branches, set with slender, small, long, narrow, greyish, or whitish leaves, somewhat hairy, and divided into three parts, many bushing together at a joint, some growing scatteringly upon the stalks, smelling somewhat strong, like unto rozin. The flowers are small, and of a pale yellow colour, growing from the joint of the stalk all along among the leaves; after which come small and round husks. The root is small and woody, perishing every year.

Place.] It grows more plentifully in Kent than any other county of this land, as namely, in many places on this side Dartford, along to Southfleet, Chatham, and Rochester, and upon Chatham down, hard by the Beacon, and half a mile from Rochester, in a field near a house called Selesys.

Time.] It flowers and gives seed in the Summer months.

Government and virtues.] Mars owns the herb. The decoction of Ground Pine drank, doth wonderfully prevail against the stranguary, or any inward pains arising from the diseases of the reins and urine, and is specially good for all obstructions of the liver and spleen, and gently opens the body; for which purpose they were wont in former times to make pills with the powder thereof, and the pulp of figs. It marvellously helps all the diseases of the mother, inwardly or outwardly applied, procuring women's courses, and expelling the dead child and after-birth; yea, it is so powerful upon those feminine parts, that it is utterly forbidden for women with child, for it will cause abortion or delivery before the time. The decoction of the herb in wine taken inwardly, or applied outwardly, or both, for some time together, is also effectual in all pains and diseases of the joints, as gouts, cramps, palsies, sciatica, and aches; for which purpose the pills made with powder of Ground Pine, and of Hermodactyls with Venice Turpentine are very effectual. The pills also, continued for some time, are special good for those that have the dropsy, jaundice, and for griping pains of the joints, belly, or inward parts. It helps also all diseases of the brain, proceeding of cold and phlegmatic humours and distillations, as also for the falling sickness. It is a special remedy for the poison of the aconites, and other poisonous herbs, as also against the stinging of any venomous creature. It is a good remedy for a cold cough, especially in the beginning. For all the purposes aforesaid, the herb being tunned up in new drink and drank, is almost as effectual, but far more acceptable to weak and dainty stomachs. The distilled water of the herb hath the same effects, but more weakly. The conserve of the flowers doth the like, which Matthiolus much commends against the palsy. The green herb, or the decoction thereof, being applied, dissolves the hardness of women's breasts, and all other hard swellings in any other part of the body. The green herb also applied, or the juice thereof with some honey, not only cleanses putrid, stinking, foul, and malignant ulcers and sores of all sorts, but heals and solders up the lips of green wounds in any part also. Let pregnant women forbear, for it works violently upon the feminine part.

PLANTAIN

THIS grows usually in meadows and fields, and by path sides, and is so well known, that it needs no description.

Time.] It is in its beauty about June, and the seed ripens shortly after.

Government and virtues.] It is true, Misaldus and others, yea, almost all astrology-physicians, hold this to be an herb of Mars, because it cures the diseases of the head and privities, which are under the houses of Mars, Aries, and Scorpio. The truth is, it is under the command of Venus, and cures the head by antipathy to Mars, and the privities by sympathy to Venus; neither is there hardly a martial disease but it cures.

The juice of Plantain clarified and drank for divers days together, either of itself, or in other drink, prevails wonderfully against all torments or excoriations in the intestines or bowels, helps the distillations of rheum from the head, and stays all manner of fluxes, even women's courses, when they flow too abundantly. It is good to stay spitting of blood and other bleedings at the mouth, or the making of foul and bloody water, by reason of any ulcers in the reins or bladder, and also stays the too free bleeding of wounds. It is held an especial remedy for those that are troubled with the phthisic, or consumption of the lungs, or ulcers of the lungs, or coughs that come of heat. The decoction or powder of the roots or seeds, is much more binding for all the purposes aforesaid than the leaves. Dioscorides saith, that three roots boiled in wine and taken, helps the tertian agues, and for the quartan agues, (but letting the number pass as fabulous) I conceive the decoction of divers roots may be effectual. The herb (but especially the seed) is held to be profitable against the dropsy, the falling-sickness, the yellow jaundice, and stoppings of the liver and reins. The roots of Plantain, and Pellitory of Spain, beaten into powder, and put into the hollow teeth, takes away the pains of them. The clarified juice, or distilled water, dropped into the eyes, cools the inflammations in them, and takes away the pain and web; and dropped into the ears, eases the pains in them, and heals and removes the heat. The same also with the juice of Houseleek is profitable against any inflammations and breakings out of the skin, and against burnings and

scaldings by fire and water. The juice or decoction made either of
itself, or other things of the like nature, is of much use and good
effect for old and hollow ulcers that are hard to be cured, and for
cankers and sores in the mouth or privy parts of man or woman;
and helps also the pains of the piles in the fundament. The juice
mixed with oil of roses, and the temples and forehead anointed
therewith, eases the pains of the head proceeding from heat, and
helps lunatic and frantic persons very much; as also the biting of
serpents, or a mad dog. The same also is profitably applied to
all hot gouts in the feet or hands, especially in the beginning. It
is also good to be applied where any bone is out of joint, to hinder
inflammations, swellings, and pains that presently rise thereupon.
The powder of the dried leaves taken in drink, kills worms of the
belly; and boiled in wine, kills worms that breed in old and foul
ulcers. One part of Plantain water, and two parts of the brine of
powdered beef, boiled together and clarified, is a most sure remedy
to heal all spreading scabs or itch in the head and body, all manner
of tetters, ring-worms, the shingles, and all other running and
fretting sores. Briefly, the Plantains are singularly good wound
herbs, to heal fresh or old wounds or sores, either inward or outward.

PLUMS

ARE so well known that they need no description.

Government and virtues.] All Plums are under Venus, and are
like women, some better, and some worse. As there is great diver-
sity of kinds, so there is in the operation of Plums, for some that are
sweet moistens the stomach, and make the belly soluble; those that
are sour quench thirst more, and bind the belly; the moist and
waterish do sooner corrupt in the stomach, but the firm do nourish
more, and offend less. The dried fruit sold by the grocers under
the names of Damask Prunes, do somewhat loosen the belly, and
being stewed, are often used, both in health and sickness, to relish
the mouth and stomach, to procure appetite, and a little to open
the body, allay choler, and cool the stomach. Plum-tree leaves
boiled in wine, are good to wash and gargle the mouth and throat,
to dry the flux of rheum coming to the palate, gums, or almonds
of the ear. The gum of the tree is good to break the stone. The
gum or leaves boiled in vinegar, and applied, kills tetters and ringworms. Matthiolus saith, The oil preserved out of the kernels of
the stones, as oil of almonds is made, is good against the inflamed
piles, the tumours or swellings of ulcers, hoarseness of the voice,
roughness of the tongue and throat, and likewise the pains in the

ears. And that five ounces of the said oil taken with one ounce of muskadel, drives forth the stone, and helps the cholic.

POLYPODY OF THE OAK

Descript.] This is a small herb consisting of nothing but roots and leaves, bearing neither stalk, flower, nor seed, as it is thought. It hath three or four leaves rising from the root, every one single by itself, of about a hand length, are winged, consisting of many small narrow leaves cut into the middle rib, standing on each side of the stalk, large below, and smaller up to the top, not dented nor notched at the edges at all, as the male fern hath, of sad green colour, and smooth on the upper side, but on the other side somewhat rough by reason of some yellowish flowers set thereon. The root is smaller than one's little finger, lying aslope, or creeping along under the upper crust of the earth, brownish on the outside and greenish within, of a sweetish harshness in taste, set with certain rough knags on each side thereof, having also much mossiness or yellow hairiness upon it, and some fibres underneath it, whereby it is nourished.

Place.] It grows as well upon old rotten stumps, or trunks of trees, as oak, beech, hazel, willow, or any other, as in the woods under them, and upon old mud walls, as also in mossy, stony, and gravelly places near unto wood. That which grows upon oak is accounted the best; but the quantity thereof is scarce sufficient for the common use.

Time.] It being always green, may be gathered for use at any time.

Government and virtues.] Polypodium of the Oak, that which grows upon the earth is best; it is an herb of Saturn, to purge melancholy; if the humour be otherwise, chuse your Polypodium accordingly. Meuse (who is called the Physician's Evangelist for the certainty of his medicines, and the truth of his opinion) saith, That it dries up thin humours, digests thick and tough, and purges burnt choler, and especially tough and thick phlegm, and thin phlegm also, even from the joints, and therefore good for those that are troubled with melancholy, or quartan agues, especially if it be taken in whey or honied water, or in barley-water, or the broth of a chicken with Epithymum, or with Beets and Mallows. It is good for the hardness of the spleen, and for pricking or stitches in the sides, as also for the cholic. Some use to put to it some Fennel seeds, or Annis seeds, or Ginger, to correct that loathing it brings to the stomach, which is more than needs, it being a safe and gentle

medicine, fit for all persons, which daily experience confirms; and an
ounce of it may be given at a time in a decoction, if there be not
Sena, or some other strong purger put with it. A dram or two of the
powder of the dried roots, taken fasting in a cup of honied water,
works gently, and for the purposes aforesaid. The distilled water
both of roots and leaves, is much commended for the quartan ague,
to be taken for many days together, as also against melancholy, or
fearful and troublesome sleeps or dreams; and with some sugar-
candy dissolved therein, is good against the cough, shortness of
breath, and wheezings, and those distillations of thin rheum upon
the lungs, which cause phthisicks, and oftentimes consumptions.
The fresh roots beaten small, or the powder of the dried roots mixed
with honey, and applied to the member that is out of joint, doth
much help it; and applied also to the nose, cures the disease called
Polypus, which is a piece of flesh growing therein, which in time
stops the passage of breath through that nostril; and it helps those
clefts or chops that come between the fingers or toes.

THE POPLAR TREE

THERE are two sorts of Poplars, which are most familiar with us,
viz. the Black and White, both which I shall here describe unto you.
   Descript.] The White Poplar grows great, and reasonably high,
covered with thick, smooth, white bark, especially the branches;
having long leaves cut into several divisions almost like a vine leaf,
but not of so deep a green on the upper side, and hoary white underneath, of a reasonable good scent, the whole form representing the
form of Coltsfoot. The catkins which it brings forth before the
leaves, are long, and of a faint reddish colour, which fall away,
bearing seldom good seed with them. The wood hereof is smooth,
soft, and white, very finely waved, whereby it is much esteemed.
   The Black Poplar grows higher and straighter than the White,
with a greyish bark, bearing broad green leaves, somewhat like ivy
leaves, not cut in on the edges like the White, but whole and
dented, ending in a point, and not white underneath, hanging by
slender long foot stalks, which with the air are continually shaken,
like as the Aspen leaves are. The catkins hereof are greater than
those of the White, composed of many round green berries, as if
they were set together in a long cluster, containing much downy
matter, which being ripe, is blown away with the wind. The clammy
buds hereof, before they spread into leaves are gathered to make
Unguentum and Populneum, and are of a yellowish green colour,
and somewhat small, sweet, but strong. The wood is smooth,

tough, and white, and easy to be cloven. On both these trees grows a sweet kind of musk, which in former times was used to put into sweet ointments.

Place.] They grow in moist woods, and by water-sides in sundry places of this land; yet the White is not so frequent as the other.

Time.] Their time is likewise expressed before. The catkins coming forth before the leaves in the end of Summer.

Government and virtues.] Saturn hath dominion over both. White Poplar, saith Galen, is of a cleansing property. The weight of an ounce in powder, of the bark thereof, being drank, saith Dioscorides, is a remedy for those that are troubled with the sciatica, or the stranguary. The juice of the leaves dropped warm into the ears, eases the pains in them. The young clammy buds or eyes, before they break out into leaves, bruised, and a little honey put to them, is a good medicine for a dull sight. The Black Poplar is held to be more cooling than the White, and therefore the leaves bruised with vinegar and applied, help the gout. The seed drank in vinegar, is held good against the falling-sickness. The water that drops from the hollow places of this tree, takes away warts, pushes, wheals, and other the like breakings-out of the body. The young Black Poplar buds, saith Matthiolus, are much used by women to beautify their hair, bruising them with fresh butter, straining them after they have been kept for some time in the sun. The ointment called Populneon, which is made of this Poplar, is singularly good for all heat and inflammations in any part of the body, and tempers the heat of wounds. It is much used to dry up the milk of women's breasts when they have weaned their children.

POPPY

OF this I shall describe three kinds, *viz.* the White and Black of the Garden, and the Erratic Wild Poppy, or Corn Rose.

Descript.] The White Poppy hath at first four or five whitish green leaves lying upon the ground, which rise with the stalk, compassing it at the bottom of them, and are very large, much cut or torn on the edges, and dented also besides. The stalk, which is usually four or five feet high, hath sometimes no branches at the top, and usually but two or three at most, bearing every one but one head wrapped up in a thin skin, which bows down before it is ready to blow, and then rising, and being broken, the flowers within it spreading itself open, and consisting of four very large, white, round leaves, with many whitish round threads in the middle, set about a small, round, green head, having a crown, or star-like cover at the head thereof, which growing ripe, becomes as large as a great apple wherein are contained a great number of small round seeds, in several partitions or divisions next unto the shell, the middle thereof remaining hollow, and empty. The whole plant, both leaves, stalks, and heads, while they are fresh, young, and green, yield a milk when they are broken, of an unpleasant bitter taste, almost ready to provoke casting, and of a strong heady smell, which being condensed, is called Opium. The root is white and woody, perishing as soon as it hath given ripe seed.

The Black Poppy little differs from the former, until it bears its flower, which is somewhat less, and of a black purplish colour, but without any purple spots in the bottom of the leaf. The head of the seed is much less than the former, and opens itself a little round about the top, under the crown, so that the seed, which is very black, will fall out, if one turn the head thereof downward.

The Wild Poppy, or Corn Rose, hath long and narrow leaves, very much cut in on the edges into many divisions, of a light green colour, sometimes hairy withal. The stalk is blackish and hairy also, but not so tall as the garden kind, having some such like leaves thereon to grow below, parted into three or four branches sometimes, whereon grow small hairy heads bowing down before the skin break, wherein the flower is inclosed, which when it is fully blown open, is of a fair yellowish red or crimson colour, and in some much paler, without any spot in the bottom of the leaves, having many black soft threads in the middle, compassing a small green head, which when it is ripe, is not bigger than one's little finger's end, wherein is contained much black seeds smaller than that of the garden. The root perishes every year, and springs again of its own sowing. Of this kind there is one lesser in all parts thereof, and differs in nothing else.

Place.] The garden kinds do not naturally grow wild in any place, but all are sown in gardens where they grow.

The Wild Poppy or Corn Rose, is plentifully enough, and many times too much so in the corn fields of all counties through this land, and also on ditch banks, and by hedge sides. The smaller wild kind is also found in corn fields, and also in some other places, but not so plentifully as the former.

Time.] The garden kinds are usually sown in the spring, which then flower about the end of May, and somewhat earlier, if they spring of their own sowing.

The wild kind flower usually from May until July, and the seed of them is ripe soon after the flowering.

Government and virtues.] The herb is Lunar, and of the juice of it is made opium; only for lucre of money they cheat you, and tell you it is a kind of tear, or some such like thing, that drops from Poppies when they weep, and that is somewhere beyond the seas, I know not where beyond the Moon. The garden Poppy heads with seeds made into a syrup, is frequently, and to good effect used to procure rest, and sleep, in the sick and weak, and to stay catarrhs and defluxions of thin rheums from the head into the stomach and lungs, causing a continual cough, the fore-runner of a consumption; it helps also hoarseness of the throat, and when one have lost their voice, which the oil of the seed doth likewise. The black seed boiled in wine, and drank, is said also to dry the flux of the belly, and women's courses. The empty shells, or poppy heads, are usually boiled in water, and given to procure rest and sleep: so doth the leaves in the same manner; as also if the head and temples be bathed with the decoction warm, or with the oil of Poppies, the green leaves or the heads bruised and applied with a little vinegar, or made into a poultice with barley-meal or hog's grease, cools and tempers all inflammations, as also the disease called St. Anthony's fire. It is generally used in treacle and mithridate, and in all other medicines that are made to procure rest and sleep, and to ease pains in the head as well as in other parts. It is also used to cool inflammations, agues, or frenzies, or to stay defluxions which cause a cough, or consumptions, and also other fluxes of the belly or women's courses; it is also put into hollow teeth, to ease the pain, and hath been found by experience to ease the pains of the gout.

The Wild Poppy, or Corn Rose (as Matthiolus saith) is good to prevent the falling-sickness. The syrup made with the flower, is with good effect given to those that have the pleurisy; and the dried flowers also, either boiled in water, or made into powder and drank, either in the distilled water of them, or some other drink, works the like effect. The distilled water of the flowers is held to be of much good use against surfeits, being drank evening and morning. It is also more cooling than any of the other Poppies, and therefore cannot but be as effectual in hot agues, frenzies, and other inflammations either inward or outward. Galen saith, The seed is dangerous to be used inwardly.

PURSLAIN

GARDEN Purslain (being used as a sallad herb) is so well known that it needs no description; I shall therefore only speak of its virtues as follows.

Government and virtues.] 'Tis an herb of the Moon. It is good to cool any heat in the liver, blood, reins, and stomach, and in hot agues nothing better. It stays hot and choleric fluxes of the belly, women's courses, the whites, and gonorrhæa, or running of the reins, the distillation from the head, and pains therein proceeding from heat, want of sleep, or the frenzy. The seed is more effectual than the herb, and is of singular good use to cool the heat and sharpness of urine, venereous dreams, and the like; insomuch that the over frequent use hereof extinguishes the heat and virtue of natural procreation. The seed bruised and boiled in wine, and given to children, expels the worms. The juice of the herb is held as effectual to all the purposes aforesaid; as also to stay vomitings, and taken with some sugar or honey, helps an old and dry cough, shortness of breath, and the phthisick, and stays immoderate thirst. The distilled water of the herb is used by many (as the more pleasing) with a little sugar to work the same effects. The juice also is singularly good in the inflammations and ulcers in the secret parts of man or woman, as also the bowels and hæmorrhoids, when they are ulcerous, or excoriations in them. The herb bruised and applied to the forehead and temples, allays excessive heat therein, that hinders rest and sleep; and applied to the eyes, takes away the redness and inflammation in them, and those other parts where pushes, wheals, pimples, St. Anthony's fire and the like, break forth; if a little vinegar be put to it, and laid to the neck, with as much of galls and linseed together, it takes away the pains therein, and the crick in the neck. The juice is used with oil of roses for the same causes, or for blasting by lightening, and burnings by gunpowder, or for women's sore breasts, and to allay the heat in all other sores or hurts; applied also to the navels of children that stick forth, it helps them; it is also good for sore mouths and gums that are swollen, and to fasten loose teeth. Camerarius saith, the distilled water used by some, took away the pain of their teeth, when all other remedies failed, and the thickened juice made into pills with the powder of gum Tragicanth and Arabic, being taken, prevails much to help those that make bloody water. Applied to the gout it eases pains thereof, and helps the hardness of the sinews, if it come not of the cramp, or a cold cause.

PRIMROSES

THEY are so well known, that they need no description. Of the leaves of Primroses is made as fine a salve to heal wounds as any that I know; you shall be taught to make salves of any herb at the latter end of the book: make this as you are taught there, and do not (you that have any ingenuity in you) see your poor neighbours go with wounded limbs when an halfpenny cost will heal them.

PRIVET

Descript.] Our common Privet is carried up with many slender branches to a reasonable height and breadth, to cover arbours, bowers and banquetting houses, and brought, wrought, and cut into so many forms, of men, horses, birds, &c. which though at first supported, grows afterwards strong of itself. It bears long and narrow green leaves by the couples, and sweet smelling white flowers in tufts at the end of the branches, which turn into small black berries that have a purplish juice with them, and some seeds that are flat on the one side, with a hole or dent therein.

Place.] It grows in this land, in divers woods.

Time.] Our Privet flowers in June and July, the berries are ripe in August and September.

Government and virtues.] The Moon is lady of this. It is little used in physic with us in these times, more than in lotions, to wash sores and sore mouths, and to cool inflammations, and dry up fluxes. Yet Matthiolus saith, it serves all the uses for which Cypress, or the East Privet, is appointed by Dioscorides and Galen. He further saith, That the oil that is made of the flowers of Privet infused therein, and set in the Sun, is singularly good for the inflammations of wounds, and for the headache, coming of a hot cause. There is a sweet water also distilled from the flowers, that is good for all those diseases that need cooling and drying, and therefore helps all fluxes of the belly or stomach, bloody-fluxes, and women's courses, being either drank or applied; as all those that void blood at the mouth, or any other place, and for distillations of rheum in the eyes, especially if it be used with them.

QUEEN OF THE MEADOWS, MEADOW SWEET, OR MEAD SWEET

Descript.] The stalks of these are reddish, rising to be three feet high, sometimes four or five feet, having at the joints thereof large winged leaves, standing one above another at distances, consisting of many and somewhat broad leaves, set on each side of a middle rib, being hard, rough, or rugged, crumpled much like unto elm leaves, having also some smaller leaves with them (as Agrimony hath) somewhat deeply dented about the edges, of a sad green colour on the upper side, and greyish underneath, of a pretty sharp scent and taste, somewhat like unto the Burnet, and a leaf hereof put into a cup of claret wine, gives also a fine relish to it. At the tops of the stalks and branches stand many tufts of small white flowers thrust thick together, which smell much sweeter than the leaves; and in their places, being fallen, come crooked and cornered seed. The root is somewhat woody, and blackish on the outside, and brownish within, with divers great strings, and lesser fibres set thereat, of a strong scent, but nothing so pleasant as the flowers and leaves, and perishes not, but abides many years, shooting forth a-new every Spring.

Place.] It grows in moist meadows that lie mostly wet, or near the courses of water.

Time.] It flowers in some places or other all the three Summer months, that is, June, July, and August, and the seed is ripe soon after.

Government and virtues.] Venus claims dominion over the herb. It is used to stay all manner of bleedings, fluxes, vomitings, and women's courses, also their whites. It is said to alter and take away the fits of the quartan agues, and to make a merry heart, for which purpose some use the flowers, and some the leaves. It helps speedily those that are troubled with the cholic; being boiled in wine, and with a little honey, taken warm, it opens the belly; but boiled in red wine, and drank, it stays the flux of the belly. Outwardly applied, it helps old ulcers that are cankerous, or hollow fistulous, for which it is by many much commended, as also for the sores in the mouth or secret parts. The leaves when they are full grown, being laid on the skin, will, in a short time, raise blisters thereon, as Tragus saith. The water thereof helps the heat and inflammation in the eyes.

THE QUINCE TREE.

Descript.] The ordinary Quince Tree grows often to the height and bigness of a reasonable apple tree, but more usually lower, and crooked, with a rough bark, spreading arms, and branches far abroad. The leaves are somewhat like those of the apple tree, but thicker, broader, and full of veins, and whiter on the under side, not dented at all about the edges. The flowers are large and white, sometimes dashed over with a blush. The fruit that follows is yellow, being near ripe, and covered with a white freeze, or cotton; thick set on the younger, and growing less as they grow to be thorough ripe, bunched out oftentimes in some places, some being like an apple, and some a pear, of a strong heady scent, and not durable to keep, and is sour, harsh, and of an unpleasant taste to eat fresh; but being scalded, roasted, baked, or preserved, becomes more pleasant.

Place and Time.] It best likes to grow near ponds and water sides, and is frequent through this land: and flowers not until the leaves be come forth. The fruit is ripe in September or October.

Government and virtues.] Old Saturn owns the Tree. Quinces when they are green, help all sorts of fluxes in men or women, and choleric lasks, casting, and whatever needs astriction, more than any way prepared by fire; yet the syrup of the juice, or the conserve, are much conducible, much of the binding quality being consumed by the fire; if a little vinegar be added, it stirs up the languishing appetite, and the stomach given to casting; some spices being added, comforts and strengthens the decaying and fainting spirits, and helps the liver oppressed, that it cannot perfect the digestion, or corrects choler and phlegm. If you would have them purging, put honey to them instead of sugar; and if more laxative, for choler, Rhubarb; for phlegm, Turbith; for watery humours, Scammony; but if more forcible to bind, use the unripe Quinces, with roses and acacia, hypocistis, and some torrified rhubarb. To take the crude juice of Quinces, is held a preservative against the force of deadly poison; for it hath been found most certainly true, that the very smell of a Quince hath taken away all the strength of the poison of white Hellebore. If there be need of any outwardly binding and cooling of hot fluxes, the oil of Quinces, or other medicines that may be made thereof, are very available to anoint the belly or other parts therewith; it likewise strengthens the stomach and belly, and the sinews that are loosened by sharp humours falling on them, and restrains immoderate sweatings. The muscilage taken from the seeds of Quinces, and boiled in a little water, is very good to cool the heat and heal the sore breasts of women. The same, with a little sugar, is good to lenify the harshness and hoarseness of the throat, and roughness of the tongue. The cotton or down of Quinces boiled and applied to plague sores, heals them up: and laid as a plaister, made up with wax, it brings hair to them that are bald, and keeps it from falling, if it be ready to shed.

RADDISH, OR HORSE-RADDISH

THE garden Raddish is so well known, that it needs no description.

Descript.] The Horse-Raddish hath its first leaves, that rise before Winter, about a foot and a half long, very much cut in or torn on the edges into many parts, of a dark green colour, with a great rib in the middle; after these have been up a while, others follow, which are greater, rougher, broader and longer, whole and not divided at first, but only somewhat rougher dented about the edges; the stalks when it bears flowers (which is seldom) is great, rising up with some few lesser leaves thereon, to three or four feet high, spreading at the top many small branches of whitish flowers, made of four leaves a-piece; after which come small pods, like those of Shepherd's Purse, but seldom with any seed in them. The root is great, long, white and rugged, shooting up divers heads of leaves, which may be parted for increase, but it doth not creep in the ground, nor run above ground, and is of a strong, sharp, and bitter taste almost like mustard.

Place.] It is found wild in some places, but is chiefly planted in gardens, and joys in moist and shadowy places.

Time.] It seldom flowers, but when it doth, it is in July.

Government and virtues.] They are both under Mars. The juice of Horse-raddish given to drink, is held to be very effectual for the scurvy. It kills the worms in children, being drank, and also laid upon the belly. The root bruised and laid to the place grieved with the sciatica, joint-ache, or the hard swellings of the liver and spleen, doth wonderfully help them all. The distilled water of the herb and root is more familiar to be taken with a little sugar for all the purposes aforesaid.

Garden Raddishes are in wantonness by the gentry eaten as a sallad, but they breed but scurvy humours in the stomach, and corrupt the blood, and then send for a physician as fast as you can; this is one cause which makes the owners of such nice palates so unhealthful; yet for such as are troubled with the gravel, stone, or stoppage of urine, they are good physic, if the body be strong that takes them; you may make the juice of the roots into a syrup if you please, for that use: they purge by urine exceedingly.

RAGWORT

It is called also St. James'-wort, and Stagger-wort, and Stammer-wort, and Segrum.

Descript.] The greater common Ragwort hath many large and long, dark green leaves lying on the ground, very much rent and torn on the sides in many places: from among which rise up sometimes but one, and sometimes two or three square or crested blackish or brownish stalks, three or four feet high, sometimes branched, bearing divers such-like leaves upon them, at several distances upon the top, where it branches forth into many stalks bearing yellow flowers, consisting of divers leaves, set as a pale or border, with a dark yellow thrum in the middle, which do abide a great while, but at last are turned into down, and with the small blackish grey seed, are carried away with the wind. The root is made of many fibres, whereby it is firmly fastened into the ground, and abides many years.

There is another sort thereof differs from the former only in this, that it rises not so high; the leaves are not so finely jagged, nor of so dark a green colour, but rather somewhat whitish, soft and woolly, and the flowers usually paler.

Place.] They grow, both of them, wild in pastures, and untilled grounds in many places, and oftentimes both in one field.

Time.] They flower in June and July, and the seed is ripe in August.

Government and virtues.] Ragwort is under the command of Dame Venus, and cleanses, digests, and discusses. The decoction of the herb is good to wash the mouth or throat that hath ulcers or sores therein: and for swellings, hardness, or imposthumes, for it thoroughly cleanses and heals them; as also the quinsy, and the king's evil. It helps to stays catarrhs, thin rheums, and defluxions from the head into the eyes, nose, or lungs. The juice is found by experience to be singularly good to heal green wounds, and to cleanse and heal all old and filthy ulcers in the privities, and in other parts of the body, as also inward wounds and ulcers; stays the malignity of fretting and running cankers, and hollow fistulas, not suffering them to spread farther. It is also much commended to help aches and pains either in the fleshy part, or in the nerves and sinews, as also the sciatica, or pain of the hips or knuckle-bone, to bathe the places with the decoction of the herb, or to anoint them with an ointment made of the herb bruised and boiled in old hog's suet, with some Mastick and Olibanum in powder added unto it after it is strained forth. In Sussex we call it Ragweed.

RATTLE GRASS

OF this there are two kinds which I shall speak of, *viz*. the red and yellow.

Descript.] The common Red Rattle hath sundry reddish, hollow stalks, and sometimes green, rising from the root, lying for the most part on the ground, some growing more upright, with many small reddish or green leaves set on both sides of a middle rib, finely dented about the edges. The flowers stand at the tops of the stalks and branches, of a fine purplish red colour, like small gaping hooks; after which come blackish seed in small husks, which lying loose therein, will rattle with shaking. The root consists of two or three small whitish strings with some fibres thereat.

The common Yellow Rattle hath seldom above one round great

stalk, rising from the foot, about half a yard, or two feet high, and but few branches thereon, having two long and somewhat broad leaves set at a joint, deeply cut in on the edges, resembling the comb of a cock, broadest next to the stalk, and smaller to the end. The flowers grow at the tops of the stalks, with some shorter leaves with them, hooded after the same manner that the others are, but of a fair yellow colour, or in some paler, and in some more white. The seed is contained in large husks, and being ripe, will rattle or make a noise with lying loose in them. The root is small and slender, perishing every year.

Place.] They grow in meadows and woods generally through this land.

Time.] They are in flower from Mid-summer until August be past, sometimes.

Government and virtues.] They are both of them under the dominion of the Moon. The Red Rattle is accounted profitable to heal up fistulas and hollow ulcers, and to stay the flux of humours in them, as also the abundance of women's courses, or any other fluxes of blood, being boiled in red wine, and drank.

The yellow Rattle, or Cock's Comb, is held to be good for those that are troubled with a cough, or dimness of sight, if the herb, being boiled with beans, and some honey put thereto, be drank or dropped into the eyes. The whole seed being put into the eyes, draws forth any skin, dimness or film, from the sight, without trouble, or pain.

REST HARROW, OR CAMMOCK

Descript.] Common Rest Harrow rises up with divers rough woody twigs half a yard or a yard high, set at the joints without order, with little roundish leaves, sometimes more than two or three at a place, of a dark green colour, without thorns while they are young; but afterwards armed in sundry places, with short and sharp thorns. The flowers come forth at the tops of the twigs and branches, whereof it is full fashioned like pease or broom blossoms, but lesser, flatter, and somewhat closer, of a faint purplish colour; after which come small pods containing small, flat, round seed. The root is blackish on the outside, and whitish within, very rough, and hard to break when it is fresh and green, and as hard as an horn when it is dried, thrusting down deep into the ground, and spreading likewise, every piece being apt to grow again if it be left in the ground.

Place.] It grows in many places of this land, as well in the arable as waste ground.

Time.] It flowers about the beginning or middle of July, and the seed is ripe in August.

Government and virtues.] It is under the dominion of Mars. It is singularly good to provoke urine when it is stopped, and to break and drive forth the stone, which the powder of the bark of the root taken in wine performs effectually. Matthiolus saith, The same helps the disease called *Herma Carnosa*, the fleshy rupture, by taking the said powder for three months together constantly, and that it hath cured some which seemed incurable by any other means than by cutting or burning. The decoction thereof made with some vinegar, gargled in the mouth, eases the tooth-ache, especially when it comes of rheum; and the said decoction is very powerful to open obstructions of the liver and spleen, and other parts. A distilled water in *Balneo Mariæ*, with four pounds of the root hereof first sliced small, and afterwards steeped in a gallon of Canary wine, is singularly good for all the purposes aforesaid, and to cleanse the urinary passages. The powder of the said root made into an electuary, or lozenges, with sugar, as also the bark of the fresh roots boiled tender, and afterwards beaten to a conserve with sugar, works the like effect. The powder of the roots strewed upon the brims of ulcers, or mixed with any other convenient thing, and applied, consumes the hardness, and causes them to heal the better.

ROCKET

IN regard the Garden Rocket is rather used as a sallad herb than to any physical purposes, I shall omit it, and only speak of the common wild Rocket. The description whereof take as follows.

Descript.] The common wild Rocket has longer and narrower leaves, much more divided into slender cuts and jags on both sides the middle rib than the garden kinds have; of a sad green colour, from among which rise up divers stalks two or three feet high, sometimes set with the like leaves, but smaller and smaller upwards, branched from the middle into divers stiff stalks, bearing sundry yellow flowers on them, made of four leaves a-piece, as the others are, which afterwards yield them small reddish seed, in small long pods, of a more bitter and hot biting taste than the garden kinds, as the leaves are also.

Place.] It is found wild in divers places of this land.

Time.] It flowers about June or July, and the seed is ripe in August.

Government and virtues.] The wild Rockets are forbidden to be used alone, in regard their sharpness fumes into the head, causing aches and pains therein, and are less hurtful to hot and choleric persons, for fear of inflaming their blood, and therefore for such we may say a little doth but a little harm, for angry Mars rules them, and he sometimes will be restive when he meets with fools. The wild Rocket is more strong and effectual to increase sperm and venerous qualities, whereunto all the seed is more effectual than the garden kind. It serves also to help digestion, and provokes urine exceedingly. The seed is used to cure the biting of serpents, the scorpion, and the shrew mouse, and other poisons, and expels worms, and other noisome creatures that breed in the belly. The herb boiled or stewed, and some sugar put thereto, helps the cough in children, being taken often. The seed also taken in drink, takes away the ill scent of the arm-pits, increases milk in nurses, and wastes the spleen. The seed mixed with honey, and used on the face, cleanses the skin from morphew, and used with vinegar, takes away freckles and redness in the face, or other parts; and with the gall of an ox, it mends foul scars, black and blue spots, and the marks of the small-pox.

WINTER-ROCKET, OR CRESSES

Descript.] Winter-Rocket, or Winter-Cresses, hath divers somewhat large sad green leaves lying upon the ground, torn or cut in divers parts, somewhat like unto Rocket or turnip leaves, with smaller pieces next the bottom, and broad at the ends, which so abide all the Winter (if it spring up in Autumn, when it is used to be eaten) from among which rise up divers small round stalks, full of branches, bearing many small yellow flowers of four leaves a-piece, after which come small pods, with reddish seed in them. The root is somewhat stringy, and perishes every year after the seed is ripe.

Place.] It grows of its own accord in gardens and fields, by the way-sides, in divers places, and particularly in the next pasture to the Conduit-head behind Gray's Inn, that brings water to Mr. Lamb's conduit in Holborn.

Time.] It flowers in May, seeds in June, and then perishes.

Government and virtues.] This is profitable to provoke urine, to help stranguary, and expel gravel and stone. It is good for the scurvy, and found by experience to be a singularly good wound herb to cleanse inward wounds; the juice or decoction being drank, or outwardly applied to wash foul ulcers and sores, cleansing them by sharpness, and hindering or abating the dead flesh from growing therein, and healing them by their drying quality.

ROSES

I HOLD it altogether needless to trouble the reader with a description of any of these, since both the garden Roses, and the Roses of the briars are well enough known: take therefore the virtues of them as follows. And first I shall begin with the garden kinds.

Government and virtues.] What a pother have authors made with Roses! What a racket have they kept! I shall add, red Roses are under Jupiter, Damask under Venus, White under the Moon, and Provence under the King of France. The white and red Roses are cooling and drying, and yet the white is taken to exceed the red in both the properties, but is seldom used inwardly in any medicine. The bitterness in the Roses when they are fresh, especially the juice, purges choler, and watery humours; but being dried, and that heat which caused the bitterness being consumed, they have then a binding and astringent quality. Those also that are not full blown, do both cool and bind more than those that are full blown, and the white Rose more than the Red. The decoction of red Roses made with wine and used, is very good for the head-ache, and pains in the eyes, ears, throat, and gums; as also for the fundament, the lower part of the belly and the matrix, being bathed or put into them. The same decoction with the Roses remaining in it, is profitably applied to the region of the heart to ease the inflammation therein; as also St. Anthony's fire, and other diseases of the stomach. Being dried and beaten to powder, and taken in steeled wine or water, it helps to stay women's courses. The yellow threads in the middle of the Roses (which are erroneously called the Rose Seed) being powdered and drank in the distilled water of Quinces, stays the overflowing of women's courses, and doth wonderfully stay the defluctions of rheum upon the gums and teeth, preserving them from corruption, and fastening them if they be loose, being washed and gargled therewith, and some vinegar of Squills added thereto. The heads with the seed being used in powder, or in a decoction, stays the lask and spitting of blood. Red Roses do strengthen the heart, the stomach and the liver, and the retentive faculty. They mitigate the pains that arise from heat, assuage inflammations, procure rest and sleep, stay both whites and reds in women, the gonorrhea, or running of the reins, and fluxes of the belly. The juice of them doth purge and cleanse the body from choler and phlegm. The husks of the Roses, with the beards and nails of the Roses, are binding and cooling, and the distilled water of either of them is good for the heat and redness in the eyes, and to stay and dry up the rheums and watering of them. Of the Red Roses are usually made many compositions, all serving to sundry good uses, viz.

Electuary of Roses, Conserve, both moist and dry, which is more usually called Sugar of roses, Syrup of dry Roses, and Honey of Roses. The cordial powder called *Diarrhoden Abbatis*, and *Aromatica Rosarum*. The distilled Water of Roses, Vinegar of Roses, Ointment, and Oil of Roses, and the Rose leaves dried, are of great use and effect. To write at large of every one of these, would make my book swell too big, it being sufficient for a volume of itself, to speak fully of them. But briefly, the Electuary is purging, whereof two or three drams taken by itself in some convenient liquor, is a purge sufficient for a weak constitution, but may be increased to six drams, according to the strength of the patient. It purges choler without trouble, it is good in hot fevers, and pains of the head arising from hot choleric humours, and heat in the eyes, the jaundice also, and joint-aches proceeding of hot humours. The moist Conserve is of much use, both binding and cordial; for until it be about two years old, it is more binding than cordial, and after that, more cordial than binding. Some of the younger Conserve taken with mithridate mixed together, is good for those that are troubled with distillations of rheum from the brain to the nose, and defluctions of rheum into the eyes; as also for fluxes and lasks of the belly; and being mixed with the powder of mastich, is very good for the gonorrhea, and for the looseness of the humours in the body. The old Conserve mixed with Aromaticum Rosarum, is a very good cordial against faintings, swoonings, weakness, and tremblings of the heart, strengthens both it and a weak stomach, helps digestion, stays casting, and is a very good preservative in the time of infection. The dry Conserve, which is called the Sugar of Roses, is a very good cordial to strengthen the heart and spirits; as also to stay defluctions. The syrup of dried red Roses strengthens a stomach given to casting, cools an over-heated liver, and the blood in agues, comforts the heart, and resists putrefaction and infection, and helps to stay lasks and fluxes. Honey of Roses is much used in gargles and lotions to wash sores, either in the mouth, throat, or other parts, both to cleanse and heal them, and to stay the fluxes of humours falling upon them. It is also used in clysters both to cool and cleanse. The cordial powders, called Diarrhoden Abbatis and Aromaticum Rosarum, do comfort and strengthen the heart and stomach, procure an appetite, help digestion, stay vomiting, and are very good for those that have slippery bowels, to strengthen them, and to dry up their moisture. Red Rose-water is well known, and of familiar use on all occasions, and better than Damask Rose-water, being cooling and cordial, refreshing, quickening the weak and faint spirits, used either in meats or broths, to wash the temples, to smell at the nose, or to smell the sweet vapours thereof out of a perfuming pot, or cast into a hot fire shovel. It is also of much good use against the redness and inflammations of the eyes to bathe them therewith, and the temples of the head; as also against pain and ache, for which purpose also Vinegar of Roses is of much good use, and to procure rest and sleep, if some thereof, and Rose-water together, be used to smell unto, or the nose and temples moistened therewith, but more usually to moisten a piece of a red Rose-cake, cut for the purpose, and heated between a double folded cloth, with a little beaten nutmeg, and poppy-seed strewed on the side that must lie next to the forehead and temples, and bound so thereto all night. The ointment of Roses is much used against heat and inflammations in the head, to anoint the forehead and temples, and being mixt with *Unguentum Populneum*, to procure rest: it is also used for the heat of the liver, the back and reins, and to cool and heal flushes, wheals, and other red pimples rising in the face or other parts. Oil of Roses is not only used by itself to cool any hot swellings or inflammations, and to bind and stay fluxes of humours unto sores, but is also put into ointments and plaisters that are cooling and binding, and restraining the flux of humours. The dried leaves of the red Roses are used both inwardly and outwardly, both cooling, binding, and cordial, for with them are made both *Aromaticum*, *Rosarum*, *Diarrhoden Abbatis*, and *Saccharum Rosarum*, each of whose properties are before declared. Rose leaves and mint, heated and applied outwardly to the stomach, stays castings, and very much strengthen a weak stomach; and applied as a fomentation to the region of the liver and heart, do much cool and temper them, and also serve instead of a Rose-cake (as is said before) to quiet the over-hot spirits, and cause rest and sleep. The syrup of Damask Roses is both simple and compound, and made with Agaric. The simple solutive syrup is a familiar, safe, gentle and easy medicine, purging choler, taken from one ounce to three or four, yet this is remarkable herein, that the distilled water of this syrup should notably bind the belly. The syrup with Agaric is more strong and effectual, for one ounce thereof by itself will open the body more than the other, and works as much on phlegm as choler. The compound syrup is more forcible in working on melancholic humours; and available against the leprosy, itch, tetters, &c. and the French disease. Also honey of Roses solutive is made of the same infusions that the syrup is made of, and therefore works the same effect, both opening and purging, but is oftener given to phlegmatic than choleric persons, and is more used in clysters than in potions, as the syrup made with sugar is. The conserve and preserved leaves of those Roses are also operative in gently opening the belly.

The simple water of Damask Roses is chiefly used for fumes to sweeten things, as the dried leaves thereof to make sweet powders, and fill sweet bags; and little use they are put to in physic, although they have some purging quality; the wild Roses also are few or none of them used in physic, but are generally held to come near the nature of the manured Roses. The fruit of the wild briar, which are called Hips, being thoroughly ripe, and made into a conserve with sugar, besides the pleasantness of the taste, doth gently bind the belly, and stay defluctions from the head upon the stomach, drying up the moisture thereof, and helps digestion. The pulp of the hips dried into a hard consistence, like to the juice of the liquorice, or so dried that it may be made into powder and taken into drink, stays speedily the whites in women. The briar ball is often used, being made into powder and drank, to break the stone, to provoke urine when it is stopped, and to ease and help the cholic; some appoint it to be burnt, and then taken for the same purpose. In the middle of the balls are often found certain white worms, which being dried and made into powder, and some of it drank, is found by experience of many to kill and drive forth the worms of the belly.

ROSA SOLIS, OR SUN DEW

It is likewise called Red-rot, and Youth-wort.

Descript.] It hath, divers small, round, hollow leaves, somewhat greenish, but full of certain red hairs, which make them seem red, every one standing upon his own foot-stalk, reddish, hairy likewise. The leaves are continually moist in the hottest day, yea, the hotter the sun shines on them, the moister they are, with a sliminess that will rope (as we say,) the small hairs always holding the moisture. Among these leaves rise up slender stalks, reddish also, three or four fingers high, bearing divers small white knobs one above another, which are flowers; after which in the heads are contained small seeds. The root is a few small hairs.

Place.] It grows usually in bogs and wet places, and sometimes in moist woods.

Time.] It flowers in June, and the leaves are then fittest to be gathered.

Government and virtues.] The Sun rules it, and it is under the sign Cancer. Rosa Solis is accounted good to help those that have a salt rheum distilling on their lungs, which breeds a consumption, and therefore the distilled water thereof in wine is held fit and profitable for such to drink, which water will be of a good yellow colour. The same water is held to be good for all other diseases of the lungs, as phthisicks, wheezings, shortness of breath, or the cough; as also to heal the ulcers that happen in the lungs; and it comforts the heart and fainting spirits. The leaves, outwardly applied to the skin will raise blisters, which has caused some to think it dangerous to be taken inwardly; but there are other things which will also draw blisters, yet nothing dangerous to be taken inwardly. There is an usual drink made thereof with aqua vitæ and spices frequently, and without any offence or danger, but to good purpose used in qualms and passions of the heart.

ROSEMARY

Our garden Rosemary is so well known, that I need not describe it.

Time.] It flowers in April and May with us, sometimes again in August.

Government and virtues.] The Sun claims privilege in it, and it is under the celestial Ram. It is an herb of as great use with us in these days as any whatsoever, not only for physical but civil purposes. The physical use of it (being my present task) is very much used both for inward and outward diseases, for by the warming and comforting heat thereof it helps all cold diseases both of the head, stomach, liver, and belly. The decoction thereof in wine, helps the cold distillations of rheum into the eyes, and all other cold diseases of the head and brain, as the giddiness or swimmings therein, drowsiness or dullness of the mind and senses like a stupidness, the dumb palsy, or loss of speech, the lethargy, and fallen-sickness, to be both drank, and the temples bathed therewith. It helps the pains in the gums and teeth, by rheum falling into them, not by putrefaction, causing an evil smell from them, or a stinking breath. It helps a weak memory, and quickens the senses. It is very comfortable to the stomach in all the cold griefs thereof, helps both retention of meat, and digestion, the decoction or powder being taken in wine. It is a remedy for the windiness in the stomach, bowels, and spleen, and expels it powerfully. It helps those that are liver-grown, by opening the obstructions thereof. It helps dim eyes, and procures a clear sight, the flowers thereof being taken all the while it is flowering every morning fasting, with bread and salt. Both Dioscorides and Galen say, That if a decoction be made thereof with water, and they that have the yellow jaundice exercise their bodies directly after the taking thereof, it will certainly cure them. The flowers and conserve made of them are singularly good to comfort the heart, and to expel the contagion of the pestilence; to burn the herb in houses and chambers, corrects the air in them. Both the flowers and leaves are very profitable for women that are troubled with the whites, if they be daily taken. The dried leaves shred small, and taken in a pipe, as tobacco is taken, helps those that have any cough, phthisic, or consumption, by warming and drying the thin distillations which cause those diseases. The leaves are very much used in bathings; and made into ointments or oil, are singularly good to help cold benumbed joints, sinews, or members. The chymical oil drawn from the leaves and flowers, is a sovereign help for all the diseases aforesaid, to touch the temples and nostrils with two or three drops for all the diseases of the head and brain spoken of before; as also to take one drop, two, or three, as the case requires, for the inward griefs. Yet must it be done with discretion, for it is very quick and piercing, and therefore but a little must be taken at a time. There is also another oil made by insolation in this manner: Take what quantity you will of the flowers, and put them into a strong glass close stopped, tie a fine linen cloth over the mouth, and turn the mouth down into another strong glass, which being set in the sun, an oil will distil down into the lower glass, to be preserved as precious for divers uses, both inward and outward, as a sovereign balm to heal the disease before-mentioned, to clear dim sights, and to take away spots, marks, and scars in the skin.

RHUBARB, OR REPHONTIC

Do not start, and say, This grows, you know not how far off: and then ask me, How it comes to pass that I bring it among our English simples? For though the name may speak it foreign, yet it grows with us in England, and that frequent enough in our gardens; and when you have thoroughly pursued its virtues, you will conclude it nothing inferior to that which is brought out of China, and by that time this hath been as much used as that hath been, the name which the other hath gotten will be eclipsed by the fame of this; take therefore a description at large of it as follows.

Descript.] At the first appearing out of the ground, when the winter is past, it hath a great round brownish head, rising from the middle or sides of the root, which opens itself into sundry leaves one after another, very much crumpled or folded together at the first, and brownish: but afterwards it spreads itself, and becomes smooth, very large and almost round, every one standing on a brownish stalk of the thickness of a man's thumb, when they are grown to their fulness, and most of them two feet and more in length, especially when they grow in any moist or good ground; and the stalk of the leaf, from the bottom thereof to the leaf itself, being also two feet, the breadth thereof from edge to edge, in the broadest place, being also two feet, of a sad or dark green colour, of a fine tart or sourish taste, much more pleasant than the garden or wood sorrel. From among these rise up some, but not every year, strong thick stalks, not growing so high as the Patience, or garden Dock, with such round leaves as grow below, but small at every joint up to the top, and among the flowers, which are white, spreading forth into many branches, consisting of five or six small leaves a-piece, hardly to be discerned from the white threads in the middle, and seeming to be all threads, after which come brownish three square seeds, like unto other Docks, but larger, whereby it may be plainly known to be a Dock. The root grows in time to be very great, with divers and sundry great spreading branches from it, of a dark brownish or reddish colour on the outside, having a pale yellow skin under it, which covers the inner substance or root, which rind and skin being pared away, the root appears of so fresh and lively a colour, with fresh coloured veins running through it, that the choicest of that Rhubarb that is brought us from beyond the seas cannot excel it, which root, if it be dried carefully, and as it ought (which must be in our country by the gentle heat of a fire, in regard the sun is not hot enough here to do it, and every piece kept from touching one another) will hold its colour almost as well as when it is fresh, and has been approved of, and commended by those who have oftentimes used them.

Place.] It grows in gardens, and flowers about the beginning and middle of June, and the seed is ripe in July.

Time.] The roots that are to be dried and kept all the year following, are not to be taken up before the stalk and leaves be quite turned red and gone, and that is not until the middle or end of October, and if they be taken a little before the leaves do spring, or when they are sprung up, the roots will not have half so good a colour in them.

I have given the precedence unto this, because in virtues also it hath the pre-eminence. I come now to describe unto you that which is called Patience, or Monk's Rhubarb; and the next unto that, the great round-leaved Dock, or Bastard Rhubarb, for the one of these may happily supply in the absence of the other, being not much unlike in their virtues, only one more powerful and efficacious than the other. And lastly, shall shew you the virtues of all the three sorts.

GARDEN-PATIENCE, OR MONK'S RHUBARB

Descript.] This is a Dock bearing the name of Rhubarb for some purging quality therein, and grows up with large tall stalks, set with somewhat broad and long, fair, green leaves, not dented at all. The tops of the stalks being divided into many small branches, bear reddish or purplish flowers, and three-square seed, like unto other Docks. The root is long, great and yellow, like unto the wild Docks, but a little redder; and if it be a little dried, shews less store of discoloured veins than the other does when it is dry.

GREAT ROUND-LEAVED DOCK, OR BASTARD RHUBARB

Descript.] This has divers large, round thin yellowish green leaves rising from the root, a little waved about the edges, every one standing upon a reasonably thick and long brownish footstalk, from among which rises up a pretty big stalk, about two feet high, with some such high leaves growing thereon, but smaller; at the top whereof stand in a long spike many small brownish flowers, which turn into a hard three square shining brown seed, like the garden Patience before described. The root grows greater than that, with many branches or great fibres thereat, yellow on the outside, and somewhat pale; yellow within, with some discoloured veins like to the Rhubarb which is first described, but much less than it, especially when it is dry.

Place and Time.] These also grow in gardens, and flower and seed at or near the same time that our true Rhubarb doth, viz. they flower in June, and the seed is ripe in July.

Government and virtues.] Mars claims predominancy over all these wholesome herbs. You cry out upon him for an unfortunate, when God created him for your good (only he is angry with fools). What dishonour is this, not to Mars, but to God himself. A dram of the dried root of Monk's Rhubarb, with a scruple of Ginger made into powder, and taken fasting in a draught or mess of warm broth, purges choler and phlegm downwards very gently and safely without danger. The seed thereof contrary doth bind the belly, and helps to stay any sort of lasks or bloody-flux. The distilled water thereof is very profitably used to heal scabs; also foul ulcerous sores, and to allay the inflammation of them; the juice of the leaves or roots or the decoction of them in vinegar, is used as the most effectual remedy to heal scabs and running sores.

The Bastard Rhubarb hath all the properties of the Monk's Rhubarb, but more effectual for both inward and outward diseases. The decoction thereof without vinegar dropped into the ears, takes away the pains; gargled in the mouth, takes away the tooth ache; and being drank, heals the jaundice. The seed thereof taken, eases the gnawing and griping pains of the stomach, and takes away the loathing thereof unto meat. The root thereof helps the ruggedness of the nails, and being boiled in wine helps the swelling of the throat, commonly called the king's evil, as also the swellings of the kernels of the ears. It helps them that are troubled with the stone, provokes urine, and helps the dimness of the sight. The roots of this Bastard Rhubarb are used in opening and purging diet-drinks, with other things, to open the liver, and to cleanse and cool the blood.

The properties of that which is called the English Rhubarb are the same with the former, but much more effectual, and hath all the properties of the true Italian Rhubarbs, except the force in purging, wherein it is but of half the strength thereof, and therefore a double quantity must be used: it likewise hath not that bitterness and astriction; in other things it works almost in an equal quantity, which are these: It purges the body of choler and phlegm, being either taken of itself, made into powder, and drank in a draught of white wine, or steeped therein all night, and taken fasting, or put among other purges, as shall be thought convenient, cleansing the stomach, liver and blood, opening obstructions, and helping those griefs that come thereof, as the jaundice, dropsy, swelling of the spleen, tertian and daily agues, and pricking pains of the sides; and also stays spitting of blood. The powder taken with cassia dissolved, and washed Venice turpentine, cleanses the reins and strengthens them afterwards, and is very effectual to stay the gonorrhea. It is also given for the pains and swellings in the head, for those that are troubled with melancholy, and helps the sciatica, gout, and the cramp. The powder of the Rhubarb taken with a little mummia and madder roots in some red wine, dissolves clotted blood in the body, happening by any fall or bruise, and helps burstings and broken parts, as well inward as outward. The oil likewise wherein it hath been boiled, works the like effects being anointed. It is used to heal those ulcers that happen in the eyes or eyelids, being steeped and strained; as also to assuage the swellings and inflammations; and applied with honey, boiled in wine, it takes away all blue spots or marks that happen therein. Whey or white wine are the best liquors to steep it in, and thereby it works more effectual in opening obstructions, and purging the stomach and liver. Many do use a little Indian Spikenard as the best corrector thereof.

MEADOW-RUE

Descript.] Meadow-rue rises up with a yellow stringy root, much spreading in the ground, shooting forth new sprouts round about, with many herby green stalks, two feet high, crested all the length of them, set with joints here and there, and many large leaves on them, above as well as below, being divided into smaller leaves, nicked or dented in the forepart of them, of a red green colour on the upper-side, and pale green underneath. Toward the top of the stalk there shoots forth divers short branches, on every one whereof stand two, three or four small heads, or buttons, which breaking the skin that incloses them, shoots forth a tuft of pale greenish yellow threads, which falling away, there come in their places small three-cornered cods, wherein is contained small, long and round seed. The whole plant has a strong unpleasant scent.

Place.] It grows in many places of this land, in the borders of moist meadows, and ditch-sides.

Time.] It flowers about July, or the beginning of August.

Government and virtues.] Dioscorides saith, That this herb bruised and applied, perfectly heals old sores, and the distilled water of the herb and flowers doth the like. It is used by some among other pot-herbs to open the body, and make it soluble; but the roots washed clean, and boiled in ale and drank, provokes to stool more than the leaves, but yet very gently. The root boiled in water, and the places of the body most troubled with vermin and lice washed therewith while it is warm, destroys them utterly. In Italy it is good against the plague, and in Saxony against the jaundice, as *Camerarius* saith.

GARDEN-RUE

GARDEN-RUE is so well known by this name, and the name Herb of Grace, that I shall not need to write any farther description of it, but shall shew you the virtue of it, as follows.

Government and virtues.] It is an herb of the Sun, and under Leo. It provokes urine and women's courses, being taken either in meat or drink. The seed thereof taken in wine, is an antidote against all dangerous medicines or deadly poisons. The leaves taken either by themselves, or with figs and walnuts, is called Mithridate's counter-poison against the plague, and causes all venomous things to become harmless; being often taken in meat and drink it abates venery. A decoction thereof with some dried dill leaves and flowers, eases all pains and torments, inwardly to be drank, and outwardly to be applied warm to the place grieved. The same being drank, helps the pains both of the chest and sides, as also coughs and hardness of breathing, the inflammations of the lungs, and the tormenting pains of the sciatica and the joints, being anointed, or laid to the places; as also the shaking fits of agues, to take a draught before the fit comes. Being boiled or infused in oil, it is good to help the wind cholic, the hardness and windiness of the mother, and frees women from the strangling or suffocation thereof, if the share and the parts thereabouts be anointed therewith. It kills and drives forth the worms of the belly, if it be drank after it is boiled in wine to the half, with a little honey; it helps the gout or pains in the joints, hands, feet or knees, applied thereunto; and with figs it helps the dropsy, being bathed therewith. Being bruised and put into the nostrils, it stays the bleeding thereof. It takes away wheals and pimples, if being bruised with a few myrtle leaves, it be made up with wax, and applied. It cures the morphew, and takes away all sorts of warts, if boiled in wine with some pepper and nitre, and the place rubbed therewith, and with almond and honey helps the dry scabs, or any tetter or ringworm. The juice thereof warmed in a pomegranate shell or rind, and dropped into the ears, helps the pains of them. The juice of it and fennel, with a little honey, and the gall of a cock put thereunto, helps the dimness of the eye-sight. An ointment made of the juice thereof with oil of roses, ceruse, and a little vinegar, and anointed, cures St. Anthony's fire and all running sores in the head: and the stinking ulcers of the nose, or other parts. The antidote used by Mithridates, every morning fasting, to secure himself from any poison or infection, was this: Take twenty leaves of rue, a little salt, a couple of walnuts, and a couple of figs, beaten together into a mess, with twenty juniper berries, which is the quantity appointed for every day. Another electuary is made thus: Take of nitre, pepper, and cummin seed, of each equal parts; of the leaves of Rue clean picked, as much in weight as all the other three weighed; beat them well together, and put as much honey as will make it up into an electuary (but you must first steep your cummin seed in vinegar twenty four hours, and then dry it, or rather roast it in a hot fire-shovel, or in an oven) and is a remedy for the pains or griefs in the chest or stomach, of the spleen, belly, or sides, by wind or stitches; of the liver by obstructions; of the reins and bladder by the stopping of urine; and helps also to extenuate fat corpulent bodies. What an infamy is cast upon the ashes of Mithridates, or Methridates (as the Augustines read his name) by unworthy people. They that deserve no good report themselves, love to give none to others, *viz.* That renowned King of Pontus fortified his body by poison against poison. (*He cast out devils by* Beelzebub, *Prince of the devils.*) What a sot is he that knows not if he had accustomed his body to cold poisons, but poisons would have dispatched him? On the contrary, if not, corrosions would have done it. The whole world is at this present time beholden to him for his studies in physic, and he that uses the quantity but of an hazel-nut of that receipt every morning, to which his name is adjoined, shall to admiration preserve his body in health, if he do but consider that Rue is an herb of the Sun, and under Leo, and gather it and the rest accordingly.

RUPTURE-WORT

Descript.] This spreads very many thready branches round about upon the ground, about a span long, divided into many other smaller parts full of small joints set very thick together, whereat come forth two very small leaves of a French yellow, green coloured branches and all, where grows forth also a number of exceedingly small yellowish flowers, scarce to be discerned from the stalks and leaves, which turn into seeds as small as the very dust. The root is very long and small, thrusting down deep into the ground. This has neither smell nor taste at first, but afterwards has a little astringent taste, without any manifest heat; yet a little bitter and sharp withal.

Place.] It grows in dry, sandy, and rocky places.

Time.] It is fresh and green all the Summer.

Government and virtues.] They say Saturn causes ruptures; if he do, he does no more than he can cure; if you want wit, he will teach you, though to your cost. This herb is Saturn's own, and is a noble antivenerean. Rupture-wort hath not its name in vain: for it is found by experience to cure the rupture, not only in children but also in elder persons, if the disease be not too inveterate, by taking a dram of the powder of the dried herb every day in wine, or a decoction made and drank for certain days together. The juice or distilled water of the green herb, taken in the same manner, helps all other fluxes either of man or woman; vomitings also, and the gonorrhea, being taken any of the ways aforesaid. It doth also most assuredly help those that have the stranguary, or are troubled with the stone or gravel in the reins or bladder. The same also helps stitches in the sides, griping pains of the stomach or belly, the obstructions of the liver, and cures the yellow jaundice; likewise it kills also the worms in children. Being outwardly applied, it conglutinates wounds notably, and helps much to stay defluctions of rheum from the head to the eyes, nose, and teeth, being bruised green and bound thereto; or the forehead, temples, or the nape of the neck behind, bathed with the decoction of the dried herb. It also dries up the moisture of fistulous ulcers, or any other that are foul and spreading.

RUSHES

ALTHOUGH there are many kinds of Rushes, yet I shall only here insist upon those which are best known, and most medicinal; as the bulrushes, and other of the soft and smooth kinds, which grow so commonly in almost every part of this land, and are so generally noted, that I suppose it needless to trouble you with any description of them. Briefly then take the virtues of them as follows.

Government and virtues.] The seed of the soft Rushes, (saith Dioscorides and Galen, toasted, saith Pliny) being drank in wine and water, stays the lask and women's courses, when they come down too abundantly: but it causes head-ache; it provokes sleep likewise, but must be given with caution. The root boiled in water, to the consumption of one third, helps the cough.

Thus you see that conveniences have their inconveniences, and virtue is seldom unaccompanied with some vices. What I have written concerning Rushes, is to satisfy my countrymen's questions: *Are our Rushes good for nothing?* Yes, and as good let them alone as taken. There are remedies enough without them for any disease, and therefore as the proverb is, I care not a rush for them; or rather they will do you as much good as if one had given you a Rush.

RYE

This is so well known in all the countries of this land, and especially to the country-population distributed thereon, that if I did describe it, they would presently say, I might as well have spared that labour. Its virtue follows.

Government and virtues.] Rye is more digesting than wheat; the bread and the leaven thereof ripens and breaks imposthumes, boils, and other swellings. The meal of Rye put between a double cloth, and moistened with a little vinegar, and heated in a pewter dish, set over a chafing dish of coals, and bound fast to the head while it is hot, doth much ease the continual pains of the head. Matthiolus saith, that the ashes of Rye straw put into water, and steeped therein a day and a night, and the chops of the hands or feet washed therewith, doth heal them.

SAFFRON

The herb needs no description, it being known generally where it grows.

Place.] It grows frequently at Walden in Essex, and in Cambridgeshire.

Government and virtues.] It is an herb of the Sun, and under the Lion, and therefore you need not demand a reason why it strengthens the heart so exceedingly. Let not above ten grains be given at one time, for the Sun, which is the fountain of light, may dazzle the eyes and make them blind; a cordial being taken in an immoderate quantity, hurts the heart instead of helping it. It quickens the brain, for the Sun is exalted in Aries, as he hath his house in Leo. It helps consumptions of the lungs, and difficulty of breathing. It is excellent in epidemical diseases, as pestilence, small-pox, and measles. It is a notable expulsive medicine, and a notable remedy for the yellow jaundice. My opinion is, (but I have no author for it) that hermodactyls are nothing else but the roots of Saffron dried; and my reason is, that the roots of all crocus, both white and yellow, purge phlegm as hermodactyls do; and if you please to dry the roots of any crocus, neither your eyes nor your taste shall distinguish them from hermodactyls.

SAGE

Our ordinary garden Sage needs no description.

Time.] It flowers in or about July.

Government and virtues.] Jupiter claims this, and bids me tell you, it is good for the liver, and to breed blood. A decoction of the leaves and branches of Sage made and drank, saith Dioscorides, provokes urine, brings down women's courses, helps to expel the dead child, and causes the hair to become black. It stays the bleeding of wounds, and cleanses foul ulcers. Three spoonfuls of the juice of Sage taken fasting, with a little honey, doth presently stay the spitting or casting of blood of them that are in a consumption. These pills are much commended: Take of spikenard, ginger, of each two drams; of the seed of Sage toasted at the fire, eight drams; of long pepper, twelve drams; all these being brought into powder, put thereto so much juice of Sage as may make them into a mass of pills, taking a dram of them every morning fasting, and so likewise at night, drinking a little pure water after them. Matthiolus saith, it is very profitable for all manner of pains in the head coming of cold and rheumatic humours: as also for all pains of the joints, whether inwardly or outwardly, and therefore helps the falling-sickness, the lethargy such as are dull and heavy of spirit, the palsy; and is of much use in all defluctions of rheum from the head, and for the diseases of the chest or breast. The leaves of Sage and nettles bruised together, and laid upon the imposthume that rises behind the ears, doth assuage it much. The juice of Sage taken in warm water, helps a hoarseness and a cough. The leaves sodden in wine, and laid upon the place affected with the palsy, helps much, if the decoction be drank. Also Sage taken with wormwood is good for the bloody-flux. Pliny saith, it procures women's courses, and stays them coming down too fast; helps the stinging and biting of serpents, and kills the worms that breed in the ear, and in sores. Sage is of excellent use to help the memory, warming and quickening the senses; and the conserve made of the flowers is used to the same purpose, and also for all the former recited diseases. The juice of Sage drank with vinegar, hath been of good use in time of the plague at all times. Gargles likewise are made with Sage, rosemary, honey-suckles, and plantain, boiled in wine or water, with some honey or allum put thereto, to wash sore mouths and throats, cankers, or the secret parts of man or woman, as need requires. And with other hot and comfortable herbs. Sage is boiled to bathe the body and the legs in the Summer time, especially to warm cold joints, or sinews, troubled with the palsy and cramp, and to comfort and strengthen the parts. It is much commended against the stitch, or pains in the side coming of wind, if the place be fomented warm with the decoction thereof in wine, and the herb also after boiling be laid warm thereunto.

WOOD-SAGE

Descript.] Wood-sage rises up with square hoary stalks, two feet high at the least, with two leaves set at every joint, somewhat like other Sage leaves, but smaller, softer, whiter, and rounder, and a little dented about the edges, and smelling somewhat stronger. At the tops of the stalks and branches stand the flowers, on a slender like spike, turning themselves all one way when they blow, and are of a pale and whitish colour, smaller than Sage, but hooded and gaping like unto them. The seed is blackish and round; four usually seem in a husk together: the root is long and stringy, with divers fibres thereat, and abides many years.

Place.] It grows in woods, and by wood-sides; as also in divers fields and bye-lanes in the land.

Time.] It flowers in June, July, and August.

Government and virtues.] The herb is under Venus. The decoction of the Wood Sage provokes urine and women's courses. It also provokes sweat, digests humours, and discusses swellings and nodes in the flesh, and is therefore thought to be good against the French pox. The decoction of the green herb, made with wine, is a safe and sure remedy for those who by falls, bruises, or blows, suspect some vein to be inwardly broken, to disperse and void the congealed blood, and to consolidate the veins. The drink used inwardly, and the herb used outwardly, is good for such as are inwardly or outwardly bursten, and is found to be a sure remedy for the palsy. The juice of the herb, or the powder thereof dried, is good for moist ulcers and sores in the legs, and other parts, to dry them, and cause them to heal more speedily. It is no less effectual also in green wounds, to be used upon any occasion.

SOLOMON'S SEAL

Descript.] The common Solomon's Seal rises up with a round stalk half a yard high, bowing or bending down to the ground, set with single leaves one above another, somewhat large, and like the leaves of the lily-convally, or May-lily, with an eye of bluish upon the green, with some ribs therein, and more yellowish underneath. At the foot of every leaf, almost from the bottom up to the top of the stalk, come forth small, long, white and hollow pendulous flowers, somewhat like the flowers of May-lily, but ending in five long points, for the most part two together, at the end of a long foot-stalk, and sometimes but one, and sometimes also two stalks, and flowers at the foot of a leaf, which are without any scent at all, and stand on the top of the stalk. After they are past, come in their places small round berries great at the first, and blackish green, tending to blueness when they are ripe, wherein lie small, white, hard, and stony seeds. The root is of the thickness of one's finger or thumb, white and knotted in some places, a flat round circle representing a Seal, whereof it took the name, lying along under the upper crust of the earth, and not growing downward, but with many fibres underneath.

Place.] It is frequent in divers places of this land; as, namely in a wood two miles from Canterbury, by Fish-Pool Hill, as also in Bushy Close belonging to the parsonage of Alderbury, near Clarendon, two miles from Salisbury: in Cheffon wood, on Chesson Hill, between Newington and Sittingbourne in Kent, and divers other places in Essex, and other counties.

Time.] It flowers about May. The root abides and shoots a-new every year.

Government and virtues.] Saturn owns the plant, for he loves his bones well. The root of Solomon's Seal is found by experience to be available in wounds, hurts, and outward sores, to heal and close up the lips of those that are green, and to dry up and restrain the flux of humours to those that are old. It is singularly good to stay vomitings and bleeding wheresoever, as also all fluxes in man or woman; also, to knit any joint, which by weakness uses to be often out of place, or will not stay in long when it is set; also to knit and join broken bones in any part of the body, the roots being bruised and applied to the places; yea, it hath been found by experience, and the decoction of the root in wine, or the bruised root put into wine or other drink, and after a night's infusion, strained forth hard and drank, hath helped both man and beast, whose bones hath been broken by any occasion, which is the most assured refuge of help to people of divers counties of the land that they can have. It is no less effectual to help ruptures and burstings, the decoction in wine, or the powder in broth or drink, being inwardly taken, and outwardly applied to the place. The same is also available for inward or outward bruises, falls or blows, both to dispel the congealed blood, and to take away both the pains and the black and blue marks that abide after the hurt. The same also, or the distilled water of the whole plant, used to the face, or other parts of the skin, cleanses it from morphew, freckles, spots, or marks whatsoever, leaving the place fresh, fair, and lovely; for which purpose it is much used by the Italian Dames.

SAMPHIRE

Descript.] Rock Samphire grows up with a tender green stalk about half a yard, or two feet high at the most, branching forth almost from the very bottom, and stored with sundry thick and almost round (somewhat long) leaves of a deep green colour, sometimes two together, and sometimes more on a stalk, and sappy, and of a pleasant, hot, and spicy taste. At the top of the stalks and branches stand umbels of white flowers, and after them come large seed, bigger than fennel seed, yet somewhat like it. The root is great, white, and long, continuing many years, and is of an hot and spicy taste likewise.

Place.] It grows on the rocks that are often moistened at the least, if not overflowed with the sea water.

Time.] And it flowers and seeds in the end of July and August.

Government and virtues.] It is an herb of Jupiter, and was in former times wont to be used more than now it is; the more is the pity. It is well known almost to every body, that ill digestions and obstructions are the cause of most of the diseases which the frail nature of man is subject to; both which might be remedied by a more frequent use of this herb. If people would have sauce to their meat, they may take some for profit as well as for pleasure. It is a safe herb, very pleasant both to taste and stomach, helps digestion, and in some sort opening obstructions of the liver and spleen: provokes urine, and helps thereby to wash away the gravel and stone engendered in the kidneys or bladder.

SANICLE

This herb is by many called Butter-wort.

Descript.] Ordinary Sanicle sends forth many great round leaves, standing upon long brownish stalks, every one somewhat deeply cut or divided into five or six parts, and some of these also cut in somewhat like the leaf of crow's-foot, or dove's-foot, and finely dented about the edges, smooth, and of a dark shining colour, and somewhat reddish about the brims; from among which arise up small, round green stalks, without any joint or leaf thereon, saving at the top, where it branches forth into flowers, having a leaf divided into three or four parts at that joint with the flowers, which are small and white, starting out of small round greenish yellow heads, many standing together in a tuft, in which afterwards are the seeds contained, which are small round burs, somewhat like the leaves of clevers, and stick in the same manner upon any thing that they touch. The root is composed of many blackish strings or fibres, set together at a little long head, which abides with green leaves all the Winter, and perishes not.

Place.] It is found in many shadowy woods, and other places of this land.

Time.] It flowers in June, and the seed is ripe shortly after.

Government and virtues.] This is one of Venus's herbs, to cure the wounds or mischiefs Mars inflicts upon the body of man. It heals green wounds speedily, or any ulcers, imposthumes, or bleedings inward, also tumours in any part of the body; for the decoction or powder in drink taken, and the juice used outwardly, dissipates the humours: and there is not found any herb that can give such present help either to man or beast, when the disease falleth upon the lungs or throat, and to heal up putrid malignant ulcers in the mouth, throat, and privities, by gargling or washing with the decoction of the leaves and roots made in water, and a little honey put thereto. It helps to stay women's courses, and all other fluxes of blood, either by the mouth, urine, or stool, and lasks of the belly; the ulcerations of the kidneys also, and the pains in the bowels, and gonorrhea, being boiled in wine or water, and drank. The same also is no less powerful to help any ruptures or burstings, used both inwardly and outwardly. And briefly, it is as effectual in binding, restraining, consolidating, heating, drying and healing, as comfrey, bugle, self-heal, or any other of the vulnerary herbs whatsoever.

SARACEN'S CONFOUND, OR SARACEN'S WOUNDWORT

Descript.] This grows sometimes, with brownish stalks, and other whiles with green, to a man's height, having narrow green leaves snipped about the edges, somewhat like those of the peach-tree, or willow leaves, but not of such a white green colour. The tops of the stalks are furnished with many yellow star-like flowers, standing in green heads, which when they are fallen, and the seed ripe, which is somewhat long, small and of a brown colour, wrapped in down, is therefore carried away with the wind. The root is composed of fibres set together at a head, which perishes not in Winter, although the stalks dry away and no leaf appears in the Winter. The taste hereof is strong and unpleasant; and so is the smell also.

Place.] It grows in moist and wet grounds, by wood-sides, and sometimes in moist places of shadowy groves, as also by the water side.

Time.] It flowers in July, and the seed is soon ripe, and carried away with the wind.

Government and virtues.] Saturn owns the herb, and it is of a sober condition, like him. Among the Germans, this wound herb is preferred before all others of the same quality. Being boiled in wine, and drank, it helps the indisposition of the liver, and freeth the gall from obstructions; whereby it is good for the yellow jaundice and for the dropsy in the beginning of it, for all inward ulcers of the reins, mouth or throat, and inward wounds and bruises, likewise for such sores as happen in the privy parts of men and women; being steeped in wine, and then distilled, the water thereof drank, is singularly good to ease all gnawings in the stomach, or other pains of the body, as also the pains of the mother: and being boiled in water, it helps continual agues; and the said water, or the simple water of the herb distilled, or the juice or decoction, are very effectual to heal any green wound, or old sore or ulcer whatsoever, cleansing them from corruption, and quickly healing them up. Briefly, whatsoever hath been said of bugle or sanicle, may be found herein.

SAUCE-ALONE, OR JACK-BY-THE-HEDGE-SIDE

Descript.] The lower leaves of this are rounder than those that grow towards the top of the stalks, and are set singly on a joint being somewhat round and broad, pointed at the ends, dented also about the edges, somewhat resembling nettle leaves for the form, but of a fresher green colour, not rough or pricking. The flowers are white, growing at the top of the stalks one above another, which being past, follow small round pods, wherein are contained round seed somewhat blackish. The root stringy and thready, perishes every year after it hath given seed, and raises itself again of its own sowing. The plant, or any part thereof, being bruised, smells of garlic, but more pleasantly, and tastes somewhat hot and sharp, almost like unto rocket.

Place.] It grows under walls, and by hedge-sides, and path-ways in fields in many places.

Time.] It flowers in June, July, and August.

Government and virtues.] It is an herb of Mercury. This is eaten by many country people as sauce to their salt fish, and helps well to digest the crudities and other corrupt humours engendered thereby. It warms also the stomach, and causes digestion. The juice thereof boiled with honey is accounted to be as good as hedge mustard for the cough, to cut and expectorate the tough phlegm. The seed bruised and boiled in wine, is a singularly good remedy for the wind colic, or the stone, being drank warm. It is also given to women troubled with the mother, both to drink, and the seed put into a cloth, and applied while it is warm, is of singularly good use. The leaves also, or the seed boiled, is good to be used in clysters to ease the pains of the stone. The green leaves are held to be good to heal the ulcers in the legs.

WINTER AND SUMMER SAVOURY

BOTH these are so well known (being entertained as constant inhabitants in our gardens) that they need no description.

Government and virtues.] Mercury claims dominion over this herb, neither is there a better remedy against the colic and iliac passion, than this herb; keep it dry by you all the year, if you love yourself and your ease, and it is a hundred pounds to a penny if you do not; keep it dry, make conserves and syrups of it for your use, and withal, take notice that the Summer kind is the best. They are both of them hot and dry, especially the Summer kind, which is both sharp and quick in taste, expelling wind in the stomach and bowels, and is a present help for the rising of the mother procured by wind; provokes urine and women's courses, and is much commended for women with child to take inwardly, and to smell often unto. It cures tough phlegm in the chest and lungs, and helps to expectorate it the more easily; quickens the dull spirits in the lethargy, the juice thereof being snuffed up into the nostrils. The juice dropped into the eyes, clears a dull sight, if it proceed of thin cold humours distilled from the brain. The juice heated with the oil of Roses, and dropped into the ears, eases them of the noise and singing in them, and of deafness also. Outwardly applied with wheat flour, in manner of a poultice, it gives ease to the sciatica and palsied members, heating and warming them, and takes away their pains. It also takes away the pains that come by stinging of bees, wasps, &c.

SAVINE

To describe a plant so well known is needless, it being nursed up almost in every garden, and abides green all the Winter.

Government and virtues.] It is under the dominion of Mars, being hot and dry in the third degree, and being of exceeding clean parts, is of a very digesting quality. If you dry the herb into powder, and mix it with honey, it is an excellent remedy to cleanse old filthy ulcers and fistulas; but it hinders them from healing. The same is excellently good to break carbuncles and plague-sores; also helps the king's evil, being applied to the place. Being spread over a piece of leather, and applied to the navel, kills the worms in the belly, helps scabs and itch, running sores, cankers, tetters, and ringworms; and being applied to the place, may haply cure venereal sores. This I thought good to speak of, as it may be safely used outwardly, for inwardly it cannot be taken without manifest danger.

THE COMMON WHITE SAXIFRAGE

Descript.] This hath a few small reddish kernels of roots covered with some skins, lying among divers small blackish fibres, which send forth divers round, faint or yellow green leaves, and greyish underneath, lying above the grounds, unevenly dented about the edges, and somewhat hairy, every one upon a little foot-stalk, from whence rises up round, brownish, hairy, green stalks, two or three feet high, with a few such like round leaves as grow below, but smaller, and somewhat branched at the top, whereon stand pretty large white flowers of five leaves a-piece, with some yellow threads in the middle, standing in a long crested, brownish green husk. After the flowers are past, there arises sometimes a round hard head, forked at the top, wherein is contained small black seed, but usually they fall away without any seed, and it is the kernels or grains of the root which are usually called the White Saxifrage-seed, and so used.

Place.] It grows in many places of our land, as well in the lowermost, as in the upper dry corners of meadows, and grassy sandy places. It used to grow near Lamb's conduit, on the backside of Gray's Inn.

Time.] It flowers in May, and then gathered, as well for that which is called the seed, as to distil, for it quickly perishes down to the ground when any hot weather comes.

Government and virtues.] It is very effectual to cleanse the reins and bladder, and to dissolve the stone engendered in them, and to expel it and the gravel by urine; to help the stranguary; for which purpose the decoction of the herb or roots in white wine, is most usual, or the powder of the small kernelly root, which is called the seed, taken in white wine, or in the same decoction made with white wine, is most usual. The distilled water of the whole herb, root and flowers, is most familiar to be taken. It provokes also women's courses, and frees and cleanses the stomach and lungs from thick and tough phlegm that trouble them. There are not many better medicines to break the stone than this.

BURNET SAXIFRAGE

Descript.] The greater sort of our English Burnet Saxifrage grows up with divers long stalks of winged leaves, set directly opposite one to another on both sides, each being somewhat broad, and a little pointed and dented about the edges, of a sad green colour. At the top of the stalks stand umbels of white flowers, after which come small and blackish seed. The root is long and whitish, abiding long. Our lesser Burnet Saxifrage hath much finer leaves than the former, and very small, and set one against another, deeply jagged about the edges, and of the same colour as the former. The umbels of the flowers are white, and the seed very small, and so is the root, being also somewhat hot and quick in taste.

Place.] These grow in moist meadows of this land, and are easy to be found being well sought for among the grass, wherein many times they lay hid scarcely to be discerned.

Time.] They flower about July, and their seed is ripe in August.

Government and virtues.] They are both of them herbs of the Moon. The Saxifrages are hot as pepper; and Tragus saith, by his experience, that they are wholesome. They have the same properties the parsleys have, but in provoking urine, and causing the pains thereof, and of the wind and colic, are much more effectual, the roots or seed being used either in powder, or in decoctions, or any other way; and likwise helps the windy pains of the mother, and to procure their courses, and to break and void the stone in the kidneys, to digest cold, viscous, and tough phlegm in the stomach, and is an especial remedy against all kind of venom. Castoreum being boiled in the distilled water thereof, is singularly good to be given to those that are troubled with cramps and convulsions. Some do use to make the seeds into comfits (as they do carraway seeds) which is effectual to all the purposes aforesaid. The juice of the herb dropped into the most grievous wounds of the head, dries up their moisture, and heals them quickly. Some women use the distilled water to take away freckles or spots in the skin or face; and to drink the same sweetened with sugar for all the purposes aforesaid.

SCABIOUS, THREE SORTS

Descript.] Common field Scabious grows up with many hairy, soft, whitish green leaves, some whereof are very little, if at all jagged on the edges, others very much rent and torn on the sides, and have threads in them, which upon breaking may be plainly seen; from among which rise up divers hairy green stalks, three or four feet high, with such like hairy green leaves on them, but more deeply and finely divided and branched forth a little. At the tops thereof, which are naked and bare of leaves for a good space, stand round heads of flowers, of a pale blueish colour, set together in a head, the outermost whereof are larger than the inward, with many threads also in the middle, somewhat flat at the top, as the head with the seed is likewise; the root is great, white and thick, growing down deep into the ground, and abides many years.

There is another sort of Field Scabious different in nothing from the former, but only it is smaller in all respects.

The Corn Scabious differs little from the first, but that it is greater in all respects, and the flowers more inclining to purple, and the root creeps under the upper crust of the earth, and runs not deep into the ground as the first doth.

Place.] The first grows more usually in meadows, especially about London every where.

The second in some of the dry fields about this city, but not so plentifully as the former.

The third in standing corn, or fallow fields, and the borders of such like fields.

Time.] They flower in June and July, and some abide flowering until it be late in August, and the seed is ripe in the mean time.

There are many other sorts of Scabious, but I take these which I have here described to be most familiar with us. The virtues of both these and the rest, being much alike, take them as follow.

Government and virtues.] Mercury owns the plant. Scabious is very effectual for all sorts of coughs, shortness of breath, and all other diseases of the breast and lungs, ripening and digesting cold phlegm, and other tough humours, voids them forth by coughing and spitting. It ripens also all sorts of inward ulcers and imposthumes; pleurisy also, if the decoction of the herb dry or green be made in wine, and drank for some time together. Four ounces of the clarified juice of Scabious taken in the morning fasting, with a dram of mithridate, or Venice treacle, frees the heart from any infection of pestilence, if after the taking of it the party sweat two hours in bed, and this medicine be again and again repeated, if need require. The green herb bruised and applied to any carbuncle or plague sore, is found by certain experience to dissolve and break it in three hours space. The same decoction also drank, helps the pains and stitches in the side. The decoction of the roots taken for forty days together, or a dram of the powder of them taken at a time in whey, doth (as Matthiolus saith) wonderfully help those that are troubled with running or spreading scabs, tetters, ringworms, yea, although they proceed from the French pox, which, he saith he hath tried by experience. The juice or decoction drank, helps also scabs and breakings-out of the itch, and the like. The juice also made up into an ointment and used, is effectual for the same purpose. The same also heals all inward wounds by the drying, cleansing and healing quality therein. And a syrup made of the juice and sugar, is very effectual to all the purposes aforesaid, and so is the distilled water of the herb and flowers made in due season, especially to be used when the green herb is not in force to be taken. The decoction of the herb and roots outwardly applied, doth wonderfully help all sorts of hard or cold swellings in any part of the body, is effectual for shrunk sinews or veins, and heals green wounds, old sores, and ulcers. The juice of Scabious, made up with the powder of Borax and Samphire, cleanses the skin of the face, or other parts of the body, not only from freckles and pimples, but also from morphew and leprosy; the head washed with the decoction, cleanses it from dandriff, scurf, sores, itch, and the like, used warm. The herb bruised and applied, doth in a short time loosen, and draw forth any splinter, broken bone, arrow head, or other such like thing lying in the flesh.

SCURVYGRASS

Descript.] The ordinary English Scurvygrass hath many thick flat leaves, more long than broad, and sometimes longer and narrower; sometimes also smooth on the edges, and sometimes a little waved; sometimes plain, smooth and pointed, of a sad green, and sometimes a blueish colour, every one standing by itself upon a long foot-stalk, which is brownish or greenish also, from among which arise many slender stalks, bearing few leaves thereon like the other, but longer and less for the most part. At the tops whereof grow many whitish flowers, with yellow threads in the middle, standing about a green head, which becomes the seed vessel, which will be somewhat flat when it is ripe, wherein is contained reddish seed, tasting somewhat hot. The root is made of many white strings, which stick deeply into the mud, wherein it chiefly delights, yet it will well abide in the more upland and drier ground, and tastes a little brackish and salt even there, but not so much as where it hath the salt water to feed upon.

Place.] It grows all along the Thames sides, both on the Essex and Kentish shores, from Woolwich round about the sea coasts to Dover, Portsmouth, and even to Bristol, where it is had in plenty;

the other with round leaves grows in the marshes in Holland, in Lincolnshire, and other places of Lincolnshire by the sea side.

Descript.] There is also another sort called Dutch Scurvygrass, which is most known, and frequent in gardens, which has fresh, green, and almost round leaves rising from the root, not so thick as the former, yet in some rich ground, very large, even twice as big as in others, not dented about the edges, or hollow in the middle, standing on a long foot-stalk; from among these rise long, slender stalks, higher than the former, with more white flowers at the tops of them, which turn into small pods, and smaller brownish seed than the former. The root is white, small and thready. The taste is nothing salt at all; it hath a hot, aromatical spicy taste.

Time.] It flowers in April and May, and gives seed ripe quickly after.

Government and virtues.] It is an herb of Jupiter. The English Scurvygrass is more used for the salt taste it bears, which doth somewhat open and cleanse; but the Dutch Scurvygrass is of better effect, and chiefly used (if it may be had) by those that have the scurvy, and is of singular good effect to cleanse the blood, liver, and spleen, taking the juice in the Spring every morning fasting in a cup of drink. The decoction is good for the same purpose, and opens obstructions, evacuating cold, clammy and phlegmatic humours both from the liver and the spleen, and bringing the body to a more lively colour. The juice also helps all foul ulcers and sores in the mouth, gargled therewith; and used outwardly, cleanses the skin from spots, marks, or scars that happen therein.

SELF-HEAL

Descript.] The common Self-heal which is called also Prunel, Carpenter's Herb, Hook-heal, and Sickle-wort, is a small, low, creeping herb, having many small, roundish pointed leaves, like leaves of wild mints, of a dark green colour, without dents on the edges; from among which rise square hairy stalks, scarce a foot high, which spread sometimes into branches with small leaves set thereon, up to the top, where stand brown spiked heads of small brownish leaves like scales and flowers set together, almost like the heads of Cassidony, which flowers are gaping, and of a blueish purple, or more pale blue, in some places sweet, but not so in others. The root consists of many fibres downward, and spreading strings also whereby it increases. The small stalks, with the leaves creeping on the ground, shoot forth fibres taking hold on the ground, whereby it is made a great tuft in a short time.

Place.] It is found in woods and fields everywhere.

Time.] It flowers in May, and sometimes in April.

Government and virtues.] Here is another herb of Venus, Self-heal, whereby when you are hurt you may heal yourself. It is a special herb for inward and outward wounds. Take it inwardly in syrups for inward wounds: outwardly in unguents, and plaisters for outward. As Self-heal is like Bugle in form, so also in the qualities and virtues, serving for all the purposes whereto Bugle is applied to with good success, either inwardly or outwardly, for inward wounds or ulcers whatsoever within the body, for bruises or falls, and such like hurts. If it be accompanied with Bugle, Sanicle, and other the like wound herbs, it will be more effectual to wash or inject into ulcers in the parts outwardly. Where there is cause to repress the heat and sharpness of humours flowing to any sore, ulcers, inflammations, swellings, or the like, or to stay the fluxes of blood in any wound or part, this is used with some good success; as also to cleanse the foulness of sores, and cause them more speedily to be healed. It is an especial remedy for all green wounds, to solder the lips of them, and to keep the place from any further inconveniencies. The juice hereof used with oil of roses to anoint the temples and forehead, is very effectual to remove head ache, and the same mixed with honey of roses, cleanses and heals all ulcers, in the mouth, and throat, and those also in the secret parts. And the proverb of the Germans, French, and others, is verified in this, *That he needs neither physician nor surgeon that hath* Self-heal *and* Sanicle *to help himself.*

THE SERVICE-TREE

It is so well known in the place where it grows, that it needs no description.

Time.] It flowers before the end of May, and the fruit is ripe in October.

Government and virtues.] Services, when they are mellow, are fit to be taken to stay fluxes, scouring, and casting, yet less than medlers. If they be dried before they be mellow, and kept all the year, they may be used in decoctions for the said purpose, either to drink, or to bathe the parts requiring it; and are profitably used in that manner to stay the bleeding of wounds, and of the mouth or nose, to be applied to the forehead and nape of the neck; and are under the dominion of Saturn.

SHEPHERD'S PURSE

It is called Whoreman's Permacety, Shepherd's Scrip, Shepherd's Pounce, Toywort, Pickpurse, and Casewort.

Descript.] The root is small, white, and perishes every year. The leaves are small and long, of a pale green colour, and deeply cut in on both sides, among which spring up a stalk which is small and round, containing small leaves upon it even to the top. The flowers are white and very small; after which come the little cases which hold the seed, which are flat, almost in the form of a heart.

Place.] They are frequent in this nation, almost by every pathside.

Time.] They flower all the Summer long; nay some of them are so fruitful, that they flower twice a year.

Government and virtues.] It is under the dominion of Saturn, and of a cold, dry, and binding nature, like to him. It helps all fluxes of blood, either caused by inward or outward wounds; as also flux of the belly, and bloody flux, spitting blood, and bloody urine, stops the terms in women; being bound to the wrists of the hands, and the soles of the feet, it helps the yellow jaundice. The herb being made into a poultice, helps inflammations and St. Anthony's fire. The juice being dropped into the ears, heals the pains, noise, and mutterings thereof. A good ointment may be made of it for all wounds, especially wounds in the head.

SMALLAGE

THIS is also very well known, and therefore I shall not trouble the reader with any description thereof.

Place.] It grows naturally in dry and marshy ground; but if it be sown in gardens, it there prospers very well.

Time.] It abides green all the Winter, and seeds in August.

Government and virtues.] It is an herb of Mercury. Smallage is hotter, drier, and much more medicinal than parsley, for it much more opens obstructions of the liver and spleen, rarefies thick phlegm, and cleanses it and the blood withal. It provokes urine and women's courses, and is singularly good against the yellow jaundice, tertian and quartan agues, if the juice thereof be taken, but especially made up into a syrup. The juice also put to honey of roses, and barley-water, is very good to gargle the mouth and throat of those that have sores and ulcers in them, and will quickly heal them. The same lotion also cleanses and heals all other foul ulcers and cankers elsewhere, if they be washed therewith. The seed is especially used to break and expel wind, to kill worms, and to help a stinking breath. The root is effectual to all the purposes aforesaid, and is held to be stronger in operation than the herb, but especially to open obstructions, and to rid away any ague, if the juice thereof be taken in wine, or the decoction thereof in wine used.

SOPEWORT, OR BRUISEWORT

Descript.] The roots creep under ground far and near, with many joints therein, of a brown colour on the outside and yellowish within, shooting forth in divers places weak round stalks, full of joints, set with two leaves a-piece at every one of them on a contrary side, which are ribbed somewhat like to plantain, and fashioned like the common field white campion leaves, seldom having any branches from the sides of the stalks, but set with flowers at the top, standing in long husks like the wild campions, made of five leaves a-piece, round at the ends, and dented in the middle, of a rose colour, almost white, sometimes deeper, sometimes paler; of a reasonable scent.

Place.] It grows wild in many low and wet grounds of this land, by brooks and the sides of running waters.

Time.] It flowers usually in July, and so continues all August, and part of September, before they be quite spent.

Government and virtues.] Venus owns it. The country people in divers places do use to bruise the leaves of Sopewort, and lay it to their fingers, hands or legs, when they are cut, to heal them up again. Some make great boast thereof, that it is diuretical to provoke urine, and thereby to expel gravel and the stone in the reins or kidneys, and do also account it singularly good to void hydropical waters: and they no less extol it to perform an absolute cure in the French pox, more than either sarsaparilla, guiacum, or China can do; which, how true it is, I leave others to judge.

SORREL

OUR ordinary Sorrel, which grows in gardens, and also wild in the fields, is so well known, that it needs no description.

Government and virtues.] It is under the dominion of Venus. Sorrel is prevalent in all hot diseases, to cool any inflammation and heat of blood in agues pestilential or choleric, or sickness and fainting, arising from heat, and to refresh the overspent spirits with the violence of furious or fiery fits of agues; to quench thirst, and procure an appetite in fainting or decaying stomachs. For it resists the putrefaction of the blood, kills worms, and is a cordial to the heart, which the seed doth more effectually, being more drying and binding, and thereby stays the hot fluxes of women's courses, or of humours in the bloody flux, or flux of the stomach. The root also in a decoction, or in powder, is effectual for all the said purposes. Both roots and seeds, as well as the herb, are held powerful to resist the poison of the scorpion. The decoction of the roots is taken to help the jaundice, and to expel the gravel and the stone in the reins or kidneys. The decoction of the flowers made with wine and drank, helps the black jaundice, as also the inward ulcers of the body and bowels. A syrup made with the juice of Sorrel and fumitory, is a sovereign help to kill those sharp humours that cause the itch. The juice thereof, with a little vinegar, serves well to be used outwardly for the same cause, and is also profitable for tetters, ringworms, &c. It helps also to discuss the kernels in the throat; and the juice gargled in the mouth, helps the sores therein. The leaves wrapt in a colewort leaf and roasted in the embers, and applied to a hard imposthume, botch, boil, or plague sore, doth both ripen and break it. The distilled water of the herb is of much good use for all the purposes aforesaid.

WOOD SORREL

Descript.] This grows upon the ground, having a number of leaves coming from the root made of three leaves like a trefoil but broad at the ends, and cut in the middle, of a yellowish green colour, every one standing on a long foot-stalk, which at their first coming up are close folded together to the stalk, but opening themselves afterwards, and are of a fine sour relish, and yielding a juice which will turn red when it is clarified, and makes a most dainty clear syrup. Among these leaves rise up divers slender, weak foot-stalks, with every one of them a flower at the top, consisting of five small pointed leaves, star-fashion, of a white colour, in most places, and in some dashed over with a small show of blueish, on the back side only. After the flowers are past, follow small round heads, with small yellowish seed in them. The roots are nothing but small strings fastened to the end of a small long piece; all of them being of a yellowish colour.

Place.] It grows in many places of our land, in woods and wood-sides, where they be moist and shadowed, and in other places not too much upon the Sun.

Time.] It flowers in April and May.

Government and virtues.] Venus owns it. Wood Sorrel serves to all the purposes that the other Sorrels do, and is more effectual in hindering putrefaction of blood, and ulcers in the mouth and body, and to quench thirst, to strengthen a weak stomach, to procure an appetite, to stay vomiting, and very excellent in any contagious sickness or pestilential fevers. The syrup made of the juice, is effectual in all the cases aforesaid, and so is the distilled water of the herb. Sponges or linen cloths wet in the juice and applied out-wardly to any hot swelling or inflammations, doth much cool and help them. The same juice taken and gargled in the mouth, and after it is spit forth, taken afresh, doth wonderfully help a foul stinking canker or ulcer therein. It is singularly good to heal wounds, or to stay the bleeding of thrusts or scabs in the body.

SOW THISTLE

Sow Thistles are generally so well known, that they need no description.

Place.] They grow in gardens and manured grounds, sometimes by old walls, pathsides of fields, and high ways.

Government and virtues.] This and the former are under the influence of Venus. Sow Thistles are cooling, and somewhat binding, and are very fit to cool a hot stomach, and ease the pains thereof. The herb boiled in wine, is very helpful to stay the dissolution of the stomach, and the milk that is taken from the stalks when they are broken, given in drink, is beneficial to those that are short winded, and have a wheezing. Pliny saith, That it hath caused the gravel and stone to be voided by urine, and that the eating thereof helps a stinking breath. The decoction of the leaves and stalks causes abundance of milk in nurses, and their children to be well coloured. The juice or distilled water is good for all hot inflammations, wheals, and eruptions or heat in the skin, itching of the hæmorrhoids. The juice boiled or thoroughly heated in a little oil of bitter almonds in the peel of a pomegranate, and dropped into the ears, is a sure remedy for deafness, singings, &c. Three spoonfuls of the juice taken, warmed in white wine, and some wine put thereto, causes women in travail to have so easy and speedy a delivery, that they may be able to walk presently after. It is wonderful good for women to wash their faces with, to clear the skin, and give it a lustre.

SOUTHERN WOOD

SOUTHERN WOOD is so well known to be an ordinary inhabitant in our gardens, that I shall not need to trouble you with any description thereof.

Time.] It flowers for the most part in July and August.

Government and virtues.] It is a gallant mercurial plant, worthy of more esteem than it hath. Dioscorides saith, That the seed bruised, heated in warm water, and drank, helps those that are bursten, or troubled with cramps or convulsions of the sinews, the sciatica, or difficulty in making water, and bringing down women's courses. The same taken in wine is an antidote, or counter-poison against all deadly poison, and drives away serpents and other venomous creatures; as also the smell of the herb, being burnt, doth the same. The oil thereof anointed on the back-bone before the fits of agues come, takes them away. It takes away inflammations in the eyes, if it be put with some part of a roasted quince, and boiled with a few crumbs of bread, and applied. Boiled with barley-meal it takes away pimples, pushes or wheals that arise in the face, or other parts of the body. The seed as well as the dried herb, is often given to kill the worms in children. The herb bruised and laid to, helps to draw forth splinters and thorns out of the flesh. The ashes thereof dries up and heals old ulcers, that are without inflammation, although by the sharpness thereof it bites sore, and puts them to sore pains; as also the sores in the privy parts of man or woman. The ashes mingled with old sallad oil, helps those that have hair fallen, and are bald, causing the hair to grow again either on the head or beard. Daranters saith, That the oil made of Southern-wood, and put among the ointments that are used against the French disease, is very effectual, and likewise kills lice in the head. The distilled water of the herb is said to help them much that are troubled with the stone, as also for the diseases of the spleen and mother. The Germans commend it for a singular wound herb, and therefore call it Stabwort. It is held by all writers, ancient and modern, to be more offensive to the stomach than worm-wood.

SPIGNEL, OR SPIKENARD

Descript.] The roots of common Spignel do spread much and deep in the ground, many strings or branches growing from one head, which is hairy at the top, of a blackish brown colour on the outside, and white within, from whence rise sundry long stalks of most fine cut leaves like hair, smaller than dill, set thick on both sides of the stalks, and of a good scent. Among these leaves rise up round stiff stalks, with a few joints and leaves on them, and at the tops an umbel of pure white flowers; at the edges whereof sometimes will be seen a shew of the reddish blueish colour, especially before they be full blown, and are succeeded by small, somewhat round seeds, bigger than the ordinary fennel, and of a brown colour, divided into two parts, and crusted on the back, as most of the umbelliferous seeds are.

Place.] It grows wild in Lancashire, Yorkshire, and other northern counties, and is also planted in gardens.

Government and virtues.] It is an herb of Venus. Galen saith,

The roots of Spignel are available to provoke urine, and women's courses; but if too much thereof be taken, it causes head-ache. The roots boiled in wine or water, and drank, helps the stranguary and stoppings of the urine, the wind, swellings and pains in the stomach, pains of the mother, and all joint-aches. If the powder of the root be mixed with honey, and the same taken as a licking medicine, it breaks tough phlegm, and dries up the rheum that falls on the lungs. The roots are accounted very effectual against the stinging or biting of any venomous creature.

SPLEENWORT, CETERACH, OR HEART'S TONGUE

Descript.] The smooth Spleenwort, from a black thready and bushy root, sends forth many long single leaves, cut in on both sides into round dents almost to the middle, which is not so hard as that of polypody, each division being not always set opposite unto the other, cut between each, smooth, and of a light green on the upper side, and a dark yellowish roughness on the back, folding or rolling itself inward at the first springing up.

Place.] It grows as well upon stone walls, as moist and shadowy places, about Bristol, and other the west parts plentifully; as also on Framlingham Castle, on Beaconsfield church in Berkshire, at Stroud in Kent, and elsewhere, and abides green all the Winter.

Government and virtues.] Saturn owns it. It is generally used against infirmities of the Spleen. It helps the stranguary, and wasteth the stone in the bladder, and is good against the yellow jaundice and the hiccough; but the juice of it in women hinders conception. Matthiolus saith, That if a dram of the dust that is on the back-side of the leaves be mixed with half a dram of amber in powder, and taken with the juice of purslain or plantain, it helps the gonorrhea speedily, and that the herb and root being boiled and taken, helps all melancholy diseases, and those especially that arise from the French diseases. Camerarius saith, That the distilled water thereof being drank, is very effectual against the stone in the reins and bladder; and that the lye that is made of the ashes thereof being drank for some time together, helps splenetic persons. It is used in outward remedies for the same purpose.

STAR THISTLE

Descript.] A common Star Thistle has divers narrow leaves lying next the ground, cut on the edges somewhat deeply into many parts, soft or a little woolly, all over green, among which rise up divers weak stalks, parted into many branches, all lying down to the ground, that it seems a pretty bush, set with divers the like divided leaves up to the tops, where severally do stand small whitish green heads, set with sharp white pricks (no part of the plant else being prickly) which are somewhat yellowish; out of the middle whereof rises the flowers composed of many small reddish purple threads; and in the heads, after the flowers are past, come small whitish round seed, lying down as others do. The root is small, long and woody, perishing every year, and rising again of its own sowing.

Place.] It grows wild in the fields about London in many places, as at Mile-End green, and many other places.

Time.] It flowers early, and seeds in July, and sometimes in August.

Government and virtues.] This, as almost all Thistles are, is under Mars. The seed of this Star Thistle made into powder, and drank in wine, provokes urine, and helps to break the stone, and drives it forth. The root in powder, and given in wine and drank, is good against the plague and pestilence; and drank in the morning fasting for some time together, it is very profitable for fistulas in any part of the body. Baptista Sardas doth much commend the distilled water thereof, being drank, to help the French disease, to open the obstructions of the liver, and cleanse the blood from corrupted humours, and is profitable against the quotidian or tertian ague.

STRAWBERRIES

THESE are so well known through this land, that they need no description.

Time.] They flower in May ordinarily, and the fruit is ripe shortly after.

Government and virtues.] Venus owns the herb. Strawberries, when they are green, are cool and dry; but when they are ripe, they are cool and moist. The berries are excellently good to cool the liver, the blood, and the spleen, or an hot choleric stomach; to refresh and comfort the fainting spirits, and quench thirst. They are good also for other inflammations; yet it is not amiss to refrain from them in a fever, lest by their putrifying in the stomach they increase the fits. The leaves and roots boiled in wine and water, and drank, do likewise cool the liver and blood, and assuage all inflammations in the reins and bladder, provoke urine, and allay the heat and sharpness thereof. The same also being drank stays the bloody flux and women's courses, and helps the swelling of the spleen. The water of the Berries carefully distilled, is a sovereign remedy and cordial in the panting and beating of the heart, and is good for the yellow jaundice. The juice dropped into foul ulcers, or they washed therewith, or the decoction of the herb and root, doth wonderfully cleanse and help to cure them. Lotions and gargles for sore mouths, or ulcers therein, or in the privy parts or elsewhere, are made with the leaves and roots thereof; which is also good to fasten loose teeth, and to heal spungy foul gums. It helps also to stay catarrhs, or defluctions of rheum in the mouth, throat, teeth, or eyes. The juice or water is singularly good for hot and red inflamed eyes, if dropped into them, or they bathed therewith. It is also of excellent property for all pushes, wheals and other break-ings forth of hot and sharp humours in the face and hands, and other parts of the body, to bathe them therewith, and to take away any redness in the face, or spots, or other deformities in the skin, and to make it clear and smooth. Some use this medicine: Take so many Strawberries as you shall think fitting, and put them into a distillatory, or body of glass fit for them, which being well closed, set it in a bed of horse dung for your use. It is an excellent water for hot inflamed eyes, and to take away a film or skin that begins to grow over them, and for such other defects in them as may be helped by any outward medicine.

SUCCORY, OR CHICORY

Descript.] The garden Succory hath long and narrower leaves than the Endive, and more cut in or torn on the edges, and the root abides many years. It bears also blue flowers like Endive, and the seed is hardly distinguished from the seed of the smooth or ordinary Endive.

The wild Succory hath divers long leaves lying on the ground, very much cut in or torn on the edges, on both sides, even to the middle rib, ending in a point; sometimes it hath a rib down to the middle of the leaves, from among which rises up a hard, round, woody stalk, spreading into many branches, set with smaller and less divided leaves on them up to the tops, where stand the flowers, which are like the garden kind, and the seed is also (only take notice that the flowers of the garden kind are gone in on a sunny day, they being so cold, that they are not able to endure the beams of the sun, and therefore more delight in the shade) the root is white, but more hard and woody than the garden kind. The whole plant is exceedingly bitter.

Place.] This grows in many places of our land in waste untilled and barren fields. The other only in gardens.

Government and virtues.] It is an herb of Jupiter. Garden Suc-cory, as it is more dry and less cold than Endive, so it opens more.

An handful of the leaves, or roots boiled in wine or water, and a draught thereof drank fasting, drives forth choleric and phlegmatic humours, opens obstructions of the liver, gall and spleen; helps the yellow jaundice, the heat of the reins, and of the urine; the dropsy also; and those that have an evil disposition in their bodies, by reason of long sickness, evil diet, &c. which the Greeks call Cachexia. A decoction thereof made with wine, and drank, is very effectual against long lingering agues; and a dram of the seed in powder, drank in wine, before the fit of the ague, helps to drive it away. The distilled water of the herb and flowers (if you can take them in time) hath the like properties, and is especially good for hot stomachs, and in agues, either pestilential or of long continuance; for swoonings and passions of the heart, for the heat and headache in children, and for the blood and liver. The said water, or the juice, or the bruised leaves applied outwardly, allay swellings, inflammations, St. Anthony's fire, pushes, wheals, and pimples, especially used with a little vinegar; as also to wash pestiferous sores. The said water is very effectual for sore eyes that are inflamed with redness, for nurses' breasts that are pained by the abundance of milk.

The wild Succory, as it is more bitter, so it is more strengthening to the stomach and liver.

STONE-CROP, PRICK-MADAM, OR SMALL-HOUSELEEK

Descript.] It grows with divers trailing branches upon the ground, set with many thick, flat, roundish, whitish green leaves, pointed at the ends. The flowers stand many of them together, somewhat loosely. The roots are small, and run creeping under ground.

Place.] It grows upon the stone walls and mud walls, upon the tiles of houses and pent-houses, and amongst rubbish, and in other gravelly places.

Time.] It flowers in June and July, and the leaves are green all the Winter.

Government and virtues.] It is under the dominion of the Moon, cold in quality, and something binding, and therefore very good to stay defluctions, especially such as fall upon the eyes. It stops bleeding, both inward and outward, helps cankers, and all fretting sores and ulcers; it abates the heat of choler, thereby preventing diseases arising from choleric humours. It expels poison much, resists pestilential fevers, being exceeding good also for tertian agues. You may drink the decoction of it, if you please, for all the foregoing infirmities. It is so harmless an herb, you can scarce use it amiss. Being bruised and applied to the place, it helps the king's evil, and any other knots or kernels in the flesh; as also the piles.

ENGLISH TOBACCO

Descript.] This rises up with a round thick stalk, about two feet high, whereon do grow thick, flat green leaves, nothing so large as the other Indian kind, somewhat round pointed also, and nothing dented about the edges. The stalk branches forth, and bears at the tops divers flowers set on great husks like the other, but nothing so large: scarce standing above the brims of the husks, round pointed also, and of a greenish yellow colour. The seed that follows is not so bright, but larger, contained in the like great heads. The roots are neither so great nor woody; it perishes every year with the hard frosts in Winter, but rises generally from its own sowing.

Place.] This came from some parts of Brazil, as it is thought, and is more familiar in our country than any of the other sorts; early giving ripe seed, which the others seldom do.

Time.] It flowers from June, sometimes to the end of August, or later, and the seed ripens in the mean time.

Government and virtues.] It is a martial plant. It is found by good experience to be available to expectorate tough phlegm from the stomach, chest, and lungs. The juice thereof made into a syrup, or the distilled water of the herb drank with some sugar, or without, if you will, or the smoak taken by a pipe, as is usual, but fainting, helps to expel worms in the stomach and belly, and to ease the pains in the head, or megrim, and the griping pains in the bowels. It is profitable for those that are troubled with the stone in the kidneys, both to ease the pains by provoking urine, and also to expel gravel and the stone engendered therein, and hath been found very effectual to expel windiness, and other humours, which cause the strangling of the mother. The seed thereof is very effectual to expel the tooth ache, and the ashes of the burnt herb to cleanse the gums, and make the teeth white. The herb bruised and applied to the place grieved with the king's evil, helps it in nine or ten days effec-tually. Monardus saith, It is a counter poison against the biting of any venomous creature, the herb also being outwardly applied to the hurt place. The distilled water is often given with some sugar before the fit of an ague, to lessen it, and take it away in three or four times using. If the distilled fæces of the herb, having been bruised before the distillation, and not distilled dry, be set in warm dung for fourteen days, and afterwards be hung in a bag in a wine cellar, the liquor that distills therefrom is singularly good to use in cramps, aches, the gout and sciatica, and to heal itches, scabs, and running ulcers, cankers, and all foul sores whatsoever. The juice is also good for all the said griefs, and likewise to kill lice in children's heads. The green herb bruised and applied to any green wounds, cures any fresh wound or cut whatsoever: and the juice put into old sores, both cleanses and heals them. There is also made hereof a singularly good salve to help imposthumes, hard tumours, and other swellings by blows and falls.

THE TAMARISK TREE

It is so well known in the place where it grows, that it needs no description.

Time.] It flowers about the end of May, or June, and the seed is ripe and blown away in the beginning of September.

Government and virtues.] A gallant Saturnine herb it is. The root, leaves, young branches, or bark boiled in wine, and drank, stays the bleeding of the hæmorrhodical veins, the spitting of blood, the too abounding of women's courses, the jaundice, the cholic, and the biting of all venomous serpents, except the asp; and outwardly applied, is very powerful against the hardness of the spleen, and the tooth-ache, pains in the ears, red and watering eyes. The decoction, with some honey put thereto, is good to stay gangrenes and fretting ulcers, and to wash those that are subject to nits and lice. Alpinus and Veslingius affirm, That the Egyptians do with good success use the wood of it to cure the French disease, as others do with lignum vitæ or guiacum; and give it also to those who have the leprosy, scabs, ulcers, or the like. Its ashes doth quickly heal blisters raised by burnings or scaldings. It helps the dropsy, arising from the hardness of the spleen, and therefore to drink out of cups made of the wood is good for splenetic persons. It is also helpful for melancholy, and the black jaundice that arise thereof.

GARDEN TANSY

Garden Tansy is so well known, that it needs no description.

Time.] It flowers in June and July.

Government and virtues.] Dame Venus was minded to pleasure women with child by this herb, for there grows not an herb, fitter for their use than this is; it is just as though it were cut out for the purpose. This herb bruised and applied to the navel, stays miscarriages. I know no herb like it for that use. Boiled in ordinary beer, and the decoction drank, doth the like; and if her womb be not as she would have it, this decoction will make it so. Let those women that desire children love this herb, it is their best companion, their husbands excepted. Also it consumes the phlegmatic humours, the cold and moist constitution of Winter most usually affects the body of man with, and that was the first reason of eating tansies in the Spring. The decoction of the common Tansy, or the juice drank in wine, is a singular remedy for all the griefs that come by stopping of the urine, helps the stranguary and those that have weak reins and kidneys. It is also very profitable to dissolve and expel wind in the stomach, belly, or bowels, to procure women's courses, and expel windiness in the matrix, if it be bruised and often smelled unto, as also applied to the lower part of the belly. It is also very profitable for such women as are given to miscarry. It is used also against the stone in the reins, especially to men. The herb fried with eggs (as it is the custom in the Spring-time) which is called a Tansy, helps to digest and carry downward those bad humours that trouble the stomach. The seed is very profitably given to children for the worms, and the juice in drink is as effectual. Being boiled in oil, it is good for the sinews shrunk by cramps, or pained with colds, if thereto applied.

WILD TANSY, OR SILVER WEED

THIS is also so well known, that it needs no description.

Place.] It grows in every place.

Time.] It flowers in June and July.

Government and virtues.] Now Dame Venus hath fitted women with two herbs of one name, the one to help conception, and the other to maintain beauty, and what more can be expected of her? What now remains for you, but to love your husbands, and not be wanting to your poor neighbours? Wild Tansy stays the lask, and all the fluxes of blood in men and women, which some say it will do, if the green herb be worn in the shoes, so it be next the skin; and it is true enough, that it will stop the terms, if worn so, and the whites too, for ought I know. It stays also spitting or vomiting of blood. The powder of the herb taken in some of the distilled water, helps the whites in women, but more especially if a little coral and ivory in powder be put to it. It is also recommended to help children that are bursten, and have a rupture, being boiled in water and salt. Being boiled in water and drank, it eases the griping pains of the bowels, and is good for the sciatica and joint-aches. The same boiled in vinegar, with honey and allum, and gargled in the mouth, eases the pains of the tooth-ache, fastens loose teeth, helps the gums that are sore, and settles the palate of the mouth in its place, when it is fallen down. It cleanses and heals ulcers in the mouth, or secret parts, and is very good for inward wounds, and to close the lips of green wounds, and to heal old, moist, and corrupt running sores in the legs or elsewhere. Being bruised and applied to the soles of the feet and hand wrists, it wonderfully cools the hot fits of agues, be they never so violent. The distilled water cleanses the skin of all discolourings therein, as morphew, sun-burnings, &c. as also pimples, freckles, and the like; and dropped into the eyes, or cloths wet therein and applied, takes away the heat and inflammations in them.

THISTLES

OF these are many kinds growing here in England which are so well known, that they need no description. Their difference is easily known on the places where they grow, *viz*.

Place.] Some grow in fields, some in meadows, and some among the corn; others on heaths, greens, and waste grounds in many places.

Time.] They flower in June and August, and their seed is ripe quickly after.

Government and virtues.] Surely Mars rules it, it is such a prickly business. All these thistles are good to provoke urine, and to mend the stinking smell thereof; as also the rank smell of the arm-pits, or the whole body; being boiled in wine and drank, and are said to help a stinking breath, and to strengthen the stomach. Pliny saith, That the juice bathed on the place that wants hair, it being fallen off, will cause it to grow speedily.

THE MELANCHOLY THISTLE

Descript.] It rises up with tender single hoary green stalks, bearing thereon four or five green leaves, dented about the edges; the points thereof are little or nothing prickly, and at the top usually but one head, yet sometimes from the bosom of the uppermost leaves there shoots forth another small head, scaly and prickly, with many reddish thrumbs or threads in the middle, which being gathered fresh, will keep the colour a long time, and fades not from the stalk a long time, while it perfects the seed, which is of a mean bigness, lying in the down. The root hath many strings fastened to the head, or upper part, which is blackish, and perishes not.

There is another sort little differing from the former, but that the leaves are more green above, and more hoary underneath, and the stalk being about two feet high, bears but one scaly head, with threads and seeds as the former.

Place.] They grow in many moist meadows of this land, as well in the southern, as in the northern parts.

Time.] They flower about July or August, and their seed ripens quickly after.

Government and virtues.] It is under Capricorn, and therefore under both Saturn and Mars, one rids melancholy by sympathy, the other by antipathy. Their virtues are but few, but those not to be despised; for the decoction of the thistle in wine being drank, expels superfluous melancholy out of the body, and makes a man as merry as a cricket; superfluous melancholy causes care, fear, sadness, despair, envy, and many evils more besides; but religion teaches to wait upon God's providence, and cast our care upon him who cares for us. What a fine thing were it if men and women could live so! And yet seven years' care and fear makes a man never the wiser, nor a farthing richer. Dioscorides saith, The root borne about one doth the like, and removes all diseases of melancholy. Modern writers laugh at him. *Let them laugh that win*: my opinion is, that it is the best remedy against all melancholy diseases that grows; they that please may use it.

OUR LADY'S THISTLE

Descript.] Our Lady's Thistle hath divers very large and broad leaves lying on the ground cut in, and as it were crumpled, but somewhat hairy on the edges, of a white green shining colour, wherein are many lines and streaks of a milk white colour, running all over, and set with many sharp and stiff prickles all about, among which rises up one or more strong, round, and prickly stalks, set full of the like leaves up to the top, where at the end of every branch, comes forth a great prickly Thistle-like head, strongly armed with prickles, and with bright purple thumbs rising out of the middle; after they are past, the seed grows in the said heads, lying in soft white down, which is somewhat flattish in the ground, and many strings and fibres fastened thereunto. All the whole plant is bitter in taste.

Place.] It is frequent on the banks of almost every ditch.

Time.] It flowers and seeds in June, July, and August.

Government and virtues.] Our Lady's Thistle is under Jupiter, and thought to be as effectual as Carduus Benedictus for agues, and to prevent and cure the infection of the plague: as also to open the obstructions of the liver and spleen, and thereby is good against the jaundice. It provokes urine, breaks and expels the stone, and is good for the dropsy. It is effectual also for the pains in the sides, and many other inward pains and gripings. The seed and distilled water is held powerful to all the purposes aforesaid, and besides, it is often applied both outwardly with cloths or spunges to the region of the liver, to cool the distemper thereof, and to the region of the heart, against swoonings and the passions of it. It cleanses the blood exceedingly: and in Spring, if you please to boil the tender plant (but cut off the prickles unless you have a mind to choak yourself) it will change your blood as the season changes, and that is the way to be safe.

THE WOOLLEN, OR COTTON THISTLE

Descript.] This has many large leaves lying upon the ground, somewhat cut in, and as it were crumpled on the edges, of a green colour on the upper side, but covered over with a long hairy wool or cotton down, set with most sharp and cruel pricks; from the middle of whose heads of flowers come forth many purplish crimson threads, and sometimes white, although but seldom. The seed that follow in those white downy heads, is somewhat large and round, resembling the seed of Lady's Thistle, but paler. The root is great and thick, spreading much, yet usually dies after seed time.

Place.] It grows in divers ditch-banks, and in the corn-fields, and highways, generally throughout the land, and is often growing in gardens.

Government and virtues.] It is a plant of Mars. Dioscorides and Pliny write, That the leaves and roots hereof taken in drink, help those that have a crick in their neck, that they cannot turn it, unless they turn their whole body. Galen saith, That the roots and leaves hereof are good for such persons that have their bodies drawn together by some spasm or convulsion, or other infirmities; as the rickets (or as the college of physicians would have it, Rachites, about which name they have quarrelled sufficiently) in children, being a disease that hinders their growth, by binding their nerves, ligaments, and whole structure of their body.

THE FULLER'S THISTLE, OR TEASLE

It is so well known, that it needs no description, being used with the cloth-workers.

The wild Teasle is in all things like the former, but that the prickles are small, soft, and upright, not hooked or stiff, and the flowers of this are of a fine blueish, or pale carnation colour, but of the manured kind, whitish.

Place.] The first grows, being sown in gardens or fields for the use of clothworkers. The other near ditches and rills of water in many places of this land.

Time.] They flower in July, and are ripe in the end of August.

Government and virtues.] It is an herb of Venus. Dioscorides saith, That the root bruised and boiled in wine, till it be thick, and kept in a brazen vessel, and after spread as a salve, and applied to the fundament, doth heal the cleft thereof, cankers and fistulas therein, also takes away warts and wens. The juice of the leaves dropped into the ears, kills worms in them. The distilled water of the leaves dropped into the eyes, takes away redness and mists in them that hinder the sight, and is often used by women to preserve their beauty, and to take away redness and inflammations, and all other heat or discolourings.

TREACLE MUSTARD

Descript.] It rises up with a hard round stalk, about a foot high, parted into some branches, having divers soft green leaves long and narrow, set thereon, waved, but not cut into the edges, broadest towards the ends, somewhat round pointed; the flowers are white that grow at the tops of the branches, spike-fashion, one above another; after which come round pouches, parted in the middle with a furrow, having one blackish brown seed on either side, somewhat sharp in taste, and smelling of garlick, especially in the fields where it is natural, but not so much in gardens. The roots are small and thready, perishing every year.

Give me leave here to add Mithridate Mustard, although it may seem more properly by the name to belong to M, in the alphabet.

MITHRIDATE MUSTARD

Descript.] This grows higher than the former, spreading more and higher branches, whose leaves are smaller and narrower, some-times unevenly dented about the edges. The flowers are small and white, growing on long branches, with much smaller and rounder vessels after them, and parted in the same manner, having smaller brown seeds than the former, and much sharper in taste. The root perishes after seed time, but abides the first Winter after springing.

Place.] They grow in sundry places in this land, as half a mile from Hatfield, by the river side, under a hedge as you go to Hatfield, and in the street of Peckham on Surrey side.

Time.] They flower and seed from May to August.

Government and virtues.] Both of them are herbs of Mars. The Mustards are said to purge the body both upwards and downwards, and procure women's courses so abundantly, that it suffocates the birth. It breaks inward imposthumes, being taken inwardly; and used in clysters, helps the sciatica. The seed applied, doth the same. It is an especial ingredient in mithridate and treacle, being of itself an antidote resisting poison, venom and putrefaction. It is also available in many cases for which the common Mustard is used, but somewhat weaker.

THE BLACK THORN, OR SLOE-BUSH

It is so well known, that it needs no description.

Place.] It grows in every county in the hedges and borders of fields.

Time.] It flowers in April, and sometimes in March, but the fruit ripens after all other plums whatsoever, and is not fit to be eaten until the Autumn frost mellow them.

Government and virtues.] All the parts of the Sloe-Bush are binding, cooling, and dry, and all effectual to stay bleeding at the nose and mouth, or any other place; the lask of the belly or stomach, or the bloody flux, the too much abounding of women's courses, and helps to ease the pains of the sides, and bowels, that come by over-much scouring, to drink the decoction of the bark of the roots, or more usually the decoction of the berries, either fresh or dried. The conserve also is of very much use, and more familiarly taken for the purposes aforesaid. But the distilled water of the flower first steeped in sack for a night, and drawn therefrom by the heat of Balneum and Anglico, a bath, is a most certain remedy, tried and approved, to ease all manner of gnawings in the stomach, the sides and bowels, or any griping pains in any of them, to drink a small quantity when the extremity of pain is upon them. The leaves also are good to make lotions to gargle and wash the mouth and throat, wherein are swellings, sores, or kernels; and to stay the defluctions of rheum to the eyes, or other parts; as also to cool the heat and in-flammations of them, and ease hot pains of the head, to bathe the forehead and temples therewith. The simple distilled water of the flowers is very effectual for the said purposes, and the condensate juice of the Sloes. The distilled water of the green berries is used also for the said effects.

THOROUGH WAX, OR THOROUGH LEAF

Descript.] Common Thorough-Wax sends forth a strait round stalk, two feet high, or better, whose lower leaves being of a bluish colour, are smaller and narrower than those up higher, and stand close thereto, not compassing it; but as they grow higher, they do not encompass the stalks, until it wholly pass through them, branching toward the top into many parts, where the leaves grow smaller again, every one standing singly, and never two at a joint. The flowers are small and yellow, standing in tufts at the heads of the branches, where afterwards grow the seed, being blackish, many thick thrust together. The root is small, long and woody, perishing every year, after seed-time, and rising again plentifully of its own sowing.

Place.] It is found growing in many corn-fields and pasture grounds in this land.

Time.] It flowers in July, and the seed is ripe in August.

Government and virtues.] Both this and the former are under the influence of Saturn. Thorough-Wax is of singular good use for all sorts of bruises and wounds either inward or outward; and old ulcers and sores likewise, if the decoction of the herb with water and wine be drank, and the place washed therewith, or the juice of the green herb bruised, or boiled, either by itself, or with other herbs, in oil or hog's grease, to be made into an ointment to serve all the year. The decoction of the herb, or powder of the dried herb, taken inwardly, and the same, or the leaves bruised, and applied outwardly, is singularly good for all ruptures and burstings, especially in children before they be too old. Being applied with a little flour and wax to children's navels that stick forth, it helps them.

THYME

It is in vain to describe an herb so commonly known.

Government and virtues.] It is a noble strengthener of the lungs, as notable a one as grows; neither is there scarce a better remedy growing for that disease in children which they commonly call the Chin-cough, than it is. It purges the body of phlegm, and is an excellent remedy for shortness of breath. It kills worms in the belly, and being a notable herb of Venus, provokes the terms, gives safe and speedy delivery to women in travail, and brings away the after birth. It is so harmless you need not fear the use of it. An ointment made of it takes away hot swellings and warts, helps the sciatica and dullness of sight, and takes away pains and hardness of the spleen. Tis excellent for those that are troubled with the gout.

It eases pains in the loins and hips. The herb taken any way inwardly, comforts the stomach much, and expels wind.

WILD THYME, OR MOTHER OF THYME

WILD Thyme also is so well known, that it needs no description.

Place.] It may be found commonly in commons, and other barren places throughout the nation.

Government and virtues.] It is under the dominion of Venus, and under the sign Aries, and therefore chiefly appropriated to the head. It provokes urine and the terms, and eases the griping pain of the belly, cramps, ruptures, and inflammation of the liver. If you make a vinegar of the herb, as vinegar of roses is made (you may find out the way in my translation of the London Dispensatory) and anoint the head with it, it presently stops the pains thereof. It is excellently good to be given either in phrenzy or lethargy, although they are two contrary diseases. It helps spitting and voiding of blood, coughing, and vomiting; it comforts and strengthens the head, stomach, reins, and womb, expels wind, and breaks the stone.

TORMENTIL, OR SEPTFOIL

Descript.] This hath reddish, slender, weak branches rising from the root, lying on the ground, rather leaning than standing upright, with many short leaves that stand closer to the stalk than cinquefoil (to which this is very like) with the foot-stalk compassing the branches in several places; but those that grow to the ground are set upon long foot stalks, each whereof are like the leaves of cinquefoil, but somewhat long and lesser dented about the edges, many of them divided into five leaves, but most of them into seven, whence it is also called Septfoil; yet some may have six, and some eight, according to the fertility of the soil. At the tops of the branches stand divers small yellow flowers, consisting of five leaves, like those of cinquefoil, but smaller. The root is smaller than bistort, somewhat thick, but blacker without, and not so red within, yet sometimes a little crooked, having blackish fibres thereat.

Place.] It grows as well in woods and shadowy places, as in the open champain country, about the borders of fields in many places of this land, and almost in every broom field in Essex.

Time.] It flowers all the Summer long.

Government and virtues.] This is a gallant herb of the Sun. Tormentil is most excellent to stay all kind of fluxes of blood or humours in man or woman, whether at nose, mouth, or belly. The juice of the herb of the root, or the decoction thereof, taken with some Venice treacle, and the person laid to sweat, expels any venom or poison, or the plague, fever, or other contagious diseases, as pox, measles, &c. for it is an ingredient in all antidotes or counter poisons. Andreas Urlesius is of opinion that the decoction of this root is no less effectual to cure the French pox than Guiacum or China; and it is not unlikely, because it so mightily resists putre-faction. The root taken inwardly is most effectual to help any flux of the belly, stomach, spleen, or blood; and the juice wonderfully opens obstructions of the liver and lungs, and thereby helps the yellow jaundice. The powder or decoction drank, or to sit thereon as a bath, is an assured remedy against abortion, if it proceed from the over flexibility or weakness of the inward retentive faculty; as also a plaster made therewith, and vinegar applied to the reins of the back, doth much help not only this, but also those that cannot hold their water, the powder being taken in the juice of plaintain, and is also commended against the worms in children. It is very powerful in ruptures and burstings, as also for bruises and falls, to be used as well outwardly as inwardly. The root hereof made up with pellitory of Spain and allum, and put into a hollow tooth, not only assuages the pain, but stays the flux of humours which causes it. Tormentil is no less effectual and powerful a remedy against outward wounds, sores and hurts, than for inward, and is therefore a special ingredient to be used in wound drinks, lotions and in-jections, for foul corrupt rotten sores and ulcers of the mouth, secrets, or other parts of the body. The juice or powder of the root put in ointments, plaisters, and such things that are to be applied to wounds or sores, is very effectual, as the juice of the leaves and the root bruised and applied to the throat or jaws, heals the king's evil, and eases the pain of the sciatica; the same used with a little vinegar, is a special remedy against the running sores of the head or other parts; scabs also, and the itch or any such eruptions in the skin, proceeding of salt and sharp humours. The same is also effectual for the piles or hæmorrhoids, if they be washed or bathed therewith, or with the distilled water of the herb and roots. It is found also helpful to dry up any sharp rheum that distills from the head into the eyes, causing redness, pain, waterings, itching, or the like, if a little prepared tutia, or white amber, be used with the distilled water thereof. And here is enough, only remember the Sun challengeth this herb.

TURNSOLE, OR HELIOTROPIUM

Descript.] The greater Turnsole rises with one upright stalk, about a foot high, or more, dividing itself almost from the bottom, into divers small branches, of a hoary colour; at each joint of the stalk and branches grow small broad leaves, somewhat white and hairy. At the tops of the stalks and branches stand small white flowers, consisting of four, and sometimes five small leaves, set in order one above another, upon a small crooked spike, which turns inwards like a bowed finger, opening by degrees as the flowers blow open; after which in their place come forth cornered seed, four for the most part standing together; the root is small and thready, perishing every year, and the seed shedding every year, raises it again the next spring.

Place.] It grows in gardens, and flowers and seeds with us, notwithstanding it is not natural to this land, but to Italy, Spain, and France, where it grows plentifully.

Government and virtues.] It is an herb of the Sun, and a good one too. Dioscorides saith, That a good handful of this, which is called the Great Turnsole, boiled in water, and drank, purges both choler and phlegm; and boiled with cummin, helps the stone in the reins, kidneys, or bladder, provokes urine and women's courses, and causes an easy and speedy delivery in child-birth. The leaves bruised and applied to places pained with the gout, or that have been out of joint and newly set, and full of pain, do give much ease; the seed and juice of the leaves also being rubbed with a little salt upon warts and wens, and other kernels in the face, eye-lids, or any other part of the body, will, by often using, take them away.

MEADOW TREFOIL, OR HONEYSUCKLES

It is so well known, especially by the name of Honeysuckles, white and red, that I need not describe them.

Place.] They grow almost every where in this land.

Government and virtues.] Mercury hath dominion over the common sort. Dodoneus saith, The leaves and flowers are good to ease the griping pains of the gout, the herb being boiled and used in a clyster. If the herb be made into a poultice, and applied to inflammations, it will ease them. The juice dropped in the eyes, is a familiar medicine, with many country people, to take away the pin and web (as they call it) in the eyes; it also allays the heat and blood shooting of them. Country people do also in many places drink the juice thereof against the biting of an adder; and having boiled the herb in water, they first wash the place with the decoction, and then lay some of the herb also to the hurt place. The herb also boiled in swine's grease, and so made into an ointment, is good to apply to the biting of any venomous creature. The herb also bruised and heated between tiles, and applied hot to the share, causes them to make water who had it stopt before. It is held likewise to be good for wounds, and to take away seed. The decoction of the herb and flowers, with the seed and root, taken for some time, helps women that are troubled with the whites. The seed and flowers boiled in water, and afterwards made into a poultice with some oil, and applied, helps hard swellings and imposthumes.

HEART TREFOIL

BESIDES the ordinary sort of Trefoil, here are two more remarkable, and one of which may be properly called Heart Trefoil, not only because the leaf is triangular, like the heart of a man, but also because each leaf contains the perfection of a heart, and that in its proper colour, viz. a flesh colour.

Place.] It grows between Longford and Bow, and beyond South-wark, by the highway and parts adjacent.

Government and virtues.] It is under the dominion of the Sun, and if it were used, it would be found as great a strengthener of the heart, and cherisher of the vital spirits as grows, relieving the body against fainting and swoonings, fortifying it against poison and pestilence, defending the heart against the noisome vapours of the spleen.

PEARL TREFOIL

IT differs not from the common sort, save only in this particular, it hath a white spot in the leaf like a pearl. It is particularly under the dominion of the Moon, and its icon shews that it is of a singular virtue against the pearl, or pin and web in the eyes.

TUSTAN, OR PARK LEAVES

Descript.] It hath brownish shining round stalks, crested the length thereof, rising two by two, and sometimes three feet high, branching forth even from the bottom, having divers joints, and at each of them two fair large leaves standing, of a dark blueish green colour on the upper side, and of a yellowish green underneath, turning reddish toward Autumn. At the top of the stalks stand large yellow flowers, and heads with seed, which being greenish at the first and afterwards reddish, turn to be of a blackish purple colour when they are ripe, with small brownish seed within them, and they yield a reddish juice or liquor, somewhat resinous, and of a harsh and stypick taste, as the leaves also and the flowers be, although much less, but do not yield such a clear claret wine colour, as some say it doth, the root is brownish, somewhat great, hard and woody, spreading well in the ground.

Place.] It grows in many woods, groves, and woody grounds, as parks and forests, and by hedge-sides in many places in this land, as in Hampstead wood, by Ratley in Essex, in the wilds of Kent, and in many other places needless to recite.

Time.] It flowers later than St. John's or St. Peter's-wort.

Government and virtues.] It is an herb of Saturn, and a most noble anti-venerean. Tustan purges choleric humours, as St. Peter's-wort is said to do, for therein it works the same effects, both to help the sciatica and gout, and to heal burning by fire; it stays all the bleedings of wounds, if either the green herb be bruised, or the powder of the dry be applied thereto. It hath been accounted, and certainly it is, a sovereign herb to heal either wound or sore, either outwardly or inwardly, and therefore always used in drinks, lotions, green wounds, ulcers, or old sores, in all balms, oils, ointments, or any other sorts of which the continual experience of former ages hath confirmed the use thereof to be admirably good, though it be not so much in use now, as when physicians and surgeons were so wise as to use herbs more than now they do.

GARDEN VALERIAN

Descript.] This hath a thick short greyish root, lying for the most part above ground, shooting forth on all other sides such like small pieces of roots, which have all of them many long green strings and fibres under them in the ground, whereby it draws nourishment. From the head of these roots spring up many green leaves, which at first are somewhat broad and long, without any divisions at all in them, or denting on the edges; but those that rise up after are more and more divided on each side, some to the middle rib, being winged, as made of many leaves together on a stalk, and those upon a stalk, in like manner more divided, but smaller towards the top than below; the stalk rises to be a yard high or more, sometimes branched at the top, with many small whitish flowers, sometimes dashed over at the edges with a pale purplish colour, of a little scent, which passing away, there follows small brownish white seed, that is easily carried away with the wind. The root smells more strong than either leaf or flower, and is of more use in medicines.

Place.] It is generally kept with us in gardens.

Time.] It flowers in June and July, and continues flowering until the frost pull it down.

Government and virtues.] This is under the influence of Mercury. Dioscorides saith, That the Garden Valerian hath a warming faculty, and that being dried and given to drink it provokes urine, and helps the stranguary. The decoction thereof taken, doth the like also, and takes away pains of the sides, provokes women's courses, and is used in antidotes. Pliny saith, That the powder of the root given in drink, or the decoction thereof taken, helps all stoppings and stranglings in any part of the body, whether they proceed in pains in the chest or sides, and takes them away. The root of Valerian boiled with liquorice, raisins, and anniseed, is singularly good for those that are short-winded, and for those that are troubled with the cough, and helps to open the passages, and to expectorate phlegm easily. It is given to those that are bitten or stung by any venomous creature, being boiled in wine. It is of a special virtue against the plague, the decoction thereof being drank, and the root being used to smell to. It helps to expel the wind in the belly. The green herb with the root taken fresh, being bruised and applied to the head, takes away the pains and prickings there, stays rheum and thin distillation, and being boiled in white wine, and a drop thereof put into the eyes, takes away the dimness of the sight, or any pin or web therein. It is of excellent property to heal any inward sores or wounds, and also for outward hurts or wounds, and drawing away splinters or thorns out of the flesh.

VERVAIN

Descript.] The common Vervain hath somewhat long broad leaves next the ground deeply gashed about the edges, and some only deeply dented, or cut all alike, of a blackish green colour on the upper side, somewhat grey underneath. The stalk is square, branched into several parts, rising about two feet high, especially if you reckon the long spike of flowers at the tops of them, which are set on all sides one above another, and sometimes two or three together, being small and gaping, of a blue colour and white intermixed, after which come small round seed, in small and somewhat long heads. The root is small and long.

Place.] It grows generally throughout this land in divers places of the hedges and way-sides, and other waste grounds.

Time.] It flowers in July, and the seed is ripe soon after.

Government and virtues.] This is an herb of Venus, and excellent for the womb to strengthen and remedy all the cold griefs of it, as

Plantain doth the hot. Vervain is hot and dry, opening obstructions, cleansing and healing. It helps the yellow jaundice, the dropsy and the gout; it kills and expels worms in the belly, and causes a good colour in the face and body, strengthens as well as corrects the diseases of the stomach, liver, and spleen; helps the cough, wheezings, and shortness of breath, and all the defects of the reins and bladder, expelling the gravel and stone. It is held to be good against the biting of serpents, and other venomous beasts, against the plague, and both tertian and quartan agues. It consolidates and heals also all wounds, both inward and outward, stays bleedings, and used with some honey, heals all old ulcers and fistulas in the legs or other parts of the body; as also those ulcers that happen in the mouth; or used with hog's grease, it helps the swellings and pains in the secret parts in man or woman, also for the piles or hæmorrhoids; applied with some oil of roses and vinegar unto the forehead and temples, it eases the inveterate pains and ache of the head, and is good for those that are frantic. The leaves bruised, or the juice of them mixed with some vinegar, doth wonderfully cleanse the skin, and takes away morphew, freckles, fistulas, and other such like inflammations and deformities of the skin in any parts of the body. The distilled water of the herb when it is in full strength, dropped into the eyes, cleanses them from films, clouds, or mists, that darken the sight, and wonderfully strengthens the optic nerves. The said water is very powerful in all the diseases aforesaid, either inward or outward, whether they be old corroding sores, or green wounds. The dried root, and peeled, is known to be excellently good against all scrophulous and scorbutic habits of body, by being tied to the pit of the stomach, by a piece of white ribband round the neck.

THE VINE

THE leaves of the English vine (I do not mean to send you to the Canaries for a medicine) being boiled, makes a good lotion for sore mouths; being boiled with barley meal into a poultice, it cools inflammations of wounds; the dropping of the vine, when it is cut in the Spring, which country people call Tears, being boiled in a syrup, with sugar, and taken inwardly, is excellent to stay women's longings after every thing they see, which is a disease many women with child are subject to. The decoction of Vine leaves in white wine doth the like. Also the tears of the Vine, drank two or three spoonfuls at a time, breaks the stone in the bladder. This is a very good remedy, and it is discreetly done, to kill a Vine to cure a man, but the salt of the leaves are held to be better. The ashes of the burnt branches will make teeth that are as black as a coal, to be as white as snow, if you but every morning rub them with it. It is a most gallant Tree of the Sun, very sympathetical with the body of men, and that is the reason spirit of wine is the greatest cordial among all vegetables.

VIOLETS

BOTH the tame and the wild are so well known, that they need no description.

Time.] They flower until the end of July, but are best in March, and the beginning of April.

Government and virtues.] They are a fine pleasing plant of Venus, of a mild nature, no way harmful. All the Violets are cold and moist while they are fresh and green, and are used to cool any heat, or distemperature of the body, either inwardly or outwardly, as inflammations in the eyes, in the matrix or fundament, in imposthumes also, and hot swellings, to drink the decoction of the leaves and flowers made with water in wine, or to apply them poultice-wise to the grieved places: it likewise eases pains in the head, caused through want of sleep; or any other pains arising of heat, being applied in the same manner, or with oil of roses. A dram weight of the dried leaves or flower of Violets, but the leaves more strongly, doth purge the body of choleric humours, and assuages the heat, being taken in a draught of wine, or any other drink; the powder of the purple leaves of the flowers, only picked and dried and drank in water, is said to help the quinsy, and the falling-sickness in children, especially in the beginning of the disease. The flowers of the white Violets ripen and dissolve swellings. The herb or flowers, while they are fresh, or the flowers when they are dry, are effectual in the pleurisy, and all diseases of the lungs, to lenify the sharpness in hot rheums, and the hoarseness of the throat, the heat also and sharpness of urine, and all the pains of the back or reins, and bladder. It is good also for the liver and the jaundice, and all hot agues, to cool the heat, and quench the thirst; but the syrup of Violets is of most use, and of better effect, being taken in some convenient liquor: and if a little of the juice or syrup of lemons be put to it, or a few drops of the oil of vitriol, it is made thereby the more powerful to cool the heat, and quench the thirst, and gives to the drink a claret wine colour, and a fine tart relish, pleasing to the taste. Violets taken, or made up with honey, do more cleanse and cool, and with sugar contrary-wise. The dried flower of Violets are accounted amongst the cordial drinks, powders, and other medicines, especially where cooling cordials are necessary. The green leaves are used with other herbs to make plaisters and poultices to inflammations and swellings, and to ease all pains whatsoever, arising of heat, and for the piles also, being fried with yolks of eggs, and applied thereto.

VIPER'S BUGLOSS

Descript.] This hath many long rough leaves lying on the ground, from among which rises up divers hard round stalks, very rough, as if they were thick set with prickles or hairs, whereon are set such like rough, hairy, or prickly sad green leaves, somewhat narrow; the middle rib for the most part being white. The flowers stand at the top of the stalk, branched forth in many long spiked leaves of flowers bowing or turning like the turnsole, all opening for the most part on the one side, which are long and hollow, turning up the brims a little, of a purplish violet colour in them that are fully blown, but more reddish while they are in the bud, as also upon their decay and withering; but in some places of a paler purplish colour, with a long pointel in the middle, feathered or parted at the top. After the flowers are fallen, the seeds growing to be ripe, are blackish, cornered and pointed somewhat like the head of a viper. The root is somewhat great and blackish, and woolly, when it grows toward seed-time, and perishes in the Winter.

There is another sort, little differing from the former, only in this, that it bears white flowers.

Place.] The first grows wild almost every where. That with white flowers about the castle-walls at Lewis in Sussex.

Time.] They flower in Summer, and their seed is ripe quickly after.

Government and virtues.] It is a most gallant herb of the Sun; it is a pity it is no more in use than it is. It is an especial remedy against the biting of the Viper, and all other venomous beasts, or serpents; as also against poison, or poisonous herbs. Dioscorides and others say, That whosoever shall take of the herb or root before they be bitten, shall not be hurt by the poison of any serpent. The root or seed is thought to be most effectual to comfort the heart, and expel sadness, or causeless melancholy; it tempers the blood, and allays hot fits of agues. The seed drank in wine, procures abundance of milk in women's breasts. The same also being taken, eases the pains in the loins, back, and kidneys. The distilled water of the herb when it is in flower, or its chief strength, is excellent to be applied either inwardly or outwardly, for all the griefs aforesaid. There is a syrup made hereof very effectual for the comforting the heart, and expelling sadness and melancholy.

WALL FLOWERS, OR WINTER GILLIFLOWERS

THE garden kind are so well known that they need no description.

Descript.] The common single Wall-flowers, which grow wild abroad, have sundry small, long, narrow, dark green leaves, set without order upon small round, whitish, woody stalks, which bear at the tops divers single yellow flowers one above another, every one bearing four leaves a-piece, and of a very sweet scent: after which come long pods, containing a reddish seed. The roots are white, hard and thready.

Place.] It grows upon church walls, and old walls of many houses, and other stone walls in divers places. The other sort in gardens only.

Time.] All the single kinds do flower many times in the end of Autumn; and if the Winter be mild, all the Winter long, but especially in the months of February, March, and April, and until the heat of the spring do spend them. But the double kinds continue not flowering in that manner all the year long, although they flower very early sometimes, and in some places very late.

Government and virtues.] The Moon rules them. Galen, in his seventh book of simple medicines, saith, That the yellow Wall-flowers work more powerfully than any of the other kinds, and are therefore of more use in physic. It cleanses the blood, and fretteth the liver and reins from obstructions, provokes women's courses, expels the secundine, and the dead child; helps the hardness and pain of the mother, and of spleen also; stays inflammations and swellings, comforts and strengthens any weak part, or out of joint; helps to cleanse the eyes from mistiness or films upon them, and to cleanse the filthy ulcers in the mouth, or any other part, and is a singular remedy for the gout, and all aches and pains in the joints and sinews. A conserve made of the flowers, is used for a remedy both for the apoplexy and palsy.

THE WALLNUT TREE

IT is so well known, that it needs no description.

Time.] It blossoms early before the leaves come forth, and the fruit is ripe in September.

Government and virtues.] This is also a plant of the Sun. Let the fruit of it be gathered accordingly, which you shall find to be of most virtues while they are green, before they have shells. The bark of the Tree doth bind and dry very much, and the leaves are much of the same temperature: but the leaves when they are older, are heating and drying in the second degree, and harder of digestion than when they are fresh, which, by reason of their sweetness, are more pleasing, and better digesting in the stomach; and taken with sweet wine, they move the belly downwards, but being old, they grieve the stomach; and in hot bodies cause the choler to abound and the head-ache, and are an enemy to those that have the cough; but are less hurtful to those that have a colder stomach, and are said to kill the broad worms in the belly or stomach. If they be taken with onions, salt, and honey, they help the biting of a mad dog, or the venom or infectious poison of any beast, &c. Caias Pompeius found in the treasury of Mithridates, king of Pontus, when he was over-thrown, a scroll of his own hand writing, containing a medicine against any poison or infection; which is this: Take two dry walnuts, and as many good figs, and twenty leaves of rue, bruised and beaten together with two or three corns of salt and twenty juniper berries, which take every morning fasting, preserves from danger of poison, and infection that day it is taken. The juice of the other green husks boiled with honey is an excellent gargle for sore mouths, or the heat and inflammations in the throat and stomach. The ker-nels, when they grow old, are more oily, and therefore not fit to be eaten, but are then used to heal the wounds of the sinews, gan-grenes, and carbuncles. The said kernels being burned, are very astringent, and will stay lasks and women's courses, being taken in red wine, and stay the falling of the hair, and make it fair, being anointed with oil and wine. The green husks will do the like, being used in the same manner. The kernels beaten with rue and wine, being applied, help the quinsy; and bruised with some honey, and applied to the ears, ease the pains and inflammation of them. A piece of the green husks put into a hollow tooth, eases the pain. The catkins hereof, taken before they fall off, dried, and given a dram thereof in powder with white wine, wonderfully helps those that are troubled with the rising of the mother. The oil that is pressed out of the kernels, is very profitable, taken inwardly like oil of almonds, to help the cholic, and to expel wind very effectually; an ounce or two thereof may be taken at any time. The young green nuts taken before they be half ripe, and preserved with sugar, are of good use for those that have weak stomachs, or defluctions there-on. The distilled water of the green husks, before they be half ripe, is of excellent use to cool the heat of agues, being drank an ounce or two at a time: as also to resist the infection of the plague, if some of the same be also applied to the sores thereof. The same also cools the heat of green wounds and old ulcers, and heals them, being bathed therewith. The distilled water of the green husks being ripe, when they are shelled from the nuts, and drank with a little vinegar, is good for the place, so as before the taking thereof a vein be opened. The said water is very good against the quinsy, being gargled and bathed therewith, and wonderfully helps deafness, the noise, and other pains in the ears. The distilled water of the young green leaves in the end of May, performs a singular cure on foul running ulcers and sores, to be bathed, with wet cloths or spunges applied to them every morning.

WOLD, WELD OR DYER'S WEED

THE common kind grows bushing with many leaves, long, narrow and flat upon the ground; of a dark blueish green colour, somewhat like unto Woad, but nothing so large, a little crumpled, and as it were round-pointed, which do so abide the first year; and the next spring from among them, rise up divers round stalks, two or three feet high, beset with many such like leaves thereon, but smaller, and shooting forth small branches, which with the stalks carry many small yellow flowers, in a long spiked head at the top of them, where afterwards come the seed, which is small and black, inclosed in heads that are divided at the tops into four parts. The root is long, white and thick, abiding the Winter. The whole herb changes to be yellow, after it hath been in flower awhile.

Place.] It grows every where by the way sides, in moist grounds, as well as dry, in corners of fields and bye lanes, and sometimes all over the field. In Sussex and Kent they call it Green Weed.

Time.] It flowers in June.

Government and virtues.] Matthiolus saith, That the root hereof cures tough phlegm, digests raw phlegm, thins gross humours, dissolves hard tumours, and opens obstructions. Some do highly commend it against the biting of venomous creatures, to be taken inwardly and applied outwardly to the hurt place; as also for the plague or pestilence. The people in some countries of this land, do use to bruise the herb, and lay it to cuts or wounds in the hands or legs, to heal them.

WHEAT

ALL the several kinds thereof are so well known unto almost all people, that it is all together needless to write a description thereof.

Government and virtues.] It is under Venus. Dioscorides saith, That to eat the corn of green Wheat is hurtful to the stomach, and breeds worms. Pliny saith, That the corn of Wheat, roasted upon an iron pan, and eaten, are a present remedy for those that are chilled with cold. The oil pressed from wheat, between two thick plates of iron, or copper heated, heals all tetters and ring-worms, being used warm; and thereby Galen saith, he hath known many to be cured. Matthiolus commends the same to be put into hollow ulcers to heal them up, and it is good for chops in the hands and feet, and to make rugged skin smooth. The green corns of Wheat being chewed, and applied to the place bitten by a mad dog, heals it; slices of Wheat bread soaked in red rose water, and applied to the eyes that are hot, red, and inflamed, or blood-shotten, helps them. Hot bread applied for an hour, at times, for three days together, perfectly heals the kernels in the throat, commonly called the king's evil. The flour of Wheat mixed with the juice of henbane, stays the flux of humours to the joints, being laid thereon. The said meal boiled in vinegar, helps the shrinking of the sinews, saith Pliny; and mixed with vinegar, and boiled together, heals all freckles, spots and pimples on the face. Wheat flour, mixed with the yolk of an egg, honey, and turpentine, doth draw, cleanse and heal any boil, plague, sore, or foul ulcer. The bran of Wheat meal steeped in sharp vinegar, and then bound in a linen cloth, and rubbed on those places that have the scurf, morphew, scabs or leprosy, will take them away, the body being first well purged and prepared. The decoction of the bran of Wheat or barley, is of good use to bathe those places that are bursten by a rupture; and the said bran boiled in good vinegar, and applied to swollen breasts, helps them, and stays all inflammations. It helps also the biting of vipers (which I take to be no other than our English adder) and all other venomous creatures. The leaves of Wheat meal applied with some salt, take away hardness of the skin, warts, and hard knots in the flesh. Wafers put in water, and drank, stays the lask and bloody flux, and are profitably used both inwardly and outwardly for the ruptures in children. Boiled in water unto a thick jelly, and taken, it stays spitting of blood; and boiled with mint and butter, it helps the hoarseness of the throat.

THE WILLOW TREE

THESE are so well known that they need no description. I shall therefore only shew you the virtues thereof.

Government and virtues.] The Moon owns it. Both the leaves, bark, and the seed, are used to stanch bleeding of wounds, and at mouth and nose, spitting of blood, and other fluxes of blood in man or woman, and to stay vomiting, and provocation thereunto, if the decoction of them in wine be drank. It helps also to stay thin, hot, sharp, salt distillations from the head upon the lungs, causing a consumption. The leaves bruised with some pepper, and drank in wine, helps much the wind cholic. The leaves bruised and boiled in wine, and drank, stays the heat of lust in man or woman, and quite extinguishes it, if it be long used. The seed also is of the same effect. Water that is gathered from the Willow, when it flowers, the bark being slit, and a vessel fitting to receive it, is very good for redness and dimness of sight, or films that grow over the eyes, and stay the rheums that fall into them; to provoke urine, being stopped, if it be drank; to clear the face and skin from spots and discolourings. Galen saith, The flowers have an admirable faculty in drying up humours, being a medicine without any sharpness or corrosion; you may boil them in white wine, and drink as much as you will, so you drink not yourself drunk. The bark works the same effect, if used in the same manner, and the Tree hath always a bark upon it, though not always flowers; the burnt ashes of the bark being mixed with vinegar, takes away warts, corns, and superfluous flesh, being applied to the place. The decoction of the leaves or bark in wine, takes away scurff and dandriff by washing the place with it. It is a fine cool tree, the boughs of which are very convenient to be placed in the chamber of one sick of a fever.

WOAD

Descript.] It hath divers large leaves, long, and somewhat broad withal, like those of the greater plantain, but larger, thicker, of a greenish colour, somewhat blue withal. From among which leaves rises up a lusty stalk, three or four feet high, with divers leaves set thereon; the higher the stalk rises, the smaller are the leaves; at the top it spreads divers branches, at the end of which appear very pretty, little yellow flowers, and after they pass away like other flowers of the field, come husks, long and somewhat flat withal; in form they resemble a tongue, in colour they are black, and they hang bobbing downwards. The seed contained within these husks (if it be a little chewed) gives an azure colour. The root is white and long.

Place.] It is sowed in fields for the benefit of it, where those that sow it, cut it three times a year.

Time.] It flowers in June, but it is long after before the seed is ripe.

Government and virtues.] It is a cold and dry plant of Saturn. Some people affirm the plant to be destructive to bees, and fluxes them, which, if it be, I cannot help it. I should rather think, unless bees be contrary to other creatures, it possesses them with the contrary disease, the herb being exceeding dry and binding. However, if any bees be diseased thereby, the cure is, to set urine by them, but set it in a vessel, that they cannot drown themselves, which may be remedied, if you put pieces of cork in it. The herb is so drying and binding, that it is not fit to be given inwardly. An ointment made thereof stanches bleeding. A plaister made thereof, and applied to the region of the spleen which lies on the left side, takes away the hardness and pains thereof. The ointment is excellently good in such ulcers as abound with moisture, and takes away the corroding and fretting humours. It cools inflammations, quenches St. Anthony's fire, and stays defluxion of the blood to any part of the body.

WOODBINE, OR HONEY-SUCKLES

IT is a plant so common, that every one that hath eyes knows it, and he that hath none, cannot read a description, if I should write it.

Time.] They flower in June, and the fruit is ripe in August.

Government and virtues.] Doctor Tradition, that grand introducer of errors, that hater of truth, lover of folly, and the mortal foe to Dr. Reason, hath taught the common people to use the leaves or flowers of this plant in mouth-water, and by long continuance of time, hath so grounded it in the brains of the vulgar, that you cannot beat it out with a beetle. All mouth-waters ought to be cooling and drying, but Honey Suckles are cleansing, consuming and digesting, and therefore fit for inflammations; thus Dr. Reason. Again if you please, we will leave Dr. Reason a while, and come to Dr. Experience, a learned gentleman, and his brother. Take a leaf and chew it in your mouth, and you will quickly find it likelier to cause a sore mouth and throat than to cure it. Well then, if it be not good for this, what is it good for? It is good for something, for God and nature made nothing in vain. It is an herb of Mercury, and appropriated to the lungs; neither is it Crab claims dominion over it; neither is it a foe to the Lion; if the lungs be afflicted by Jupiter, this is your cure. It is fitting a conserve made of the flowers of it were kept in every gentlewoman's house; I know no better cure for an asthma than this: besides, it takes away the evil of the spleen, provokes urine, procures speedy delivery of women in travail, helps cramps, convulsions, and palsies, and whatsoever griefs come of cold or stopping; if you please to make use of it as an ointment, it will clear your skin of morphew, freckles, and sun-burnings, or whatsoever else discolours it, and then the maids will love it. Authors say, The flowers are of more effect than the leaves, and that is true; but they say the seeds are least effectual of all. But Dr. Reason told me, That there was a vital spirit in every seed to beget its like; and Dr. Experience told me, That there was a greater heat in the seed than there was in any other part of the plant: and withal, That heat was the mother of action, and then judge if old Dr. Tradition (who may well be honoured for his age, but not for his goodness) hath not so poisoned the world with errors before I was born, that it was never well in its wits since, and there is a great fear it will die mad.

WORMWOOD

THREE Wormwoods are familiar with us; one I shall not describe, another I shall describe, and the third be critical at; and I care not greatly if I begin with the last first.

Sea Wormwood hath gotten as many names as virtues, (and perhaps one more) Seriphian, Santomeon, Belchion, Narbinense, Hantonicon, Misneule, and a matter of twenty more which I shall not blot paper withal. A papist got the toy by the end, and he called it Holy Wormwood; and in truth I am opinion, their giving so much holiness to herbs, is the reason there remains so little in themselves. The seed of this Wormwood is that which women usually give their children for the worms. Of all Wormwoods that grow here, this is the weakest, but Doctors commend it, and apothecaries sell it; the one must keep his credit, and the other get money, and that is the key of the work. The herb is good for something, because God made nothing in vain. Will you give me leave to weigh things in the balance of reason, then thus: The seeds of the common Wormwood are far more prevalent than the seed of this, to expel worms in children, or people of ripe age; of both some are weak, some are strong. The Seriphian Wormwood is the weakest, and haply may prove to be fittest for the weak bodies, (for it is weak enough of all conscience.) Let such as are strong take the common Wormwood, for the others will do but little good. Again, near the sea many people live, and Seriphian grows near them, and therefore is more fitting for their bodies, because nourished by the same air; and this I had from Dr. Reason. In whose body Dr. Reason dwells not, dwells Dr. Madness, and he brings in his brethren, Dr. Ignorance, Dr. Folly, and Dr. Sickness, and these together make way for Death, and the latter end of that man is worse than the beginning. Pride was the cause of Adam's fall; pride begat a daughter, I do not know the father of it, unless the devil, but she christened it, and called it Appetite, and sent her daughter to taste these wormwoods, who finding this the least bitter, made the squeamish wench extol it to the skies, though the virtues of it never reached the middle region of the air. Its due praise is this: It is weakest, therefore fittest for weak bodies, and fitter for those bodies that dwell near it, than those that dwell far from it; my reason is, the sea (those that live far from it, know when they come near it) casts not such a smell as the land doth. The tender mercies of God being over all his works, hath by his eternal Providence, planted Seriphian by the seaside, as a fit medicine for the bodies of those that live near it. Lastly, it is known to all that know any thing in the course of nature, that the liver delights in sweet things, if so, it abhors bitter; then if your liver be weak, it is none of the wisest courses to plague it with an enemy. If the liver be weak, a consumption follows; would you know the reason? It is this, A man's flesh is repaired by blood, by a third concoction, which transmutes the blood into flesh, it is well I said, (concoction) say I, if I had said (boiling) every cook would have understood me. The liver makes blood, and if it be weakened that if it makes not enough, the flesh wastes; and why must flesh always be renewed? Because the eternal God, when he made the creation, made one part of it in continual dependency upon another; and why did he so? Because himself only is permanent; to teach us, That we should not fix our affections upon what is transitory, but what endures for ever. The result of this is, if the liver be weak, and cannot make blood enough, I would have said, Sanguify, if I had written only to scholars, the Seriphian, which is the weakest of Wormwoods, is better than the best. I have been critical enough, if not too much.

Place.] It grows familiarly in England, by the sea-side.

Descript.] It starts up out of the earth, with many round, woody, hairy stalks from one root. Its height is four feet, or three at least. The leaves in longitude are long, in latitude narrow, in colour white, in form hoary, in similitude like Southernwood, only broader and longer; in taste rather salt than bitter, because it grows so near the salt-water; at the joints, with the leaves toward the tops it bears little yellow flowers; the root lies deep, and is woody.

Common Wormwood I shall not describe, for every boy that can eat an egg knows it.

Roman Wormwood; and why Roman, seeing it grows familiarly in England? It may be so called, because it is good for a stinking breath, which the Romans cannot be very free from, maintaining so many bad houses by authority of his Holiness.

Descript.] The stalks are slender, and shorter than the common Wormwood by one foot at least; the leaves are more finely cut and divided than they are, but something smaller; both leaves and stalks are hoary, the flowers of a pale yellow colour; it is altogether like the common Wormwood, save only in bigness, for it is smaller; in taste, for it is not so bitter; in smell, for it is spicy.

Place.] It grows upon the tops of the mountains (it seems 'tis aspiring) there 'tis natural, but usually nursed up in gardens for the use of the apothecaries in London.

Time.] All Wormwoods usually flower in August, a little sooner or later.

Government and virtues.] Will you give me leave to be critical a little? I must take leave. Wormwood is an herb of Mars, and if Pontanus say otherwise, he is beside the bridge; I prove it thus: What delights in martial places, is a martial herb; but Wormwood delights in martial places (for about forges and iron works you may gather a cart-load of it,) *ergo*, it is a martial herb. It is hot and dry in the first degree, viz. just as hot as your blood, and no hotter. It remedies the evils choler can inflict on the body of man by sympathy. It helps the evils Venus and the wanton Boy produce, by antipathy; and it doth something else besides. It cleanses the body of choler (who dares say Mars doth no good?) It provokes urine, helps surfeits, or swellings in the belly: it causes appetite to meat, because Mars rules the attractive faculty in man. The sun never shone upon a better herb for the yellow jaundice than this. Why should men cry out so much upon Mars for an infortunate, (or Saturn either?) Did God make creatures to do the creation a mischief? This herb testifies, that Mars is willing to cure all diseases he causes; the truth is, Mars loves no cowards, nor Saturn fools, nor I neither. Take of the flowers of Wormwood, Rosemary, and Black Thorn, of each a like quantity, half that quantity of saffron; boil this in Rhenish wine, but put it not in saffron till it is almost boiled. This is the way to keep a man's body in health, appointed by Camerarius, in his book intitled *Hortus Medicus*, and it is a good one too. Besides all this, Wormwood provokes the terms. I would willingly teach astrologers, and make them physicians (if I knew how) for they are most fitting for the calling; if you will not believe me, ask Dr. Hippocrates, and Dr. Galen, a couple of gentlemen that our college of physicians keep to vapour with, not to follow. In this our herb, I shall give the pattern of a ruler, the sons of art rough cast, yet as near the truth as the men of Benjamin could throw a stone. Whereby, my brethren, the astrologers may know by a penny how a shilling is coined. As for the college of physicians, they are too stately to college or too proud to continue. They say a mouse is under the dominion of the Moon, and that is the reason they feed in the night; the house of the Moon is Cancer; rats are of the same nature with mice, but they are a little bigger; Mars receives his fall in Cancer, *ergo*, Wormwood being an herb of Mars, is a present remedy for the biting of rats and mice. Mushrooms (I cannot give them the title of Herba, Frutex, or

Arbor) are under the dominion of Saturn, (and take one time with another, they do as much harm as good;) if any have poisoned himself by eating them, Wormwood, an herb of Mars, cures him, because Mars is exalted in Capricorn, the house of Saturn, and this it doth by sympathy, as it did the other by antipathy. Wheals, pushes, black and blue spots, coming either by bruises or beatings. Wormwood, an herb of Mars, helps, because Mars, (as bad you love him, and as you hate him) will not break your head, but he will give you a plaister. If he do but teach you to know yourselves, his courtesy is greater than his discourtesy. The greatest antipathy between the planets, is between Mars and Venus: one is hot, the other cold; one diurnal, the other nocturnal; one dry, the other moist; their houses are opposite, one masculine, the other feminine; one public, the other private; one is valiant, the other effeminate: one loves the light, the other hates it; one loves the field, the other sheets: then the throat is under Venus, the quinsy lies in the throat, and is an inflammation there; Venus rules the throat, (it being under Tamus her sign.) Mars eradicates all diseases in the throat by his herbs (for wormwood is one) and sends them to Egypt on an errand never to return more, this done by antipathy. The eyes are under the Luminaries; the right eye of a man, and the left eye of a woman the Sun claims dominion over: the left eye of a man, and the right eye of a woman, are privileges of the Moon, Wormwood, an herb of Mars cures both; what belongs to the Sun by sympathy, because he is exalted in his house; but what belongs to the Moon by antipathy, because he hath his fall in her's. Suppose a man be bitten or stung by a martial creature, imagine a wasp, a hornet, a scorpion, Wormwood, an herb of Mars, gives you a present cure; that Mars, choleric as he is, hath learned that patience, to pass by your evil speeches of him, and tells you by my pen, That he gives you no affliction, but he gives you a cure; you need not run to Apollo, nor Æsculapius; and if he was so choleric as you make him to be, he would have drawn his sword for anger, to see the ill conditions of these people that can spy his vices, and not his virtues. The eternal God, when he made Mars, made him for public good, and the sons of men shall know it in the latter end of the world. *Et cælum Mars solus babet.* You say Mars is a destroyer; mix a little Wormwood, an herb of Mars, with your ink, neither rats nor mice touch the paper written with it, and then Mars is a preserver. Astrologers think Mars causes scabs and itch, and the virgins are angry with him, because wanton Venus told them he deforms their skins; but, quoth Mars, my only desire is, they should know themselves; my herb Wormwood will restore them to the beauty they formerly had, and in that I will not come an inch behind my opposite, Venus: for which doth the greatest evil, he that takes away an innate beauty, and when he has done, knows how to restore it again? Or she that teaches a company of wanton lasses to paint their faces? If Mars be in a Virgin, in the nativity, they say he causes the cholic (it is well God hath set some body to pull down the pride of man.) He in the Virgin troubles none with the cholic, but them that know not themselves (for who knows himself, may easily know all the world.) Wormwood, an herb of Mars, is a present cure for it; and whether it be most like a Christian to love him for his good, or hate him for his evil, judge ye. I had almost forgotten, that charity thinks no evil. I was once in the Tower and viewed the wardrobe, and there was a great many fine clothes. I can give them no other title (for I was never either linen or woolen draper), yet as brave as they looked, my opinion was that the moths might consume them; moths are under the dominion of Mars; this herb Wormwood being laid among cloaths, will make a moth scorn to meddle with the cloaths, as much as a lion scorns to meddle with a mouse, or an eagle with a fly. You say Mars is angry, and it is true enough he is angry with many countrymen, for being such fools to be led by the noses by the college of physicians, as they lead bears to Paris garden. Melancholy men cannot endure to be wronged in point of good fame, and that doth sorely trouble old Saturn, because they call him the greatest infortunate; in the body of man he rules the spleen, (and that makes covetous man so splenetic) the poor old man lies crying out of his left side. Father Saturn's angry, Mars comes to him. Come, brother, I confess thou art evil spoken of, and so am I; thou knowest I have my exaltation in thy house, I give him an herb of mine, Wormwood, to cure the old man. Saturn consented, but spoke little, and so Mars cured him by sympathy. When Mars was free from war, (for he loves to be fighting, and is the best friend a soldier hath) I say, when Mars was free from war, he called a council of war in his own brain, to know how he should do poor sinful man good, desiring to forget his abuses in being called an infortunate. He musters up his own forces, and places them in battalia. Oh! quoth he, why do I hurt a poor silly man or woman? His angel answers him, It is because they have offended their God, (Look back to Adam:) Well, says Mars, though they speak evil of me, I will do good to them; Death's cold, my herb shall heat them: they are full of ill humours (else they would never have spoken ill of me;) my herb shall cleanse them, and dry them; they are poor weak creatures, my herb shall strengthen them; they are dull witted, my herb shall fortify their apprehensions; and yet among astrologers all this does not deserve a good word. Oh the patience of Mars!

Felix qui potuit rerum cognoscere caucas,
Inque domus superum scandere cura facit.
O happy he that can the knowledge gain,
To know the eternal God made nought in vain.

To this I add,

I know the reason causeth such a dearth
Of knowledge; 'tis because men love the earth.

The other day Mars told me he met with Venus, and he asked her, What was the reason that she accused him for abusing women? He never gave them the pox. In the dispute they fell out, and in anger parted, and Mars told me that his brother Saturn told him, that an antivenerean medicine was the best against the pox. Once a month he meets with the Moon. Mars is quick enough of speech, and the Moon not much behind hand, (neither are most women.) The Moon looks much after children, and children are much troubled with the worms; she desired a medicine of him, he bid her take his own herb, Wormwood. He had no sooner parted with the Moon, but he met with Venus, and she was as drunk as a hog. Alas! poor Venus, quoth he; What! thou a fortune, and be drunk? I'll give thee antipathetical cure. Take my herb Wormwood, and thou shall never get a surfeit by drinking. A poor silly countryman hath got an ague, and cannot go about his business: he wishes he had it not, and so do I; but I will tell him a remedy, whereby he shall prevent it. Take the herb of Mars, Wormwood, and if infortunes will do good, what will fortunes do? Some think the lungs are under Jupiter; and if the lungs then the breath; and though sometimes a man gets a stinking breath, and yet Jupiter is a fortune, forsooth; up comes Mars to him. Come brother Jupiter, thou knowest I sent thee a couple of trines to thy house last night, the one from Aries, and the other from Scorpio; give me thy leave by sympathy to cure this poor man with drinking a draught of Wormwood beer every morning. The Moon was weak the other day, and she gave a man two terrible mischiefs, a dull brain and a weak sight; Mars laid by his sword, and comes to her. Sister Moon, said he, this man hath angered thee, but I beseech thee take notice he is but a fool; prithee be patient, I will with my herb wormwood cure him of both infirmities by antipathy, for thou knowest thou and I cannot agree; with that the Moon began to quarrel; Mars (not delighting much in women's tongues) went away, and did it whether she would or no.

He that reads this, and understands what he reads, hath a jewel of more worth than a diamond; he that understands it not, is as little fit to give physick. There lies a key in these words which will unlock, (if it be turned by a wise hand) the cabinet of physick. I have delivered it as plain as I durst; it is not only upon Wormwood as I wrote, but upon all plants, trees, and herbs, he that understands it not, is unfit (in my opinion) to give physic. This shall live when I am dead. And thus I leave it to the world, not caring a farthing whether they like it or dislike it. The grave equals all men, and therefore shall equal me with all princes; until which time the eternal Providence is over me. Then the ill tongue of a prating fellow, or one that hath more tongue than wit, or more proud than honest, shall never trouble me. *Wisdom is justified by her children*. And so much for Wormwood.

YARROW, CALLED NOSE-BLEED, MILFOIL AND THOUSALD-LEAL

Descript.] It hath many long leaves spread upon the ground, finely cut, and divided into many small parts. Its flowers are white, but not all of a whiteness and stayed in knots, upon divers green stalks which rise from among the leaves.

Place.] It is frequent in all pastures.

Time.] It flowers late, even in the latter end of August.

Government and virtues.] It is under the influence of Venus. An ointment of them cures wounds, and is most fit for such as have inflammations, it being an herb of Dame Venus; it stops the terms in women, being boiled in white wine, and the decoction drank; as also the bloody flux; the ointment of it is not only good for green wounds, but also for ulcers and fistulas, especially such as abound with moisture. It stays the shedding of hair, the head being bathed with the decoction of it; inwardly taken it helps the retentive faculty of the stomach: it helps the gonorrhea in men, and the whites in women, and helps such as cannot hold their water; and the leaves chewed in the mouth eases the tooth-ache, and these virtues being put together, shew the herb to be drying and binding. Achilles is supposed to be the first that left the virtues of this herb to posterity, having learned them of this master Chiron, the Centaur; and certainly a very profitable herb it is in cramps, and therefore called Militaris.

Directions for making Syrups, Conserves, &c. &c.

HAVING in divers places of this Treatise promised you the way of making Syrups, Conserves, Oils, Ointments, &c, of herbs, roots, flowers, &c. whereby you may have them ready for your use at such times when they cannot be had otherwise; I come now to perform what I promised, and you shall find me rather better than worse than my word.

That this may be done methodically, I shall divide my directions into two grand sections, and each section into several chapters, and then you shall see it look with such a countenance as this is.

SECTION I

Of gathering, drying, and keeping Simples, and their juices

SECTION II

Of making and keeping Compounds

Of all these in order.

CHAPTER I

Of Leaves of Herbs, or Trees

1. Of leaves, choose only such as are green, and full of juice; pick them carefully, and cast away such as are any way declining, for they will putrify the rest. So shall one handful be worth ten of those you buy at the physic herb shops.

2. Note what places they most delight to grow in, and gather them there; for Betony that grows in the shade, is far better than that which grows in the Sun, because it delights in the shade; so also such herbs as delight to grow near the water, shall be gathered near it, though happily you may find some of them upon dry ground. The Treatise will inform you where every herb delights to grow.

3. The leaves of such herbs as run up to seed, are not so good when they are in flower as before (some few excepted, the leaves of which are seldom or never used). In such cases, if through ignorance they were not known, or through negligence forgotten, you had better take the top and the flowers, then the leaf.

4. Dry them well in the Sun, and not in the shade, as the saying of physicians is; for if the sun draw away the virtues of the herb, it must need do the like by hay, by the same rule, which the experience of every country farmer will explode for a notable piece of nonsense.

5. Such as are artists in astrology, (and indeed none else are fit to make physicians) such I advise: Let the planet that governs the herb be angular, and the stronger the better; if they can, in herbs of Saturn, let Saturn be in the ascendant; in the herbs of Mars, let Mars be in the mid heaven, for in those houses they delight; let the Moon apply to them by good aspect, and let her not be in the houses of her enemies; if you cannot well stay till she apply to them, let her apply to a planet of the same triplicity; if you cannot wait that time neither, let her be with a fixed star of their nature.

6. Having well dried them, put them up in brown paper, sewing the paper up like a sack, and press them not too hard together, and keep them in a dry place near the fire.

7. As for the duration of dried herbs, a just time cannot be given, let authors prate their pleasure; for,

1st. Such as grow upon dry grounds will keep better than such as grow on moist.

2dly. Such herbs as are full of juice, will not keep so long as such as are drier.

3dly. Such herbs as are well dried, will keep longer than such as are slack dried. Yet you may know when they are corrupted, by their loss of colour, or smell, or both; and if they be corrupted, reason will tell you that they must needs corrupt the bodies of those people that take them.

4. Gather all leaves in the hour of that planet that governs them.

CHAPTER II

Of Flowers

1. The flower, which is the beauty of the plant, and of none of the least use in physick, grows yearly, and is to be gathered when it is in its prime.

2. As for the time of gathering them, let the planetary hour, and the planet they come of, be observed, as we shewed you in the foregoing chapter: as for the time of the day, let it be when the sun shine upon them, that so they may be dry; for, if you gather either flowers or herbs when they are wet or dewy, they will not keep.

3. Dry them well in the sun, and keep them in papers near the fire, as I shewed you in the foregoing chapter.

4. So long as they retain the colour and smell, they are good; either of them being gone, so is the virtue also.

CHAPTER III

Of Seeds

1. The seed is that part of the plant which is endowed with a vital faculty to bring forth its like, and it contains potentially the whole plant in it.

2. As for place, let them be gathered from the place where they delight to grow.

3. Let them be full ripe when they are gathered; and forget not the celestial harmony before mentioned, for I have found by experience that their virtues are twice as great at such times as others: "There is an appointed time for every thing under the sun."

4. When you have gathered them, dry them a little, and but a little in the sun, before you lay them up.

5. You need not be so careful of keeping them so near the fire, as the other beforementioned, because they are fuller of spirit, and therefore not so subject to corrupt.

6. As for the time of their duration, it is palpable they will keep

a good many years; yet, they are best the first year, and this I make appear by a good argument. They will grow sooner the first year they be set, therefore then they are in their prime; and it is an easy matter to renew them yearly.

CHAPTER IV

Of Roots

1. Of roots, chuse such as are neither rotten nor worm-eaten, but proper in their taste, colour, and smell; such as exceed neither in softness nor hardness.

2. Give me leave to be a little critical against the vulgar received opinion, which is, That the sap falls down into the roots in the Autumn, and rises again in the Spring, as men go to bed at night, and rise in the morning; and this idle talk of untruth is so grounded in the heads, not only of the vulgar, but also of the learned, that a man cannot drive it out by reason. I pray let such sapmongers answer me this argument: If the sap falls into the roots in the fall of the leaf, and lies there all the Winter, then must the root grow only in the Winter. But the root grows not at all in the Winter, as experience teaches, but only in the Summer. Therefore, if you set an apple-kernel in the Spring, you shall find the root to grow to a pretty bigness in the Summer, and be not a whit bigger next Spring. What doth the sap do in the root all that while? Pick straws? 'Tis as rotten as a rotten post.

The truth is, when the sun declines from the tropic of Cancer, the sap begins to congeal both in root and branch; when he touches the tropic of Capricorn, and ascends to us-ward, it begins to wax thin again, and by degrees, as it congealed. But to proceed.

3. The drier time you gather the roots in, the better they are; for they have the less excrementitious moisture in them.

4. Such roots as are soft, your best way is to dry in the sun, or else hang them in the chimney corner upon a string; as for such as are hard, you may dry them any where.

5. Such roots as are great, will keep longer than such as are small; yet most of them will keep a year.

6. Such roots as are soft, it is your best way to keep them always near the fire, and to take this general rule for it: If in Winter-time you find any of your roots, herbs or flowers begin to be moist, as many times you shall (for it is your best way to look to them once a month) dry them by a very gentle fire; or, if you can with convenience keep them near the fire, you may save yourself the labour.

7. It is in vain to dry roots that may commonly be had, as Parsley, Fennel, Plantain, &c. but gather them only for present need.

CHAPTER V

Of Barks

1. Barks, which physicians use in medicine, are of these sorts: Of fruits, of roots, of boughs.

2. The barks of fruits are to be taken when the fruit is full ripe, as Oranges, Lemons, &c. but because I have nothing to do with exotics here, I pass them without any more words.

3. The barks of trees are best gathered in the Spring, if of oaks, or such great trees; because then they come easier off, and so you may dry them if you please; but indeed the best way is to gather all barks only for present use.

4. As for the barks of roots, 'tis thus to be gotten. Take the roots of such herbs as have a pith in them, as parsley, fennel, &c. slit them in the middle, and when you have taken out the pith (which you may easily do) that which remains is called (tho' improperly) the bark, and indeed is only to be used.

CHAPTER VI

Of Juices

1. Juices are to be pressed out of herbs when they are young and tender, out of some stalks and tender tops of herbs and plants, and also out of some flowers.

2. Having gathered the herb, would you preserve the juice of it, when it is very dry (for otherwise the juice will not be worth a button) bruise it very well in a stone mortar with a wooden pestle, then having put it into a canvas bag, the herb I mean, not the mortar, for that will give but little juice, press it hard in a press, then take the juice and clarify it.

3. The manner of clarifying it is this: Put it into a pipkin or skillet, or some such thing, and set it over the fire; and when the scum rises, take it off; let it stand over the fire till no more scum arise; when you have your juice clarified, cast away the scum as a thing of no use.

4. When you have thus clarified it, you have two ways to preserve it all the year.

(1) When it is cold, put it into a glass, and put so much oil on it as will cover it to the thickness of two fingers; the oil will swim at the top, and so keep the air from coming to putrify it. When you intend to use it, pour it into a porringer, and if any oil come out with it, you may easily scum it off with a spoon, and put the juice you use not into the glass again, it will quickly sink under the oil. This is the first way.

(2) The second way is a little more difficult, and the juice of fruits is usually preserved this way. When you have clarified it, boil it over the fire, till (being cold) it be of the thickness of honey. This is most commonly used for diseases of the mouth, and is called Roba and Saba. And thus much for the first section, the second follows.

SECTION II

The way of making and keeping all necessary Compounds

CHAPTER V

Of distilled Waters

HITHERTO we have spoken of medicines which consist in their own nature, which authors vulgarly call Simples, though sometimes improperly; for in truth, nothing is simple but pure elements; all things else are compounded of them. We come now to treat of the artificial medicines, in the form of which (because we must begin somewhere) we shall place distilled waters; in which consider:

1. Waters are distilled of herbs, flowers, fruits, and roots.

2. We treat not of strong waters, but of cold, as being to act Galen's part, and not Paracelsus's.

3. The herbs ought to be distilled when they are in the greatest vigour, and so ought the flowers also.

4. The vulgar way of distillations which people use, because they know no better, is in a pewter still; and although distilled waters are the weakest of artificial medicines, and good for little but mixtures of other medicines, yet they are weaker by many degrees, than they would be were they distilled in sand. If I thought it not impossible, to teach you the way of distilling in sand, I would attempt it.

5. When you have distilled your water, put it into a glass, covered over with a paper pricked full of holes, so that the excrementitious and fiery vapours may exhale, which cause that settling

in distilled waters called the Mother, which corrupt them, then cover it close, and keep it for your use.

6. Stopping distilled waters with a cork, makes them musty, and so does paper, if it but touch the water: it is best to stop them with a bladder, being first put in water, and bound over the top of the glass.

Such cold waters as are distilled in a pewter still (if well kept) will endure a year; such as are distilled in sand, as they are twice as strong, so they endure twice as long.

CHAPTER II

Of Syrups

1. A syrup is a medicine of a liquid form, composed of infusion, decoction and juice. And, 1. For the more grateful taste. 2. For the better keeping of it: with a certain quantity of honey or sugar, hereafter mentioned, boiled to the thickness of new honey.

2. You see at the first view, that this aphorism divides itself into three branches, which deserve severally to be treated of, viz.

1. Syrups made by infusion.
2. Syrups made by decoction.
3. Syrups made by juice.

Of each of these, (for your instruction-sake, kind countrymen and women) I speak a word or two apart.

1st, Syrups made by infusion, are usually made of flowers, and of such flowers as soon lose their colour and strength by boiling, as roses, violets, peach flowers, &c. They are thus made: Having picked your flowers clean, to every pound of them add three pounds or three pints, which you will (for it is all one) of spring water, made boiling hot; first put your flowers into a pewter-pot, with a cover, and pour the water on them; then shutting the pot, let it stand by the fire, to keep hot twelve hours, and strain it out: (in such syrups as purge) as damask roses, peach flowers, &c. the usual, and indeed the best way, is to repeat this infusion, adding fresh flowers to the same liquor divers times, that so it may be the stronger) having strained it out, put the infusion into a pewter bason, or an earthen one well glazed, and to every pint of it add two pounds of sugar, which being only melted over the fire, without boiling, and scummed, will produce you the syrup you desire.

2dly, Syrups made by decoction are usually made of compounds, yet may any simple herb be thus converted into syrup: Take the herb, root, or flowers you would make into a syrup, and bruise it a little; then boil it in a convenient quantity of spring water; the more water you boil it in, the weaker it will be; a handful of the herb or root is a convenient quantity for a pint of water, boil it till half the water be consumed, then let it stand till it be almost cold, and strain it through a woollen cloth, letting it run out at leisure: without pressing. To every pint of this decoction add one pound of sugar, and boil it over the fire till it come to a syrup, which you may know, if you now and then cool a little of it with a spoon. Scum it all the while it boils, and when it is sufficiently boiled, whilst it is hot, strain it again through a woollen cloth, but press it not. Thus you have the syrup perfected.

3dly, Syrups made of juice, are usually made of such herbs as are full of juice, and indeed they are better made into a syrup this way than any other; the operation is thus: Having beaten the herb in a stone mortar, with a wooden pestle, press out the juice, and clarify it, as you are taught before in the juices; then let the juice boil away till about a quarter of it be consumed; to a pint of this add a pound of sugar, and when it is boiled, strain it through a woollen cloth, as we taught you before, and keep it for your use.

3. If you make a syrup of roots that are any thing hard, as parsley, fennel, and grass roots, &c. when you have bruised them, lay them in steep some time in that water which you intend to boil them in hot, so will the virtue the better come out.

4. Keep your syrups either in glasses or stone pots, and stop them not with cork nor bladder, unless you would have the glass break, and the syrup lost, only bind paper about the mouth.

5. All syrups, if well made, continue a year with some advantage; yet such as are made by infusion, keep shortest.

CHAPTER III

Of Juleps

1. Juleps were first invented, as I suppose, in Arabia; and my reason is, because the word Julep is an Arabic word.

2. It signifies only a pleasant potion, as is vulgarly used by such as are sick, and want help, or such as are in health, and want no money to quench thirst.

3. Now-a-day it is commonly used—
    1. To prepare the body for purgation.
    2. To open obstructions and the pores.
    3. To digest tough humours.
    4. To qualify hot distempers, &c.

4. Simple Juleps, (for I have nothing to say to compounds here) are thus made: Take a pint of such distilled water, as conduces to the cure of your distemper, which this treatise will plentifully furnish you with, to which add two ounces of syrup, conducing to the same effect; (I shall give you rules for it in the next chapter) mix them together, and drink a draught of it at your pleasure. If you love tart things, add ten drops of oil of vitriol to your pint, and shake it together, and it will have a fine grateful taste.

5. All juleps are made for present use; and therefore it is vain to speak of their duration.

CHAPTER IV

Of Decoctions

1. All the difference between decoctions, and syrups made by decoction, is this: Syrups are made to keep, decoctions only for present use; for you can hardly keep a decoction a week at any time; if the weather be hot, not half so long.

2. Decoctions are made of leaves, roots, flowers, seeds, fruits or barks, conducing to the cure of the disease you make them for; are made in the same manner as we shewed you in syrups.

3. Decoctions made with wine last longer than such as are made with water; and if you take your decoction to cleanse the passages of the urine, or open obstructions, your best way is to make it with white wine instead of water, because this is penetrating.

4. Decoctions are of most use in such diseases as lie in the passages of the body, as the stomach, bowels, kidneys, passages of urine and bladder, because decoctions pass quicker to those places than any other form of medicines.

5. If you will sweeten your decoction with sugar, or any syrup fit for the occasion you take it for, which is better, you may, and no harm.

6. If in a decoction, you boil both roots, herbs, flowers, and seed together, let the roots boil a good while first, because they retain their virtue longest; then the next in order by the same rule, *viz.* 1. Barks. 2. The herbs. 3. The seeds. 4. The flowers. 5. The spices, if you put any in, because their virtues come soonest out.

7. Such things as by boiling cause sliminess to a decoction, as figs, quince-seed, linseed, &c. your best way is, after you have bruised them, to tie them up in a linen rag, as you tie up calf's brains, and so boil them.

8. Keep all decoctions in a glass close stopped, and in the cooler place you keep them, the longer they will last ere they be sour.

Lastly, the usual dose to be given at one time, is usually two, three, four, or five ounces, according to the age and strength of the patient, the season of the year, the strength of the medicine, and the quality of the disease.

CHAPTER V

Of Oils

1. Oil Olive, which is commonly known by the name of Sallad Oil, I suppose because it is usually eaten with sallads by them that love it, if it be pressed out of ripe olives, according to Galen, is temperate, and exceeds in no one quality.

2. Of oils, some are simple, and some are compound.

3. Simple oils, are such as are made of fruits or seeds by expression, as oil of sweet and bitter almonds, linseed and rape-seed oil, &c. of which see in my Dispensatory.

4. Compound oils, are made of oil of olives, and other simples, imagine herbs, flowers, roots, &c.

5. The way of making them is this: Having bruised the herbs of flowers you would make your oil of, put them into an earthen pot, and to two or three handfuls of them pour a pint of oil, cover the pot with a paper, set it in the sun about a fortnight or so, according as the sun is in hotness; then having warmed it very well by the fire, press out the herb, &c. very hard in a press, and add as many more herbs to the same oil; bruise the herbs (I mean not the oil) in like manner, set them in the sun as before; the oftener you repeat this, the stronger your oil will be. At last when you conceive it strong enough, boil both herbs and oil together, till the juice be consumed, which you may know by its bubbling, and the herbs will be crisp; then strain it while it is hot, and keep it in a stone or glass vessel for your use.

6. As for chymical oils, I have nothing to say here.

7. The general use of these oils, is for pains in the limbs, roughness of the skin, the itch, &c. as also for ointments and plaisters.

8. If you have occasion to use it for wounds, or ulcers, in two ounces of oil, dissolve half an ounce of turpentine, the heat of the fire will quickly do it; for oil itself is offensive to wounds, and the turpentine qualifies it.

CHAPTER VI

Of Electuaries

PHYSICIANS make more a quoil than needs by half, about electuaries. I shall prescribe but one general way of making them up; as for ingredients, you may vary them as you please, and as you find occasion, by the last chapter.

1. That you may make electuaries when you need them, it is requisite that you keep always herbs, roots, flowers, seeds, &c. ready dried in your house, that so you may be in a readiness to beat them into powder when you need them.

2. It is better to keep them whole than beaten; for being beaten, they are more subject to lose their strength; because the air soon penetrates them.

3. If they be not dry enough to beat into powder when you need them, dry them by a gentle fire till they are so.

4. Having beaten them, sift them through a fine tiffany searce, that no great pieces may be found in your electuary.

5. To one ounce of your powder add three ounces of clarified honey; this quantity I hold to be sufficient. If you would make more or less electuary, vary your proportion accordingly.

6. Mix them well together in a mortar, and take this for a truth, you cannot mix them too much.

7. The way to clarify honey, is to set it over the fire in a convenient vessel, till the scum rise, and when the scum is taken off, it is clarified.

8. The usual dose of cordial electuaries, is from half a dram to two drams; of purging electuaries, from half an ounce to an ounce.

9. The manner of keeping them is in a pot.

10. The time of taking, is either in a morning fasting, and fasting an hour after them; or at night going to bed, three or four hours after supper.

CHAPTER VII

Of Conserves

1. The way of making conserves is twofold, one of herbs and flowers, and the other of fruits.

2. Conserves of herbs and flowers, are thus made: if you make your conserves of herbs, as of scurvy-grass, wormwood, rue, and the like, take only the leaves and tender tops (for you may beat

your heart out before you can beat the stalks small) and having beaten them, weigh them, and to every pound of them add three pounds of sugar, you cannot beat them too much.

3. Conserves of fruits, as of barberries, sloes and the like, is thus made: First, Scald the fruit, then rub the pulp through a thick hair sieve made for the purpose, called a pulping sieve; you may do it for a need with the back of a spoon: then take this pulp thus drawn, and add to it its weight of sugar, and no more; put it into a pewter vessel, and over a charcoal fire; stir it up and down till the sugar be melted, and your conserve is made.

4. Thus you have the way of making conserves; the way of keeping them is in earthen pots.

5. The dose is usually the quantity of a nutmeg at a time morning and evening, or (unless they are purging) when you please.

6. Of conserves, some keep many years, as conserves of roses: other but a year, as conserves of Borage, Bugloss, Cowslips and the like.

7. Have a care of the working of some conserves presently after they are made; look to them once a day, and stir them about, conserves of Borage, Bugloss, Wormwood, have got an excellent faculty at that sport.

8. You may know when your conserves are almost spoiled by this; you shall find a hard crust at top with little holes in it, as though worms had been eating there.

CHAPTER VIII

Of Preserves

OF Preserves are sundry sorts, and the operation of all being somewhat different, we will handle them all apart. These are preserved with sugar:

1. Flowers   3. Roots
2. Fruits   4. Barks

1. Flowers are very seldom preserved; I never saw any that I remember, save only cowslip flowers, and that was a great fashion in Sussex when I was a boy. It is thus done: Take a flat glass, we call them jat glasses; strew on a laying of fine sugar, on that a laying of flowers, and on that another laying of sugar, on that another laying of flowers, so do till your glass be full; then tie it over with a paper, and in a little time, you shall have very excellent and pleasant preserves.

There is another way of preserving flowers; namely, with vinegar and salt, as they pickle capers and broom-buds; but as I have little skill in it myself, I cannot teach you.

2. Fruits, as quinces, and the like, are preserved two ways:

(1) Boil them well in water, and then pulp them through a sieve, as we shewed you before; then with the like quantity of sugar, boil the water they were boiled in into a syrup, viz. a pound of sugar to a pint of liquor; to every pound of this syrup, add four ounces of the pulp; then boil it with a very gentle fire to their right consistence, which you may easily know if you drop a drop of it upon a trencher; if it be enough, it will not stick to your fingers when it is cold.

(2) Another way to preserve fruits is this: First, pare off the rind; then cut them in halves, and take out the core: then boil them in water till they are soft; if you know when beef is boiled enough, you may easily know when they are. Then boil the water with its like weight of sugar into a syrup; put the syrup into a pot, and put the boiled fruit as whole as you left it when you cut it into it, and let it remain until you have occasion to use it.

3. Roots are thus preserved. First, scrape them very clean, and cleanse them from the pith, if they have any, for some roots have not, as Eringo and the like. Boil them in water till they be soft, as we shewed you before in the fruits; then boil the water you boiled the root in into a syrup, as we shewed you before; then keep the root whole in the syrup till you use them.

4. As for barks, we have but few come to our hands to be done, and of those the few that I can remember, are, oranges, lemons, citrons, and the outer bark of walnuts, which grow without side the shell, for the shells themselves would make but scurvy preserves; these be they I can remember, if there be any more put them into the number.

The way of preserving these, is not all one in authors, for some are bitter, some are hot; such as are bitter, say authors, must be soaked in warm water, oftentimes changing till their bitter taste be fled. But I like not this way and my reason is this: because I doubt when their bitterness is gone, so is their virtue also. I shall then prescribe one common way, namely, the same with the former, viz.: First, boil them whole till they be soft, then make a syrup with sugar and the liquor you boil them in, and keep the barks in the syrup.

5. They are kept in glasses or in glazed pots.

6. The preserved flowers will keep a year, if you can forbear eating of them; the roots and barks much longer.

7. This art was plainly and first invented for delicacy, yet came afterwards to be of excellent use in physic; For,

(1) Hereby medicines are made pleasant for sick and squeamish stomachs, which else would loathe them.

(2) Hereby they are preserved from decaying a long time.

CHAPTER IX

Of Lohocks

1. That which the Arabians call Lohocks, and the Greeks Eclegma, the Latins call Linctus, and in plain English signifies nothing else but a thing to be licked up.

2. They are in body thicker than a syrup, and not so thick as an electuary.

3. The manner of taking them is, often to take a little with a liquorice stick, and let it go down at leisure.

4. They are easily thus made; Make a decoction of pectoral herbs, and the treatise will furnish you with enough, and when you have strained it, with twice its weight of honey or sugar, boil it to a lohock; if you are molested with much phlegm, honey is better than sugar; and if you add a little vinegar to it, you will do well; if not, I hold sugar to be better than honey.

5. It is kept in pots, and may be kept a year and longer.

6. It is excellent for roughness of the wind-pipe, inflammations and ulcers of the lungs, difficulty of breathing, asthmas, coughs, and distillation of humours.

CHAPTER X

Of Ointments

1. Various are the ways of making ointments, which authors have left to posterity, which I shall omit, and quote one which is easiest to be made, and therefore most beneficial to people that are ignorant in physic, for whose sake I write this. It is thus done.

Bruise those herbs, flowers, or roots, you will make an ointment of, and to two handfuls of your bruised herbs add a pound of hog's grease dried, or cleansed from the skins, beat them very well together in a stone mortar with a wooden pestle, then put it into a stone pot, (the herb and grease I mean, not the mortar,) cover it with a paper and set it either in the sun, or some other warm place; three, four, or five days, that it may melt; then take it out and boil it a little; then whilst it is hot, strain it out, pressing it out very hard in a press: to this grease add as many more herbs bruised as before;

let them stand in like manner as long, then boil them as you did the former. If you think your ointment is not strong enough, you may do it the third and fourth time; yet this I will tell you, the fuller of juice the herbs are, the sooner will your ointment be strong; the last time you boil it, boil it so long till your herbs be crisp, and the juice consumed, then strain it pressing it hard in a press, and to every pound of ointment add two ounces of turpentine, and as much wax, because grease is offensive to wounds, as well as oil.

2. Ointments are vulgarly known to be kept in pots, and will last above a year, some above two years.

CHAPTER XI

Of Plaisters

1. The Greeks made their plaisters of divers simples, and put metals into the most of them, if not all; for having reduced their metals into powder, they mixed them with that fatty substance whereof the rest of the plaister consisted, whilst it was thus hot, continually stirring it up and down, lest it should sink to the bottom; so they continually stirred it till it was stiff; then they made it up in rolls, which when they needed for use, they could melt by the fire again.

2. The Arabians made up theirs with oil and fat, which needed not so long boiling.

3. The Greeks emplaisters consisted of these ingredients, metals, stones, divers sorts of earth, feces, juices, liquors, seeds, roots, herbs, excrements of creatures, wax, rosin, gums.

CHAPTER XII

Of Poultices

1. Poultices are those kind of things which the Latins call *Cataplasmata*, and our learned fellows, that if they can read English, that's all, call them Cataplasms, because 'tis a crabbed word few understand; it is indeed a very fine kind of medicine to ripen sores.

2. They are made of herbs and roots, fitted for the disease, and members afflicted, being chopped small, and boiled in water almost to a jelly; then by adding a little barleymeal, or meal of lupins, and a little oil, or rough sweet suet, which I hold to be better, spread upon a cloth and apply to the grieved places.

3. Their use is to ease pain, to break sores, to cool inflammations, to dissolve hardness, to ease the spleen, to concoct humours, and dissipate swellings.

4. I beseech you take this caution along with you: Use no poultices (if you can help it) that are of an healing nature, before you have first cleansed the body, because they are subject to draw the humours to them from every part of the body.

CHAPTER XIII

Of Troches

1. The Latins call them *Placentula*, or little cakes, and the Greeks *Prochikois*, *Kukliscoi*, and *Artiscoi*; they are usually little round flat cakes, or you may make them square if you will.

2. Their first invention was, that powders being so kept might resist the intermission of air, and so endure pure the longer.

3. Besides, they are easier carried in the pockets of such as travel; as many a man (for example) is forced to travel whose stomach is too cold, or at least not so hot as it should be, which is most proper, for the stomach is never cold till a man be dead; in such a case, it is better to carry troches of wormwood, or galangal, in a paper in his pocket, than to lay a gallipot along with him.

4. They are made thus: At night when you go to bed, take two drams of fine gum tragacanth; put it into a gallipot, and put half a quarter of a pint of any distilled water fitting for the purpose you would make your troches for to cover it, and the next morning you shall find it in such a jelly as the physicians call mucilage. With this you may (with a little pains taken) make a powder into a paste, and that paste into cakes called troches.

5. Having made them, dry them in the shade, and keep them in a pot for your use.

CHAPTER XIV

Of Pills

1. They are called *Pilulæ*, because they resemble little balls; the Greeks call them *Catapotia*.

2. It is the opinion of modern physicians, that this way of making medicines, was invented only to deceive the palate, that so by swallowing them down whole, the bitterness of the medicine might not be perceived, or at least it might not be unsufferable: and indeed most of their pills, though not all, are very bitter.

3. I am of a clean contrary opinion to this. I rather think they were done up in this hard form, that so they might be the longer in digesting; and my opinion is grounded upon reason too, not upon fancy, or hearsay. The first invention of pills was to purge the head, now, as I told you before, such infirmities as lie near the passages were best removed by decoctions, because they pass to the grieved part soonest; so here, if the infirmity lies in the head, or any other remote part, the best way is to use pills, because they are longer in digestion, and therefore the better able to call the offending humour to them.

4. If I should tell you here a long tale of medicine working by sympathy and antipathy, you would not understand a word of it. They that are set to make physicians may find it in the treatise. All modern physicians know not what belongs to a sympathetical cure, no more than a cuckow what belongs to flats and sharps in music, but follow the vulgar road, and call it a hidden quality, because 'tis hidden from the eyes of dunces, and indeed none but astrologers can give a reason for it; and physic without reason is like a pudding without fat.

5. The way to make pills is very easy, for with the help of a pestle and mortar, and a little diligence, you may make any powder into pills, either with syrup, or the jelly I told you before.

CHAPTER XV

The way of mixing Medicines according to the Cause of the Disease, and Parts of the Body afflicted

THIS being indeed the key of the work, I shall be somewhat the more diligent in it. I shall deliver myself thus;

1. To the Vulgar.

2. To such as study Astrology; or such as study physic astrologically.

1st, To the Vulgar. Kind souls, I am sorry it hath been your hard mishap to have been so long trained in such Egyptian darkness which to your sorrow may be felt. The vulgar road of physic is not my practice, and I am therefore the more unfit to give you advice. I have now published a little book, (*Galen's Art of Physic*,) which will fully instruct you, not only in the knowledge of your own bodies, but also in fit medicines to remedy each part of it when afflicted; in the mean season take these few rules to stay your stomachs.

1. With the disease, regard the cause, and the part of the body

afflicted; for example, suppose a woman be subject to miscarry, through wind, thus do;

(1) Look Abortion in the table of diseases, and you shall be directed by that, how many herbs prevent miscarriage.

(2) Look Wind in the same table, and you shall see how many of these herbs expel wind.

These are the herbs medicinal for your grief.

2. In all diseases strengthen the part of the body afflicted.

3. In mixed diseases there lies some difficulty, for sometimes two parts of the body are afflicted with contrary humours, as sometimes the liver is afflicted with choler and water, as when a man hath both the dropsy and the yellow-jaundice; and this is usually mortal.

In the former, suppose the brain be too cool and moist, and the liver be too hot and dry; thus do;

1. Keep your head outwardly warm.

2. Accustom yourself to the smell of hot herbs.

3. Take a pill that heats the head at night going to bed.

4. In the morning take a decoction that cools the liver, for that quickly passes the stomach, and is at the liver immediately.

You must not think, courteous people, that I can spend time to give you examples of all diseases. These are enough to let you see so much light as you without art are able to receive. If I should set you to look at the sun, I should dazzle your eyes, and make you blind.

2dly, To such as study Astrology, who are the only men I know that are fit to study physic, physic without astrology being like a lamp without oil: you are the men I exceedingly respect, and such documents as my brain can give you at present (being absent from my study) I shall give you.

1. Fortify the body with herbs of the nature of the Lord of the Ascendant, 'tis no matter whether he be a Fortune or Infortune in this case.

2. Let your medicine be something antipathetical to the Lord of the sixth.

3. Let your medicine be something of the nature of the sign ascending.

4. If the Lord of the Tenth be strong, make use of his medicines.

5. If this cannot well be, make use of the medicines of the Light of Time.

6. Be sure always to fortify the grieved part of the body by sympathetical remedies.

7. Regard the heart, keep that upon the wheels, because the Sun is the foundation of life, and therefore those universal remedies, *Aurum Potabile*, and the Philosopher's Stone, cure all diseases by fortifying the heart.

The English Physician and Family Dispensatory

AN ASTROLOGO-PHYSICAL DISCOURSE OF THE HUMAN VIRTUES IN THE BODY OF MAN; BOTH PRINCIPAL AND ADMINISTERING

Human virtues are either PRINCIPAL for *procreation, and conservation*; or ADMINISTERING, for *Attraction, Digestion, Retention, or Expulsion*.

Virtues *conservative*, are Vital, Natural, and Animal.

By the *natural* are bred Blood, Choler, Flegm, and Melancholy.

The *animal virtue* is Intellective, and Sensitive.

The *Intellective* is Imagination, Judgment, and Memory.

The *sensitive* is Common, and Particular.

The *particular* is Seeing, Hearing, Smelling, Tasting, and Feeling.

The scope of this discourse is, to preserve in soundness and vigour, the mind and understanding of man; to strengthen the brain, preserve the body in health, to teach a man to be an able co-artificer, or helper of nature, to withstand and expel Diseases.

I shall touch only the principal faculties both of body and mind; which being kept in a due decorum, preserve the body in health, and the mind in vigour.

I shall in this place speak of them only in the general, as they are laid down to your view in the *Synopsis*, in the former pages, and in the same order.

Virtue Procreative.] The first in order, is the Virtue Procreative: for natural regards not only the conservation of itself, but to beget its like, and conserve in *Species*.

The seat of this is the Member of Generation, and is governed principally by the influence of *Venus*.

It is augmented and encreased by the strength of *Venus*, by her Herbs, Roots, Trees, Minerals, &c.

It is diminished and purged by those of *Mars*, and quite extinguished by those of *Saturn*.

Observe the hour and Medicines of *Venus*, to fortify; of *Mars*, to cleanse this virtue; of *Saturn*, to extinguish it.

Conservative.] The conservative virtue is Vital, Natural, Animal.

Vital.] The Vital spirit hath its residence in the heart, and is dispersed from it by the Arteries; and is governed by the influence of the Sun. And it is to the body, as the Sun is to the Creation; as the heart is in the *Microcosm*, so is the Sun in the *Megacosm*: for as the Sun gives life, light, and motion to the Creation, so doth the heart to the body; therefore it is called *Sol Corporis*, as the Sun is called *Cor Cæli*, because their operations are similar.

Inimical and destructive to this virtue, are *Saturn* and *Mars*.

The Herbs and Plants of *Sol*, wonderfully fortify it.

Natural.] The natural faculty or virtue resides in the liver, and is generally governed by *Jupiter*, *Quasi Juvans Pater*; its office is to nourish the body, and is dispersed through the body by the veins.

From this are bred four particular humours, *Blood*, *Choler*, *Flegm*, and *Melancholy*.

Blood is made of meat perfectly concocted, in quality hot and moist, governed by *Jupiter*. It is by a third concoction transmuted into flesh, the superfluity of it into seed, and its receptacle is the veins, by which it is dispersed through the body.

Choler is made of meat more than perfectly concocted; and it is the spume or froth of blood: it clarifies all the humours, heats the body, nourishes the apprehension, as blood doth the judgment. It is in quality hot and dry; fortifies the attractive faculty, as blood doth the digestive; moves man to activity and valour: its receptacle is the gall, and it is under the influence of *Mars*.

Flegm is made of meat not perfectly digested; it fortifies the virtue expulsive, makes the body slippery, fit for ejection; it fortifies the brain by its consimilitude with it; yet it spoils apprehension by its antipathy to it. It qualifies choler, cools and moistens the heart, thereby sustaining it, and the whole body, from the fiery effects, which continual motion would produce. Its receptacle is the lungs, and is governed by *Venus*, some say by the *Moon*, perhaps it may be governed by them both, it is cold and moist in quality.

Melancholy is the sediment of blood, cold and dry in quality, fortifying the retentive faculty, and memory; makes men sober, solid, and staid, fit for study; stays the unbridled toys of lustful blood, stays the wandering thoughts, and reduces them home to the centre: its receptacle is in the spleen, and it is governed by *Saturn*.

Of all these humours blood is the chief, all the rest are superfluities of blood; yet are they necessary superfluities, for without any of them, man cannot live.

Namely; Choler is the fiery superfluities, Flegm, the Watery; Melancholy, the Earthly.

Animal.] The third principal virtue remains, which is Animal; its residence is in the brain, and *Mercury* is the general significator of it. *Ptolomy* held the *Moon* signified the Animal virtue; and I am of opinion, both *Mercury* and the *Moon* dispose it; and my reason is, 1, Because both of them in nativities, either fortify, or impedite it. 2, Ill directions to either, or from either afflict it, as good ones help it. Indeed the *Moon* rules the bulk of it, as also the sensitive part of it: *Mercury* the rational part: and that's the reason, if in a nativity the *Moon* be stronger than *Mercury*, sense many times over-powers reason; but if *Mercury* be strong, and the *Moon* weak, reason will be master ordinarily in despite of sense.

It is divided into Intellective, and Sensitive.

1. *Intellective.*] The Intellectual resides in the brain, within the *Pia mater*, is governed generally by *Mercury*.

It is divided into Imagination, Judgment, and Memory.

Imagination is seated in the forepart of the brain; it is hot and dry in quality, quick, active, always working; it receives vapours from the heart, and coins them into thoughts: it never sleeps, but always is working, both when the man is sleeping and waking; only when Judgment is awake it regulates the Imagination, which runs at random when Judgment is asleep, and forms any thought according to the nature of the vapour sent up to it. *Mercury* is out of question the disposer of it.

A man may easily perceive his Judgment asleep before himself many times, and then he shall perceive his thoughts run at random.

Judgment always sleeps when men do, Imagination never sleeps; Memory sometimes sleeps when men sleep, and sometimes it doth not: so then when memory is awake, and the man asleep, then memory remembers what apprehension coins, and that is a dream. The thoughts would have been the same, if memory had not been awake to remember it.

These thoughts are commonly (I mean in sleep, when they are purely natural,) framed according to the nature of the humour, called complexion, which is predominate in the body; and if the humour be peccant it is always so.

So that it is one of the surest rules to know a man's own complexion, by his dreams, I mean a man void of distractions, or deep studies: (this most assuredly shews *Mercury* to dispose of the Imagination, as also because it is mutable, applying itself to any object, as *Mercury's* nature is to do;) for then the imagination will follow its old bent; for if a man be bent upon a business, his apprehension will work as much when he is asleep, and find out as many truths by study, as when the man is awake; and perhaps more too, because then it is not hindered by ocular objects.

And thus much for imagination, which is governed by *Mercury*, and fortified by his influence; and is also strong or weak in man, according as *Mercury* is strong or weak in the nativity.

Judgment is seated in the midst of the brain, to shew that it ought to bear rule over all the other faculties: it is the judge of the little world, to approve of what is good, and reject what is bad; it is the seat of reason, and the guide of actions; so that all failings are committed through its infirmity, it not rightly judging between a real and an apparent good. It is hot and moist in quality, and under the influence of *Jupiter*.

Memory is seated in the hinder cell of the brain, it is the great register to the little world; and its office is to record things either done and past, or to be done.

It is in quality cold and dry, melancholic, and therefore generally melancholic men have best memories, and most tenacious every way. It is under the dominion of *Saturn*, and is fortified by his influence, but purged by the luminaries.

2. *Sensitive*.] The second part of the animal virtue, is sensitive, and it is divided into two parts, common and particular.

Common sense is an imaginary term, and that which gives virtue to all the particular senses, and knits and unites them together within the *Pia Mater*. It is regulated by *Mercury*, (perhaps this is one reason why men are so fickle-headed) and its office is to preserve a harmony among the senses.

Particular senses are five, *viz. seeing, hearing, smelling, tasting, and feeling*.

These senses are united in one, in the brain, by the common sense, but are operatively distinguished into their several seats, and places of residence.

The *sight* resides in the eyes, and particularly in the christaline humour. It is in quality cold and moist, and governed by the luminaries. They who have them weak in their genesis, have always weak sights; if one of them be so, the weakness possesses but one eye.

The *hearing* resides in the ears; is in quality, cold and dry, melancholy, and under the dominion of *Saturn*.

The *smelling* resides in the nose, is in quality hot and dry, choleric, and that is the reason choleric creatures have so good smells, as dogs. It is under the influence of *Mars*.

The *taste* resides in the palate, which is placed at the root of the tongue on purpose to discern what food is congruous for the stomach, and what not; as the meseraik veins are placed to discern what nourishment is proper for the liver to convert into blood. In some very few men, and but a few, and in those few, but in few instances these two tasters agree not, and that is the reason some men covet meats that make them sick, *viz.* the taste craves them, and the meseraik veins reject them. In quality hot and moist, and is ruled by *Jupiter*.

The *feeling* is deputed to no particular organ, but is spread abroad, over the whole body; is of all qualities, hot, cold, dry, and moist, and is the index of all tangible things; for if it were only hot alone, it could not feel a quality contrary, *viz.* cold, and this might be spoken of other qualities. It is under the dominion of *Venus*, some say, *Mercury*. A thousand to one, but it is under *Mercury*.

The four ADMINISTERING VIRTUES are, *attractive, digestive, retentive, and expulsive*.

The *attractive* virtue is hot and dry, hot by quality, active, or principal, and that appears because the fountain of all heat is attractive, *viz.* the sun. Dry by a quality passive, or an effect of its heat; its office is to remain in the body, and call for what nature wants.

It is under the influence of the *Sun*, say authors, and not under *Mars*, because he is of a corrupting nature, yet if we cast an impartial eye upon experience, we shall find, that martial men call for meat none of the least, and for drink the most of all other men, although many times they corrupt the body by it, and therefore I see no reason why *Mars* being of the same quality with the *Sun*, should not have a share in the dominion. It is in vain to object, that the influence of *Mars* is evil, and therefore he should have no dominion over this virtue; for then,

1. By the same rule, he should have no dominion at all in the body of man.

2. All the virtues in man are naturally evil, and corrupted by *Adam's* fall.

This *attractive* virtue ought to be fortified when the *Moon* is in fiery signs, *viz. Aries* and *Sagitary*, but not in *Leo*, for the sign is so violent, that no physic ought to be given when the *Moon* is there: (and why not *Leo*, seeing that is the most attractive sign of all; and that's the reason such as have it ascending in their genesis, are such greedy eaters.) If you cannot stay till the *Moon* be in one of them, let one of them ascend when you administer the medicine.

The *digestive* virtue is hot and moist, and is the principal of them all, the other like handmaids attend it.

The *attractive* virtue draws that which it should digest, and serves continually to feed and supply it.

The *retentive* virtue, retains the substance with it, till it be perfectly digested.

The *expulsive* virtue casteth out, expels what is superfluous by digestion. It is under the influence of *Jupiter*, and fortified by his herbs and plants, &c. In fortifying it, let your *Moon* be in *Gemini*, *Aquary*, or the first half of *Libra*, or if matters be come to that extremity, that you cannot stay till that time, let one of them ascend, but both of them together would do better, always provided that the *Moon* be not in the ascendent. I cannot believe the *Moon* afflicts the ascendent so much as they talk of, if she be well dignified, and in a sign she delights in.

The *retentive* virtue is in quality cold and dry; cold, because the nature of cold is to compress, witness the ice; dry, because the nature of dryness, is to keep and hold what is compressed. It is under the influence of *Saturn*, and that is the reason why usually Saturnine men are so covetous and tenacious. In fortifying of it, make use of the herbs and plants, &c. of *Saturn*, and let the *Moon* be in *Taurus* or *Virgo*, *Capricorn* is not so good, say authors, (I can give no reason for that neither;) let not *Saturn* nor his ill aspect molest the ascendent.

The *expulsive* faculty is cold and moist; cold because that compasses the superfluities; moist, because that makes the body slippery and fit for ejection, and disposes it to it. It is under the dominion of *Luna*, with whom you may join *Yerus*, because she is of the same nature.

Also in whatsoever is before written, of the nature of the planets, take notice, that fixed stars of the same nature, work the same effect.

In fortifying this, (which ought to be done in all purgations,) let the *Moon* be in *Cancer*, *Scorpio*, or *Pisces*, or let one of these signs ascend.

Although I did what I could throughout the whole book to express myself in such a language as might be understood by all, and therefore avoided terms of art as much as might be, Yet, 1. *Some words of necessity fall in which need explanation.* 2. *It would be very tedious at the end of every receipt to repeat over and over again, the way of administration of the receipt, or ordering your bodies after it, or to instruct you in the mixture of medicines, and indeed would do nothing else but stuff the book full of tautology.*

To answer to both these is my task at this time.

To the first: The words which need explaining, such as are obvious to my eye, are these that follow.

1. *To distil in* Balno Mariæ, *is the usual way of distilling in water. It is no more than to place your glass body which holds the matter to be distilled in a convenient vessel of water, when the water is cold (for fear of breaking) put a wisp of straw, or the like under it, to keep it from the bottom, then make the water boil, that so the spirit may be distilled forth; take not the glass out till the water be cold again, for fear of*

breaking. It is impossible for a man to learn how to do it, unless he saw it done.

2. *Manica Hippocrates.* Hippocrates's sleeve, is a piece of woolen cloth, new and white, sewed together in form of a sugar-loaf. Its use is, to strain any syrup or decoction through, by pouring it into it, and suffering it to run through without pressing or crushing it.

3. *Calcination,* is a burning of a thing in a crucible or other such convenient vessel that will endure the fire. A crucible is such a thing as goldsmiths melt silver in, and founders metals; you may place it in the midst of the fire, with coals above, below, and on every side of it.

4. *Filtration,* is straining of a liquid body through a brown paper: make up the paper in form of a funnel, the which having placed in a funnel, and the funnel and the paper in it in an empty glass, pour in the liquor you would filter, and let it run through at its leisure.

5. *Coagulation,* is curdling or hardening: it is used in physic for reducing a liquid body to hardness by the heat of the fire.

6. Whereas you find *vital, natural,* and *animal spirits* often mentioned in the virtues or receipts, I shall explain what they be, and what their operation is in the body of man.

The actions or operations of the animal virtues, are, 1. *sensitive,* 2. *motive.*

The sensitive is, 1. *external,* 2. *internal.*

The external senses are, 1. *seeing,* 2. *hearing,* 3. *tasting,* 4. *smelling,* 5. *feeling.*

The internal senses are, 1. *the Imagination, to apprehend a thing.* 2. *Judgment, to judge of it.* 3. *Memory, to remember it.*

The seat of all these is in the brain.

The *vital spirits* proceed from the heart, and cause in man *mirth, joy, hope, trust, humanity, mildness, courage, &c.* and their opposite: *viz. sadness, fear, care, sorrow, despair, envy, hatred, stubbornness, revenge, &c.* by heat natural or not natural.

The *natural spirit* nourishes the body throughout (as the vital quickens it, and the animal gives it sense and motion) its office is to alter or concoct food into chile, chile into blood, blood into flesh, to form, engender, nourish, and increase the body.

7. *Infusion,* is to steep a gross body into one more liquid.

8. *Decoction,* is the liquor in which any thing is boiled.

As for the manner of using or ordering the body after any sweating, or purging medicines, or pills, or the like, they will be found in different parts of the work, as also in page 307.

The different forms of making up medicines, as some into syrups, others into electuaries, pills, troches, &c. was partly to please the different palates of people, that so medicines might be more delightful, or at least less burdensome. You may make the mixtures of them in what form you please, only for your better instruction at present accept of these few lines.

1. Consider, that all diseases are cured by their contraries, but all parts of the body maintained by their likes: then if heat be the cause of the disease, give the cold medicine appropriated to it; if wind, see how many medicines appropriated to that disease expel wind, and use them.

2. Have a care you use not such medicines to one part of your body which are appropriated to another, for if your brain be over heated, and you use such medicines as cool the heart or liver, you may make bad work.

3. The distilled water of any herb you would take for a disease, is a fit mixture for the syrup of the same herb, or to make any electuary into a drink, if you affect such liquid medicines best; if you have not the distilled water, make use of the decoction.

4. Diseases that lie in the parts of the body remote from the stomach and bowels, it is in vain to think to carry away the cause at once, and therefore you had best do it by degrees; pills, and such like medicines which are hard in the body, are fittest for such a business, because they are longest before they digest.

5. Use no strong medicines, if weak will serve the turn, you had better take one too weak by half, than too strong in the least.

6. Consider the natural temper of the part of the body afflicted, and maintain it in that, else you extinguish nature, as the heart is hot, the brain cold, or at least the coldest part of the body.

7. Observe this general rule: That such medicines as are hot in the first degree are most habitual to our bodies, because they are just of the heat of our blood.

8. All opening medicines, and such as provoke urine or the menses, or break the stone, may most conveniently be given in white wine, because white wine of itself is of an opening nature, and cleanses the reins.

9. Let all such medicines as are taken to stop fluxes or looseness, be taken before meat, about an hour before, more or less, that so they may strengthen the digestion and retentive faculty, before the food come into the stomach, but such as are subject to vomit up their meat, let them take such medicines as stay vomiting presently after meat, at the conclusion of their meals, that so they may close up the mouth of the stomach; and that is the reason why usually men eat a bit of cheese after meat, because by its sourness and binding it closes the mouth of the stomach, thereby staying belching and vomiting.

10. In taking purges be very careful, and that you may be so, observe these rules.

(1) Consider what the humour offending is, and let the medicine be such as purges that humour, else you will weaken nature, not the disease.

(2) Take notice, if the humour you would purge out be thin, then gentle medicines will serve the turn, but if it be tough and viscous, then such medicines as are cutting and opening, the night before you would take the purge.

(3) In purging tough humours, forbear as much as may be such medicines as leave a binding quality behind them.

(4) Have a care of taking purges when your body is astringent; your best way, is first to open it by a clyster.

(5) In taking opening medicines, you may safely take them at night, eating but a little supper three or four hours before, and the next morning drinking a draught of warm posset-drink, and you need not fear to go about your business. In this manner you may take *Lenitive Electuary*, *Diacatholicon*, *Pulp of Cassia*, and the like gentle electuaries, as also all pills that have neither *Diagrydium* nor *Colocynthus*, in them. But all violent purges require a due ordering of the body; such ought to be taken in the morning after you are up, and not to sleep after them before they are done working, at least before night: two hours after you have taken them, drink a draught of warm posset-drink, or broth, and six hours after eat a bit of mutton, often walking about the chamber; let there be a good fire in the chamber, and stir not out of the chamber till the purge have done working, or not till next day.

Lastly, take sweating medicines when you are in bed, covered warm, and in the time of your sweating drink posset-drink as hot as you can. If you sweat for a fever, boil sorrel and red sage in your posset-drink, sweat an hour or longer if your strength will permit, then (the chamber being kept very warm) shift yourself all but your head, about which (the cap which you sweat in being still kept on) wrap a napkin very hot, to repel the vapours back.

I confess these, or many of these directions may be found in one place of the book or other, and I delight as little to write tautology as another, but considering it might make for the public good, I inserted them in this place: if, notwithstanding, any will be so mad as to do themselves a mischief, the fault is not mine.

ROOTS

Acanths, Brancæ Ursinæ. Of bearsbreech, or brankursine, it is meanly hot and dry, helps aches and numbness of the joints, and is of a binding quality, good for wounds and broken bones. *Dioscorides* saith, They are profitable for ruptures, or such as are bursten, or burnt with fire, a dram of the root in powder being taken in the morning fasting, in a decoction made with the same root and water.

Acori, Veri, Perigrini, vulgaris, &c. See *Calamus Aromaticus.* I shall not speak concerning the several sorts of it, one of which is Water-flag, or Flower-de-luce, which is hot and dry in the second degree, binds, strengthens, stops fluxes of the belly, and immoderate flowing of the menses, a dram being taken in red wine every morning.

Allium. Garlic. It is hot and dry in the fourth degree, breeds corrupt blood, yet is an enemy to all poisons, and such as are bitten by cold venomous beasts, viz. Adders, Toads, Spiders, &c. it provokes urine, and expels wind.

Alcannæ. Of privet. See the leaves.

Althææ. Of Marsh mallows, are meanly hot, of a digesting, softening nature, ease pains, help bloody fluxes, the stone, and gravel; being bruised and boiled in milk, and the milk drank, is a good remedy for gripings of the belly, and the bloody flux. If a fever accompany the disease, boil a handful of common mallow leaves with a handful of these roots.

Angelicæ. Of Angelica; is hot and dry in the third degree, strengthens the heart, and is good against pestilence and poison, half a dram taken in the morning fasting.

Anchusæ. Of Alkanet; cold and dry, binding, good for old ulcers.

Anthoræ. A foreign root, the counter-poison for Monkshood, it is an admirable remedy for the wind cholic, and resists poison.

Apii. Of smallage. See the barks.

Aristolochiæ. Of birthwort; of which are three sorts, long, round, and climing. All hot and dry in the third degree. The long, being drank in wine, brings away both birth and after-birth, and whatsoever a careless midwife hath left behind. *Dioscorides, Galen.* The round, being drank with wine, helps (besides the former) stuffings of the lungs, hardness of the spleen, ruptures, convulsions; both of them resist poison. I never read any use of the climing birthwort.

Artanitæ, Cyclaminis, &c. Of Sowbread, hot and dry in the third degree, a most violent purge, dangerous; outwardly applied to the place, it profits much in the bitings of venomous beasts, also being hung about women in labour, it causes speedy deliverance. See the Herb.

Arundinis, Vallanoriæ, and Saccharinæ. Of common reeds and sugar reeds. The roots of common reeds applied to the place draw out thorns, and ease sprains; the ashes of them mixed with vinegar, take scurf, or dandrif off from the head, and prevent the falling off of the hair, they are hot and dry in the second degree, according to *Galen*. I never read any virtue of the root of sugar cane.

Ari, &c. Of Cuckow-points, or Wake-Robin, hot and dry in the third degree, I know no great good they do inwardly taken, unless to play the rogue withal, or make sport: outwardly applied, they take off scurf, morphew, or freckles from the face, clear the skin, and ease the pains of the gout.

Asclepiadis, vincetoxici. Of Swallow-wort, hot and dry, good against poison, and gripings of the belly, as also against the bitings of mad dogs, taken inwardly.

Asari. Of Asarabacca: the roots are a safer purge than the leaves, and not so violent, they purge by vomit, stool, and urine; they are profitable for such as have agues, dropsies, stoppings of the liver, or spleen, green sickness.

Asparagi. Of Asparagus, or sperage: they are temperate in quality, opening, they provoke urine, and cleanse the reins and bladder, being boiled in white wine, and the wine drank.

Asphodeli, Hastæ Reigæ fœm. Of Kings Spear, or Female Asphodel. I know no physical use of the roots, probably there is, for I do not believe God created any thing of no use.

Asphodeli, Albuci, muris. Of male Asphodel. Hot and dry in the second degree, inwardly taken, they provoke vomit, urine, and the menses: outwardly used in ointments, they cause hair to grow, cleanse ulcers, and take away morphew and freckles from the face.

Bardanæ, &c. Of Bur, Clot-bur, or Burdock, temperately hot and dry. Helps such as spit blood and matter; bruised and mixed with salt and applied to the place, helps the bitings of mad dogs. It expels wind, eases pains of the teeth, strengthens the back, helps the running of the reins, and the whites, being taken inwardly. *Dioscorides, Apuleius.*

Behen. alb. rub. Of Valerian, white and red. *Mesue, Serapio,* and other Arabians, say they are hot and moist in the latter end of the first, or beginning of the second degree, and comfort the heart, stir up lust. The Grecians held them to be dry in the second degree, that they stop fluxes, and provoke urine.

Bellidis. Of Dasies. See the Leaves.

Betæ, nigræ, albæ, rubræ. Of Beets, black, white, and red; as for black Beets I have nothing to say, I doubt they are as rare as black swans. The red Beet root boiled and preserved in vinegar, makes a fine, cool, pleasing, cleansing, digesting sauce. See the leaves.

Bistortæ, &c. Of Bistort, or snakeweed, cold and dry in the third degree, binding: half a dram at a time taken inwardly, resists pestilence and poison, helps ruptures and bruises, stays fluxes, vomiting, and immoderate flowing of the menses, helps inflammations and soreness of the mouth, and fastens loose teeth, being bruised and boiled in white wine, and the mouth washed with it.

Borraginis. Of Borrage, hot and moist in the first degree, cheers the heart, helps drooping spirits. *Dioscorides.*

Broniæ, &c. Of Briony both white and black: they are both hot and dry, some say in the third degree, and some say but in the first; they purge flegm and watery humours, but they trouble the stomach much, they are very good for dropsies, the white is most in use, and is good for the fits of the mother: both of them externally used, take away freckles, sunburning, and morphew from the face, and cleanse filthy ulcers. It is but a churlish purge, but being let alone, can do no harm.

Buglossi. Of Bugloss. Its virtues are the same with Borrage, and the roots of either seldom used.

Bulbus Vomitorius. A Vomiting Root: I never read of it elsewhere by this general name.

Calami Aromatici. Of Aromatical Reed, or sweet garden flag: it provokes urine, strengthens the lungs, helps bruises, resists poison, &c. being taken inwardly in powder, the quantity of half a dram at a time. You may mix it with syrup of violets, if your body be feverish.

Capparum. Capper Roots. Are hot and dry in the second degree, cutting and cleansing: they provoke menses, help malignant ulcers, ease the toothache, assuage swelling, and help the rickets. *See Oil of Cappers.*

Cariophillatæ, &c. Of Avens, or Herb Bennet. The roots are dry, and something hot, of a cleansing quality, they keep garments from being moth-eaten. See the leaves.

Caulium. Of Colewort. I know nothing the roots are good for, but only to bear the herbs and flowers.

Centrurii majoris. Of Centaury the Greater. The roots help such as are bursten, such as spit blood, shrinking of sinews, shortness of wind, coughs, convulsions, cramps: half a dram in powder being taken inwardly, either in muskadel, or in a decoction of the same roots. They are either not at all, or very scarce in *England*, our centaury is the small centaury.

Cepæ. Of Onions. Are hot and dry (according to *Galen*) in the fourth degree: they cause dryness, and are extremely hurtful for choleric people, they breed but little nourishment, and that little is naught: they are bad meat, yet good physic for phlegmatic people, they are opening, and provoke urine and the menses, if cold be the cause obstructing: bruised and outwardly applied, they cure the bitings of mad dogs, roasted and applied, they help boils, and aposthumes: raw, they take the fire out of burnings, but ordinarily eaten, they cause headache, spoil the sight, dull the senses, and fill the body full of wind.

Chameleontis albi nigri, &c. Of Chameleon, white and black. *Tragus* calls the carline thistle by the name of white chameleon, the root whereof is hot in the second degree, and dry in the third, it provokes sweat, kills worms, resists pestilence and poison; it is given with success in pestilential fevers, helps the toothache by being chewed in the mouth, opens the stoppings of the liver and spleen, provokes urine, and the menses: give but little of it at a time, by reason of its heat. As for the black chameleon, all physicians hold it to have a kind of venomous quality, and unfit to be used inwardly, *Galen, Clusius, Nicander, Dioscorides, and Ægineta*. Outwardly in ointments, it is profitable for scabs, morphew, tetters, &c. and all things that need cleansing.

Chelidonij majoris, minoris. Of celandine, the greater and lesser. The greater is that which we usually call Celandine: the root is hot and dry, cleansing and scouring, proper for such as have the yellow jaundice, it opens obstructions of the liver, being boiled in white wine, and the decoctions drank; and if chewed in the mouth it helps the tooth-ache. Celandine the lesser is that which usually we call Pilewort, which with us is hot in the first degree; the juice of the root mixed with honey and snuffed up in the nose, purges the head, helps the hemorrhoids or piles being bathed with it, as also doth the root only carried about one: being made into an ointment, it helps the king's evil or *Scrophula*.

China, wonderfully extenuates and dries, provokes sweat, resists putrefaction; it strengthens the liver, helps the dropsy and malignant ulcers, leprosy, itch, and venereal, and is profitable in diseases coming of fasting. It is commonly used in diet drinks for the premises.

Cichorii. Of Succory; cool and dry in the second degree, strengthens the liver and veins, it opens obstructions, stoppings in the liver and spleen, being boiled in white wine and the decoction drank.

Colchici. Of Meadow Saffron. The roots are held to be hurtful to the stomach, therefore I let them alone.

Consolidæ, majoris, minoris. Consolida Major, is that which we ordinarily call Comfry, it is of a cold quality, yet pretty temperate, so glutinous, that, according to *Dioscorides*, they will join meat together that is cut in sunder, if they be boiled with it; it is excellent for all wounds, both internal and external, for spitting of blood, ruptures or burstness, pains in the back, it strengthens the reins, it stops the menses and helps hemorrhoids. The way to use them is to boil them in water and drink the decoction. Consolida minor, is that we call Self-heal, and the latins *Prunella*. See the herb.

Costi utriusque. Of Costus both sorts, being roots coming from beyond sea, hot and dry, break wind, being boiled in oil, it is held to help the gout by anointing the grieved place with it.

Cucumeris a grestis. Of wild Cucumber roots; they purge flegm, and that with such violence, that I would advise the country man that knows not how to correct them, to let them alone.

Cinaræ, &c. Of Artichokes. The roots purge by urine, whereby the rank savour of the body is much amended.

Cynoglossæ, &c. Of Hounds-tongue, Cold and dry: being roasted and laid to the fundament, helps the hemorrhoids, is also good for burnings and scaldings.

Curcumæ. Of Turmerick, hot in the third degree, opens obstructions, is profitable against the yellow jaundice, and cold distemper of the liver and spleen, half a dram being taken at night going to bed in the pulp of a roasted apple, and if you add a little saffron to it, it will be the better by far.

Cyperi utriusque, longi, rotundi. Of Cyprus Grass, or English Galanga, both sorts, long and round: is of a warm nature, provokes urine, breaks the stone, provokes the menses; the ashes of them (being burnt) are used for ulcers in the mouth, cankers, &c.

Dauci. Of Carrots. Are moderately hot and moist, breed but little nourishment, and are windy.

Dentaria majoris, &c. Of Toothwort, toothed violets, or corral-wort: they are drying, binding, and strengthening; are good to ease pains in the sides and bowels; also being boiled, the decoction is said to be good to wash green wounds and ulcers with.

Dictiamni. Of Dittany: is hot and dry in the third degree, hastens travail in women, provokes the menses. (See the leaves.)

Doronici. Of Doronicum, a supposed kind of Wolf's bane. It is hot and dry in the third degree, strengthens the heart, is a sovereign cordial, and preservative against the pestilence: it helps the vertigo or swimming of the head, is admirable against the bitings of venomous beasts, and such as have taken too much opium, as also for lethargies, the juice helps hot rheums in the eyes; a scruple of the root in powder is enough to take at one time.

Dracontii, Dracunculi. Divers authors attribute divers herbs to this name. It is most probable that they mean dragons, the roots of which cleanse mightily, and take away proud, or dead flesh, the very smell of them is hurtful for pregnant women: outwardly in ointments, they take away scurf, morphew, and sun-burning; I would not wish any, unless very well read in physic, to take them inwardly. *Matthiolus, Dioscorides.*

Ebuli. Of Dwarf Elder, Walwort, or Danewort; hot and dry in the third degree, the roots are as excellent a purge for the dropsy as any under the sun. You may take a dram or two drams (if the patient be strong) in white wine at a time.

Echij. Of Viper's Bugloss, or wild Bugloss. *This root is cold and dry, good for such as are bitten by venemous beasts, either being boiled in wine and drank, or bruised and applied to the place: being boiled in wine and drank, it encreaseth milk in nurses.*

Ellebori, Veratri, albi nigri. *Of Hellebore white and black. The root of white Hellebore, or sneezewort, being grated and snuffed up the nose, causeth sneezing; kills rats and mice being mixed with their meat.*

Black Hellebore, Bears-foot or Christmas flower: both this and the former are hot and dry in the third degree. This is neither so violent nor dangerous as the former.

Enulæ Campanæ Helenij. *Of Elecampane. It is hot and dry in the third degree, wholesome for the stomach, resists poison, helps old coughs, and shortness of breath, helps ruptures, and provokes lust; in ointments, it is good against scabs and itch.*

Endivæ, &c. *Of Endive, Garden Endive, which is the root here specified, is held to be somewhat colder, though not so dry and cleansing as that which is wild; it cools hot stomachs, hot livers, amends the blood corrupted by heat, and therefore is good in fevers, it cools the reins, and therefore prevents the stone, it opens obstructions, and provokes urine: you may bruise the root, and boil it in white wine, 'tis very harmless.*

Eringij. *Of Eringo or Sea-holly: the roots are moderately hot, something drying and cleansing, bruised and applied to the place; they help the* Scrophula, *or disease in the throat called the King's Evil, they break the stone, encrease seed, stir up lust, provoke the terms, &c.*

Esulæ, majoris, minoris. *Of Spurge the greater and lesser, they are both (taken inwardly) too violent for common use; outwardly in ointments they cleanse the skin, take away sunburning.*

Filicis, &c. *Fearn, of which are two grand distinctions,* viz. *male and female. Both are hot and dry, and good for the rickets in children, and diseases of the spleen, but dangerous for pregnant women.*

Filipendulæ. *Of Dropwort. The roots are hot and dry in the third degree, opening, cleansing, yet somewhat binding; they provoke urine, ease pains in the bladder, and are a good preservative against the falling-sickness.*

Fœniculi. *Of Fennel. The root is hot and dry, some say in the third degree, opening; it provokes urine, and menses, strengthens the liver, and is good against the dropsy.*

Fraxini. *Of Ash-tree. I know no great virtues in physic of the roots.*

Galangæ, majoris, minoris. *Galanga, commonly called Galingal, the greater and lesser. They are hot and dry in the third degree, and the lesser are accounted the hotter, it strengthens the stomach exceedingly, and takes away the pains thereof coming of cold or wind; the smell of it strengthens the brain, it relieves faint hearts, takes away windiness of the womb, heats the reins, and provokes amorous diseases. You may take half a dram at a time.* Matthiolus.

Gentiana. *Of Gentian; some call it Felwort, and Baldmoney. It is hot, cleansing, and scouring, a notable counterpoison, it opens obstructions, helps the biting of venemous beasts, and mad dogs, helps digestion, and cleanseth the body of raw humours; the root is profitable for ruptures, or such as are bursten.*

Glycyrrhizæ. *Of Liquorice; the best that is grows in* England: *it is hot and moist in temperature, helps the roughness of the windpipe, hoarsness, diseases in the kidneys and bladder, and ulcers in the bladder, it concocts raw humours in the stomach, helps difficulty of breathing, is profitable for all salt humours, the root dried and beaten into powder, and the powder put into the eye, is a special remedy for a pin and web.*

Gramminis. *Of Grass, such as in* London *they call couch grass, and Squitch-grass; in* Sussex *Dog-grass. It gallantly provokes urine, and easeth the kidneys oppressed with gravel, gripings of the belly, and difficulty of urine. Let such as are troubled with these diseases, drink a draught of white wine, wherein these roots (being bruised) have been boiled, for their morning's draught, bruised and applied to the place, they speedily help green wounds.* Galen, Dioscorides.

Hermodactyli. *Of Hermodactils. They are hot and dry, purge flegm, especially from the joints, therefore are good for gouts, and other diseases in the joints. Their vices are corrected with long pepper, ginger, cinnamon, or mastich. I would not have unskilful people too busy with purges.*

Hyacinthi. *Of Jacinths. The roots are dry in the first degree, and cold in the second, they stop looseness, bind the belly.*

Iridis, vulgaris, *and* Florentine, &c. Orris, or Flower-de-luce, both that which grows with us, and that which comes from *Florence.* They are hot and dry in the third degree, resist poison, help shortness of the breath, provoke the menses; the Root being green and bruised, takes away blackness and blueness of a stroke, being applied thereto.

Imperitoriæ, &c. Of Master-wort. The root is hot and dry in the third degree; mitigates the rigour of agues, helps dropsies, provokes sweat, breaks carbuncles, and plague-sores, being applied to them; it is very profitable being given inwardly in bruises.

Isotidis, Glasti. Of Woad. I know no great physical virtue in the root. See the Herb.

Labri Veneris, Dipsaci. Fullers-Thistle, Teazle. The root being boiled in wine till it be thick (quoth *Dioscorides*) helps by unction the clefts of the fundament, as also takes away warts and wens. *Galen* saith, they are dry in the second degree: and I take it all

Authors hold them to be cold and dry. Unslacked lime beaten into powder, and mixed with black soap, takes away a wen being anointed with it.

Lactucæ. Of Lettice. I know no physical virtue residing in the roots.

Lauri. Of the Bay-tree. The Bark of the root drunk with wine, provokes urine, breaks the stone, opens obstructions of the liver and spleen. But according to *Dioscorides* is naught for pregnant women. *Galen.*

Lapathi acuti, Oxylapathi. Sorrel, according to *Galen*; but Sharp-pointed Dock, according to *Dioscorides.* The roots of Sorrel are held to be profitable against the jaundice. Of Sharp-pointed Dock; cleanse, and help scabs and itch.

Levistici. Of Lovage. They are hot and dry, and good for any diseases coming of wind.

Lillij albi. Of white Lillies. The root is something hot and dry, helps burnings, softens the womb, provokes the menses, if boiled in wine, is given with good success in rotten Fevers, Pestilences, and all diseases that require suppuration: outwardly applied, it helps ulcers in the head, and amends the ill colour of the face.

Malvæ. Of Mallows. They are cool, and digesting, resist poison, and help corrosions, or gnawing of the bowels, or any other part; as also ulcers in the bladder. See Marsh-mallows.

Mandragoræ. Of Mandrakes. A root dangerous for its coldness, being cold in the fourth degree: the root is dangerous.

Mechoachanæ. Of Mechoacah. It is corrected with Cinnamon, is temperate yet drying, purges flegm chiefly from the head and joints, it is good for old diseases in the head, and may safely be given even to feverish bodies, because of its temperature: it is also profitable against coughs and pains in the reins; as also against venereal complaints; the strong may take a dram at a time.

Mei, &c. Spignel. The roots are hot and dry in the second or third degree, and send up unwholesome vapours to the head.

Mezerei, &c. Of Spurge, Olive, or Widow-wail. See the Herb, if you think it worth the seeing.

Merorum Celci. Of Mulberry Tree. The bark of the root is bitter, hot and dry, opens stoppings of the liver and spleen, purges the belly, and kills worms, boiled in vinegar, helps the tooth-ache.

Morsus Diaboli, Succisæ, &c. Devil's-bit. See the herb.

Norpi Spicæ, Indicæ, Celticæ, &c. Of Spikenard, Indian, and Cheltic. Cheltic Nard wonderfully provokes urine. They are both hot and dry. The Indian, also provokes urine, and stops fluxes, helps windiness of the stomach, resists the pestilence, helps gnawing pains of the stomach, and dries up rheums that molest the head.

The Celtic Spikenard performs the same offices, though in a weaker measure.

Nenupharis, Nymphæ. Of Water-lilies. They are cold and dry, and stop lust: I never dived so deep to find what virtue the roots have.

Ononidis, Arrestæ Bovis, &c. Of Cammock, or Rest-harrow, so called because it makes oxen stand still when they are ploughing. The roots are hot and dry in the third degree; it breaks the stone (viz. the bark of it). The root itself, according to *Pliny*, helps the falling-sickness; according to *Matthiolus*, helps ruptures: you may take half a dram at a time.

Ostrutij. Masterwort, given once before under the name of *Imperitoria.* But I have something else to do than to write one thing twice as they did.

Pastinatæ, Sativæ, and *silvestris.* Garden and Wild Parsnips. They are of a temperate quality, inclining something to heat. The Garden Parsnips provoke lust, and nourish as much and more too, than any root ordinarily eaten: the wild are more physical, being cutting, cleansing, and opening: they resist the bitings of venomous beasts, ease pains and stitches in the sides, and are a sovereign remedy against the wind cholic.

Pentafylli. Of Cinqfyl, commonly called Five-leaved, or Five-finger'd grass: the root is very drying, but moderately hot. It is admirable against all fluxes, and stops blood flowing from any part of the body: it helps infirmities of the liver and lungs, helps putrified ulcers of the mouth, the root boiled in vinegar is good against the shingles, and appeases the rage of any fretting sores. You may safely take half a dram at a time in any convenient liquor.

Petacitæ. Of Butter-bur. The roots are hot and dry in the second degree, they are exceeding good in violent and pestilential fevers, they provoke the menses, expel poison, and kill worms.

Peucedani, Fœniculi porcini. Of Sulphurwort, Hogs-fennel, or Hore-strange. It is very good applied to the navels of children that stick out, and ruptures: held in the mouth, it is a present remedy for the fits of the mother: being taken inwardly, it gives speedy deliverance to women in travail, and brings away the placenta.

Pœoniœ, maris, fœmellæ. Of Peony male and female. They are meanly hot, but more drying. The root helps women not sufficiently purged after travail, it provokes the menses, and helps pains in the belly, as also in the reins and bladder, falling sickness, and convulsions in children, being either taken inwardly, or hung about their necks. You may take half a dram at a time, and less for children.

Phu, Valerinæ, majoris, minoris. *Valerian, or Setwal, greater and lesser. They are temperately hot, the greater provokes urine and the menses, helps the stranguary, stays rheums in the head, and takes away the pricking pains thereof. The lesser resist poison, assuages the swelling of the testicles, coming either through wind or cold, helps cold taken after sweating or labour, wind cholic: outwardly it draws out thorns, and cures both wounds and ulcers.*

Pimpinellæ, &c. *Of Burnet. It doth this good, to bring forth a gallant physical herb.*

Plantaginis. *Of Plantane. The root is something dryer than the leaf, but not so cold, it opens stoppages of the liver, helps the jaundice, and ulcers of the reins and bladder. A little bit of the root being eaten, instantly stays pains in the head, even to admiration.*

Polypodij. Of Polypodium, or Fern of the Oak. It is a gallant though gentle purger of melancholy. Also in the opinion of *Mesue* (as famous a physician as ever I read for a Galenist), it dries up superfluous humours, takes away swellings from the hands, feet, knees, and joints, stitches and pains in the sides, infirmities of the spleen, rickets; correct it with a few Annis seeds, or Fennel seeds, or a little ginger, and then the stomach will not loath it. Your best way of taking it, is to bruise it well, and boil it in white wine till half be consumed, you may put in much, or little, according to the strength of the diseased, it works very safely.

Poligonati, sigilli Solomonis, &c. Of Solomon's Seal. Stamped and boiled in wine it speedily helps (being drank) all broken bones, and is of incredible virtue that way; as also being stamped and applied to the place, it soon heals all wounds, and quickly takes away the black and blue marks of blows, being bruised and applied to the place, and for these, I am persuaded there is not a better medicine under the sun.

Porri. Of Leeks. They say they are hot and dry in the fourth degree; they breed ill-favoured nourishment at the best, they spoil the eyes, heat the body, cause troublesome sleep, and are noisome to the stomach: yet are they good for something else, for the juice of them dropped into the ears takes away the noise of them, mixed with a little vinegar and snuffed up the nose, it stays the bleeding of it, they are better of the two boiled than raw, but both ways exceedingly hurtful for ulcers in the bladder: and so are onions and garlic.

Prunellorum Silvestrium. Of Sloe-bush, or Sloe-tree. I think the college set this amongst the roots only for fashion sake, and I did it because they did.

Pyrethri Salivaris, &c. Pelitory of Spain. It is hot and dry in the fourth degree, chewed in the mouth, it draws away rheum in the tooth-ache; bruised and boiled in oil, it provokes sweat by unction; inwardly taken, they say it helps palsies and other cold effects in the brain and nerves.

Rhapontici. Rhupontick, or Rhubarb of Pontus. It takes away windiness and weakness of the stomach, sighings, sobbings, spittings of blood, diseases of the liver and spleen, rickets, &c. if you take a dram at a time it will purge a little but bind much, and therefore fit for foul bodies that have fluxes.

Rhabarbari. Of Rhubarb. It gently purges choler from the stomach and liver, opens stoppings, withstands the dropsy, Hypocondriac Melancholly; a little boiling takes away the virtue of it, and therefore it is best given by infusion only; If your body be any thing strong, you may take two drams of it at a time being sliced thin and steeped all night in white wine, in the morning strain it out and drink the white wine; it purges but gently, it leaves a binding quality behind it, therefore dried a little by the fire and beaten into powder, it is usually given in fluxes.

Rhaphani, Domesticæ and Sylvestris. Of Raddishes, garden and wild. Garden Raddishes provoke urine, break the stone, and purge by urine exceedingly, yet breed very bad blood, are offensive to the stomach, and hard of digestion, hot and dry in quality. Wild, or Horse Raddishes, such as grow in ditches, are hotter and drier than the former, and more effectual.

Rhodie Rad. Rose Root. Stamped and applied to the head it mitigates the pains thereof, being somewhat cool in quality.

Rhabarbari Monachorum. Monks Rhubarb, or Bastard-Rhubarb, it also purges, and cleanses the blood, and opens obstructions of the liver.

Rubiæ tinctorum. Of Madder. It is both drying and binding, yet not without some opening quality, for it helps the yellow jaundice, and therefore opens obstructions of the liver and gall; it is given with good success, to such as have had bruises by falls, stops looseness, the hemorrhoids, and the menses.

Rusci. Of Knee-holly or Butchers-broom, or Bruscus. They are meanly hot and dry, provoke urine, break the stone, and help such as cannot evacuate urine freely. Use them like grass roots.

Sambuci. Of Elder. I know no wonders the root will do.

Sarsæ-Parigliæ. Of Sarsa-Parilla, or Bind-weed; somewhat hot and dry, helpful against pains in the head, and joints; they provoke sweat, and are used familiarly in drying diet drinks.

Satyrij utriusque. Of Satyrion, each sort. They are hot and moist in temper, provoke venery, and increase seed; each branch bears two roots, both spongy, yet the one more solid than the other, which is of most virtue, and indeed only to be used, for some say the most spongy root is quite contrary in operation to the other, as the one increaseth, the other decreaseth.

Saxifragiæ albæ. Of white Saxifrage, in *Sussex* we call them

Lady-smocks. The roots powerfully break the stone, expel wind, provoke urine, and cleanse the reins.

Sanguisorbæ. A kind of Burnet.

Scabiosa. Of Scabious. The roots either boiled, or beaten into powder, and so taken, help such as are extremely troubled with scabs and itch, are medicinal in the french disease, hard swellings, inward wounds, being of a drying, cleansing, and healing faculty.

Scordij. Of Scordium, or Water-Germander. See the herb.

Scillæ. Of Squills. See vinegar, and wine of Squills, in the compound.

Scropulariæ, &c. Of Figwort. The roots being of the same virtue with the herb, I refer you thither.

Scorzoneræ. Of Vipers grass. The root cheers the heart, and strengthens the vital spirits, resists poison, helps passions and tremblings of the heart, faintness, sadness, and melancholy, opens stoppings of the liver and spleen, provokes the menses, ease women of the fits of the mother, and helps swimmings in the head.

Seseleos. Of Seseli, or Hartwort. The roots provoke urine, and help the falling-sickness.

Sisari, secacul. Of Scirrets. They are hot and moist, of good nourishment, something windy, as all roots are; by reason of which, they provoke venery, they stir up appetite, and provoke urine.

Sconchi. Of Sow-thistles. See the herb.

Spinæ albæ, Bedeguar. The Arabians called our Ladies-thistles by that name; the roots of which are drying and binding, stop fluxes, bleeding, take away cold swellings, and ease the pains of the teeth.

Spatulæ fœtidæ. Stinking Gladon, a kind of Flower-de-luce, called so for its unsavory smell. It is hot and dry in the third degree; outwardly they help the king's evil, soften hard swellings, draw out broken bones: inwardly taken, they help convulsions, ruptures, bruises, infirmities of the lungs.

Tamarisci. Of Tamaris. See the herbs, and barks.

Tanaceti. Of Tansie. The root eaten, is a singular remedy for the gout: the rich may bestow the cost to preserve it.

Thapsi, &c. A venomous foreign root: therefore no more of it.

Tormentillæ. Of Tormentil. A kind of Sinqfoil; dry in the third degree, but moderately hot; good in pestilences, provokes sweat, stays vomiting, cheers the heart, expels poison.

Trifolij. Of Trefoil. See the herb.

Tribuli Aquatici. Of Water Caltrops. The roots lie too far under water for me to reach to.

Trachellij. Of Throat-wort: by some called Canterbury Bells: by some Coventry Bells. They help diseases and ulcers in the throat.

Trinitatis herbæ. Hearts-ease, or Pansies, I know no great virtue they have.

Tunicis. I shall tell you the virtue when I know what it is.

Tripolij. The root purges flegm, expels poison.

Turbith. The root purges flegm, (being hot in the third degree) chiefly from the exterior parts of the body: it is corrected with ginger, or Mastich. Let not the vulgar be too busy with it.

Tuburnum. Or Toad-stools. Whether these be roots or no, it matters not much; for my part I know but little need of them, either in food or physic.

Victorialis. A foreign kind of Garlick. They say, being hung about the neck of cattle that are blind suddenly, it helps them; and defends those that bear it, from evil spirits.

Swallow-wort, and teazles were handled before.

Ulmariæ, Reginæ, prati, &c. Mead-sweet. Cold and dry, binding, stops fluxes, and the immoderate flowing of the menses: you may take a dram at a time.

Urticæ. Of Nettles. See the leaves.

Zedoariæ. Of Zedoary, or Setwall. This and *Zurumbet,* according to *Rhasis,* and *Mesue,* are all one; *Avicenna* thinks them different: I hold with *Mesue*; indeed they differ in form, for the one is long, the other round; they are both hot and dry in the second degree, expel wind, resist poison, stop fluxes, and the menses, stay vomiting, help the cholic, and kill worms; you may take half a dram at a time.

Zingiberis. Of Ginger. Helps digestion, warms the stomach, clears the sight, and is profitable for old men: heats the joints, and therefore is profitable against the gout, expels wind; it is hot and dry in the second degree.

BARKS

A Pil Rad. Of the roots of Smallage. Take notice here, that the Barks both of this root, as also of Parsley, Fennel, &c. is all of the root which is in use, neither can it properly be called bark, for it is all the root, the hard pith in the middle excepted, which is always thrown away, when the roots are used. It is something hotter and drier than Parsley, and more medicinal; it opens stoppings, provokes urine, helps digestion, expels wind, and warms a cold stomach: use them like grass roots.

Avellanarum. Of Hazel. The rind of the tree provokes urine, breaks the stone; the husks and shells of the nuts, dried and given in powder, stay the immoderate flux of the menses.

Aurantiorum. Of Oranges. Both these, and also Lemons and Citrons, are of different qualities: the outward bark, *viz.* what looks red, is hot and dry, the white is cold and moist, the juice colder than it, the seeds hot and dry; the outward bark is that which here I am to speak to, it is somewhat hotter than either that of Lemons or Citrons, therefore it warms a cold stomach more, and expels wind better, but strengthens not the heart so much.

Berber, &c. Barberries. The Rind of the tree according to *Clæsius*, being steeped in wine, and the wine drank, purges choler, and is a singular remedy for the yellow jaundice. Boil it in white wine and drink it. See the directions at the beginning.

Cassia Lignea, &c. It is something more oily than Cinnamon, yet the virtues being not much different, I refer you thither.

Capparis Rad. Of Caper roots. See the roots.

Castanearum. Of Chesnuts. The bark of the Chesnut tree is dry and binding, and stops fluxes.

Cinnamonum. Cinnamon, and Cassia Lignea, are hot and dry in the second degree, strengthens the stomach, help digestion, cause a sweet breath, resist poison, provoke urine, and the menses, cause speedy delivery to women in travail, help coughs and defluxions of humours upon the lungs, dropsy, and difficulty of urine. In ointments it takes away red pimples, and the like deformities from the face. There is scarce a better remedy for women in labour, than a dram of Cinnamon newly beaten into powder, and taken in white wine.

Citrij. Of Pome Citrons. The outward pill, which I suppose is that which is meant here: It strengthens the heart, resists poison, amends a stinking breath, helps digestion, comforts a cold stomach.

Ebuli Rad. Of the roots of Dwarf-Elder, or Walwort. See the herbs.

Enulæ. Of Elecampane. See the roots.

Esulæ Rad. See the roots.

Fabarum. Of Beans. Bean Cods (or Pods, as we in *Sussex* call them) being bruised, the ashes are a sovereign remedy for aches in the joints, old bruises, gouts, and sciaticas.

Fœniculi Rad. Of Fennel roots. See the roots, and remember the observation given in Smallage at the beginning of the barks.

Fraxini Rad. Of the bark of Ash-tree roots. The bark of the tree, helps the rickets, is moderately hot and dry, stays vomiting; being burnt, the ashes made into an ointment, helps leprosy and other deformity of the skin, eases pains of the spleen. You may lay the bark to steep in white wine for the rickets, and when it hath stood so for two or three days, let the diseased child drink now and then a spoonful of it.

Granatorum. Of Pomegranates. The rind cools, and forcibly binds, stays fluxes, and the menses, helps digestion, strengthens weak stomachs, fastens the teeth, and are good for such whose gums waste. You may take a dram of it at a time inwardly. Pomegranate flowers are of the same virtue.

Gatrujaci. See the wood.

Juglandium Virid. Of green Walnuts. As for the outward green bark of Walnuts, I suppose the best time to take them is before the Walnuts be shelled at all, and then you may take nuts and all (if they may properly be called nuts at such a time) you shall find them exceeding comfortable to the stomach, they resist poison, and are a most excellent preservative against the plague, inferior to none: they are admirable for such as are troubled with consumptions of the lungs.

Lauri. Of the Bay-tree. See the root.

Limonum. Of Lemons. The outward peel is of the nature of Citron, but helps not so effectually; however, let the poor country man that cannot get the other, use this.

Mandragora Rad. Be pleased to look back to the root.

Myrobalanorum. Of Myrobalans. See the fruits.

Macis. Of Mace. It is hot in the third degree, strengthens the stomach and heart exceedingly, and helps concoction.

Maceris, &c. It is held to be the inner bark of Nutmeg-tree, helps fluxes and spitting of blood.

Petroselini Rad. Of Parsley root: opens obstructions, provokes urine and the menses, warms a cold stomach, expels wind, and breaks the stone. Use them as grass roots, and take out the inner pith as you were taught in smallage roots.

Prunelli Silvestris. Of Sloe-tree. I know no use of it.

Pinearum putaminae. Pine shucks, or husks. I suppose they mean of the cones that hold the seeds; both those and also the bark of the tree, stop fluxes, and help the lungs.

Querci. Of Oak-tree. Both the bark of the oak, and Acorn Cups are drying and cold, binding, stop fluxes and the menses, as also the running of the reins; have a care how you use them before due purging.

Rhaphani. Of Radishes. I could never see any bark they had.

Suberis. Of Cork. It is good for something else besides to stop bottles: being dry and binding, stanches blood, helps fluxes, especially the ashes of it being burnt. *Paulus.*

Sambuci, &c. Of Elder roots and branches; purges water, helps the dropsy.

Cort. Medius Tamaricis. The middle Bark of Tameris, eases the spleen, helps the rickets. Use them as Ash-tree bark.

Tilliæ. Of Line-tree. Boiled, the water helps burnings.

Thuris. Of Frankinsenses. I must plead *Ignoramus.*

Ulmi. Of Elm. Moderately hot and cleansing good for wounds, burns, and broken bones, *viz.* boiled in water and the grieved place bathed with it.

WOODS AND THEIR CHIPS, OR RASPINGS

A Gallochus, Lignum Aloes. Wood of Aloes; is moderately hot and dry: a good cordial: a rich perfume, a great strengthener to the stomach.

Aspalathus. Rose-wood. It is moderately hot and dry, stops looseness, provokes urine, and is excellent to cleanse filthy ulcers.

Bresilium. Brasil. All the use I know of it is, to die cloth, and leather, and make red ink.

Buxus. Box. Many Physicians have written of it, but no physical virtue of it.

Cypressus. Cypress. The Wood laid amongst cloaths, secures them from moths. See the leaves.

Ebenum. Ebony. It is held to clear the sight, being either boiled in wine, or burnt to ashes.

Guajacum, Lignum vitæ. Dries, attenuates, causes sweat, resists putrefaction, is good for the French disease, as also for ulcers, scabs, and leprosy: it is used in diet drinks.

Juniperus. Juniper. The smoak of the wood, drives away serpents; the ashes of it made into lie, cures itch, and scabs.

Nephriticum. It is a light wood and comes from *Hispaniola*; being steeped in water, will soon turn it blue, it is hot and dry in the first degree, and so used as before, is an admirable remedy for the stone, and for obstructions of the liver and spleen.

Rhodium. Encreases milk in nurses.

Santalum, album, Rubrum, citrinum. White, red, and yellow Sanders. They are all cold and dry in the second or third degree: the red stops defluxions from any part, and helps inflammations: the white and yellow (of which the yellow is best) cool the heat of fevers, strengthen the heart, and cause cheerfulness.

Sassafras. Is hot and dry in the second degree, it opens obstructions or stoppings, it strengthens the breast exceedingly; if it be weakened through cold, it breaks the stone, stays vomiting, provokes urine, and is very profitable in the venereal, used in diet drinks.

Tamaris. Is profitable for the rickets, and burnings.

Xylobalsamum. Wood of the Balsam tree, it is hot and dry in the second degree, according to *Galen.* I never read any great virtues of it.

HERBS AND THEIR LEAVES

A Brotanum, mas, fœmina. Southernwood, male and female. It is hot and dry in the third degree, resists poison, kills worms; outwardly in plaisters, it dissolves cold swellings, and helps the bitings of venomous beasts, makes hair grow: take not above half a dram at a time in powder.

Absinthium, &c. Wormwood. Its several sorts, are all hot and dry in the second or third degrees, the common Wormwood is thought to be hottest, they all help weakness of the stomach, cleanse choler, kill worms, open stoppings, help surfeits, clear the sight, resist poison, cleanse the blood, and secure cloaths from moths.

Abugilissa, &c. Alkanet. The leaves are something drying and binding, but inferior in virtue to the roots, to which I refer you.

Acetosa. Sorrel. Is moderately cold, dry and binding, cuts tough humours, cools the brain, liver and stomach, cools the blood in fevers, and provokes appetite.

Acanthus. Bears-breech, or Branks ursine, is temperate, something moist. See the root.

Adiantum, Album, nigrum. Maiden hair, white and black. They are temperate, yet drying. White Maiden hair is that we usually call Wall-rue; they both open obstructions, cleanse the breast and lungs of gross slimy humours, provoke urine, help ruptures and shortness of wind.

Adiantum Aurcum Politrycum. Golden Maiden-hair. Its temperature and virtues are the same with the former; helps the spleen; burned, and lye made with the ashes, keeps the hair from falling off the head.

Agrimonia. Agrimony. *Galen's Eupatorium.* It is hot and dry in the first degree, binding, it amends the infirmities of the liver, helps such as evacuate blood instead of water, helps inward wounds, opens obstructions. Outwardly applied it helps old sores, ulcers, &c. Inwardly, it helps the jaundice and the spleen. Take a dram of this or that following, inwardly in white wine, or boil the herb in white wine, and drink the decoction. *Galen, Pliny, Dioscorides, Serapio.*

Ageretum. Hot and dry in the second degree, provokes urine and the menses, dries the brain, opens stoppings, helps the green sickness, and profits such as have a cold, weak liver; outwardly applied, it takes away the hardness of the matrix, and fills hollow ulcers with flesh.

Agnus Castus, &c. Chast-tree. The leaves are hot and dry in the third degree; expel wind, consume the seed, cause chastity being only borne about one; it dissolves swellings of the testicles, being applied to them, head-ache, and lethargy.

Allajula, Lujula, &c. Wood Sorrel. It is of the temperature of other Sorrel, and held to be more cordial, cools the blood, helps ulcers in the mouth; hot defluxions upon the lungs, wounds, ulcers, &c.

Alcea. Vervain Mallow. The root helps fluxes and burstness. *Ætius, Dioscorides.*

Allium. Garlick. Hot and dry in the fourth degree, troublesome to the stomach: it dulls the sight, spoils a clear skin, resists poison, eases the pains of the teeth, helps the bitings of mad dogs, and venomous beasts, helps ulcers, leprosies, provokes urine, is exceedingly opening, and profitable for dropsies.

Althæa, &c. Marsh-Mallows. Are moderately hot and drier than other Mallows; they help digestion, and mitigate pain, ease the pains of the stone, and in the sides. Use them as you were taught in the roots, whose virtues they have, and both together will do better.

Alsine. Chickweed. Is cold and moist without any binding, assuages swelling, and comforts the sinews much; therefore it is good for such as are shrunk up; it dissolves aposthumes, hard swellings, and helps mange in the hands and legs, outwardly applied in a pultis. *Galen.*

Alchymilla. Ladies-Mantle. Is hot and dry, some say in the second degree, some say in the third: outwardly it helps wounds, reduces women's breasts that hang down: inwardly, helps bruises, and ruptures, stays vomiting, and the Fluor Albus, and is very profitable for such women as are subject to miscarry through cold and moisture.

Alkanna. Privet hath a binding quality, helps ulcers in the mouth, is good against burnings and scaldings, cherishes the nerves and sinews; boil it in white wine to wash the mouth, and in hog's grease for burnings and scaldings.

Amaracus, Majorana. Marjoram. Some say 'tis hot and dry in the second degree, some advance it to the third. Sweet Marjoram, is an excellent remedy for cold diseases in the brain, being only smelled to helps such as are given to much sighing, easeth pains in the belly, provokes urine, being taken inwardly: you may take a dram of it at a time in powder. Outwardly in oils or salves, it helps sinews that are shrunk; limbs out of joint, all aches and swellings coming of a cold cause.

Angelica. Is hot and dry in the third degree; opens, digests, makes thin, strengthens the heart, helps fluxes, and loathsomeness of meat. It is an enemy to poison and pestilence, provokes menses, and brings away the placanta. You may take a dram of it at a time in powder.

Anagallis, mas, femina. Pimpernel, male and female. They are something hot and dry, and of such a drying quality that they draw thorns and splinters out of the flesh, amend the sight, cleanse ulcers, help infirmities of the liver and reins. *Galen.*

Anethum. Dill. Is hot and dry in the second degree. It stays vomiting, eases hiccoughs, assuages swellings, provokes urine, helps such as are troubled with fits of the mother, and digests raw humours.

Apium. Smallage. So it is commonly used; but indeed all Parsley is called by the name of Apium, of which this is one kind. It is something hotter and dryer than Parsley, and more efficacious; it opens stoppings of the liver, and spleen, cleanses the blood, provokes the menses, helps a cold stomach to digest its meat, and is good against the yellow jaundice. Both Smallage and Clevers, may be well used in pottage in the morning instead of herbs.

Aparine. Goose-grass, or Clevers. They are meanly hot and dry, cleansing, help the bitings of venomous beasts, keep men's bodies from growing too fat, help the yellow jaundice, stay bleeding, fluxes, and help green wounds. *Dioscorides, Pliny, Galen, Tragus.*

Aspergula odorata. Wood-roof. Cheers the heart, makes men merry, helps melancholy, and opens the stoppings of the liver.

Aquilegia. Columbines: help sore throats, are of a drying, binding quality.

Argentina. Silver-weed, or Wild Tansy, cold and dry almost in the third degree; stops lasks, fluxes, and the menses, good against ulcers, the stone, and inward wounds: easeth gripings in the belly, fastens loose teeth: outwardly it takes away freckles, morphew, and sunburning, it takes away inflammations, and bound to the wrists stops the violence of the fits of the ague.

Artanita. Sow-bread: hot and dry in the third degree, it is a dangerous purge: outwardly in ointments it takes away freckles, sunburning, and the marks which the small pox leaves behind them: dangerous for pregnant women.

Aristolochia, longa, rotunda. Birth-wort long and round. See the roots.

Artemisia. Mugwort: is hot and dry in the second degree: binding: an herb appropriated to the female sex; it brings down the menses, brings away both birth and placenta, eases pains in the matrix. You may take a dram at a time.

Asparagus. See the roots.

Asarum, &c. Asarabacca: hot and dry; provokes vomiting and urine, and are good for dropsies. They are corrected with mace or cinnamon.

Atriplex, &c. Orach, or Arrach. It is cold in the first degree, and moist in the second, saith *Galen*, and makes the belly soluble. It is an admirable remedy for the fits of the mother, and other infirmities of the matrix, and therefore the Latins called it *Vulvaria*.

Aricula muris, major. Mouse-ear: hot and dry, of a binding quality, it is admirable to heal wounds, inward or outward, as also ruptures or burstness. Edge-tools quenched in the juice of it, will cut iron without turning the edge, as easy as they will lead. And, lastly, it helps the swelling of the spleen, coughs and consumptions, of the lungs.

Attractivis hirsuta. Wild Bastard-saffron, Distaff-thistle, or Spindle-thistle. Is dry and moderately digesting, helps the biting of venomous beasts. *Mesue* saith, It is hot in the first degree, and dry in the second, and cleanseth the breast and lungs of tough flegm.

Balsamita, &c. Costmary, Alecost. See Maudlin.

Barbajovis, sedum majus. Houseleek or Sengreen: cold in the third degree, profitable against the Shingles, and other hot creeping ulcers, inflammations, *St. Anthony's* fire, frenzies; it cools and takes away corns from the toes, being bathed with the juice of it, and a skin of the leaf laid over the place; stops fluxes, helps scalding and burning.

Bardana. Clot-bur, or Bur-dock: temperately dry and wasting, something cooling; it is held to be good against the shrinking of the sinews; eases pains in the bladder, and provokes urine. Also *Mizaldus* saith, That a leaf applied to the top of the head of a woman draws the matrix upwards, but applied to the soles of the feet draws it downwards, and is therefore an admirable remedy for suffocations, precipitations, and dislocations of the matrix, if a wise man have but the using of it.

Beta, alba, nigra, rubra. Beets, white, black, and red; black Beets I have no knowledge of. The white are something colder and moister than the red, both of them loosen the belly, but have little or no nourishment. The white provoke to stool, and are more cleansing, open stoppings of the liver and spleen, help the vertigo or swimming in the head. The red stay fluxes, help the immoderate flowing of the menses, and are good in the yellow jaundice.

Benedicta Cariphyllara. Avens: hot and dry, help the cholic and rawness of the stomach, stitches in the sides, and take away clotted blood in any part of the body.

Betonica vulgaris. Common Wood Betony: hot and dry in the second degree, helps the falling sickness and all head-aches coming of cold, cleanses the breast and lungs, opens stoppings of the liver and spleen, as the rickets, &c. procures appetite, helps sour belchings, provokes urine, breaks the stone, mitigates the pains of the reins and bladder, helps cramps, and convulsions, resists poison, helps the gout, such as evacuate blood, madness and head-ache, kills worms, helps bruises, and cleanseth women after labour. You may take a dram of it at a time in white wine, or any other convenient liquor proper against the disease you are afflicted with.

Betonica Pauli, &c. Paul's Betony, or Male Lluellin, to which add *Elative*, or Female Lluellin, which comes afterwards; they are pretty temperate, stop defluxions of humours that fall from the head into the eyes, are profitable in wounds, help filthy foul eating cankers.

Betonica Coronaria, &c. Is Clove Gilliflowers. See the flowers.

Bellis. Dasies: are cold and moist in the second degree, they ease all pains and swellings coming of heat, in clysters they loose the belly, are profitable in fevers and inflammations of the testicles, they take away bruises, and blackness and blueness; they are admirable in wounds and inflammations of the lungs or blood.

Blitum. Blites. Some say they are cold and moist, others cold and dry: none mention any great virtues of them.

Borrago. Borrage: hot and moist, comforts the heart, cheers the spirits, drives away sadness and melancholy, they are rather laxative than binding; help swooning and heart-qualms, breed good blood, help consumptions, madness, and such as are much weakened by sickness.

Bonus Henricus. Good Henry, or all good; hot and dry, cleansing and scouring, inwardly taken it loosens the belly; outwardly it cleanseth old sores and ulcers.

Botrys. Oak of Jerusalem: hot and dry in the second degree, helps such as are short-winded, cuts and wastes gross and tough flegm, laid among cloaths they preserve them from moths, and give them a sweet smell.

Branca ursina. Bears-breech.

Brionia, &c. Briony, white and black; both are hot and dry in the third degree, purge violently, yet are held to be wholesome physic for such as have dropsies, vertigo, or swimming in the head, falling-sickness, &c. Certainly it is a strong, troublesome purge, therefore not to be tampered with by the unskilful, outwardly in ointments it takes away freckles, wrinkles, morphew, scars, spots, &c. from the face.

Bursa pastoris. Shepherd's Purse, is manifestly cold and dry, though *Lobel* and *Pena* thought the contrary; it is binding and stops blood, the menses; and cools inflammations.

Buglossom. Buglosse. Its virtues are the same with Borrage.

Bugula. Bugle, or Middle Comfrey; is temperate for heat, but very drying, excellent for falls or inward bruises, for it dissolves congealed blood, profitable for inward wounds, helps the rickets and other stoppings of the liver; outwardly it is of wonderful force in curing wounds and ulcers, though festered, as also gangreens and fistulas, it helps broken bones, and dislocations. Inwardly you may take it in powder a dram at a time, or drink the decoction of it in white-wine: being made into an ointment with hog's grease, you shall find it admirable in green wounds.

Buphthalmum, &c. Ox eye. *Matthiolus* saith they are commonly used for black Hellebore, to the virtues of which I refer.

Buxus. Boxtree: the leaves are hot, dry, and binding, they are profitable against the biting of mad dogs; both taken inwardly boiled and applied to the place: besides they are good to cure horses of the bots.

Calamintha, Montana, Palustris. Mountain and Water Calamint. For the Water Calamint see mints, than which it is accounted stronger. Mountain Calamint is hot and dry in the third degree, provokes urine and the menses, hastens the birth in women, brings away the placenta, helps cramps, convulsions, difficulty of breathing, kills worms, helps the dropsy: outwardly used, it helps such as hold their necks on one side: half a dram is enough at one time. *Galen, Dioscorides, Apuleius.*

Calendula, &c. Marigolds. The leaves are hot in the second degree, and something moist, loosen the belly: the juice held in the mouth, helps the toothache, and takes away any inflammation or hot swelling being bathed with it, mixed with a little vinegar.

Callitricum. Maiden-hair. See *Adianthum.*

Caprisolium. Honey-suckles. The leaves are hot, and therefore naught for inflammations of the mouth and throat, for which the ignorant people oftentime give them: and *Galen* was true in this, let modern writers write their pleasure. If you chew but a leaf of it in your mouth, experience will tell you that it is likelier to cause, than to cure a sore throat, they provoke urine, and purge by urine, bring speedy delivery to women in travail, yet procure barrenness and hinder conception, outwardly they dry up foul ulcers, and cleanse the face from morphew, sun-burning and freckles.

Carduncellus, &c. Groundsell. Cold and moist according to *Tragus,* helps the cholic, and gripings in the belly, helps such as cannot make water, cleanses the reins, purges choler and sharp humours: the usual way of taking it is to boil it in water with currants, and so eat it. I hold it to be a wholesome and harmless purge. Outwardly it easeth women's breasts that are swollen and inflamed; as also inflammations of the joints, nerves, or sinews. *Ægineta.*

Carduus B. Mariæ. Our Ladies Thistles. They are far more

temperate than *Carduus Benedictus*, open obstructions of the liver, help the jaundice and dropsy, provoke urine, break the stone.

Carduus Benedictus. Blessed Thistle, but better known by the Latin name: it is hot and dry in the second degree, cleansing and opening, helps swimming and giddiness in the head, deafness, strengthens the memory, helps griping pains in the belly, kills worms, provokes sweat, expels poison, helps inflammation of the liver, is very good in pestilence and venereal: outwardly applied, it ripens plague-sores, and helps hot swellings, the bitings of mad dogs and venomous beasts, and foul filthy ulcers. Every one that can but make a Carduus posset, knows how to use it. *Camerarius, Arnuldus vel anovanus.*

Chalina. See the roots, under the name of white Chameleon.

Corallina. A kind of Sea Moss: cold, binding, drying, good for hot gouts, inflammations: also they say it kills worms, and therefore by some is called Maw-wormseed.

Cussutha, cascuta, potagralini. Dodder. See *Epithimum.*

Caryophyllata. Avens, or Herb Bennet, hot and dry: they help the cholic, rawness of the stomach, stitches in the sides, stoppings of the liver, and bruises.

Cataputia minor. A kind of Spurge. See *Tythymalus.*

Cattaria, Nepeta. Nep, or Catmints. The virtues are the same with Calaminth.

Cauda Equina. Horse-tail; is of a binding drying quality, cures wounds, and is an admirable remedy for sinews that are shrunk: it is a sure remedy for bleeding at the nose, or by wound, stops the menses, fluxes, ulcers in the reins and bladder, coughs, ulcers in the lungs, difficulty of breathing.

Caulis, Brassica hortensis, silvestris. Colewort, or Cabbages, garden and wild. They are drying and binding, help dimness of the sight: help the spleen, preserve from drunkenness, and help the evil effects of it; provoke the menses.

Centaurium, majus, minus. Centaury the greater and less. They say the greater will do wonders in curing wounds: see the root. The less is a present remedy for the yellow jaundice, opens stoppings of the liver, gall, and spleen: purges choler, helps gout, clears the sight, purgeth the stomach, helps the dropsy and green sickness. It is only the tops and flowers which are useful, of which you may take a dram inwardly in powder, or half a handful boiled in posset-drink at a time.

Centinodium, &c. Knotgrass: cold in the second degree, helps spitting and other evacuations of blood, stops the menses and all other fluxes of blood, vomiting of blood, gonorrhæa, or running of the reins, weakness of the back and joints, inflammations of the privities, and such as make water by drops, and it is an excellent remedy for hogs that will not eat their meat. Your only way is to boil it, it is in its prime about the latter end of *July* or beginning of *August*: at which time being gathered it may be kept dry all the year. *Brassavolus, Camerarius.*

Caryfolium vulgare et Myrrhis. Common and great chervil. Take them both together, and they are temperately hot and dry, provoke urine, stir up venery, comfort the heart, and are good for old people; help pleurises and pricking in the sides.

Cæpea, Anagallis aquatica. Brooklime, hot and dry, but not so hot and dry as Water cresses; they help mangy horses; see Water cresses.

Ceterach, &c. Spleenwort: moderately hot, waste and consumes the spleen, insomuch that *Vitruvius* affirms he hath known hogs that have fed upon it, that have had (when they were killed) no spleens at all. It is excellently good for melancholy people, helps the stranguary, provokes urine, and breaks the stone in the bladder, boil it and drink the decoction; but because a little boiling will carry away the strength of it in vapours, let it boil but very little, and let it stand close stopped till it be cold before you strain it out; this is the general rule for all simples of this nature.

Chamapitys. Ground-pine; hot in the second degree, and dry in the third, helps the jaundice, sciatica, stopping of the liver, and spleen, provokes the menses, cleanses the entrails, dissolves congealed blood, resists poison, cures wounds and ulcers. Strong bodies may take a dram, and weak bodies half a dram of it in powder at a time.

Chamæmelum, sativum, sylvestre. Garden and Wild Chamomel. Garden Chamomel, is hot and dry in the first degree, and as gallant a medicine against the stone in the bladder as grows upon the earth, you may take it inwardly, I mean the decoction of it, being boiled in white wine, or inject the juice of it into the bladder with a syringe. It expels wind, helps belchings, and potently provokes the menses: used in baths, it helps pains in the sides, gripings and gnawings in the belly.

Chamædris, &c. Germander: hot and dry in the third degree; cuts and brings away tough humours, opens stoppings of the liver and spleen, helps coughs and shortness of breath, stranguary and stopping of urine, and provokes the menses; half a dram is enough to take at a time.

Chelidonium utrumque. Celandine both sorts. Small Celandine is usually called Pilewort; it is something hotter and dryer than the former, it helps the hemorrhoids or piles, bruised and applied to the grief. Celandine the greater is hot and dry (they say in the third degree) any way used; either the juice or made into an oil or ointment, it is a great preserver of the sight, and an excellent help for the eyes.

Cinara, &c. Artichokes. They provoke venery, and purge by urine.

Cichorium. Succory, to which add Endive which comes after. They are cold and dry in the second degree, cleansing and opening; they cool the heats of the liver, and are profitable in the yellow jaundice, and burning fevers; help excoriations in the privities, hot stomachs; and outwardly applied, help hot rheums in the eyes.

Cicuta. Hemlock: cold in the fourth degree, poisonous: outwardly applied, it helps *Priapismus*, the shingles, *St. Anthony's fire*, or any eating ulcers.

Clematis Daphnoides, Vinca provinca. Periwinkle. Hot in the second degree, something dry and binding; stops lasks, spitting of blood, and the menses.

Consolida major. Comfrey, I do not conceive the leaves to be so virtuous as the roots.

Consolida media. Bugles, of which before.

Consolida minima. Dasies.

Consolida rubra. Golden Rod: hot and dry in the second degree, cleanses the reins, provokes urine, brings away the gravel; an admirable herb for wounded people to take inwardly, stops blood, &c.

Consolida Regalis, Delphinium. Lark heels: resist poison, help the bitings of venomous beasts.

Saracenica Solidago. Saracens Confound. Helps inward wounds, sore mouths, sore throats, wasting of the lungs, and liver.

Coronepus. Buchorn Plantane, or Sea-plantain; cold and dry, helps the bitings of venomous beasts, either taken inwardly or applied to the wound: helps the cholic, breaks the stone. *Ægineta.*

Coronaria. Hath got many English names. Cottonweed, Cudweed, Chaffweed, and Petty Cotton. Of a drying and binding nature; boiled in lye, it keeps the head from nits and lice; being laid among clothes, it keeps them safe from moths, kills worms, helps the bitings of venomous beasts; taken in a tobacco-pipe, it helps coughs of the lungs, and vehement headaches.

Cruciata. Crosswort: (there is a kind of Gentian called also by this name, which I pass by) is drying and binding, exceeding good for inward or outward wounds, either inwardly taken, or outwardly applied: and an excellent remedy for such as are bursten.

Crassula. Orpine. Very good: outwardly used with vinegar, it clears the skin; inwardly taken, it helps gnawings of the stomach and bowels, ulcers in the lungs, bloody-flux, and quinsy in the throat, for which last disease it is inferior to none, take not too much of it at a time, because of its coolness.

Crithamus, &c. Sampire. Hot and dry, helps difficulty of urine, the yellow jaundice, provokes the menses, helps digestion, opens stoppings of the liver and spleen. *Galen.*

Cucumis Asininus. Wild Cucumbers. See *Elaterium.*

Cyanus major, minor. Blue bottle, great and small, a fine cooling herb, helps bruises, wounds, broken veins; the juice dropped into the eye, helps the inflammations thereof.

Cygnoglossam. Hound's-Tongue, cold and dry: applied to the fundament helps the hemorrhoids, heals wounds and ulcers, and is a present remedy against the bitings of dogs, burnings and scaldings.

Cypressus, Chamœ Cyparissus. Cypress-tree. The leaves are hot and binding, help ruptures, and *Polypus* or flesh growing on the nose.

Chamæ cyparissus. Is Lavender Cotton. Resists poison, and kills worms.

Disetamnus Cretensis. Dictamny, or Dittany of *Creet,* hot and dry, brings away dead children, hastens delivery, brings away the placenta, the very smell of it drives away venomous beasts, so deadly an enemy it is to poison; it is an admirable remedy against wounds and gunshot, wounds made with poisoned weapons, it draws out splinters, broken bones, &c. The dose from half a dram to a dram.

Dipsacus, sativ. sylv. Teazles, garden and wild, the leaves bruised and applied to the temples, allay the heat in fevers, qualify the rage in frenzies; the juice dropped into the ears, kills worms in them, dropped into the eyes, clears the sight, helps redness and pimples in the face, being anointed with it.

Ebulus. Dwarf Elder, or Walwort. Hot and dry in the third degree; waste hard swellings, being applied in form of a poultice; the hair of the head anointed with the juice of it turns it black; the leaves being applied to the place, help inflammations, burnings, scaldings, the bitings of mad dogs; mingled with bulls suet is a present remedy for the gout; inwardly taken, is a singular purge for the dropsy and gout.

Echium. Viper's-bugloss, Viper's-herb, Snake bugloss, Wal-bugloss, Wild-bugloss, several counties give it these several names. It is a singular remedy being eaten, for the biting of venomous beasts: continually eating of it makes the body invincible against the poison of serpents, toads, spiders, &c. however it be administered; it comforts the heart, expels sadness and melancholy. The rich may make the flowers into a conserve, and the herb into a syrup, the poor may keep it dry, both may keep it as a jewel.

Empetron, Calcifragra, Herniaria, &c. Rupture-wort, or Burst-wort. The English name tells you it is good against ruptures, and so such as are bursten shall find it, if they please to make trial of it, either inwardly taken, or outwardly applied to the place, or both. Also the Latin names hold it forth to be good against the stone, which whoso tries shall find true.

Enula Campana. Elicampane. Provokes urine. See the root.

Epithimum. Dodder of Time, to which add common Dodder, which is usually that which grows upon flax: indeed every Dodder retains a virtue of that herb or plant it grows upon, as Dodder that grows upon Broom, provokes urine forcibly, and loosens the belly, and is moister than that which grows upon flax; that which grows upon time, is hotter and dryer than that which grows upon flax, even in the third degree, opens obstructions, helps infirmities of the spleen, purgeth melancholy, relieves drooping spirits, helps the rickets. That which grows on flax, is excellent for agues in young children, strengthens weak stomachs, purgeth choler, provokes urine, opens stoppings in the reins and bladder. That which grows upon nettles, provokes urine exceedingly. The way of using it is to boil it in white wine, or other convenient decoction, and boil it very little. *Ætias, Mesue, Actuarius, Serapio, Avicenna.*

Eruch. Rocket, hot and dry in the third degree, being eaten alone, causeth head-ache, by its heat procures urine. *Galen.*

Eupatorium. See *Ageratum.*

Euphragia. Eyebright is something hot and dry, the very sight of it refresheth the eyes; inwardly taken, it restores the sight, and makes old men's eyes young, a dram of it taken in the morning is worth a pair of spectacles, it comforts and strengthens the memory, outwardly applied to the place, it helps the eyes.

Filix fœmina.
Filicula, polypidium. } See the roots.
Filipendula.

Malahathram. Indian leaf, hot and dry in the second degree, comforts the stomach exceedingly, helps digestion, provokes urine, helps inflammations of the eyes, secures cloaths from moths.

Fœniculum. Fennel, encreaseth milk in nurses, provokes urine, breaks the stone, easeth pains in the reins, opens stoppings, breaks wind, provokes the menses; you may boil it in white wine.

Fragaria. Strawberry leaves, are cold, dry, and binding, a singular remedy for inflammations and wounds, hot diseases in the throat; they stop fluxes and the terms, cool the heat of the stomach, and the inflammations of the liver. The best way is to boil them in barley water.

Fraxinus, &c. Ash-trees, the leaves are moderately hot and dry, cure the bitings of Adders, and Serpents; they stop looseness, and stay vomiting, help the rickets, open stoppages of the liver and spleen.

Fumaria. Fumitory: cold and dry, it opens and cleanses by urine, helps such as are itchy, and scabbed, clears the skin, opens stoppings of the liver and spleen, helps rickets, hypochondriac melancholy, madness, frenzies, quartan agues, loosens the belly, gently purgeth melancholy, and addust choler: boil it in white wine, and take this one general rule. *All things of a cleansing or opening nature may be most commodiously boiled in white wine.* Remember but this, and then I need not repeat it.

Galega. Goat's-rue. Temperate in quality, resists poison, kills worms, helps the falling-sickness, resists the pestilence. You may take a dram of it at a time in powder.

Galion. Ladies-bed straw: dry and binding, stanches blood, boiled in oil, the oil is good to anoint a weary traveller; inwardly it provokes venery.

Gentiana. See the root.

Genista. Brooms: hot and dry in the second degree, cleanse and open the stomach, break the stone in the reins and bladder, help the green sickness. Let such as are troubled with heart-qualms or faintings, forbear it, for it weakens the heart and spirit vital. See the flowers.

Geranium. Cranebill, the divers sorts of it, one of which is that which is called Muscata; it is thought to be cool and dry, helps hot swellings, and by its smell amends a hot brain.

Geranium Columbinum. Doves-foot; helps the wind cholic, pains in the belly, stone in the reins and bladder, and is good in ruptures, and inward wounds. I suppose these are the general virtues of them all.

Gramen. Grass. See the root.

Gratiola. Hedge-Hyssop, purges water and flegm, but works very churlishly. *Gesner* commends it in dropsies.

Asphodelus fœm. See the root.

Hepatica, Lichen. Liverwort, cold and dry, good for inflammations of the liver, or any other inflammations, yellow jaundice.

Hedera Arborea, Terrostris. Tree and Ground-Ivy. Tree-Ivy helps ulcers, burnings, scaldings, the bad effects of the spleen; the juice snuffed up the nose, purges the head, it is admirable for surfeits or headache, or any other ill effects coming of drunkenness. Ground-Ivy is that which usually is called Alehoof, hot and dry, the juice helps noise in the ears, fistulas, gouts, stoppings of the liver, it strengthens the reins and stops the menses, helps the yellow jaundice, and other diseases coming of stoppings of the liver, and is excellent for wounded people.

Herba Camphorata. Stinking Groundpine, is of a drying quality, and therefore stops defluxions either in the eyes or upon the lungs, the gout, cramps, palsies, aches: strengthens the nerves.

Herba Paralysis, *Primula veris*. Primroses, or Cowslips, which you will. The leaves help pains in the head and joints; see the flowers which are most in use.

Herba Paris. Herb True-love, or One-berry. It is good for wounds, falls, bruises, aposthumes, inflammations, ulcers in the privities. Herb True-love, is very cold in temperature. You may take half a dram of it at a time in powder.

Herba Roberti. A kind of Cranebill.

Herba venti, *Anemone*. Wind-flower. The juice snuffed up in the nose purgeth the head, it cleanses filthy ulcers, encreases milk in nurses, and outwardly by ointment, helps leprosies.

Herniaria. The same with *Empetron*.

Helxine. Pellitory of the wall. Cold, moist, cleansing, helps the stone and gravel in the kidnies, difficulty of urine, sore throats, pains in the ears, the juice being dropped in them; outwardly it helps the shingles and *St. Anthony's fire*.

Hyppoglossum. Horse-tongue, Tongue-blade or Double-Tongue. The roots help the stranguary, provoke urine, ease the hard labour of women, provoke the menses, the herb helps ruptures and the fits of the mother: it is hot in the second degree, dry in the first: boil it in white wine.

Hyppolapathum. Patience, or Monk's Rhubarb. See the Root.

Hypposclinum. Alexanders, or Alisanders: provoke urine, expel the placenta, help the stranguary, expel wind.

Sage either taken inwardly or beaten and applied plaister-wise to the matrix, draws forth both menses and placenta.

Horminum. Clary: hot and dry in the third degree; helps the weakness in the back, stops the running of the reins, and the Fluor Albus, provokes the menses, and helps women that are barren through coldness or moisture, or both: causes fruitfulness, but is hurtful for the memory. The usual way of taking it is to fry it with butter, or make a tansy with it.

Hydropiper. Arsmart. Hot and dry, consumes all cold swellings and blood congealed by bruises, and stripes; applied to the place, it helps that aposthume in the joints, commonly called a felon: strewed in a chamber, kills all the fleas there: this is hottest Arsmart, and is unfit to be given inwardly: there is a milder sort, called *Persicaria*, which is of a cooler and milder quality, drying, excellently good for putrified ulcers, kills worms. I had almost forgot that the former is an admirable remedy for the gout, being roasted between two tiles and applied to the grieved place, and yet I had it from Dr. *Butler* too.

Hysopus. Hysop. Helps coughs, shortness of breath, wheezing, distillations upon the lungs: it is of a cleansing quality: kills worms in the body, amends the whole colour of the body, helps the dropsy and spleen, sore throats, and noise in the ears. See Syrup of Hysop.

Hyosciamus, &c. Henbane. The white Henbane is held to be cold in the third degree, the black or common Henbane and the yellow, in the fourth. They stupify the senses, and therefore not to be taken inwardly, outwardly applied, they help inflammations, hot gouts: applied to the temples they provoke sleep.

Hypericon. St. John's Wort. It is as gallant a wound-herb as any is, either given inwardly, or outwardly applied to the wound: it is hot and dry, opens stoppings, helps spitting and vomiting of blood, it cleanses the reins, provokes the menses, helps congealed blood in the stomach and meseraic veins, the falling-sickness, palsy, cramps and aches in the joints; you may give it in powder or any convenient decoction.

Hypoglottis, Laurus, Alexandrina. Laurel of Alexandria, provokes urine and the menses, and is held to be a singular help to women in travail.

Hypoglossum, the same with *Hypoglossum* before, only different names given by different authors, the one deriving his name from the tongue of a horse, of which form the leaf is; the other the form of the little leaf, because small leaves like small tongues grow upon the greater.

Iberis Cardamantice. Sciatica-cresses. I suppose so called because they help the Sciatica, or Huckle-bone Gout.

Ingunialis, Asther. Setwort or Shartwort: being bruised and applied, they help swellings, botches, and venerous swellings in the groin, whence they took their name, as also inflammation and falling out of the fundament.

Iris. See the roots.

Isatis, Glastum. Woad. Drying and binding; the side being bathed with it, it easeth pains in the spleen, cleanseth filthy corroding gnawing ulcers.

Iva Arthritica. The same with *Camæpytis.*

Iuncus oderatus. The same with *Schœnanthus.*

Labrum veneris. The same with *Dipsacus.*

Lactuca. Lettice. Cold and moist, cools the inflammation of the stomach, commonly called heart-burning: provokes sleep, resists drunkenness, and takes away the ill effects of it; cools the blood, quenches thirst, breeds milk, and is good for choleric bodies, and such as have a frenzy, or are frantic. It is more wholesome eaten boiled than raw.

Logabus, Herba Leporina. A kind of Trefoil growing in *France* and *Spain.* Let them that live there look after the virtues of it.

Lavendula. Lavender. Hot and dry in the third degree: the

temples and forehead bathed with the juice of it; as also the smell of the herb helps swoonings, catalepsis, falling-sickness, provided it be not accompanied with a fever. See the flowers.

Laureola. Laurel. The leaves purge upward and downward: they are good for rheumatic people to chew in their mouths, for they draw forth much water.

Laurus. Bay-tree. The leaves are hot and dry, resist drunkenness, they gently bind and help diseases in the bladder, help the stinging of bees and wasps, mitigate the pain of the stomach, dry and heal, open obstructions of the liver and spleen, resist the pestilence.

Lappa Minor. The lesser Burdock.

Lentiscus. Mastich-tree. Both the leaves and bark of it stop fluxes (being hot and dry in the second degree) spitting and evacuations of blood, and the falling out of the fundament.

Lens palustris. Duckmeat. Cold and moist in the second degree, helps inflammations, hot swellings, and the falling out of the fundament, being warmed and applied to the place.

Lepidium Piperites. Dittander, Pepperwort, or Scar-wort. A hot fiery sharp herb, admirable for the gout being applied to the place: being only held in the hand, it helps the tooth-ache, and withall leaves a wan colour in the hand that holds it.

Livisticum. Lovage. Clears the sight, takes away redness and freckles from the face.

Libanotis Coronaria. See Rosemary.

Linaria. Toad-flax, or Wild-flax: hot and dry, cleanses the reins and bladder, provokes urine, opens the stoppings of the liver and spleen, and helps diseases coming thereof: outwardly it takes away yellowness and deformity of the skin.

Lillium convallium. Lilly of the Valley. See the flowers.

Lingua Cervina. Hart's-tongue: drying and binding, stops blood, the menses and fluxes, opens stoppings of the liver and spleen, and diseases thence arising. The like quantity of Hart's-tongue, Knotgrass and Comfrey Roots, being boiled in water, and a draught of the decoction drunk every morning, and the materials which have boiled applied to the place, is a notable remedy for such as are bursten.

Limonium. Sea-bugloss, or Marsh-bugloss, or Sea-Lavender; the seeds being very drying and binding, stop fluxes and the menses, help the cholic and stranguary.

Lotus urbana. Authors make some flutter about this herb. I conceive the best take it to be *Trisolium Odoratum*, Sweet Trefoyl, which is of a temperate nature, cleanses the eyes gently of such things as hinder the sight, cures green wounds, ruptures, or burstness, helps such as urine blood or are bruised, and secures garments from moths.

Lupulus. Hops. Opening, cleansing, provoke urine, the young sprouts open stoppings of the liver and spleen, cleanse the blood, clear the skin, help scabs and itch, help agues, purge choler: they are usually boiled and taken as they eat asparagus, but if you would keep them, for they are excellent for these diseases, you may make them into a conserve, or into a syrup.

Lychnitis Coronaria: or as others write it, *Lychnis*. Rose Campion. I know no great physical virtue it hath.

Macis. See the barks.

Magistrantia, &c. Masterwort. Hot and dry in the third degree: it is good against poison, pestilence, corrupt and unwholesome air, helps windiness in the stomach, causeth an appetite to one's victuals, very profitable in falls and bruises, congealed and clotted blood, the bitings of mad-dogs; the leaves chewed in the mouth, cleanse the brain of superfluous humours, thereby preventing lethargies, and apoplexes.

Malva. Mallows. The best of Authors account wild Mallows to be best, and hold them to be cold and moist in the first degree, they are profitable in the bitings of venomous beasts, the stinging of bees and wasps, &c. Inwardly they resist poison, provoke to stool; outwardly they assuage hard swellings of the privities or other places; in clysters they help roughness and fretting of the entrails, bladder, or fundament; and so they do being boiled in water, and the decoction drank, as I have proved in the bloody flux.

Majorana. See *Amaraeus.*

Mandragora. Mandrakes. Fit for no vulgar use, but only to be used in cooling ointments.

Marrubium, album, nigrum, fœtidum.

Marrubium album, is common Horehound. Hot in the second degree, and dry in the third, opens the liver and spleen, cleanses the breast and lungs, helps old coughs, pains in the sides, ptisicks, or ulceration of the lungs, it provokes the menses, eases hard labour in child-bearing, brings away the placenta. See the syrups.

Marrubium, nigrum, et fœtidum. Black and stinking Horehound, I take to be all one. Hot and dry in the third degree; cures the bitings of mad dogs, wastes and consumes hard knots in the fundament and matrix, cleanses filthy ulcers.

Marum. Herb Mastich. Hot and dry in the third degree, good against cramps and convulsions.

Matricaria. Feverfew. Hot in the third degree, dry in the second; opens, purges; a singular remedy for diseases incident to the matrix, and other diseases incident to women, eases their travail, and infirmities coming after it; it helps the vertigo or dissiness of the head, melancholy sad thoughts: you may boil it either alone, or with other herbs fit for the same purpose, with which this treatise will furnish you: applied to the wrists, it helps the ague.

Matrisylva. The same with *Caprifolium.*

Meliotus. Melilot. Inwardly taken, provokes urine, breaks the Stone, cleanses the reins and bladder, cutteth and cleanses the lungs of tough flegm, the juice dropped into the eyes, clears the sight, into the ears, mitigates pain and noise there; the head bathed with the juice mixed with vinegar, takes away the pains thereof: outwardly in pultisses, it assuages swellings in the privities and elsewhere.

Mellissa. Balm. Hot and dry: outwardly mixed with salt and applied to the neck, helps the King's-evil, bitings of mad dogs, venomous beasts, and such as cannot hold their neck as they should do; inwardly it is an excellent remedy for a cold and moist stomach, cheers the heart, refreshes the mind, takes away griefs, sorrow, and care, instead of which it produces joy and mirth. See the syrup. *Galen, Avicenna.*

Mentha sativa. Garden Mints, Spear Mints. Are hot and dry in the third degree, provoke hunger, are wholesome for the stomach, stay vomiting, stop the menses, help sore heads in children, strengthen the stomach, cause digestion; outwardly applied, they help the bitings of mad-dogs. Yet they hinder conception.

Mentha aquatica. Water Mints. Ease pains of the belly, headache, and vomiting, gravel in the kidnies and stone.

Methastrum. Horse-mint. I know no difference between them and water mints.

Mercurialis, mas, fæmina. Mercury male and female, they are both hot and dry in the second degree, cleansing, digesting, they purge watery humours, and further conception.

Mezereon. Spurge-Olive, or Widdow-wail. A dangerous purge, better let alone than meddled with.

Millefolium. Yarrow. Meanly cold and binding, an healing herb for wounds, stanches bleeding; and some say the juice snuffed up the nose, causeth it to bleed, whence it was called, Nose-bleed; it stops lasks, and the menses, helps the running of the reins, helps inflammations and excoriations of the priapus, as also inflammations of wounds. *Galen.*

Muscus. Mosse. Is something cold and binding, yet usually retains a smatch of the property of the tree it grows on; therefore that which grows upon oaks is very dry and binding. *Serapio* saith that it being infused in wine, and the wine drank, it stays vomiting and fluxes, as also the Fluor Albus.

Myrtus. Myrtle-tree. The leaves are of a cold earthly quality, drying and binding, good for fluxes, spitting and vomiting of blood; stop the Fluor Albus and menses.

Nardus. See the root.

Nasturtium, Aquaticum, Hortense. Water-cresses, and Garden-cresses. Garden-cresses are hot and dry in the fourth degree, good for the scurvy, sciatica, hard swellings; yet do they trouble the belly, ease pains of the spleen, provoke lust. *Dioscorides.* Water-cresses are hot and dry, cleanse the blood, help the scurvy, provoke urine and the menses, break the stone, help the green-sickness, cause a fresh lively colour.

Nasturtium Alhum, Thlaspie. Treacle-mustard. Hot and dry in the third degree, purges violently, dangerous for pregnant women. Outwardly it is applied with profit to the gout.

Nicorimi. Tobacco. It is hot and dry in the second degree, and of a cleansing nature: the leaves warmed and applied to the head, are excellently good in inveterate head-aches and megrims, if the diseases come through cold or wind, change them often till the diseases be gone, help such whose necks be stiff: it eases the faults of the breast: Asthmas or head-flegm in the lappets of the lungs: eases the pains of the stomach and windiness thereof: being heated by the fire, and applied hot to the side, they loosen the belly, and kill worms being applied unto it in like manner: they break the stone being applied in like manner to the region of the bladder: help the rickets, being applied to the belly and sides: applied to the navel, they give present ease to the fits of the mother: they take away cold aches in the joints applied to them: boiled, the liquor absolutely and speedily cures scabs and itch: neither is there any better salve in the world for wounds than may be made of it: for it cleanses, fetches out the filth though it lie in the bones, brings up the flesh from the bottom, and all this it doth speedily: it cures wounds made with poisoned weapons, and for this *Clusius* brings many experiences too tedious here to relate. It is an admirable thing for carbuncles and plague-sores, inferior to none: green wounds 'twill cure in a trice: ulcers and gangreens very speedily, not only in men, but also in beasts, therefore the Indians dedicated it to their god. Taken in a pipe, it hath almost as many virtues; it easeth weariness, takes away the sense of hunger and thirst, provokes to stool: he saith, the Indians will travel four days without either meat or drink, by only chewing a little of this in their mouths. It eases the body of superfluous humours, opens stoppings. See the ointment of Tobacco.

Nummularia. Money-wort, or Herb Two-pence; cold, dry, binding, helps fluxes, stops the menses, helps ulcers in the lungs; outwardly it is a special herb for wounds.

Nymphea. See the flowers.

Ocynum. Basil, hot and moist. The best use that I know of it, is, it gives speedy deliverance to women in travail. Let them not take above half a dram of it at a time in powder, and be sure also the birth be ripe, else it causes abortion.

Oleæ folia. Olive leaves: they are hard to come by here.

Ononis. Restharrow. See the roots.

Ophioglossum. Adder's-tongue. The leaves are very drying: being boiled in oil they make a dainty green balsam for green wounds: taken inwardly, they help inward wounds.

Origanum. Origany: a kind of wild Marjoram; hot and dry in the third degree, helps the bitings of venomous beasts, such as have taken Opium, Hemlock, or Poppy; provokes urine, brings down the menses, helps old coughs; in an ointment it helps scabs and itch.

Oxylapathum. Sorrel. See *Acetosa.*

Papaver, &c. Poppies, white, black, or erratick. I refer you to the syrups of each.

Parietaria. Given once before under the name of *Helxine.*

Pastinæa. Parsnips. See the roots.

Persicaria. See *Hydropiper.* This is the milder sort of Arsmart I described there. If ever you find it amongst the compounds, take it under that notion.

Pentaphyllium. Cinquefoil: very drying, yet but meanly hot, if at all; helps ulcers in the mouth, roughness of the wind-pipe (whence comes hoarseness and coughs, &c.), helps fluxes, creeping ulcers, and the yellow jaundice; they say one leaf cures a quotidian ague, three a tertain, and four a quartan. I know it will cure agues without this curiosity, if a wise man have the handling of it; otherwise a cart load will not do it.

Petroselinum. Parsley. See Smallage.

Per Columbinus. See *Geranium.*

Persicarium folia. Peach Leaves: they are a gentle, yet a complete purger of choler, and disease coming from thence; fit for children because of their gentleness. You may boil them in white wine: a handfull is enough at a time.

Pilosella. Mouse-ear: once before and this is often enough.

Pithyusa. A new name for Spurge of the last Edition.

Plantago. Plantain. Cold and dry; an herb, though common, yet let none despise it, for the decoction of it prevails mightily against tormenting pains and excoriations of the entrails, bloody fluxes, it stops the menses, and spitting of blood, phthisicks, or consumptions of the lungs, the running of the reins, and the Fluor Albus, pains in the head, and frenzies: outwardly it clears the sight, takes away inflammations, scabs, itch, the shingles, and all spreading sores, and is as wholesome an herb as can grow about any an house. *Tragus, Dioscorides.*

Poliam, &c. Polley, or Pellamountain. All the sorts are hot in the second degree, and dry in the third: helps dropsies, the yellow jaundice, infirmities of the spleen, and provokes urine. *Dioscorides.*

Polygonum. Knotgrass.

Polytricum. Maidenhair.

Portulaca. Purslain. Cold and moist in the second or third degree: cools hot stomachs, and it is admirable for one that hath his teeth on edge by eating sour apples, it cools the blood, liver, and is good for hot diseases, or inflammations in any of these places, stops fluxes, and the menses, and helps all inward inflammations whatsoever.

Porrum. Leeks. See the roots.

Primula Veris. See Cowslips, or the Flowers, which you will.

Prunella. Self-heal, Carpenter's-herb, and Sicklewort. Moderately hot and dry, binding. See Bugle, the virtues being the same.

Pulegium. Pennyroyal; hot and dry in the third degree; provokes urine, breaks the stone in the reins, strengthens women's backs, provokes the menses, easeth their labour in child-bed, brings away the placenta, stays vomiting, strengthens the brain, breaks wind, and helps the vertigo.

Pulmonaria, arborea, et Symphytum maculosum. Lung-wort. It helps infirmities of the lungs, as hoarseness, coughs, wheezing, shortness of breath, &c. You may boil it in Hyssop-water, or any other water that strengthens the lungs.

Pulicaria. Fleabane; hot and dry in the third degree, helps the biting of venomous beasts, wounds and swellings, the yellow jaundice, the falling sickness, and such as cannot make water; being burnt, the smoak of it kills all the gnats and fleas in the chamber; it is dangerous for pregnant women.

Pyrus sylvestris. Wild Pear-tree. I know no virtue in the leaves.

Pyrola. Winter-green. Cold and dry, and very binding, stops fluxes, and the menses, and is admirably good in green wounds.

Quercus folia. Oak Leaves. Are much of the nature of the former, stay the Fluor Albus. See the bark.

Ranunculus. Hath got a sort of English Names: Crowfoot, King-kob, Gold-cups, Gold-knobs, Butter-flowers, &c. they are of a notable hot quality, unfit to be taken inwardly. If you bruise the roots and apply them to a plague-sore, they are notable things to draw the venom to them.

Raparum folia. If they do mean Turnip leaves, when they are young and tender, they are held to provoke urine.

Rosmarirum. Rosemary, hot and dry in the second degree, binding, stops fluxes, helps stuffings in the head, the yellow jaundice, helps the memory, expels wind. See the flowers. *Serapio, Dioscorides.*

Rosa solis. See the water.

Rosa alba, rubra, Damascena. White, Red, and Damask Roses.

Rumex. Dock. All the ordinary sort of Docks are of a cool and drying substance, and therefore stop fluxes; and the leaves are seldom used in physic.

Rubus Idæus. Raspis, Raspberries, or Hind-berries. I know no great virtues in the leaves.

Ruta. Rue, or Herb of Grace; hot and dry in the third degree, consumes the seed, and is an enemy to generation, helps difficulty of breathing, and inflammations of the lungs, pains in the sides, inflammations of the priapus and matrix, naught for pregnant women: no herb resists poison more. It strengthens the heart exceedingly, and no herb better than this in pestilential times, take it what manner you will or can.

Ruta Muraria. See *Adianthum.*

Sabina. Savin: hot and dry in the third degree, potently provokes the menses, expels both birth and afterbirth, they (boiled in oil and used in ointments) stay creeping ulcers, scour away spots, freckles and sunburning from the face; the belly anointed with it kills worms in children.

Salvia. Sage: hot and dry in the second or third degree, binding, it stays abortion in such women as are subject to come before their times, it causes fruitfulness, it is singularly good for the brain, strengthens the senses and memory, helps spitting and vomiting of blood: outwardly, heat hot with a little vinegar and applied to the side, helps stitches and pains in the sides.

Salix. Willow leaves, are cold, dry, and binding, stop spitting of blood, and fluxes; the boughs stuck about a chamber, wonderfully cool the air, and refresh such as have fevers; the leaves applied to the head, help hot diseases there, and frenzies.

Sampsucum. Marjoram.

Sunicula. Sanicle; hot and dry in the second degree, cleanses wounds and ulcers.

Saponaria. Sope-wort, or Bruise-wort, vulgarly used in bruises and cut fingers, and is of notable use in the veneral disease.

Satureia. Savory. Summer savory is hot and dry in the third degree, Winter savory is not so hot, both of them expel wind.

Sazifragia alba. White Saxifrage, breaks wind, helps the cholic and stone.

Scabiosa. Scabious: hot and dry in the second degree, cleanses the breast and lungs, helps old rotten coughs, and difficulty of breathing, provokes urine, and cleanses the bladder of filthy stuff, breaks aposthumes, and cures scabs and itch. Boil it in white wine.

Scariola. An Italian name for Succory.

Schœnanthus. Schœnanth, Squinanth, or Chamel's hay; hot and binding. It digests and opens the passages of the veins: surely it is as great an expeller of wind as any is.

Scordium. Water-Germander, hot and dry, cleanses ulcers in the inward parts, it provokes urine and the menses, opens stopping of the liver, spleen, reins, bladder, and matrix, it is a great counter poison, and eases the breast oppressed with flegm. See Diascordium.

Scrophularia. Figwort, so called of *Scrophula*, the King's Evil, which it cures they say, by being only hung about the neck. If not, bruise it, and apply it to the place, it helps the piles or hemorrhoids.

Sedum. And all his sorts. See *Barba Jovis.*

Senna. It heats in the second degree and dries in the first, cleanses, purges and digests; it carries downward both choler, flegm, and melancholy, it cleanses the brain, heart, liver, spleen; it cheers the senses, opens obstructions, takes away dullness of sight, helps deafness, helps melancholy and madness, resists resolution of the nerves, pains of the head, scabs, itch, falling-sickness, the windiness of it is corrected with a little ginger. You may boil half an ounce of it at a time, in water or white wine, but boil it not too much; half an ounce is a moderate dose to be boiled for any reasonable body.

Serpillum. Mother-of-Time, with Time; it is hot and dry in the third degree, it provokes the menses, and helps the stranguary or stoppage of urine, gripings in the belly, ruptures, convulsions, inflammation of the liver, lethargy, and infirmities of the spleen, boil it in white wine. *Ætius, Galen.*

Sigillum Solomonis. Solomon's seal. See the root.

Smyrnium. Alexander of *Crete.*

Solanum. Night-shade: very cold and dry, binding; it is somewhat dangerous given inwardly, unless by a skilful hand; outwardly it helps the Shingles, *St. Anthony's* fire, and other hot inflammations.

Soldanella. Bindweed, hot and dry in the second degree, it opens obstructions of the liver, and purges watery humours, and is therefore very profitable in dropsies, it is very hurtful to the stomach, and therefore if taken inwardly it had need be well corrected with cinnamon, ginger, or annis-seed, &c.

Sonchus levis Asper. Sow-thistles smooth and rough, they are of a cold, watery, yet binding quality, good for frenzies, they increase milk in nurses, and cause the children which they nurse to have a good colour, help gnawings of the stomach coming of a hot cause; outwardly they help inflammations, and hot swellings, cool the heat of the fundament and privities.

Sophi Chirurgorum. Fluxweed: drying without any manifest heat or coldness; it is usually found about old ruinous buildings; it is so called because of its virtue in stopping fluxes.

Shinachia. Spinage. I never read any physical virtues of it.

Spina Alba. See the root.

Spica. See *Nardus.*

Stæbe. Silver Knapweed. The virtues be the same with Scabious, and some think the herbs too; though I am of another opinion.

Stæchas. French Lavender. Cassidony, is a great counterpoison, opens obstructions of the liver and spleen, cleanses the matrix and bladder, brings out corrupt humours, provokes urine.

Succisa, Marsus Diaboli. Devil's-bit. Hot and dry in the second degree: inwardly taken, it eases the fits of the mother, and breaks wind, takes away swellings in the mouth, and slimy flegm that stick to the jaws, neither is there a more present remedy in the world for those cold swellings in the neck which the vulgar call the almonds of the ears, than this herb bruised and applied to them.

Suchaha. An Egyptian Thorn. Very hard, if not impossible to come by here.

Tanacetum. Tansy: hot in the second degree and dry in the third; the very smell of it stays abortion, or miscarriages in women; so it doth being bruised and applied to their navels, provokes urine, and is a special help against the gout.

Taraxacon. Dandelion, or to write better French, Dent-de-lion, for in plain English, it is called lyon's tooth; it is a kind of Succory, and thither I refer you.

Tamariscus. Tamiris. It hath a dry cleansing quality, and hath a notable virtue against the rickets, and infirmities of the spleen, provokes the menses. *Galen, Dioscorides.*

Telephium. A kind of Opine.

Thlaspi. See *Nasturtium.*

Thymbra. A wild Savory.

Thymum. Thyme. Hot and dry in the third degree; helps coughs and shortness of breath, provokes the menses, brings away dead children and the after birth; purges flegm, cleanses the breast and lungs, reins and matrix; helps the sciatica, pains in the breast, expels wind in any part of the body, resists fearfulness and melancholy, continual pains in the head, and is profitable for such as have the falling-sickness to smell to.

Thymælea. The Greek name for Spurge-Olive: *Mezereon* being the Arabick name.

Tithymallus, Esula, &c. Spurge. Hot and dry in the fourth degree: a dogged purge, better let alone than taken inwardly: hair anointed with the juice of it will fall off: it kills fish, being mixed with any thing that they will eat: outwardly it cleanses ulcers, takes away freckles, sunburning and morphew from the face.

Tormentilla. See the root.

Trinitatis herba. Pansies, or Heart's-ease. They are cold and moist, both herbs and flowers, excellent against inflammations of the breast or lungs, convulsions or falling-sickness, also they are held to be good for venereal complaints.

Trifolium. Trefoil: dry in the third degree, and cold. The ordinary Meadow Trefoil, cleanses the bowels of slimy humours that stick to them, being used either in drinks or clysters; outwardly they take away inflammations.

Tussilago. Colt's-foot: something cold and dry, and therefore good for inflammations, they are admirably good for coughs, and consumptions of the lungs, shortness of breath, &c. It is often used and with good success taken in a tobacco-pipe, being cut and mixed with a little oil of annis seeds. See the Syrup of Colt's-foot.

Valeriana. Valerian, or Setwall. See the roots.

Verbascum, Thapsus Barbatus. Mullin, or Higtaper. It is something dry, and of a digesting, cleansing quality, stops fluxes and the hemorrhoids, it cures hoarseness, the cough, and such as are broken winded.

Verbena. Vervain: hot and dry, a great opener, cleanser, healer, it helps the yellow jaundice, defects in the reins and bladder, pains in the head; if it be but bruised and hung about the neck, all diseases in the privities; made into an ointment it is a sovereign remedy for old head-aches, as also frenzies, it clears the skin, and causes a lovely colour.

Voronica. See *Betonica Pauli.*

Violaria. Violet Leaves: they are cool, ease pains in the head proceeding of heat and frenzies, either inwardly taken or outwardly applied; heat of the stomach, or inflammation of the lungs.

Vitis Viniseria. The manured Vine: the leaves are binding and cool withal; the burnt ashes of the sticks of a vine, scour the teeth and make them as white as snow; the leaves stop bleeding, fluxes, heart-burnings, vomitings; as also the longings of pregnant women. The coals of a burnt Vine, in powder, mixed with honey, doth make the teeth as white as ivory, which are rubbed with it.

Vincitoxicum. Swallow-wort. A pultis made with the leaves helps sore breasts, and also soreness of the matrix.

Virga Pastoris. A third name for Teazles. See *Dipsatus.*

Virga Aurea. See *Consolida.*

Ulmaria. See the root. *Meadsweet.*

Umbilicus Veneris. Navil-wort. Cold, dry, and binding, therefore helps all inflammations; they are very good for kibed heels, being bathed with it and a leaf laid over the sore.

Urtica. Nettles: an herb so well known, that you may find them by the feeling in the darkest night: they are something hot, not very hot; the juice stops bleeding; they provoke lust, help difficulty of breathing, pleurisies, inflammations of the lung; that troublesome cough that women call the Chincough; they exceedingly break the stone, provoke urine, and help such as cannot hold their necks upright. Boil them in white wine.

Usnea. Moss; once before.

FLOWERS

BORAGE, and Bugloss flowers strengthen the brain, and are profitable in fevers.

Chamomel flowers, heat and assuage swellings, inflammation of the bowels, dissolve wind, are profitably given in clysters or drink, to such as are troubled with the cholic, or stone.

Stæchea, opens stoppings in the bowels, and strengthens the whole body.

Saffron powerfully concocts, and sends out whatever humour offends the body, drives back inflammations; applied outwardly, encreases venery, and provokes urine.

Clove-Gilliflowers, resist the pestilence, strengthen the heart, liver, and stomach, and provoke venery.

Schænanth (which I touched slightly amongst the herbs) provokes urine potently, provokes the menses, breaks wind, helps such as spit or vomit blood, eases pains of the stomach, reins, and spleen, helps dropsies, convulsions, and inflammations of the womb.

Lavender-flowers, resist all cold afflictions of the brain, convulsions, falling-sickness, they strengthen cold stomachs, and open obstructions of the liver, they provoke urine and the menses, bring forth the birth and placenta.

Hops, open stoppings of the bowels, and for that cause beer is better than ale.

Balm-flowers, cheer the heart and vital spirits, strengthen the stomach.

Rosemary-flowers, strengthen the brain exceedingly, and resist madness; clear the sight.

Winter-Gilliflowers, or Wall-flowers, help inflammation of the womb, provoke the menses, and help ulcers in the mouth.

Honey-suckles, provoke urine, ease the pains of the spleen, and such as can hardly fetch their breath.

Mallows, help coughs.

Red Roses, cool, bind, strengthen both vital and animal virtue, restore such as are in consumptions, strengthen. There are so many compositions of them which makes me more brief in the simples.

Violets, (to wit, the blue ones,) cool and moisten, provoke sleep, loosen the belly, resist fevers, help inflammations, correct the heat of choler, ease the pains in the head, help the roughness of the wind-pipe, diseases in the throat, inflammations in the breast and sides, plurisies, open stoppings of the liver, and help the yellow jaundice.

Chicory, (or Succory as the vulgar call it) cools and strengthens the liver, so doth Endive.

Water lilies ease pains of the head coming of choler and heat, provoke sleep, cool inflammations, and the heat in fevers.

Pomegranate-flowers, dry and bind, stop fluxes, and the menses.

Cowslips, strengthen the brain, senses, and memory, exceedingly, resist all diseases there, as convulsions, falling-sickness, palsies, &c.

Centaury, purges choler and gross humours, helps the yellow jaundice, opens obstructions of the liver, helps pains of the spleen, provokes the menses, brings away birth and afterbirth.

Elder flowers, help dropsies, cleanse the blood, clear the skin, open stoppings of the liver and spleen, and diseases arising therefrom.

Bean-flowers, clear the skin, stop humours flowing into the eyes.

Peach-tree flowers, purge choler gently.

Broom-flowers, purge water, and are good in dropsies.

The temperature of all these differ either very little or not at all from the herbs.

The way of using the flowers I did forbear, because most of them may, and are usually made into conserves, of which you may take the quantity of a nutmeg in the morning; all of them may be kept dry a year, and boiled with other herbs conducing to the cures they do.

FRUITS AND THEIR BUDS

Green Figs, are held to be of ill juice, but the best is, we are not much troubled with them in *England*; dry figs help coughs, cleanse the breast, and help infirmities of the lungs, shortness of wind, they loose the belly, purge the reins, help inflammations of the liver and spleen; outwardly they dissolve swellings.

Pine-nuts, restore such as are in consumptions, amend the failings of the lungs, concoct flegm, and yet are naught for such as are troubled with the head-ache.

Dates, are binding, stop eating ulcers being applied to them; they are very good for weak stomachs, for they soon digest, and breed good nourishment, they help infirmities of the reins, bladder, and womb.

Sebestens, cool choler, violent heat of the stomach, help roughness of the tongue and wind-pipe, cool the reins and bladder.

Raisins of the Sun, help infirmities of the breast and liver, restore consumptions, gently cleanse and move to stool.

Walnuts, kill worms, resist the pestilence, (I mean the green ones, not the dry).

Capers eaten before meals, provoke hunger.

Nutmegs, strengthen the brain, stomach, and liver, provoke urine, ease the pains of the spleen, stop looseness, ease pains of the head, and pains in the joints, strengthen the body, take away weakness coming of cold, and cause a sweet breath.

Cloves, help digestion, stop looseness, provoke lust, and quicken the sight.

Pepper, binds, expels wind, helps the cholic, quickens digestion oppressed with cold, heats the stomach.

Quinces. See the Compositions.

Pears are grateful to the stomach, drying, and therefore help fluxes.

All plums that are sharp or sour, are binding, the sweet are loosening.

Cucumbers, cool the stomach, and are good against ulcers in the bladder.

Galls, are exceeding binding, help ulcers in the mouth, wasting of the gums, ease the pains of the teeth, help the falling out of the womb and fundament, make the hair black.

Pompions are a cold and moist fruit, of small nourishment, they provoke urine, outwardly applied; the flesh of them helps inflammations and burnings; applied to the forehead they help inflammations of the eyes.

Melons, have few other virtues.

Apricots, are very grateful to the stomach, and dry up the humours thereof. *Peaches* are held to do the like.

Cubebs, are hot and dry in the third degree, they expel wind, and cleanse the stomach of tough and viscous humours, they ease the pains of the spleen, and help cold diseases of the womb, they cleanse the head of flegm and strengthen the brain, they heat the stomach and provoke venery.

Bitter Almonds, are hot in the first degree and dry in the second, they cleanse and cut thick humours, cleanse the lungs, and eaten every morning, they are held to preserve from drunkenness.

Bay-berries, heat, expel wind, mitigate pain; are excellent for cold infirmities of the womb, and dropsies.

Cherries are of different qualities according to their different taste, the sweet are quickest of digestion, but the sour are more pleasing to a hot stomach, and procure appetite to one's meat.

Medlars, are strengthening to the stomach, binding, and the green are more binding than the rotten, and the dry than the green.

Olives, cool and bind.

English-currants, cool the stomach, and are profitable in acute fevers, they quench thirst, resist vomiting, cool the heat of choler, provoke appetite, and are good for hot complexions.

Services, or Chockers are of the nature of Medlars, but something weaker in operation.

Barberries, quench thirst, cool the heat of choler, resist the pestilence, stay vomiting and fluxes, stop the menses, kill worms, help spitting of blood, fasten the teeth, and strengthen the gums.

Strawberries, cool the stomach, liver, and blood, but are very hurtful for such as have agues.

Winter-Cherries, potently provoke urine, and break the stone.

Cassia-fistula, is temperate in quality, gently purgeth choler and flegm, clarifies the blood, resists fevers, cleanses the breast and lungs, it cools the reins, and thereby resists the breeding of the stone, it provokes urine, and therefore is exceeding good for the running of the reins in men, and the Fluor Albus in women.

All the sorts or *Myrobalans*, purge the stomach; the Indian Myrobalans, are held to purge melancholy most especially, the other flegm; yet take heed you use them not in stoppings of the bowels: they are cold and dry, they all strengthen the heart, brain, and sinews, strengthen the stomach, relieve the senses, take away tremblings and heart-qualms. They are seldom used alone.

Prunes, are cooling and loosening.

Tamarinds, are cold and dry in the second degree, they purge choler, cool the blood, stay vomiting, help the yellow jaundice, quench thirst, cool hot stomachs, and hot livers.

I omit the use of these also as resting confident a child of three years old, if you should give it Raisins of the sun or Cherries, would not ask how it should take them.

SEEDS OR GRAINS

Coriander seed, hot and dry, expels wind, but is hurtful to the head; sends up unwholesome vapours to the brain, dangerous for mad people.

Fenugreek seeds, are of a softening, discussing nature, they cease inflammations, be they internal or external: bruised and mixed with vinegar they ease the pains of the spleen: being applied to the sides, help hardness and swellings of the matrix, being boiled, the decoction helps scabby heads.

Lin-seed hath the same virtues with Fenugreek.

Gromwell seed, provokes urine, helps the cholic, breaks the stone, and expels wind. Boil them in white wine; but bruise them first.

Lupines, ease the pains of the spleen, kill worms and cast them out: outwardly, they cleanse filthy ulcers, and gangrenes, help scabs, itch, and inflammations.

Dill seed, encreases milk in nurses, expels wind, stays vomitings, provokes urine; yet it dulls the sight, and is an enemy to generation.

Smallage seed, provokes urine and the menses, expels wind, resists poison, and eases inward pains, it opens stoppings in any part of the body, yet it is hurtful for such as have the falling-sickness, and for pregnant women.

Rocket seed, provokes urine, stirs up lust, encreases seed, kills worms, eases pains of the spleen. Use all these in like manner.

Basil seed. If we may believe *Dioscorides* and *Crescentius*, cheers the heart, and strengthens a moist stomach, drives away melancholy, and provokes urine.

Nettle seed, provokes venery, opens stoppages of the womb, helps inflammations of the sides and lungs; purgeth the breast: boil them (being bruised) in white wine also.

The seeds of *Ammi,* or *Bishop's-weed,* heat and dry, help difficulty of urine, and the pains of the cholic, the bitings of venomous beasts; they provoke the menses, and purge the womb.

Annis seeds, heat and dry, ease pain, expel wind, cause a sweet breath, help the dropsy, resist poison, breed milk, and stop the Fluor Albus in women, provoke venery, and ease the head-ache.

Cardamoms, heat, kill worms, cleanse the reins, and provoke urine.

Fennel seed, breaks wind, provokes urine and the menses, encreases milk in nurses.

Cummin seed, heat, bind, and dry, stop blood, expel wind, ease pain, help the bitings of venomous beasts: outwardly applied (viz. in Plaisters) they are of a discussing nature.

Carrot seeds, are windy, provoke lust exceedingly, and encrease seed, provoke urine and the menses, cause speedy delivery to women in travail, and bring away the placenta. All these also may be boiled in white wine.

Nigella seeds, boiled in oil, and the forehead anointed with it, ease pains in the head, take away leprosy, itch, scurf, and help scaly heads. Inwardly taken they expel worms, they provoke urine, and the menses, help difficulty of breathing.

Stavesacre, kills lice in the head. I hold it not fitting to be given inwardly.

Olibanum mixed with as much Barrow's Grease (beat the Olibanum first in powder) and boiled together, make an ointment which will kill the lice in children's heads, and such as are subject to breed them, will never breed them. A Medicine cheap, safe, and sure, which breeds no annoyance to the brain.

The seeds of *Water-cresses*, heat, yet trouble the stomach and belly; ease the pains of the spleen, are very dangerous for pregnant women, yet they provoke lust; outwardly applied, they help leprosies, scaly heads, and the falling off of hair, as also carbuncles, and cold ulcers in the joints.

Mustard seed, heats, extenuates, and draws moisture from the brain: the head being shaved and anointed with Mustard, is a good remedy for the lethargy, it helps filthy ulcers, and hard swellings in the mouth, it helps old aches coming of cold.

French Barley, is cooling, nourishing, and breeds milk.

Sorrel seeds, potently resist poison, help fluxes, and such stomachs as loath their meat.

Succory seed, cools the heat of the blood, extinguishes lust, opens stoppings of the liver and bowels, it allays the heat of the body, and produces a good colour, it strengthens the stomach, liver, and reins.

Poppy seeds, ease pain, provoke sleep. Your best way is to make an emulsion of them with barley water.

Mallow seeds, ease pains in the bladder.

Chich-pease, are windy, provoke lust, encrease milk in nurses, provoke the menses, outwardly, they help scabs, itch, and inflammations of the testicles, ulcers, &c.

White Saxifrage seeds, provoke urine, expel wind, and break the stone. Boil them in white wine.

Rue seeds, helps such as cannot hold their water.

Lettice seed, cools the blood, restrains venery.

Also *Gourds, Citruls, Cucumbers, Melons, Purslain, and Endive* seeds, cool the blood, as also the stomach, spleen, and reins, and allay the heat of fevers. Use them as you were taught to do poppy-seeds.

Wormseed, expels wind, kills worms.

Ash-tree Keys, ease pains in the sides, help the dropsy, relieve men weary with labour, provoke venery, and make the body lean.

Piony seeds, help the *Ephialtes*, or the disease the vulgar call the Mare, as also the fits of the mother, and other such like infirmities of the womb, stop the menses, and help convulsions.

Broom seed, potently provoke urine, break the stone.

Citron seeds, strengthen the heart, cheer the vital spirit, resist pestilence and poison.

TEARS, LIQUORS, AND ROZINS

Laudanum, is of a heating, mollifying nature, it opens the mouth of the veins, stays the hair from falling off, helps pains in the ears, and hardness of the womb. It is used only outwardly in plaisters.

Assafœtida. Is commonly used to allay the fits of the mother by smelling to it; they say, inwardly taken, it provokes lust, and expels wind.

Benzoin, or *Benjamin*, makes a good perfume.

Sanguis Draconis, cools and binds exceedingly.

Aloes, purges choler and flegm, and with such deliberation that it is often given to withstand the violence of other purges; it preserves the senses and betters the apprehension, it strengthens the liver, and helps the yellow-jaundice. Yet is naught for such as are troubled with the hemorrhoids, or have agues. I do not like it taken raw. See Aloe Rosata, which is nothing but it washed with the juice of roses.

Manna, is temperately hot, of a mighty dilative quality, windy, cleanses choler gently, also it cleanses the throat and stomach. A child may take an ounce of it at a time melted in milk, and the dross strained out, it is good for them when they are scabby.

Scamony, or *Diagridium*, call it by which name you please, is a desperate purge, hurtful to the body by reason of its heat, windiness, corroding, or gnawing, and violence of working. I would advise my countrymen to let it alone; it will gnaw their bodies as fast as doctors gnaw their purses.

Opopanax, is of a heating, molifying, digesting quality.

Gum Elemi, is exceeding good for fractures of the skull, as also in wounds, and therefore is put in plaisters for that end. See *Arceus* his Liniment.

Tragacanthum, commonly called Gum Traganth, and Gum Dragon, helps coughs, hoarseness, and distillations on the lungs.

Bdellium, heats and softens, helps hard swellings, ruptures, pains in the sides, hardness of the sinews.

Galbanum. Hot and dry, discussing; applied to the womb, it hastens both birth and after-birth, applied to the navel it stays the strangling of the womb, commonly called the fits of the mother, helps pains in the sides, and difficulty of breathing, being applied to it, and the smell of it helps the vertigo or diziness in the head.

Myrh, heats and dries, opens and softens the womb, provokes the birth and after-birth; inwardly taken, it helps old coughs and hoarseness, pains in the sides, kills worms, and helps a stinking breath, helps the wasting of the gums, fastens the teeth: outwardly it helps wounds, and fills up ulcers with flesh. You may take half a dram at a time.

Mastich, strengthens the stomach exceedingly, helps such as vomit or spit blood, it fastens the teeth and strengthens the gums, being chewed in the mouth.

Frankinsense, and *Olibanum,* heat and bind, fill up old ulcers with flesh, stop bleeding, but is extremely bad for mad people.

Turpentine, purges, cleanses the reins, helps the running of them.

Styrax Calamitis, helps coughs, and distillations upon the lungs, hoarseness, want of voice, hardness of the womb, but it is bad for head-aches.

Ammoniacum, applied to the side, helps the hardness and pains of the spleen.

Camphire, eases pains of the head coming of heat, takes away inflammations, and cools any place to which it is applied.

JUICES

THAT all juices have the same virtues with the herbs or fruits whereof they are made, I suppose few or none will deny, therefore I shall only name a few of them, and that briefly.

Sugar is held to be hot in the first degree, strengthens the lungs, takes away the roughness of the throat, succours the reins and bladder.

The juice of *Citrons* cools the blood, strengthens the heart, mitigates the violent heat of fevers.

The juice of *Lemons* works the same effect, but not so powerfully.

Juice of *Liquorice,* strengthens the lungs, helps coughs and colds.

THINGS BRED FROM PLANTS

These have been treated of before, only two excepted. The first of which is :

Agaricus. *Agarick: It purges flegm, choler, and melancholy, from the brain, nerves, muscles, marrow (or more properly brain) of the back, it cleanses the breast, lungs, liver, stomach, spleen, reins, womb, joints; it provokes urine, and the menses, kills worms, helps pains in the joints, and causes a good colour: it is very seldom or never taken alone. See Syrup of Roses with Agarick.*

Lastly, Vicus Quircinus, *or Misleto of the Oak, helps the falling-sickness being either taken inwardly, or hung about one's neck.*

LIVING CREATURES

Millepedes (*so called from the multitude of their feet, though it cannot be supposed they have a thousand*) sows, hog-lice, wood-lice, *being bruised and mixed with wine, they provoke urine, help the yellow jaundice; outwardly being boiled in oil, help pains in the ears, a drop being put into them.*

The flesh of vipers *being eaten, clear the sight, help the vices of the nerves, resist poison exceedingly, neither is there any better remedy under the sun for their bitings than the head of the viper that bit you, bruised and applied to the place, and the flesh eaten, you need not eat above a dram at a time, and make it up as you shall be taught in troches of vipers. Neither any comparable to the stinging of bees and wasps, &c. than the same that sting you, bruised and applied to the place.*

Land Scorpions *cure their own stingings by the same means; the ashes of them (being burnt) potently provokes urine, and breaks the stone.*

Earth-worms, *are an admirable remedy for cut nerves being applied to the place; they provoke urine; see the oil of them, only let me not forget one notable thing quoted by* Mizaldus, *which is, That the powder of them put into an hollow tooth, makes it drop out.*

To draw a tooth without pain, *fill an earthen crucible full of Emmets, Ants, or Pismires, eggs and all, and when you have burned them, keep the ashes, with which if you touch a tooth it will fall out.*

Eels, *being put into wine or beer, and suffered to die in it, he that drinks it will never endure that sort of liquor again.*

Oysters *applied alive to a pestilential swelling, draw the venom to them.*

Crab-fish, *burnt to ashes, and a dram of it taken every morning helps the bitings of mad dogs, and all other venomous beasts.*

Swallows, *being eaten, clear the sight, the ashes of them (being burnt) eaten, preserves from drunkenness, helps sore throats being applied to them, and inflammations.*

Grass-hoppers, *being eaten, ease the cholic, and pains in the bladder.*

Hedge Sparrows, *being kept in salt, or dried and eaten raw, are an admirable remedy for the stone.*

Young Pigeons *being eaten, help pains in the reins, and the disease called Tenesmus.*

PARTS OF LIVING CREATURES,
AND EXCREMENTS

THE brain of *Sparrows* being eaten, provokes lust exceedingly.

The brain of an *Hare* being roasted, helps trembling, it makes children breed teeth easily, their gums being rubbed with it, it also helps scald heads, and falling off of hair, the head being anointed with it.

The head of a young *Kite*, being burnt to ashes and the quantity of a drachm of it taken every morning in a little water, is an admirable remedy against the gout.

Crab-eyes break the stone, and open stoppings of the bowels.

The lungs of a *Fox*, well dried (but not burned) is an admirable strengthener to the lungs. See the Lohoch of Fox lungs.

The liver of a *Duck*, stops fluxes, and strengthens the liver exceedingly.

The liver of a *Frog*, being dried and eaten, helps the quartan agues, or as the vulgar call them, *third-day agues.*

Castoreum resists poison, the bitings of venomous beasts; it provokes the menses, and brings forth birth and after-birth; it expels wind, eases pains and aches, convulsions, sighings, lethargies; the smell of it allays the fits of the mother; inwardly given, it helps tremblings, falling-sickness, and other such ill effects of the brain and nerves. A scruple is enough to take at a time, and indeed spirit of Castorium is better than Castorium, raw, to which I refer you.

A *Sheep's* or *Goat's* bladder being burnt, and the ashes given inwardly, helps the *Diabetes.*

A flayed *Mouse* dried and beaten into powder, and given at a time, helps such as cannot hold their water, or have a *Diabetes*, if you do the like three days together.

Ivory, or *Elephant's tooth*, binds, stops the *Whites*, it strengthens the heart and stomach, helps the yellow jaundice, and makes women fruitful.

Those small bones which are found in the fore-feet of an *Hare*, being beaten into powder and drank in wine, powerfully provoke urine.

Goose grease, and Capons grease, are both softening, help gnawing sores, stiffness of the womb, and mitigate pain.

I am of opinion that the suet of a *Goat* mixed with a little saffron, is as excellent an ointment for the gout, especially the gout in the knees, as any is.

Bears grease stays the falling off of the hair.

Fox grease helps pains in the ears.

Elk's claws or hoofs are a sovereign remedy for the falling sickness, though it be but worn in a ring, much more being taken inwardly; but saith *Mizaldus*, it must be the hoof of the right foot behind.

Milk is an extreme windy meat; therefore I am of the opinion of *Dioscorides*, *viz.* that it is not profitable in head-aches; yet this is for certain, that it is an admirable remedy for inward ulcers in any part of the body, or any corrosions, or excoriations, pains in the reins and bladder; but it is very bad in diseases of the liver, spleen, the falling-sickness, vertigo, or dissiness in the head, fevers and head-aches. Goat's milk is held to be better than Cow's for Hectic fevers, phthisick, and consumptions, and so is Ass's also.

Whey, attenuates and cleanses both choler and melancholy: wonderfully helps melancholy and madness coming of it; opens stoppings of the bowels; helps such as have the dropsy and are troubled with the stoppings of the spleen, rickets and hypochondriac melancholy: for such diseases you may make up your physic with whey. Outwardly it cleanses the skin of such deformities as come through choler or melancholy, as scabs, itch, morphew, leprosies, &c.

Honey is of a gallant cleansing quality, exceeding profitable in all inward ulcers in what part of the body soever; it opens the veins, cleanses the reins and bladder. I know no vices belonging to it, but only it is soon converted into choler.

Wax, softens, heats, and meanly fills sores with flesh, it suffers not the milk to curdle in women's breasts; inwardly it is given (ten grains at a time) against bloody-fluxes.

Raw-silk, heats and dries, cheers the heart, drives away sadness, comforts all the spirits, both natural, vital and animal.

BELONGING TO THE SEA

Sperma Cæti, is well applied outwardly to eating ulcers, the marks which the small pox leaves behind them; it clears the sight, provokes sweat: inwardly it troubles the stomach and belly, helps bruises, and stretching of the nerves, and therefore is good for women newly delivered.

Amber-grease, heats and dries, strengthens the brain and nerves exceedingly, if the infirmity of them come of cold, resists pestilence.

Sea-sand, a man that hath the dropsy, being set up to the middle in it, it draws out all the water.

Red Coral, is cold, dry and binding, stops the immoderate flowing of the menses, bloody-fluxes, the running of the reins, and the Fluor Albus, helps such as spit blood; it is an approved remedy for the falling sickness. Also if ten grains of red Coral be given to a child in a little breast-milk so soon as it is born, before it take any other food, it will never have the falling-sickness, nor convulsions. The common dose is from ten grains to thirty.

Pearls, are a wonderful strengthener to the heart, encrease milk in nurses, and amend it being naught, they restore such as are in consumptions; both they and the red Coral preserve the body in health, and resist fevers. The dose is ten grains or fewer; more, I suppose, because it is dear, than because it would do harm.

Amber, (*viz.* yellow Amber) heats and dries, therefore prevails against moist diseases of the head; it helps violent coughs, helps consumption of the lungs, spitting of blood, the Fluor Albus; it stops bleeding at the nose, helps difficulty of urine. You may take ten or twenty grains at a time.

The Froth of the *Sea*, it is hot and dry, helps scabs, itch, and leprosy, scald heads, &c. it cleanses the skin, helps difficulty of urine, makes the teeth white, being rubbed with it, the head being washed with it, it helps baldness, and trimly decks the head with hair.

METALS, MINERALS, AND STONES

Gold is temperate in quality, it wonderfully strengthens the heart and vital spirits, which one perceiving, very wittily inserted these verses:

> For Gold is cordial; and that's the reason,
> Your raking Misers live so long a season.

However, this is certain, in cordials, it resists melancholy, faintings, swoonings, fevers, falling-sickness, and all such like infirmities, incident either to the vital or animal spirit.

Alum. Heats, binds, and purges; scours filthy ulcers, and fastens loose teeth.

Brimstone, or flower of brimstone, which is brimstone refined, and the better for physical uses; helps coughs and rotten flegm; outwardly in ointments it takes away leprosies, scabs, and itch; inwardly it helps yellow jaundice, as also worms in the belly, especially being mixed with a little Saltpetre: it helps lethargies being snuffed up in the nose.

Litharge, both of gold and silver; binds and dries much, fills up ulcers with flesh, and heals them.

Lead is of a cold dry earthly quality, of an healing nature; applied to the place it helps any inflammation, and dries up humours.

Pompholix, cools, dries and binds.

Jacynth, strengthens the heart being either beaten into powder, and taken inwardly, or only worn in a ring.

Sapphire, quickens the senses, helps such as are bitten by venomous beasts, ulcers in the bowels.

Emerald, called a chaste stone because it resists lust: being worn in a ring, it helps, or at least mitigates the falling sickness and vertigo; it strengthens the memory, and stops the unruly passions of men.

Ruby (or *carbuncle*, if there be such a stone) restrains lust; resists pestilence; takes away idle and foolish thoughts, makes men cheerful. *Cardanus*.

Granite. Strengthens the heart, but hurts the brain, causes anger, takes away sleep.

Diamond, is reported to make him that bears it unfortunate.

Amethist, being worn, makes men sober and steady, keeps men from drunkenness and too much sleep, it quickens the wit, is profitable in huntings and fightings, and repels vapours from the head.

Bezoar, is a notable restorer of nature, a great cordial, no way hurtful nor dangerous, is admirably good in fevers, pestilences, and consumptions, *viz.* taken inwardly; for this stone is not used to be worn as a jewel; the powder of it put upon wounds made by venomous beasts, draws out the poison.

Topaz (if *Epiphanius* spake truth) if you put it into boiling water, it doth so cool it that you may presently put your hands into it without harm; if so, then it cools inflammations of the body by touching them.

Toadstone, being applied to the place helps the bitings of venomous beasts, and quickly draws all the poison to it; it is known to be a true one by this; hold it near to any toad, and she will make proffer to take it away from you if it be right; else not. *Lemnius*.

Nephritichus lapis, helps pains in the stomach, and is of great force in breaking and bringing away the stone and gravel.

Jasper, being worn, stops bleeding, eases the labour in women, stops lust, resists fevers and dropsies. *Mathiolus*.

Atites, or the stone with child, because being hollow in the middle, it contains another little stone within it, is found in an Eagle's nest, and in many other places; this stone being bound to the left arm of women with child, stays their miscarriage or abortion, but when the time of their labour comes, remove it from their arm, and bind it to the inside of their thigh, and it brings forth the child, and that (almost) without any pain at all. *Dioscorides*, *Pliny*.

Lapis Lazuli, purges melancholy being taken inwardly; outwardly worn as a jewel, it makes men cheerful, fortunate and rich.

And thus I end the stones, the virtues of which if any think incredible, I answer, 1. I quoted the authors where I had them. 2. I know nothing to the contrary but why it may be as possible as the sound of a trumpet is to incite a man to valour; or a fiddle to dancing: and if I have added a few simples which the Colledge left out, I hope my fault is not much, or at a leastwise, venial.

A Catalogue of Simples in the New Dispensatory

ROOTS

College.] *Sorrel, Calamus Aromaticus, Water-flag, Privet, Garlick, Marsh-mallows, Alcanet, Angelica, Anthora, Smallage, Aron, Birthwort long and round, Sowbread, Reeds, Asarabacca, Virginian Snakeweed, Swallwort, Asparagus, Asphodel, male and female.* Burdocks great and small, Behen, or Bazil, Valerian, white and red. Daisies, Beets, white, red, and black. Marsh-mallows, *Bistort, Borrage, Briony, white and black, Bugloss, garden and wild.* Calamus Aromaticus, Our Lady's thistles, *Avens, Coleworts, Centaury the less.* Onions, Chameleon, white and black. Celandine, *Pilewort, China, Succory, Artichokes.* Virginian Snakeroot, *Comfry greater and lesser, Contra yerva, Costus, sweet and bitter. Turmerick, wild Cucumbers, Sowbread, Hound's-tongue, Cypres, long and round.* Toothwort, white Dittany, *Doronicum, Dragons, Woody Nightshade, Vipers Bugloss, Smallage, Hellebore, white and black, Endive, Elicampane, Eringo, Colt's-foot, Fearn, male and female, Filipendula or Drop-wort, Fennel,* white Dittany, *Galanga, great and small, Gentian, Liquorice, Doggrass, Hermodactils.* Swallow wort, *Jacinth, Henbane, Jallap, Master-wort, Orris or Flower-de-luce, both English and Florentine, sharp pointed Dock, Burdock greater and lesser, Lovage, Privet, white Lilies, Liquorice, Mallows, Mechoacan, Jallap, Spignel, Mercury, Devil's bit, sweet Navew, Spikenard, Celtic and Indian, Water lilies, Rest-harrow, sharp pointed Dock, Peony, male and female, Parsnips, garden and wild, Cinquefoil, Butter-Bur, Parsley, Hog's Fennel, Valerian, greater and lesser, Burnet, Land and Water Plantain, Polypodium of the Oak, Solomon's Seal, Leeks, Pellitory of Spain, Cinquefoil, Turnips, Raddishes, garden and wild, Rhapontick, common Rhubarb, Monk's Rhubarb, Rose Root, Madder Bruscus. Sopewort, Sarsaparilla, Satyrion, male and female, White Saxifrage, Squills, Figwort, Scorzonera, English and Spanish, Virginian Snake weed, Solomon's Seal, Cicers, stinking Gladon, Devil's bit, Dandelion, Thapsus, Tormentil, Turbith, Colt's-foot, Valerian, greater and lesser, Vervain, Swallow-wort, Nettles, Zedoary long and round, Ginger.*

Culpeper.] These be the roots the college hath named, and but only named, and in this order I have set them down. It seems the college holds a strange opinion, viz. that it would do an Englishman a mischief to know what the herbs in his garden are good for.

But my opinion is, that those herbs, roots, plants, &c. which grow near a man, are far better and more congruous to his nature than any outlandish rubbish whatsoever, and this I am able to give a reason of to any that shall demand it of me, therefore I am so copious in handling of them, you shall observe them ranked in this order:

1. The temperature of the roots, herbs, flowers, &c. viz. hot, cold, dry, moist, together with the degree of each quality.

2. What part of the body each root, herb, flower, is appropriated to, viz. head, throat, breast, heart, stomach, liver, spleen, bowels, reins, bladder, womb, joints, and in those which heat those places, and which cool them.

3. The property of each simple, as they bind, open, mollify, harden, extenuate, discuss, draw out, suppure, cleanse, glutinate, break wind, breed seed, provoke or stop the menses, resist poison, abate swellings, ease pain.

This I intend shall be my general method throughout the simples, which, having finished I shall give you a paraphrase explaining these terms, which rightly considered, will be the key of *Galen's* way of administering physic.

Temperature of the Roots

Roots hot in the first degree. Marsh-mallows, Bazil, Valerian, Spattling, Poppy, Burdocks, Borrage, Bugloss, Calamus Aromaticus, Avens, Pilewort, China, Self-heal, Liquorice, Dog-grass, white Lilies, Peony, male and female, wild Parsnips, Parsley, Valerian, great and small, Knee-holly, Satyrion, Scorzonera, Skirrets.

Hot in the second degree. Water-flag, Reeds, Swallow-wort, Asphodel, male, Carline Thistle, Cypress, long and round, Fennel, Lovage, Spignel, Mercury, Devil's bit, Butter Bur, Hog's Fennel, Sarsaparilla, Squils, Zedoary.

Hot in the third degree. Angelica, Aron, Birthwort long and round, Sowbread, Asarabacca, Briony, white and black, Sallendine, Virginian snakeroot, Hemeric, White Dittany, Doronicum, Hellebore, white and black, Elicampane, Fillipendula, Galanga greater and lesser, Masterwort, Orris English and Florentine, Restharrow, stinking Gladen, Turbith, Ginger.

Hot in the fourth degree. Garlick, Onions, Leeks, Pellitory of Spain.

Roots temperate in respect of heat, are Bear's breech, Sparagus, our Lady's Thistle, Eringo, Jallap, Mallows, Mechoacan, garden Parsnips, Cinquefoil, Tormentil.

Roots cold in the first degree. Sorrel, Beets, white and red, Comfrey the greater, Plantain, Rose Root, Madder.

Cold in the second degree. Alcanet, Daisies, Succory, Hound's tongue, Endive, Jacinth.

Cold in the third degree. Bistort and Mandrakes are cold in the third degree, and Henbane in the fourth.

Roots dry in the first degree. Bears-breech, Burdocks, Redbeets, Calamus Aromaticus, Pilewort, Self-heal, Endive, Eringo, Jacinth, Madder, Kneeholly.

Dry in the second degree. Waterflag, Marshmallows, Alkanet, Smallage, Reeds, Sorrel, Swallow-wort, Asphodel male, Bazil, Valerian and Spatling Poppy, according to the opinion of the Greeks. Our Lady's Thistles, Avens, Succory, Hound's tongue, Cypress long and round, Fennel, Lovage, Spignel, Mercury, Devil's bit, Butter-bur, Parsley, Plantain, Zedoary.

Dry in the third degree. Angelica, Aron, Birthwort, long and round, Sowbread, Bistort, Asarabacca, Briony, white and black, Carline Thistle, China, Sallendine, Virginian Snake-root, white Dittany, Doronicum, Hellebore white and black, Elicampane, Fillipendula, Galanga greater and lesser, Masterwort, Orris, English and Florentine, Restharrow, Peony male and female, Cinquefoil, Hog's Fennel, Sarsaparilla, stinking Gladen, Tormentil, Ginger.

Dry in the fourth degree. Garlick, Onions, Costus, Leeks, Pellitory of Spain.

Roots moist are, Bazil, Valerian, and Spatling-poppy, according to the Arabian Physicians, Daisies, white Beets, Borrage, Bugloss, Liquorice, Dog grass, Mallows, Satyrion, Scorzonera, Parsnips, Skirrets.

Roots appropriated to several parts of the body

Heat the head. Doronicum, Fennel, Jallap, Mechoacan, Spikenard, Celtic and Indian. Peony male and female.

Neck and throat. Pilewort, Devil's bit.

Breast and lungs. Birthwort long and round, Elicampane, Liquorice, Orris English and Florentine, Calamus Aromaticus, Cinquefoil, Squills.

Heart. Angelica, Borrage, Bugloss, Carline Thistle, Doronicum, Butter bur, Scorzonera, Tormentil, Zedoary, Bazil, Valerian white and red.

Stomach. Elicampane, Galanga greater and lesser, Spikenard, Celtic and Indian, Ginger, Fennel, Avens, Raddishes.

Bowels. Valerian great and small, Zedoary, Ginger.

Liver. Smallage, Carline Thistle, Sullendine, China, Turmerick,

Fennel, Gentian, Dog-grass, Cinquefoil, Parsley, Smallage, Asparagus, Rhubarb, Rhapontic, Kneeholly.

Spleen. Smallage, Carline Thistle, Fern male and female, Parsley, Water-flag, Asparagus, round Birthwort, Fennel, Capers, Ash, Gentian.

Reins and Bladder. Marshmallows, Smallage, Asparagus, Burdock, Bazil, Valerian, Spatling Poppy, Carline Thistle, China, Cyprus long and round, Fillipendula, Dog grass, Spikenard, Celtic and Indian, Parsly, Knee-holly, white Saxifrage.

Womb. Birthwort long and round, Galanga greater and lesser, Peony male and female, Hog's Fennel.

Fundament. Pilewort.

Joints. Bear's-breech, Hermodactils, Jallap, Mecoacan, Ginger, Costus.

Roots cool the head. Rose root.

Stomach. Sow Thistles, Endive, Succory, Bistort.

Liver. Madder, Endive, Chicory.

Properties of the Roots

Although I confess the properties of the simples may be found out by the ensuing explanation of the terms, and I suppose by that means they were found out at first; and although I hate a lazy student from my heart, yet to encourage young students in the art, I shall quote the chief of them. I desire all lovers of physic to compare them with the explanation of these rules, so shall they see how they agree, so may they be enabled to find out the properties of all simples to their own benefit in physic.

Roots, bind. Cypress, Bistort, Tormentil, Cinquefoil, Bear's breech, Water-flag, Alkanet, Toothwort, &c.

Discuss. Birthwort, Asphodel, Briony, Capers, &c.

Cleanse. Birthwort, Aron, Sparagus, Grass, Asphodel, Celandine, &c.

Open. Asarabacca, Garlic, Leeks, Onions, Rhapontick, Turmerick, Carline Thistle, Succory, Endive, Fillipendula, Fennel, Parsly, Bruscus, Sparagus, Smallage, Gentian, &c.

Extenuate. Orris English and Florentine, Capers, &c.

Burn. Garlick, Onions, Pellitory of Spain, &c.

Mollify. Mallows, Marshmallows, &c.

Suppur. Marshmallows, Briony, white Lillies, &c.

Glutinate. Comfrey, Solomon's Seal, Gentian, Birthwort, Daisies, &c.

Expel Wind. Smallage, Parsly, Fennel, Water-flag, Garlick,

Costus, Galanga, Hog's Fennel, Zedoary, Spikenard Indian, and Celtic, &c.

Breed Seed. Waterflag, Eringo, Satyrian, Galanga, &c.

Provoke the menses. Birthwort, Asarabacca, Aron, Waterflag, white Dittany, Asphodel, Garlick, Centaury the less, Cyperus long and round, Costus, Capers, Calamus Aromaticus, Dittany of Crete, Carrots, Eringo, Fennel, Parsly, Smallage, Grass, Elicampane, Peony, Valerian, Kneeholly, &c.

Stop the menses. Comfrey, Tormentil, Bistort, &c.

Provoke sweat. Carolina Thistle, China, Sarsaparilla, &c.

Resist poison. Angelica, Garlick, long Birthwort, Smallage, Doronicum, Costus, Zedoary, Cyprus, Gentian, Carolina Thistle, Bistort, Tormentil, Swallow-wort, Viper's Bugloss, Elicampane, &c.

Help burnings. Asphodel, Jacinth, white Lilies, &c.

Ease pains. Waterflag, Eringo, Orris, Restharrow, &c.

Purge choler. Asarabacca, Rhubarb, Rhapontick, Fern, &c.

Relieve melancholy. Hellebore, white and black, Polipodium.

Purge flegm and watery humours. Squills, Turbith, Hermodactils, Jallap, Mecoacan, wild Cucumbers, Sowbread, male Asphodel, Briony white and black, Elder, Spurge great and small.

I quoted some of these properties to teach you the way how to find the rest, which the explanation of these terms will give you ample instructions in. I quoted not all because I would fain have you studious: be diligent gentle reader.

How to use your bodies in, and after taking purges, you shall be taught by and by.

Barks mentioned by the College are these

College.] *Hazel Nuts, Oranges, Barberries, Birch-tree, Caper roots, Cassia Lignea, Chestnuts, Cinnamon, Citron Pills, Dwarf-Elder, Spurge roots, Alder, Ash, Pomegranates, Guajacum, Walnut tree, green Walnuts, Laurel, Bay, Lemon, Mace, Pomegranates, Mandrake roots, Mezereon, Mulberry tree roots, Sloe tree roots, Pinenuts, Fisticknuts, Poplar tree, Oak, Elder, Sassafras, Cork, Tamerisk, Lime tree, Frankincense, Elm, Capt. Winter's Cinnamon.*

Culpeper.] Of these, Captain Winter's Cinnamon, being taken as ordinary spice, or half a dram taken in the morning in any convenient liquor, is an excellent remedy for the scurvy; the powder of it being snuffed up in the nose, cleanses the head of rheum gallantly.

The bark of the black Alder tree purges choler and flegm if you make a decoction with it. Agrimony, Wormwood, Dodder, Hops,

Endive and Succory roots: Parsly and Smallage roots, or you may bruise a handful of each of them, and put them in a gallon of ale, and let them work together: put the simples into a boulter-bag, and a draught, (half a pint, more or less, according to the age of him that drinks it,) being drunk every morning, helps the dropsy, jaundice, evil disposition of the body; also helps the rickets, strengthens the liver and spleen; makes the digestion good, troubles not the stomach at all, causes appetite, and helps such as are scabby and itchy.

The rest of the barks that are worth the noting, and the virtues of them, are to be found in the former part of the book.

Barks are hot in the first degree. Guajacum, Tamarisk, Oranges, Lemons, Citrons.

In the second. Cinnamon, Cassia, Lignea, Captain Winter's Cinnamon, Frankincense, Capers.

In the third. Mace.

Cold in the first. Oak, Pomegranates.

In the third. Mandrakes.

Appropriated to parts of the body

Heat the head. Captain Winter's Cinnamon.

The heart. Cinnamon, Cassia, Lignea, Citron Pills, Walnuts, Lemon pills, Mace.

The stomach. Orange pills, Cassia Lignea, Cinnamon, Citron pills, Lemon pills, Mace, Sassafras.

The lungs. Cassia Lignea, Cinnamon, Walnuts.

The liver. Barberry-tree, Bay-tree, Captain Winter's Cinnamon.

The spleen. Caper bark, Ash tree bark, Bay tree.

The reins and bladder. Bay-tree, Sassafras.

The womb. Cassia Lignea, Cinnamon.

Cool the stomach. Pomegranate pills.

Purge choler. The bark of Barberry tree.

Purge flegm and water. Elder, Dwarf-Elder, Spurge, Laurel.

WOODS

College.] *Firr, Wood of Aloes, Rhodium, Brazil, Box, Willow, Cypress, Ebony, Guajacum, Juniper, Lentisk, Nephriticum, Rhodium, Rosemary, Sanders, white, yellow, and red, Sassafras, Tamarisk.*

Of these some are hot. Wood of Aloes, Rhodium, Box, Ebony, Guajacum, Nephriticum, Rosemary, Sassafras, Tamarisk.

Some cold. As Cypress, Willow, Sanders white, red, and yellow.

Rosemary is appropriated to the head, wood of Aloes to the heart and stomach, Rhodium to the bowels and bladder, Nephriticum to the liver, spleen, reins and bladder, Sassafras to the breast, stomach and bladder, Tamarisk to the spleen, Sanders cools the heart and spirits in fevers.

For the particular virtues of each, see that part of the book preceding.

HERBS

College.] *Southernwood male and female. Wormwood, common, Roman, and such as bear Wormseed, Sorrel, wood Sorrel, Maiden-hair common, white or wall Rue, black and golden Maudlin, Agremony, Vervain, Mallow, Ladies Mantle, Chickweed, Marshmallows, and Pimpernel both male and female, Water Pimpernel, Dill, Angelica, Smallage, Goose-grass, or Cleavers, Columbine, wild Tansie, or Silver Weed, Mugwort, Asarabacca, Woodroofe, Arach, Distaff Thistle, Mousear, Costmary, or Alcost, Burdock greater and lesser, Brooklime, or water Pimpernel, Beets white, red, and black, Betony of the wood and water. Daisies greater and lesser, Blite, Mercury, Borrage, Oak of Jerusalem, Cabbages, Sodonella, Briony white and black, Bugloss, Buglesse, Shepherd's Purse, Ox-eye, Box leaves, Calaminth of the Mountains and Fens, Ground Pine, Wood-bine, or Honey-suckles, Lady-smocks, Marygolds, Our Lady's Thistle, Carduus Benedictus, Avens, small Spurge, Horse-tail, Coleworts, Centaury the less, Knotgrass, Cervil, Germander, Camomile, Chamepytis female Southernwood, Chelene, Pilewort, Chicory, Hemlock, garden and sea Scurvy-grass, Fleawort, Comfry great, middle, or bugle, least or Daisies, Sarasens, Confound, Buck-horn, Plantain, May weed, (or Margweed, as we in Sussex call it) Orpine, Sampeer, Crosewort, Dodder, Blue Bottle great and small, Artichokes, Houndstone, Cypress leaves, Dandelion, Dittany of Treet, Box leaves, Teazles garden and wild, Dwarff Elder, Viper's Bugloss, Lluellin, Smallage, Endive, Elecampane, Horsetail, Epithimum, Groundsel, Hedge-mustard, Spurge, Agrimony, Maudlin, Eye-bright, Orpine, Fennel, Sampeer, Fillipendula, Indian leaf, Strawberry leaves, Ash tree leaves, Fumitory, Goat's Rue, Lady's Bedstraw, Broom, Muscatu, Herb Robert, Doves Foot, Cottonweed, Hedge Hyssop, Tree Ivy, Ground Ivy, or Alehoof, Elecampane, Pellitory of the wall, Liver-wort, Cowslips, Rupture-wort, Hawkweed, Monk's Rhubarb, Alexan-ders, Clary garden and wild, Henbane, St. John's-wort, Horsetongue, or double tongue, Hysop, Sciatica cresses, small Sengreen, Sharewort, Woad, Reeds, Schænanth, Chamepitys, Glasswort, Lettice, Lagobus, Arch-angel, Burdock great and small, Lavender, Laurel, Bay leaves, English and Alexandrian, Duckweed, Dittander, or Pepper-wort,*

Lovage, Privet, Sea bugloss, Toad flax, Harts-tongue, sweet Trefoil, Wood-sorrel, Hops, Willow-herb, Marjoram, common and tree Mallows, Mandrake, Horehound white and black, Herb Mastich, Featherfew, Woodbine, Melilot, Bawm garden and water, Mints, Horse-mints, Mercury, Mezereon, Yarrow, Devil's-bit, Moss, sweet Chivil, Mirtle leaves, Garden and water Cresses, Nep, Tobacco, Money-wort, Water Lilies, Bazil, Olive Leaves, Rest-harrow, Adder's Tongue, Origanum, sharp-pointed Dock, Poppy, white, black, and red, or Erratick, Pellitory of the Wall, Cinquefoil, Ars-smart spotted and not spotted, Peach Leaves, Thoroughwax, Parsley, Hart's Tongue, Valerian, Mouse-ear, Burnet, small Spurge, Plantain common and narrow leaved, Mountain and Cretick Poley, Knotgrass, Golden Maidenhair, Poplar leaves and buds, Leeks, Purslain, Silverweed, or wild Tansy, Horehound white and black, Primroses, Self-heal, Field Pellitory, or Sneezewort, Penny-royal, Fleabane, Lungwort, Winter-green, Oak leaves and buds, Docks, common Rue, Wall Rue or white Maidenhair, wild Rue, Savin, Osier Leaves, Garden Sage the greater and lesser, Wild Sage, Elder leaves and buds, Marjorum, Burnet, Sanicle, Sopewort, Savory, White Saxi-frage, Scabious, Chicory, Schænanth, Clary, Scordium, Figwort, House-leek, or Sengreen the greater and lesser, Groundsel, Senna leaves and pods, Mother of Time, Solomon's Seal, Alexanders, Nightshade, Solda-nela, Sow-thistles, smooth and rough, Flixweed, common Spike, Spinach, Hawthorn, Devil's-bit, Comfry, Tamarisk leaves, Tansy, Dandelyon, Mullen or Higcaper, Time, Lime tree leaves, Spurge, Tormentil, common and golden Trefoil, Wood-sorrel, sweet Trefoil, Colt's-foot, Valerian, Mullen, Vervain, Paul's Bettony, Lluellin, Violets, Tansy, Perewinkles, Swallow-wort, golden Rod, Vine leaves, Mead-sweet, Elm leaves, Navel-wort, Nettles, common and Roman, Archangel, or dead Nettles, white and red.

Culpeper.] These be the herbs as the college set down to look upon, we will see if we can translate them in another form to the benefit of the body of man.

Herbs temperate in respect of heat, are common Maiden-hair, Wall-rue, black and golden Maiden-hair, Woodroof, Bugle, Goat's Rue, Hart's-tongue, sweet Trefoil, Flixweed, Cinquefoil, Trefoil, Paul's Bettony, Lluellin.

Intemperate and hot in the first degree, are Agrimony, Marsh-mallows, Goose-grass or Cleavers, Distaff Thistle, Borrage, Bug-loss, or Lady's Thistles, Avens, Cetrach, Chervil, Chamomel, Eye-bright, Cowslips, Melilot, Bazil, Self-heal.

In the second. Common and Roman Wormwood, Maudlin, Lady's Mantle, Pimpernel male and female, Dill, Smallage, Mug-wort, Costmary, Betony, Oak of Jerusalem, Marigold, Cuckoo-flowers, Carduus Benedictus, Centaury the less, Chamepitys,

Scurvy-grass, Indian Leaf, Broom, Alehoof, Alexanders, Double-tongue, or Tongue-blade, Archangel, or dead Nettles, Bay Leaves, Marjoram, Horehound, Bawm, Mercury, Devil's-bit, Tobacco, Parsley, Poley mountain, Rosemary, Sage, Sanicle, Scabious, Senna, Soldanella, Tansy, Vervain, Perewinkle.

In the third degree. Southernwood male and female, Brooklime, Angelica, Briony white and black, Calaminth, Germander, Sullendine, Pilewort, Fleabane, Dwarf Elder, Epithimun, Bank-cresses, Clary, Glasswort, Lavender, Lovage, Herb Mastich, Featherfew, Mints, Water-cresses, Origanum, biting Arsmart, called in Latin Hydropiper (the college confounds this with *Persicaria*, or mild Arsmart, which is cold), Sneezewort, Pennyroyal, Rue, Savin, summer and winter Savory, Mother of Time, Lavender, Spike, Time, Nettles.

In the fourth degree. Sciatica-cresses, Stone-crop, Dittany, or Pepper-wort, garden-cresses, Leeks, Crowfoot, Rosa Solis, Spurge.

Herbs cold in the first degree. Sorrel, Wood-sorrel, Arach, Burdock, Shepherd's-purse, Pellitory of the wall, Hawk-weed, Mallows, Yarrow, mild Arsmart, called *Persicaria*, Burnet, Coltsfoot, Violets.

Cold in the second degree. Chickweed, wild Tansy, or Silverweed, Daisies, Knotgrass, Succory, Buck-horn, Plantain, Dandelyon, Endive, Fumitory, Strawberry leaves, Lettice, Duck-meat, Plantain, Purslain, Willow leaves.

In the third degree. Sengreen, or Houseleek, Nightshade.

In the fourth degree. Hemlock, Henbane, Mandrakes, Poppies.

Herbs dry in the first degree. Agrimony, Marsh-mallows, Cleavers, Burdocks, Shepherds-purse, our Lady's Thistle, Chervil, Chamomel, Eye-bright, Cowslips, Hawkweed, Tongue-blade, or double tongue, Melilot, mild Arsmart, Self-heal, Senna, Flixweed, Coltsfoot, Perewinkle.

Dry in the second degree. Common and Roman Wormwood, Sorrel, Wood-sorrel, Maudlin, Lady's mantle, Pimpernel male and female, Dill, Smallage, wild Tansy, or Silverweed, Mugwort, Distaff Thistle, Costmary, Betony, Bugle, Cuckooflowers, Carduus Benedictus, Avens, Centaury the less, Chicory, commonly called Succory, Scurvy-grass, Buckhorn, Plantain, Dandelyon, Endive, Indian Leaf, Strawberry leaves, Fumitory, Broom, Alehoof, Alexanders, Archangel, or Dead Nettles, white and red, Bay Leaves, Marjoram, Featherfew, Bawm, Mercury, Devil's-bit, Tobacco, Parsley, Burnet, Plantain, Rosemary, Willow Leaves, Sage, Santicle, Scabious, Soldanella, Vervain.

Dry in the third degree. Southernwood, male and female, Brooklime, Angelica, Briony, white and black, Calamint, Germander,

Chamepitys, Selandine, Pilewort, Fleabane, Epithinum, Dwarf-Elder, Bank cresses, Clary, Glasswort, Lavender, Lovage, Horehound, Herb Mastic, Mints, Watercresses, Origanum, Cinquefoil, hot Arsmart, Poley mountain, Sneezewort, Penny-royal, Rue, or herb of Grace, Savin winter and summer Savory, Mother of Time, Lavender, Silk, Tansy, Time, Trefoil.

In the fourth degree. Garden-cresses, wild Rue, Leeks, Onions, Crowfoot, Rosa Solis, Garlic, Spurge.

Herbs moist in the first degree. Borrage, Bugloss, Marigolds, Pellitory of the wall, Mallows, Bazil.

In the fourth degree. Chickweed, Arach, Daisies, Lettice, Duckmeat, Purslain, Sow Thistles, Violets, Water-lilies.

Herbs appropriated to certain parts of the body of man

Heat the head. Maudlin, Costmary, Betony, Carduus Benedictus, Sullendine, Scurvy-grass, Eye-bright, Goat's Rue, Cowslips, Lavender, Laurel, Lovage, herb Mastich, Feather-few, Melilot, Sneezewort, Penny-royal, Senna, Mother of Time, Vervain, Rosemary.

Heat the throat. Archangel white and red, otherwise called dead Nettles, Devil's-bit.

Heat the breast. Maiden-hair, white, black, common and golden, Distaff Thistle, Time, Betony, Calaminth, Chamomel, Fennel, Indian-leaf, Bay leaves, Hyssop, Bawm, Horehound, Oak of Jerusalem, Germander, Melilot, Origanum, Rue, Scabious, Periwinkles, Nettles.

Heat the heart. Southernwood male and female, Angelica, Wood-roof, Bugloss, Carduus Benedictus, Borrage, Goat's Rue, Senna, Bazil, Rosemary, Elecampane.

Heat the stomach. Wormwood common and Roman, Smallage, Avens, Indian leaf, Broom, Schenanth, Bay leaves, Bawm, Mints, Parsley, Fennel, Time, Mother of Time, Sage.

Heat the liver. Agrimony, Maudlin, Pimpernel, male and female, Smallage, Costmary, or Ale cost, our Lady's Thistles, Centaury the less, Germander, Chamepytis, Selandine, Sampier, Fox Gloves, Ash-tree leaves, Bay leaves, Toad-flax, Hops, Horehound, Water-cresses, Parsley, Poley Mountain, Sage, Scordium, Senna, Mother of Time, Soldanella, Asarabacca, Fennel, Hyssop, Spikenard.

Heat the bowels. Chamomel, Alehoofe, Alexanders.

Heat the spleen. All the four sorts of Maiden-hair, Agrimony, Smallage, Centaury the less, Cetrach, Germander, Chamepitys, Samphire, Fox-glove, Epithimum, Ash-tree, Bay leaves, Toad-flax,

Hops, Horehound, Parsley, Poley, Mountain Sage, Scordium, Senna, Mother of Time, Tamarisk, Wormwood, Water-cresses, Hart's-tongue.

Heat the reins and bladder. Agrimony, Maudlin, Marsh-mallows, Pimpernel male and female, Brooklime, Costmary, Bettony, Chervil, Germander, Chamomel, Samphire, Broom, Rupture-wort, Clary, Schenanth, Bay-leaves, Toad-flax, Hops, Melilot, Water-cresses, Origanum, Pennyroyal, Scordium, Vervain, Mother of Time, Rocket, Spikenard, Saxifrage, Nettles.

Heat the womb. Maudlin, Angelica, Mugwort, Costmary, Calaminth, Flea-bane, May-weed, Ormarg-weed, Dittany of Crete, Schenanth, Arch-angel or Dead Nettles, Melilot, Feather-few, Mints, Devil's-bit, Origanum, Bazil, Pennyroyal, Savin, Sage, Scordium, Tansy, Time, Vervain, Periwinkles, Nettles.

Heat the joints. Cowslips, Sciatica-cresses, hot Arsmart, Garden-cresses, Costmary, Agrimony, Chamomel, Saint John's-wort, Melilot, Water-cresses, Rosemary, Rue, Sage Stechas.

Herbs cooling the head. Wood-sorrel, Teazles, Lettice, Plantain, Willow-leaves, Sengreen or Houseleek, Strawberry-leaves, Violet-leaves, Fumitory, Water Lilies.

Cool the throat. Orpine, Strawberry leaves, Privet, Bramble leaves.

Breast. Mulberry leaves, Bramble leaves, Violet leaves, Strawberry leaves, Sorrel, Wood-sorrel, Poppies, Orpine, Moneywort, Plantain, Colt's-foot.

Heart. Sorrel, Wood sorrel, Viper's Bugloss, Lettice, Burnet, Violet leaves, Strawberry leaves, and Water-Lilies.

Stomach. Sorrel, Wood sorrel, Succory, Orpine, Dandelyon, Endive, Strawberry leaves, Hawkweed, Lettice, Purslain, Sow Thistles, Violet leaves.

Liver. Sorrel, Woodsorrel, Dandelyon, Endive, Succory, Strawberry leaves, Fumitory, Liverwort, Lettice, Purslain, Nightshade, Water Lilies.

Bowels. Fumitory, Mallows, Buckthorn, Plantain, Orpine, Plantain, Burnet.

Spleen. Fumitory, Endive, Succory, Lettice.

Reins and bladder. Knotgrass, Mallows, Yarrow, Moneywort, Plantain, Endive, Succory, Lettice, Purslain, Water Lilies, Houseleek or Sengreen.

The womb. Wild Tansy, Arrach, Burdocks, Willow herb, Mirtle leaves, Moneywort, Purslain, Sow Thistles, Endive, Succory, Lettice, Water Lilies, Sengreen.

The joints. Willow leaves, Vine leaves, Lettice, Henbane, Nightshade, Sengreen or Houseleek.

Herbs altering according to property, in operation, some bind, as

Amomus, Agnus Castus, Shepherd's purse, Cypress, Horsetail, Ivy, Bay leaves, Melilot, Bawm, Mirtles, Sorrel, Plantain, Knotgrass, Comfry, Cinquefoil, Fleawort, Purslain, Oak leaves, Willow leaves, Sengreen or Houseleek, &c.

Open, as, Garlick, Onions, Wormwood, Mallows, Marsh-mallows, Pellitory of the Wall, Endive, Succory, &c.

Soften. Mallows, Marsh-mallows, Beets, Pellitory of the Wall, Violet leaves, Strawberry leaves, Arrach, Cypress leaves, Bay leaves, Fleawort, &c.

Harden. Purslain, Nightshade, Houseleek or Sengreen, Duckmeat, and most other herbs that are very cold.

Extenuate. Mugwort, Chamomel, Hysop, Pennyroyal, Stœchas, Time, Mother of Time, Juniper, &c.

Discuss. Southernwood male and female, all the four sorts of Maidenhair, Marshmallows, Dill, Mallows, Arrach, Beets, Chamomel, Mints, Melilot, Pelitory of the Wall, Chickweed, Rue, Stœchas, Marjoram.

Draw. Pimpernel, Birthwort, Dittany, Leeks, Onions, Garlick, and also take this general rule, as all cold things bind and harden, so all things very hot are drying.

Suppure. Mallows, Marsh-mallows, White Lily leaves, &c.

Cleanse. Pimpernel, Southernwood, Sparagus, Cetrach, Arrach, Wormwood, Beet, Pellitory of the Wall, Chamepitis, Dodder, Liverwort, Horehound, Willow leaves, &c.

Glutinate. Marsh-mallows, Pimpernel, Centaury, Chamepitis, Mallows, Germander, Horsetail, Agrimony, Maudlin, Strawberry leaves, Woad-chervil, Plantain, Cinquefoil, Comfry, Bugle, Selfheal, Woundwort, Tormentil, Rupture-wort, Knot-grass, Tobacco.

Expel wind. Wormwood, Garlick, Dill, Smallage, Chamomel, Epithimum, Fennel, Juniper, Marjoram, Origanum, Savory both winter and summer. Tansy is good to cleanse the stomach and bowels of rough viscous flegm, and humours that stick to them, which the flegmatic constitution of the winter usually infects the body of man with, and occasions gouts and other diseases of like nature and lasting long. This was the original of that custom to eat Tansys in the spring: the herb may be made into a conserve with sugar, or boil it in wine and drink the decoction, or make the juice into a syrup with sugar, which you will.

Herbs breed seed. Clary, Rocket, and most herbs that are hot and moist, and breed wind.

Provoke the terms. Southernwood, Garlick, all the sorts of Maiden hair, Mugwort, Wormwood, Bishops-weed, Cabbages, Bettony,

Centaury, Chamomel, Calaminth, Germander, Dodder, Dittany, Fennel, St. John's Wort, Marjoram, Horehound, Bawm, Water-cresses, Origanum, Bazil, Pennyroyal, Poley mountain, Parsley, Smallage, Rue, Rosemary, Sage, Savin, Hartwort, Time, Mother of Time, Scordium, Nettles.

Stop the terms. Shepherd's purse, Strawberries, Mirtles, Water Lilies, Plantain, Houseleek or Sengreen, Comfry, Knotgrass.

Resist poison. Southernwood, Wormwood, Garlick, all sorts of Maiden hair, Smallage, Bettony, Carduus Benedictus, Germander, Calaminth, Alexanders, Carline Thistle, Agrimony, Fennel, Juniper, Horehound, Origanum, Pennyroyal, Poleymountain, Rue, Scordium, Plantain.

Discuss swellings. Maiden-hair, Cleavers, or Goosegrass, Mallows, Marsh-mallows, Docks, Bawm, Water-cresses, Cinquefoil, Scordium, &c.

Ease pain. Dil, Wormwood, Arach, Chamomel, Calaminth, Chamepitis, Henbane, Hops, Hog's Fennel, Parsley, Rosemary, Rue, Marjoram, Mother of Time.

Herbs purging

Choler. Groundsel, Hops, Peach leaves, Wormwood, Centaury, Mallows, Senna.

Melancholy. Ox-eye, Epithimum, Fumitory, Senna, Dodder.

Flegm and water. Briony, white and black, Spurge, both work most violently and are not fit for a vulgar use, Dwarf Elder, Hedge Hyssop, Laurel leaves, Mercury, Mezereon also purges violently, and so doth Sneezewort, Elder leaves, Senna.

For the particular operations of these, as also how to order the body after purges, the quantity to be taken at a time, you have been in part instructed already, and shall be more fully hereafter.

FLOWERS

College.] *Wormwood, Agnus Castus, Amaranthus, Dill, Rosemary, Columbines, Orrenges, Balaustins, or Pomegranate Flowers, Bettony, Borrage, Bugloss, Marigolds, Woodbine or Honey-suckles, Clove Gilliflowers, Centaury the less, Chamomel, Winter Gilliflowers, Succory, Comfry the greater, Saffron, Bluebottle great and small,* (Synosbatus, Tragus, *and* Dedonæus *hold our white thorn to be it,* Cordus *and* Marcelus *think it to be Bryars,* Lugdunensis *takes it for the sweet Bryar, but what our College takes it for, I know not*) *Cytinus,* (Dioscorides *calls the flowers of the Manured Pomegranates, Cytinus, but*

Pliny *calls the flowers of the wild kind by that name,*) Fox-glove, Viper's Bugloss, Rocket, Eyebright, Beans, Fumitory, Broom, Cowslips, St. John's Wort, Hysop, Jessamine or Shrub, Trefoil, Archangel, or Dead Nettles white and red, Lavender, Wall-flowers, or Winter-Gilliflowers, Privet, Lilies white, and of the valley, Hops, Common and tree Mallows, Feather-few, Woodbine, or Honey-suckles, Melilot, Bawm, Walnuts, Water-Lilies white and yellow, Origanum, Poppies white and red, or Erraticks, Poppies, or corn Roses, so called because they grow amongst Corn, Peony, Honey-suckles, or Woodbine, Peach-flowers, Primroses, Self-heal, Sloebush, Rosemary flowers, Roses, white, damask and red, Sage, Elder, white Saxifrage, Scabious, Siligo, (*I think they mean wheat by it, Authors are not agreed about it*) Steches, Tamarisk, Tansy, Mullen or Higtaper, Limetree, Clove Gilliflowers, Colt's-foot, Violets, Agnus Castus, Dead Nettles white and red.

Culpeper.] That these may be a little explained for the public good: be pleased to take notice.

Some are hot in the first degree, as Borrage, Bugloss, Bettony, Ox-eye, Melilot, Chamomel, Stœchas.

Hot in the second degree. Amomus, Saffron, Clove-gilliflowers, Rocket, Bawm, Spikenard, Hops, Schenanth, Lavender, Jasmine, Rosemary.

In the third degree. Agnus Castus, Epithimum, Winter-gilliflowers, or Wallflowers, Woodbine, or Honey-suckles.

Cold in the first degree. Mallows, Roses, red, white, and damask, Violets.

In the second. Anemone, or Wind-flower, Endive, Succory, Water-lilies, both white and yellow.

In the third. Balaustins, or Pomegranate flowers.

In the fourth. Henbane, and all the sorts of Poppies, only whereas authors say, field Poppies, which some call red, others erratick, and corn Roses, are the coldest of all the others: yet my opinion is, that they are not cold in the fourth degree.

Moist in the first degree. Borrage, Bugloss, Mallows, Succory, Endive.

In the second. Water-lilies, Violets.

Dry in the first degree. Ox-eye, Saffron, Chamomel, Melilot, Roses.

In the second. Wind-flower, Amomus, Clove-gilliflowers, Rocket, Lavender, Hops, Peony, Rosemary, Spikenard.

In the third. Woodbine, or Honeysuckles, Balaustines, Epithimum, Germander, Chamepitis.

The temperature of any other flowers not here mentioned are of the same temperature with the herbs, you may gain skill by searching there for them, you can loose none.

For the parts of the body, they are appropriated to, some heat

The head; as, Rosemary flowers, Self-heal, Chamomel, Bettony, Cowslips, Lavender, Melilot, Peony, Sage, Stœchas.

The breast. Bettony, Bawm, Scabious, Schœnanth.

The heart. Bawm, Rosemary flowers, Borrage, Bugloss, Saffron, Spikenard.

The stomach. Rosemary-flowers, Spikenard, Schœnanth.

The liver. Centaury, Schœnanth, Elder, Bettony, Chamomel, Spikenard.

The spleen. Bettony, Wall-flowers.

The reins and bladder. Bettony, Marsh-mallows, Melilot, Schœnanth, Spikenard.

The womb. Bettony, Squinanth or Schœnanth, Sage, Orris or Flower-de-luce.

The joints. Rosemary-flowers, Cowslips, Chamomel, Melilot.

Flowers, as they are cooling, so they cool

The head. Violets, Roses, the three sorts of Poppies, and Water-lilies.

The breast and heart. Violets, Red Roses, Water-lilies.

The stomach. Red Roses, Violets.

The liver and spleen. Endive, and Succory.

Violets, Borrage, and Bugloss, moisten the heart, Rosemary-flowers, Bawm and Bettony, dry it.

According to property, so they bind

Balaustins, Saffron, Succory, Endive, red-roses, Melilot, Bawm, Clove-gilliflowers, Agnus Castus.

Discuss. Dill, Chamomel, Marsh-mallows, Mallows, Melilot, Stœchas, &c.

Cleanse. Damask-roses, Elder flowers, Bean flowers, &c.

Extenuate. Orris, or Flower-de-luce, Chamomel, Melilot, Stœchas, &c.

Mollify. Saffron, white Lilies, Mallows, Marsh-mallows, &c.

Suppure. Saffron, white Lilies, &c.

Glutinate. Balaustines, Centaury, &c.

Provoke the terms. Bettony, Centaury, Chamomel, Schœnanth, Wall-flowers, Bawm, Peony, Rosemary, Sage.

Stop the terms. Balaustines, or Pomegranate flowers, Water Lilies.

Expel wind. Dill, Chamomel, Schœnanth, Spikenard.

Help burnings. White Lilies, Mallows, Marsh-mallows.

Resist poison. Bettony, Centaury.

Ease pain. Dill, Chamomel, Centaury, Melilot, Rosemary.

Flowers purge choler. Peach flowers, Damask Roses, Violets.

Flegm. Broom flowers, Elder flowers.

If you compare but the quality of the flowers with the herbs, and with the explanation of these terms at the latter end, you may easily find the temperature and property of the rest.

The flowers of Ox-eye being boiled into a poultice with a little barley meal, take away swellings and hardness of the flesh, being applied warm to the place.

Chamomel flowers heat, discuss, loosen and rarify, boiled in Clysters, they are excellent in the wind cholic, boiled in wine, and the decoction drunk, purges the reins, break the stone, opens the pores, cast out choleric humours, succours the heart, and eases pains and aches, or stiffness coming by travelling.

The flowers of Rocket used outwardly, discuss swellings, and dissolve hard tumours, you may boil them into a poultice, but inwardly taken they send but unwholesome vapours up to the head.

Hops open obstructions of the bowels, liver, and spleen, they cleanse the body of choler and flegm, provoke urine.

Jasmine flowers boiled in oil, and the grieved place bathed with it, takes away cramps and stitches in the sides.

The flowers of Woodbine, or Honeysuckles, being dryed and beaten into powder, and a dram taken in white wine in the morning, helps the rickets, difficulty of breathing; provoke urine, and help the stranguary.

The flowers of Mallows being bruised and boiled in honey (two ounces of the flowers is sufficient for a pound of honey; and having first clarified the honey before you put them in) then strained out; this honey taken with a liquorice stick, is an excellent remedy for Coughs, Asthmas, and consumptions of the lungs.

FRUITS

College.] *Winter-cherries, Love Apples, Almonds sweet and bitter, Anacardia, Oranges, Hazel Nuts, the oily Nut Ben, Barberries, Capers, Guinny Pepper, Figs, Carpobalsamum, Cloves, Cassia Fistula, Chestnuts, Cherries, black and red, Cicers, white, black and red, Pome Citrons, Coculus Indi, Colocynthis, Currants, Cornels, or Cornelian*

Cherries, Cubebs, Cucumbers garden and wild, Gourds, Cynosbatus, Cypress, Cones, Quinces, Dates, Dwarf-Elder, Green Figs, Strawberries, common and Turkey Galls, Acorns, Acorn Cups, Pomegranates, Gooseberries, Ivy, Herb True-Love, Walnuts, Jujubes, Juniper berries, Bayberries, Lemons, Oranges, Citrons, Quinces, Pomegranates, Lemons, Mandrakes, Peaches, Stramonium, Apples, garden and wild, or Crabs and Apples, Musk Melons, Medlars, Mulberries, Myrobalans, Bellericks, Chebs, Emblicks, Citron and Indian, Mirtle, Berries, water Nuts, Hazel Nuts, Chestnuts, Cypress Nuts, Walnuts, Nutmegs, Fistick Nuts, Vomiting Nuts, Olives pickled in brine, Heads of white and black Poppies, Pompions, Peaches, French or Kidney Beans, Pine Cones, white black and long Pepper, Fistick Nuts, Apples and Crabs, Prunes, French and Damask, Sloes, Pears, English Currants, Berries of Purging Thorn, black Berries, Raspberries, Elder berries, Sebastens, Services, or Checkers, Hawthorn berries, Pine Nuts, Water Nuts, Grapes, Gooseberries, Raisins, Currants.

Culpeper.] That you may reap benefit by these, be pleased to consider, that they are some of them.

Temperate in respect of heat. Raisins of the sun, Currants, Figs, Pine Nuts, Dates, Sebastens.

Hot in the first degree. Sweet Almonds, Jujubes, Cypress Nuts, green Hazel Nuts, green Walnuts.

Hot in the second degree. The Nut Ben, Capers, Nutmegs, dry Walnuts, dry Hazel Nuts, Fistick Nuts.

In the third degree. Juniper Berries, Cloves Carpobalsamum, Cubebs, Anacardium, bitter Almonds.

In the fourth degree. Pepper, white, black and long, Guinny Pepper.

Cold in the first degree. The flesh of Citrons, Quinces, Pears, Prunes, &c.

In the second. Gourds, Cucumbers, Melons, Pompions, Oranges, Lemons, Citrons, Pomegranates, viz. the juice of them, Peaches, Prunes, Galls, Apples.

In the third. Mandrakes.

In the fourth. Stramonium.

Moist in the first degree. The flesh of Citrons, Lemons, Oranges, viz. the inner rhind which is white, the outer rhind is hot.

In the second. Gourds, Melons, Peaches, Prunes, &c.

Dry in the first degree. Juniper Berries.

In the second. The Nut Ben, Capers, Pears, Fistick Nuts, Pine Nuts, Quinces, Nutmegs, Bay berries.

In the third. Cloves, Galls, &c.

In the fourth. All sorts of Pepper.

As appropriated to the body of Man, so they heat the head: as

Anacardia, Cubebs, Nutmegs.

The breast. Bitter Almonds, Dates, Cubebs, Hazel Nuts, Pine Nuts, Figs, Raisins of the sun, Jujubes.

The heart. Walnuts, Nutmegs, Juniper berries.

The stomach. Sweet Almonds, Cloves, Ben, Juniper berries, Nutmegs, Pine Nuts, Olives.

The spleen. Capers.

The reins and bladder. Bitter Almonds, Juniper Berries, Cubebs, Pine Nuts, Raisins of the sun.

The womb. Walnuts, Nutmegs, Bay-berries, Juniper berries.

Cool the breast. Sebastens, Prunes, Oranges, Lemons.

The heart. Oranges, Lemons, Citrons, Pomegranates, Quinces, Pears.

The stomach. Quinces, Citruls, Cucumbers, Gourds, Musk Melons, Pompions, Cherries, Gooseberries, Cornelian Cherries, Lemons, Apples, Medlars, Oranges, Pears, English Currants, Cervices or Checkers.

The liver. Those that cool the stomach and Barberries.

The reins and womb. Those that cool the stomach, and Strawberries.

By their several operations, some

Bind. As the berries of Mirtles, Barberries, Chestnuts, Cornels, or Cornelian Cherries, Quinces, Galls, Acorns, Acorn-cups, Medlars, Checkers or Cervices, Pomegranates, Nutmegs, Olives, Pears, Peaches.

Discuss. Capers, all the sorts of Pepper.

Extenuate. Sweet and bitter Almonds, Bayberries, Juniper berries.

Glutinate. Acorns, Acorn Cups, Dates, Raisins of the sun, Currants.

Expel Wind. Bay berries, Juniper berries, Nutmegs, all the sorts of Pepper.

Breed Seed. Raisins of the sun, sweet Almonds, Pine Nuts, Figs, &c.

Provoke urine. Winter Cherries.

Provoke the terms. Ivy berries, Capers, &c.

Stop the terms. Barberries, &c.

Resist poison. Bay berries, Juniper berries, Walnuts, Citrons, commonly called Pome Citrons, all the sorts of Pepper.

Ease pain. Bay berries, Juniper berries, Ivy berries, Figs, Walnuts, Raisins, Currants, all the sorts of Pepper.

Fruits purging

Choler. Cassia Fistula, Citron Myrobalans, Prunes, Tamarinds, Raisins.

Melancholy. Indian Myrobalans.

Flegm. Colocynthis and wild Cucumbers purge violently, and therefore not rashly to be meddled withal. I desire my book should be beneficial, not hurtful to the vulgar, but Myrobalans of all sorts, especially Chebs, Bellericks and Emblicks, purge flegm very gently, and without danger.

Of all these give me leave to commend only one to you as of special concernment, which is Juniper berries.

SEEDS

College.] *Sorrel, Agnus Castus, Marsh-mallows, Bishop's weed true and common, Amomus, Dill, Angellica, Annis, Rose-seed, Smallage, Columbines, Sparagus, Arach, Oats, Oranges, Burdocks, Bazil, Barberries, Cotton, Bruscus or Knee-holly, Hemp, Cardamoms greater and lesser, Carduus Benedictus, our Lady's Thistles, Bastard, Saffron, Caraway, Spurge greater and lesser, Coleworts, Onions, the Kernels of Cherry stones, Chervil, Succory, Hemlock, Citrons, Citruls, Garden Scurvy-grass, Colocynthis, Coriander, Samphire, Cucumbers, garden and wild, Gourds, Quinces, Cummin, Cynosbatus, Date-stones, Carrots, English, and cretish, Dwarf-Elder, Endive, Rocket, Hedge Mustard, Orobus, Beans, Fennel, Fenugreek, Ash-tree keys, Fumitory, Brooms, Grains of Paradise, Pomegranates, wild Rue, Alexanders, Barley, white Henbane, St. John's Wort, Hyssop, Lettice, Sharp-pointed-Dock, Spurge, Laurel, Lentils, Lovage, Lemons, Ash-tree-keys, Linseed, or Flaxweed, Gromwell, Darnel, Sweet Trefoil, Lupines, Masterwort, Marjoram, Mallows, Mandrakes, Melons, Medlars, Mezereon, Gromwell, sweet Navew, Nigella, the kernels of Cherries, Apricots, and Peaches, Bazil, Orobus, Rice, Panick, Poppies white and black, Parsnips garden and wild. Thorough Wax, Parsley, English and Macedonian, Burnet, Pease, Plantain, Peony, Leeks, Purslain, Fleawort, Turnips, Radishes, Sumach, Spurge, Roses, Rue, garden and wild, Wormseed, Saxifrage, Succory, Sesami, Hartwort, common and cretish, Mustard-seed, Alexanders, Nightshade, Steves Ager, Sumach, Treacle Mustard, sweet Trefoil, Wheat, both the fine flour and the bran, and that which starch is made of, Vetches or Tares, Violets, Nettles, common and Roman, the stones of Grapes, Greek Wheat, or Spelt Wheat.*

Culpeper.] That you may receive a little more benefit by these, than the bare reading of them, which doth at the most but tell you

what they are; the following method may instruct you what they
are good for.

Seeds are hot in the first degree

Linseed, Fenugreek, Coriander, Rice, Gromwell, Lupines.

In the second. Dill, Smallage, Orobus, Rocket, Bazil, Nettles.

In the third. Bishop's Weed, Annis, Amomus, Carraway, Fennel,
(and so I believe Smallage too, let authors say what they will, for
if the herb of Smallage be somewhat hotter than Parsley; I know
little reason why the seed should not be so hot) Cardamoms, Parsley,
Cummin, Carrots, Nigella, Navew, Hartwort, Staves Ager.

In the fourth. Water-cresses, Mustard-seed.

Cold in the first degree. Barley, &c.

In the second. Endive, Lettice, Purslain, Succory, Gourds, Cucumbers, Melons, Citruls, Pompions, Sorrel, Nightshade.

In the third. Henbane, Hemlock, Poppies white and black.

Moist in the first degree. Mallows, &c.

Dry in the first degree. Beans, Fennel, Fenugreek, Barley, Wheat,
&c.

In the second. Orobus, Lentils, Rice, Poppies, Nightshade, and
the like.

In the third. Dill, Smallages, Bishop's Weed, Annis, Caraway,
Cummin, Coriander, Nigella, Gromwell, Parsley.

Appropriated to the body of man, and so they

Heat the head. Fennel, Marjoram, Peony, &c.

The breast. Nettles.

The heart. Bazil, Rue, &c. Mustard seed, &c.

The stomach. Annis, Bishop's weed, Amomus, Smallage, Cummin, Cardamoms, Cubebs, Grains of Paradise.

The liver. Annis, Fennel, Bishop's weed, Amomus, Smallage,
Sparagus, Cummin, Caraway, Carrots.

The spleen. Annis, Caraway, Watercresses.

The reins and bladder. Cicers, Rocket, Saxifrage, Nettles, Gromwell.

The womb. Peony, Rue.

The joints. Water-cresses, Rue, Mustard-seed.

Cool the head. Lettice, Purslain, white Poppies.

The breast. White Poppies, Violets.

The heart. Orange, Lemon, Citron and Sorrel seeds.

Lastly, the four greater and four lesser cold seeds, which you
may find in the beginning of the compositions, as also the seed of
white and black Poppies cool the liver and spleen, reins and bladder,
womb and joints.

According to operation some seeds

Bind, as Rose-seeds, Barberries, Shepherd's purse, Purslain, &c.

Discuss. Dill, Carrots, Linseeds, Fenugreek, Nigella, &c.

Cleanse. Beans, Orobus, Barley, Lupines, Nettles, &c.

Mollify. Linseed, or Flax seed, Fenugreek seed, Mallows, Nigella.

Harden. Purslain seed, &c.

Suppure. Linseed, Fenugreek seed, Darnel, Barley husked, commonly called French Barley.

Glutinate. Orobus, Lupines, Darnel, &c.

Expel wind. Annis, Dill, Smallage, Caraway, Cummin, Carrots, Fennel, Nigella, Parsley, Hartwort, Wormseed.

Breed Seed. Rocket, Beans, Cicers, Ash-tree keys.

Provoke the menses. Amomus, Sparagus, Annis, Fennel, Bishop's weed, Cicers, Carrots, Smallage, Parsley, Lovage, Hartwort.

Break the stone. Mallows, Marsh-mallows, Gromwell, &c.

Stop the terms. Rose seeds, Cummin, Burdock, &c.

Resist poison. Bishop's weed, Annis, Smallage, Cardamoms, Oranges, Lemons, Citrons, Fennel, &c.

Ease pain. Dill, Amomus, Cardamoms, Cummin, Carrots, Orobus, Fenugreek, Linseed, Gromwell, Parsley, Panick.

Assuage swellings. Linseed, Fenugreek seeds, Marsh-mallows, Mallows, Coriander, Barley, Lupines, Darnel, &c.

*　　　*　　　*

The College tells you a tale that there are such things in Rerum Natura, as these, Gums, Rozins, Balsams, and Juices made thick, viz.

College.] *Juices of Wormwood and Maudlin, Acacia, Aloes, Lees of Oil, Assa-fœtida, Balsam of Peru and India; Bdellium, Benzoin, Camphire, Caranna, Colophonia, Juice of Maudlin, Euphorbium, Lees of Wine, Lees of Oil, Gums of Galbanum, Amoniacum, Anime, Arabick, Cherry Trees, Copal, Elemy, Juniper, Ivy, Plumb Trees, Cambuge, Hypocystis, Labdanum, Lacca, Liquid Amber, Manna, Mastich, Myrrh, Olibanum, Opium, Opopanax, Pice-bitumen, Pitch of the Cedar of Greece, Liquid and dry Rozins of Fir-tree, Larch-tree, Pine tree, Pine-fruit, Mastich, Venice and Cyprus Turpentine. Sugar, white, red, and Christaline, or Sugar Candy white and red, Sagapen, Juniper, Gum, Sanguis Draconis, Sarcocolla, Scamony, Styrax, Liquid and Calamitis, Tacha, Mahacca, Tartar, Frankincense, Olibanum, Tragaganth, Birdlime.*

Culpeper.] That my country may receive more benefit than ever the college of Physicians intended them from these, I shall treat of them severally.

　　1. Of the Juices.　　2. Of the Gums and Rosins.

Concrete Juices, or Juices made thick, are either

Temperate, as, Juice of Liquorice, white starch.
Hot in the first degree. Sugar.
In the second. Labdanum.
In the third. Benzoin, Assafœtida.
Cold in the third degree. Sanguis Draconis, Acacia.
In the third. Hypocistis.
In the fourth. Opium, and yet some authors think Opium is hot because of its bitter taste.

Aloes and Manna purge choler gently, and Scamony doth purge choler violently, that it is no ways fit for a vulgar man's use, for it corrodes the Bowels. Opopoanax purges flegm very gently.

White starch gently levigates or makes smooth such parts as are rough, syrup of Violets being made thick with it and so taken on the point of a knife, helps coughs, roughness of the throat, wheezing, excoriations of the bowels, the bloody-flux.

Juice of *Liquorice* helps roughness of the *Trachea Arteria,* which is in plain English called the windpipe, the roughness of which causes coughs and hoarseness, difficulty of breathing, &c. It allays the heat of the stomach and liver, eases pains, soreness and roughness of the reins and bladder, it quencheth thirst, and strengthens the stomach exceedingly. It may easily be carried about in one's pocket, and eat a little now and then.

Sugar cleanses and digests, takes away roughness of the tongue, it strengthens the reins and bladder, being weakened: being beaten into fine powder, and put into the eyes, it takes away films that grow over the sight.

Labdanum is in operation, thickening, heating and mollifying, it opens the passage of the veins, and keeps the hair from falling off; the use of it is usually external; being mixed with wine, myrrh, and oil of mirtles, and applied like a plaister, it takes away filthy scars, and the deformity the small pox leaves behind them; being mixed with oil of Roses, and dropped into the ears, it helps pains there; being used as a pessary, it provokes the menses, and helps hardness or stiffness of the womb. It is sometimes used inwardly in such medicines as ease pains and help the cough: if you mix a little of it with old white wine and drink it, it both provokes urine and stops looseness or fluxes.

Dragons blood, cools, binds, and repels.
Acasia, and *Hyposistis,* do the like.

The juice of *Maudlin,* or, for want of it Costmary, which is the same in effect, and better known to the vulgar, the juice is made thick for the better keeping of it; first clarify the juice before you boil it to its due thickness, which is something thicker than honey.

It is appropriated to the liver, and the quantity of a dram taken every morning, helps the *Cachexia*, or evil disposition of the body proceeding from coldness of the liver: it helps the rickets and worms in children, provokes urine, and gently (without purging) disburdens the body of choler and flegm; it succours the lungs, opens obstructions, and resists putrefaction of blood.

Gums are either temperate, as, Lacca, Elemi, Tragacanth, &c.

Intemperate, and so are hot in the first degree, as Bdellium, Gum of Ivy.

In the second, Galbanum, Myrrh, Mastich, Frankincense, Olibanum, Pitch, Rozin, Styrax.

In the third. Amoniacum.

In the fourth. Euphorbium.

Gum Arabick is cold.

Colophonia and Styrax soften.

Gum Arabick and Tragacanth, Sandarack or Juniper Gum, and Sarcocolla bind.

Gum of Cherry trees, breaks the stone.

Styrax provokes the menses.

Opopanax gently purges flegm.

From the prickly *Cedar* when it is burned comes forth that which, with us, is usually known by the name of Tar, and is excellently good for unction either for scabs, itch, or manginess, either in men or beasts, as also against the leprosy, tetters, ringworms, and scald heads.

All sorts of *Rozins* fill up hollow ulcers, and relieve the body sore pressed with cold griefs.

The *Rozin* of Pitch-tree, is that which is commonly called Burgundy pitch, and is something hotter and sharper than the former, being spread upon a cloth is excellently good for old aches coming of former bruises or dislocations.

Pitch mollifies hard swellings, and brings boils and sores to suppuration, it breaks carbuncles, disperses aposthumes, cleanses ulcers of corruption and fills them with flesh.

Bdellium heats and mollifies, and that very temperately, being mixed with any convenient ointment or plaister, it helps kernels in the neck and throat, *Scrophula*, or that disease which was called the King's Evil. Inwardly taken in any convenient medicine, it provokes the menses, and breaks the stone, it helps coughs and bitings of venomous beasts: it helps windiness of the spleen, and pains in the sides thence coming. Both outwardly applied to the place and inwardly taken, it helps ruptures or such as are burst, it softens the hardness of the womb, dries up the moisture thereof and expels the dead child.

Bitumen Jadaicum is a certain dry pitch which the dead sea, or lake of *Sodom in India* casts forth at certain times, the inhabitants thereabouts pitch their ships with it. It is of excellent use to mollify the hardness of swellings and discuss them, as also against inflammations; the smoke of it burnt is excellently good for the fits of the mother, and the falling-sickness. Inwardly taken in wine it provokes the menses, helps the bitings of venomous beasts, and dissolves congealed blood in the body.

Ambergreese is hot and dry in the second degree, I will not dispute whether it be a Gum or not. It strengthens nature much which way soever it be taken, there are but few grains usually given of it at a time: mixed with a little ointment of Orange flowers, and the temples and forehead anointed with it, it eases the pains of the head and strengthens the brain exceedingly; the same applied to the privities helps the fits of the mother; inwardly taken it strengthens the brain and memory, the heart and vital spirit, warms cold stomachs, and is an exceeding strengthener of nature to old people, adding vigour to decayed and worn-out spirits: it provokes venery, and makes barren women fruitful, if coldness and moisture or weakness be the cause impediting.

Assafœtida being smelled to, is vulgarly known to repress the fits of the mother; a little bit put into an aching tooth, presently eases the pain, ten grains of it taken before dinner, walking half an hour after it, provokes appetite, helps digestion, strengthens the stomach, and takes away loathing of meat, it provokes lust exceedingly and expels wind as much.

Borax, besides the virtues it has to solder Gold, Silver, Copper, &c. inwardly given in small quantities, it stops fluxes, and the running of the reins; being in fine powder, and put into green wounds, it cures them at once dressing.

Gambuge, which the College calls *Gutta Gamba*. I know no good of it.

Caranna outwardly applied, is excellent for aches and swellings in the nerves and joints. If you lay it behind the ears, it draws back humours from the eyes; applied to the temples as they usually do Mastich, it helps the tooth-ache.

Gum Elimi, authors appropriate to fractures in the skull and head. See *Arceus'* liniment.

Gum Lacca being well purified, and the quantity of half a dram taken in any convenient liquor, strengthens the stomach and liver, opens obstructions, helps the yellow jaundice and dropsy; provokes urine, breaks the stone in the reins and bladder.

Liquid *Amber* is not much unlike liquid *Styrax*: by unction it warms and comforts a cold and moist brain, it eases all griefs coming of a cold cause, it mightily comforts and strengthens a weak stomach, being anointed with it, and helps digestion exceedingly, it dissolves swellings. It is hot in the third degree, and moist in the first.

I think it would do the commonwealth no harm if I should speak a word or two of *Manna* here, although it be no Gum. I confess authors make some flutter about it, what it is, some holding it to be the juice of a tree; I am confident it is the very same condensated that our honey-dews here are, only the countries whence it comes being far hotter, it falls in great abundance. Let him that desires reason for it, be pleased to read *Butler's* book of Bees, a most excellent experimental work, there he shall find reason enough to satisfy any reasonable man. Choose the driest and whitest; it is a very gentle purger of choler, quenches thirst, provokes appetite, eases the roughness of the throat, helps bitterness in the throat, and often proneness to vomit, it is very good for such as are subject to be costive to put it into their drink instead of sugar, it hath no obnoxious quality at all in it, but may be taken by a pregnant woman without any danger; a child of a year old may take an ounce of it at a time dissolved in milk, it will melt like sugar, neither will it be known from it by the taste.

Myrrh is hot and dry in the second degree, dangerous for pregnant women, it is bitter and yet held to be good for the roughness of the throat and wind-pipe; half a dram of it taken at a time helps rheumatic distillations upon the lungs, pains in the sides; it stops fluxes, provokes the menses, brings away both birth and after-birth, softens the hardness of the womb; being taken two hours before the fit comes, it helps agues. *Mathiolus* saith he seldom used any other medicine for the quartan ague than a dram of myrrh given in Muskadel an hour before the fit usually came; if you make it up into pills with treacle, and take one of them every morning fasting, it is a sovereign preservative against the pestilence, against the poison of serpents, and other venomous beasts; a singular remedy for a stinking breath if it arise from putrefaction of the stomach, it fastens loose teeth, and stays the shedding off of the hair, outwardly used it breeds flesh in deep wounds, and covers the naked bones with flesh.

Olibanum is hot in the second degree, and dry in the first, you may take a dram of it at a time, it stops looseness and the running of the reins; it strengthens the memory exceedingly, comforts the heart, expels sadness and melancholy, strengthens the heart, helps coughs, rheums and pleurises; your best way (in my opinion), to take it is to mix it with conserve of roses, and take it in the morning fasting.

Tachamacha is seldom taken inwardly, outwardly spread upon leather, and applied to the navel; it stays the fits of the mother, applied to the side, it mitigates speedily, and in little time quite takes away the pain and windiness of the spleen; the truth is, whatsoever ache or swelling proceeds of wind or cold raw humours, I know no better plaister coming from beyond sea than this gum. It strengthens the brain and memory exceedingly, and stops all such defluctions thence as trouble the eyes, ears, or teeth, it helps the gout and sciatica.

Gum Coopal, and Gum Anime, are very like one another both in body and operation, the former is hard to come by, the last not very easy. It stops defluctions from the head, if you perfume your cap with the smoke of it, it helps the headache and megrim, strengthens the brain, and therefore the sinews.

Gum Tragaganth, which the vulgar call Gum Dragon, being mixed with pectoral Syrups, (which you shall find noted in their proper places) it helps coughs and hoarseness, salt and sharp distillations upon the lungs, being taken with a liquorice stick, being dissolved in sweet wine, it helps (being drank) gnawing in the bowels, sharpness and freetings of the urine, which causes excoriations either in the reins or bladder, being dissolved in milk and the eyes washed with it, it takes away weals and scabs that grow on the eyelids, it is excellently good to be put in poultice to fodder wounds, especially if the nerves or sinews be hurt.

Sagapen, dissolved in juice of rue and taken, wonderfully breaks the stone in the bladder, expels the dead child and afterbirth, clears the sight; dissolved in wine and drank, it helps the cough, and distillation upon the lungs, and the fits of the mother; outwardly in oils or ointments, it helps such members as are out of joint or over-stretched.

Galbanum is of the same operation, and also taken from the same plant, *viz.* Fennel, Giant.

Gum Arabic, thickens and cools, and corrects choleric sharp humours in the body, being dissolved in the white of an egg, well beaten, it helps burnings, and keeps the place from blistering.

Mastich stays fluxes, being taken inwardly any way. Three or four small grains of Mastich, swallowed at night going to bed, is a remedy for pains in the stomach; being beaten into powder, and mixed with conserve of Roses, it strengthens the stomach, stops distillations upon the lungs, stays vomiting, and causes a sweet breath; being mixed with white wine and the mouth washed with it, it cleanses the gums of corruption, and fastens loose teeth.

Frankincense being used outwardly in the way of a plaister, heats and binds; being applied to the temples, stops the rheums that flow to the eyes, helps green wounds, and fills hollow ulcers with flesh, stops the bleeding of wounds, though the arteries be cut; being made into an ointment with Vinegar and Hog's-grease, helps the itch, pains in the ears, inflammations in women's breasts commonly called agues in the breast; beware of taking it inwardly, lest it cause madness.

Turpentine is hot in the second degree, it heals, softens, it discusses and purges, cleanses the reins, provokes urine.

Styrax Calamitis is hot and dry in the second degree, it heals, mollifies, and concocts; being taken inwardly helps the cough, and distillations of the lungs, hoarseness and loss of voice, helps the hardness of the womb, and provokes the menses.

Ammoniacum, hot and dry in the third degree, softens, draws, and heats; being dissolved in vinegar, strained and applied plaisterwise, it takes away carbuncles and hardness in the flesh, it is one of the best remedies that I know for infirmities of the spleen, being applied to the left side; being made into an ointment with oil, it is good to anoint the limbs of such as are weary: a scruple of it being taken in the form of a pill loosens the belly, gives speedy delivery to women in travail, helps diseases of the spleen, the sciatica and all pains in the joints, and have any humour afflicting their breast.

Camphire, it is held by all authority to be cold and dry in the third degree, it is of very thin subtile parts, insomuch that being beaten into very fine powder it will vanquish away into the air, being beaten into powder and mixed with oil, and the temples anointed therewith, eases headaches proceeding of heat, all inflammations whatsoever, the back being anointed with the same, cools the reins, and seminal vessels, stops the running of the reins and Fluor Albus, the moderate use of Venery, the like it doth if it be drank inwardly with Bettony-water, take but a small quantity of it at a time inwardly, it resists poison and bitings by venomous beasts; outwardly, applied as before, and the eyes anointed with it, stops hot rheums that flow thither.

Opopanax purges thick flegm from the most remote parts of the body, *viz.* the brain, joints, hands, and feet, the nerves and breast, and strengthens all those parts when they are weak, if the weakness proceed of cold, as usually it doth; it helps weakness of the sight, old rotten coughs, and gouts of all sorts, dropsies, and swellings of the spleen, it helps the stranguary and difficulty of making urine, provokes the menses, and helps all cold afflictions of the womb; have a care you give it not to any pregnant women. The dose is one dram at most, corrected with a little Mastich, dissolved in Vinegar and outwardly applied helps the passions of the spleen.

*   *   *

In the next place the College tells you a tale concerning Liquid, Juices, and Tears, which are to be kept for present use, *viz.*

College.] *Vinegar, Juice of Citrons, Juice of sour Grapes, Oranges, Barberries, Tears of a Birch-tree, Juice of Chermes, Quinces, Pomegranates, Lemons, Wood sorrel, Oil of unripe Olives, and ripe Olives, both new and cold, Juice of red and Damask Roses, Wine Tears of a Vine.*

Culpeper.] The virtues of the most of these may be found in the Syrups, and are few of them used alone.

Then the College tells you there are things bred of PLANTS.

College.] *Agarick, Jew's-ears, the berries of Chermes, the Spungy substance of the Briar, Moss, Viscus Quercinus, Oak, Apples.*

Culpeper.] As the College would have you know this, so would I know what the chief of them are good for.

Jew's-ears boiled in milk and drank, helps sore throats.

Moss is cold, dry, and binding, therefore good for fluxes of all sorts.

Misleto of the Oak, it helps the falling sickness and the convulsions, being discreetly gathered and used.

Oak Apples are dry and binding; being boiled in milk and drank, they stop fluxes and the menses, and being boiled in vinegar, and the body anointed with the vinegar, cures the itch.

* * *

Then the College acquaints you, That there are certain living Creatures called:

College.] *Bees, Woodlice, Silkworms, Toads, Crabs of the River, little Puppy Dogs, Grass-hoppers, Cantharides, Cothanel, Hedgehogs,* Emmets or Ants, Larks, Swallows, and their young ones, Horse-leeches, Snails, Earthworms, Dishwashers or Wagtails, House Sparrows and Hedge Sparrows, Frogs, Scineus, Land Scorpions, Moles, or Monts, Tortoise of the Woods, Tenches, Vipers and Foxes.

Culpeper.] That part of this crew of Cattle and some others which they have not been pleased to learn, may be made beneficial to your sick bodies, be pleased to understand, that

Bees being burnt to ashes, and a lye made with the ashes, trimly decks a bald head being washed with it.

Snails with shells on their backs, being first washed from the dirt, then the shells broken, and they boiled in spring water, but not scummed at all, for the scum will sink of itself, and the water drank for ordinary drink is a most admirable remedy for consumption; being bruised and applied to the place they help the gout, draw thorns out of the flesh, and held to the nose help the bleeding thereof.

* * *

Therefore consider that the College gave the Apothecaries a catalogue of what *Parts of Living creatures* and *Excrements* they must keep in their shops.

College.] *The fat, grease, or suet, of a Duck, Goose, Eel, Boar, Herron, Thymallows* (if you know where to get it) *Dog, Capon, Beaver, wild Cat, Stork, Coney, Horse, Hedge-hog, Hen, Man, Lion, Hare, Pike, or Jack,* (if they have any fat, I am persuaded 'tis worth twelve-pence a grain) *Wolf, Mouse of the mountains,* (if you can catch them) *Pardal, Hog, Serpent, Badger, Grey or brock Fox, Vulture,* (if you can catch them) *Album Græcum, Anglice, Dog's dung, the hucklebone of a Hare and a Hog, East and West Bezoar, Butter not salted and salted, stone taken out of a man's bladder, Vipers flesh, fresh Cheese, Castorium, white, yellow, and Virgin's Wax, the brain of Hares and Sparrows, Crabs' Claws, the Rennet of a Lamb, a Kid, a Hare, a Calf, and a Horse, the heart of a Bullock, a Stag, Hog, and a Wether, the horn of an Elk, a Hart, a Rhinoceros, an Unicorn, the skull of a man killed by a violent death, a Cockscomb, the tooth of a Bore, an Elephant, and a Sea-horse, Ivory, or Elephant's Tooth, the skin a Snake hath cast off, the gall of a Hawk, Bullock, a she Goat, a Hare, a Kite, a Hog, a Bull, a Bear, the cases of Silk-worms, the liver of a Wolf, an Otter, a Frog, Isinglass, the guts of a Wolf and a Fox, the milk of a she Ass, a she Goat, a Woman, an Ewe, a Heifer, East and West Bezoar, the stone in the head of a Crab, and a Perch, if there be any stone in an Ox Gall, stone in the bladder of a Man, the Jaw of a Pike or Jack, Pearls, the marrow of the Leg of a Sheep, Ox, Goat, Stag, Calf, common and virgin Honey, Musk, Mummy, a Swallow's nest, Crabs Eyes, the Omentum or call of a Lamb, Ram, Wether, Calf, the whites, yolks, and shells of Hen's Eggs, Emmet's Eggs, bone of a Stag's heart, an Ox leg, Ossepiæ, the inner skin of a Hen's Gizzard, the wool of Hares, the feathers of Partridges, that which Bees make at the entrance of the hive, the pizzle of a Stag, of a Bull, Fox Lungs, fasting spittle, the blood of a Pigeon, of a Cat, of a he Goat, of a Hare, of a Partridge, of a Sow, of a Bull, of a Badger, of a Snail, Silk, Whey, the suet of a Bullock, of a Stag, of a he Goat, of a Sheep, of a Heifer, Spermaceti, a Bullock's spleen, the skin a Snake hath cast off, the excrements of a Goose, of a Dog, of a Goat, of Pigeons, of a stone Horse, of a Hen, of Swallows, of a Hog, of a Heifer, the ancle of a Hare, of a Sow, Cobwebs, Water thells, as Blatta Bazantia, Buccinæ, Crabs, Cockles, Dentalis, Entalis, Mother of Pearl, Mytuli Purpuræ, Os sepiæ, Umbilious Marinus, the testicles of a Horse, a Cock, the hoof of an Elk, of an Ass, a Bullock, of a Horse, of a Lyon, the urine of a Boar, of a she Goat.*

Culpeper.] The liver of an Hedge-hog being dried and beaten into powder and drank in wine, strengthens the reins exceedingly, and helps the dropsy, convulsions, and the falling sickness, together with all fluxes of the bowels.

The liver being in like manner brought into powder, strengthens the liver exceedingly, and helps the dropsy.

* * *

Then the College tells you these things may be taken from the SEA, as College.] *Amber-grease, Sea-water, Sea-sand, Bitumen, Amber white and yellow, Jet, Carlinæ, Coral, white and red, Foam of the Sea, Spunge, Stone Pumice, Sea salt, Spunges, Amber.*

METALS, STONES, SALTS, AND OTHER MINERALS

Ver-de-grease, Scales of Brass, Ætitis, Alana Terra, Alabaster, Alectorions, Alum Seisile and Roach Amethist, Amianth, Amphelites, Antimony, leaves and filings of Silver, Quick Silver, Lapis, Armenius, native Arsenic, both white and red, artificial Arsenic, white and realgar, Argilla, Asteria, leaves and filings of Gold, Belemites, Berril, Bole-armenick, Borrax, Toad-stone, Lapis Calaminatis, Cadmia, Lime quick and quenched, Vitriol, white, blue, and green, Steel, Borrax, Chrisolite, Chrisopus, Cynabris, native and artificial, Whetstones, Chalk, white and green, Crystal, Diphriges, the rust, dust, scales, and flakes of Iron, Granite, Mortar, such as walls are daubed with, Hema-titis, Heliotropium, Jacinth, Hyber, Nicius, Jasper, Lapis Judacious, Tiles, Lapis Lazuly, Lapis Lincis, Lithanthrax, Litharge of Silver and Gold, Loadstone, Marchasite, or fire stone Marble, Red Lead, native and artificial, Miss, Naptha, Lapis Nephriticus, Nitre, Oaker yellow and red, Onyx, Opalus, Ophytes, Ostcocolla Lead white and black, Plumbago, Pompholix, Marchasite, Realgar, Ruby, red Oaker, Sal Armoniach, Sal Gem, and salt Nitre, Saphyr and Sardine, Seleni-tis, Flints, Emerald, Smiris, Sori, Spodium, Pewter, Brimstone, quick and common, Talth, Earth of Cimolia, Sames, Lemnos, Sylesia, Topas, Alana, Terra, Tutty, Vitriol, white, blue, and green.

Precious stones alter by a way manifest or hidden

By a way manifest, they are hot, in the first degree. Hemetitis, Pyritis, Lopis Asius, Thyitis, Smyres, Lapis Schistus.

Precious stones cold, are in the first degree. Jacinth, Saphyr, Emerald, Cristal, Lapis Samius, Lapis Phrigius.

In the second degree. Ruby, Carbuncle, Granite, Sardony.

In the fourth degree. Diamond.

In respect of property, they bind, as Lapis Asius, Nectius, Geodes, Pumice-stone.

Emolient, as Alabaster, Jet, Lapis Thrasius.

Stupify, as Memphitis, Jasper, Ophites.

Clease, as Lapis Arabicus.

Glutinate, as Galactitis, Melites.

Scarify, as Morochtus.

Break the stone, as Lapis Lyncis, Lapis Judaicus, Lapis Sponge.

Retain the fruit in the womb, as Ætitis, Jasper.

Provoke the menses. Ostracites.

Stones altering by a hidden property (as they call it,) are

Bezoar, Topaz, Lapis Colubrinus, Toad-stone, Emerald, Alectorius, Calcidonius, Amethist, Saphyr, Jasper, Lapis Nephriticus, Lapis Tibernum, Lapis Spongites, the stone found in the maw of a Swallow, Load-stone, Lapis Vulturis, Merucius, Coral, Lynturius, Jet, Ætites, the stones of Crabs, Amber, Crystal, &c.

The *Load-stone* purges gross humours.

Lapis Armenius and *Lapis Lazuli,* purge melancholy.

Pyrites heat and cleanse, take away dimness of sight. *Dioscorides.* Lapis Asius binds and moderately corrodes and cleanses filthy ulcers, and fills them up with flesh; being mixed with honey, and applied to the place, is an admirable remedy for the gout.

Chrystal being beaten into very fine powder, and a dram of it taken at a time helps the bloody-flux, stops the Fluor Albus, and increases milk in Nurses. *Mathiolus.*

Lapis Samius is cooling and binding, it is very comfortable to the stomach, but it dulls the senses, helps fluxes of the eyes and ulcers.

Geodetes binds and drys, being beaten into powder and mixed with water, and applied to the place, takes away inflammations of the Testicles.

Pumice-stone being beaten into powder and the teeth rubbed with it, cleanses them. *Dioscorides.*

Jet, it is of a softening and discussing nature, it resists the fits of the mother.

Lapis Arabicus being beaten into powder, and made into an ointment helps the hemorrhoids.

Ostracites, a dram of it taken in powder provokes the menses; being taken after that purgation, causes conception, also being made into an ointment, helps inflammations of the breast.

Myexis being borne about one takes away pains in the reins, and hinders the breeding of the stone.

Lapis Armenius purges melancholy, and also causes vomiting, I hold it not very safe for our English bodies, and therefore I will speak no more of it.

Explanation of certain Vacuations

The five opening Roots.
Smallage, Sparagus, Fennel, Parsley, Knee-holly.
The two opening Roots.
Fennel, Parsley.
The five emolient Herbs.
Marsh-mallows, Mallows, Beets, Mercury, Pellitory of the Wall, Violet Leaves.
The five Capillary Herbs.
Maidenhair, Wall Rue, Cetrach, Hart's-tongue, Politricum.
The four cordial Flowers.
Borrage, Bugloss, Roses, Violets.
The four greater hot Seeds, Carminative, or breaking wind.
Annis, Carraway, Cummin, Fennel.
The four lesser hot seeds.
Bishop's weed, Amomus, Smallage, Carrots.
The four greater cold seeds.
Citrul, Cucumber, Gourds, Melon.
The four lesser cold seeds.
Succory, Endive, Lettice, Purslain.
Five fragments of precious stones.
Granite, Jacinth, Sapphire, Sardine, Emerald.

The right worshipful, the College of Physicians of *London* in their New Dispensatory give you free leave to distil these common waters that follow, but they never intend you should know what they are good for.

SIMPLE DISTILLED WATERS

Of fresh Roots of

Briony, Onions, Elecampane, Orris, or Flower-de-luce, Turnips.

Of flowers and buds of

Southernwood, both sorts of Wormwood, Wood Sorrel, Lady's-Mantle, Marsh-mallows, Angelica, Pimpernel with purple flowers, Smallage, Columbines, Sparagus, Mouse-ear, Borrage, Shepherd's Purse, Calaminth, Woodbine or Honey-suckles, Carduus Benedictus, our Lady's Thistles, Knotgrass, Succory, Dragons, Colt's-foot, Fennel, Goat's Rue, Grass, Hyssop, Lettice, Lovage, Toad-flax, Hops, Marjoram, Mallows, Horehound, Featherfew, Bawm, Mints, Horse-mints, Water Cresses, English Tobacco, white Poppies, Pellatory of the Wall, Parsley, Plantain, Purslain, Self-heal, Pennyroyal, Oak leaves, Sage, Scabious, Figwort or Throatwort, Houseleek, or Sengreen, the greater and lesser Mother of Time, Nightshade, Tansy, Tormentil, Valerian.

Of Flowers of

Oranges, (if you can get them) *Blue-bottle the greater, Beans, Water-Lilies, Lavender, Nut-tree, Cowslips, Sloes, Rosemary, Roses white, damask, and red, Satyrien, Lime-tree, Clove-gilliflowers, Violets.*

Of Fruits of

Oranges, Black Cherries, Pome Citrons, Quinces, Cucumbers, Strawberries, Winter Cherries, Lemons, Rasberries, unripe Walnuts, Apples.

Of parts of living Creatures and their excrements

Lobsters, Cockles, or Snails, Hartshorn, Bullocks dung made in May, Swallows, Earthworms, Magpies, Spawn of Frogs.

SIMPLE WATERS DISTILLED

being digested before-hand

Of the fresh Roots of Nettles

Of the leaves of Agrimony, wild Tansy, or Silverweed, Mugwort, Bettony, Marigolds, Chamomel, Chamepitys, Celandine, Pilewort, Scurvy-grass, Comfry the greater, Dandelyon, Ash-tree leaves, Eyebright, Fumitory, Alehoof, or ground Ivy, Horsetail, St. John's Wort, Yarrow, Moneywort, Restharrow, Solomon's Seal, Res solis, Rue, Savin, Saxifrage, Hart's tongue, Scordium, Tamarisk, Mullin, Vervain, Paul's Bettony, Mead-sweet, Nettles.

Of the Flowers of Mayweed, Broom, Cowslips, Butter-bur, Peony, Elder.

Of the berries of Broom, Elder.

Culpeper.] Then the College gives you an admonition concerning these, which being converted into your native language, is as follows.

We give you warning that these common waters be better prepared for time to come, either in common stills, putting good store of ashes underneath, the roots and herbs being dryer, &c. or if they be full of Juice, by distilling the juice in a convenient bath, that so burning may be avoided, which hitherto hath seldom been. But let the other Herbs, Flowers, or Roots, be bruised, and by adding Tartar, common salt, or leven be digested, then putting spring water to them, distil them in an Alembick with its refrigeratory, or Worm, till the change of the taste shew the virtue to be drawn off; then let the oil (if any) be separated from the water according to art.

Into the number of these waters may be ascribed.

The Tears of Vines, the liquor of the Birch-tree, May dew.

Culpeper.] That my country may receive the benefit of these waters, I shall first shew the temperatures, secondly, the virtues of the most usual and most easy to come by. If any should take exceptions that I mention not all, I answer first, I mention enough.

Secondly, who ever makes this objection, they shew extreme ingratitude, for had I mentioned but only one, I had revealed more to them than ever the College intended they should know, or give me thanks for doing.

The qualities and appropriation of the simple Distilled Waters

Simple distilled waters either cool or heat: such as cool, either cool the blood or choler.

Waters cooling the blood. Lettice, Purslain, Water Lilies, Violets, Sorrel Endive, Succory, Fumitory.

Waters cooling and repressing choleric humours, or vapours in the head

Nightshade, Lettice, Water Lilies, Plantain, Poppies, *viz.* The flowers both of white black and red Poppies, black Cherries.

The breast and lungs. Violets, Poppies all three sorts, Colt's-foot.

In the heart. Sorrel, Quinces, Water Lilies, Roses, Violets, green or unripe Walnuts.

In the stomach. Quinces, Roses, Violets, Nightshade, House-leeks, or Sengreen, Lettice, Purslain.

In the liver. Endive, Succory, Night-shade, Purslain, Water Lilies.

In the reins and bladder. Endive, Succory, Winter Cherries, Plantain, Water Lilies, Strawberries, Houseleek or Sengreen, black Cherries.

In the womb. Endive, Succory, Lettice, Water Lilies, Purslain, Roses.

Simple waters which are hot, concoct either flegm or melancholy.

Waters concocting flegm in the head, are

Bettony, Sage, Marjoram, Chamomel, Fennel, Calaminth, Rosemary-flowers, Primroses, Eye-bright.

In the breast and lungs. Maiden-hair, Bettony, Hysop, Horehound, Carduus Benedictus, Scabious, Orris, or Flower-de-luces, Bawm, Self-heal, &c.

In the heart. Bawm, Rosemary.

In the stomach. Wormwood, Mints, Fennel, Chervil, Time, Mother of Time, Marigolds.

In the liver. Wormwood, Centaury, Origanum, Marjoram, Maudlin, Costmary, Agrimony, Fennel.

In the spleen. Water-cresses, Wormwood, Calaminth.

In the reins and bladder. Rocket, Nettles, Saxifrage, Pellitory of the Wall, Alicampane, Burnet.

In the womb. Mugwort, Calaminth, Penny-royal, Savin, Mother of Time, Lovage.

Waters concocting Melancholy in the head, are

Hops, Fumitory.

The breast. Bawm, Carduus Benedictus.

The heart. Borrage, Bugloss, Bawm, Rosemary.

The liver. Endive, Chicory, Hops.

The spleen. Dodder, Hart's-tongue, Tamarisk, Time.

Having thus ended the appropriation, I shall speak briefly of the virtues of distilled waters.

Lettice water cools the blood when it is over-heated, for when it is not, it needs no cooling: it cools the head and liver, stays hot vapours ascending to the head, and hinders sleep; it quenches immoderate thirst, and breeds milk in nurses, distil it in *May*.

Purslain water cools the blood and liver, quenches thirst, helps such as spit blood, have hot coughs, or pestilences.

The distilled water of *water Lily-flower*, cools the blood and the bowels, and all internal parts of the body; helps such as have the yellow jaundice, hot coughs and pleurisies, the head-ache, coming of heat, fevers pestilential and not pestilential, as also hectic fevers.

The water of *Violet flowers*, cools the blood, the heart, liver and lungs, over-heated, and quenches an insatiable desire of drinking, they are in their prime about the latter end of *March*, or beginning of *April*, according as the year falls out.

The water of *Sorrel* cools the blood, heart, liver, and spleen. If Venice Treacle be given with it, it is profitable in pestilential fevers, distil it in *May*.

Endive and *Succory* water are excellent against heat in the stomach; if you take an ounce of either (for their operation is the same) morning and evening, four days one after another, they cool the liver, and cleanse the blood: they are in their prime in *May*.

Fumitory water is usual with the city dames to wash their faces with, to take away morphew, freckles, and sun-burning; inwardly taken, it helps the yellow jaundice and itch, cleanses the blood, provokes sweat, strengthens the stomach, and cleanses the body of adust humours: it is in its prime in *May* and *June*.

The water of *Nightshade* helps pains in the head coming of heat. Take heed you distil not the deadly Nightshade instead of the common, if you do, you may make mad work. Let such as have not wit enough to know them asunder, have wit enough to let them both alone till they do.

The water of *white Poppies* extinguishes all heat against nature, helps head-aches coming of heat, and too long standing in the sun. Distil them in *June* or *July*.

Colt's-foot water is excellent for burns to wash the place with it; inwardly taken it helps Phthisicks and other diseases incident to the lungs, distil them in *May* or *June*.

The water of *Distilled Quinces* strengthens the heart and stomach exceedingly, stays vomiting and fluxes, and strengthens the retentive faculty in man.

Damask Rose water cools, comforts, and strengthens the heart, so doth Red Rose-water, only with this difference, the one is binding, the other loosening; if your body be costive, use Damask Rose water, because it is loosening: if loose, use red, because it is binding.

White Rose water is generally known to be excellent against hot rheums, and inflammations in the eyes, and for this it is better than the former.

The water of *Red Poppy flowers*, called by many Corn-roses, because they grow so frequently amongst corn, cools the blood and spirits over-heated by drinking or labour, and is therefore excellent in surfets.

Green Walnuts gathered about the latter end of *June* or *July*, and bruised, and so stilled, strengthen the heart, and resist the pestilence.

Plantain water helps the headache; being dropped into the ear it helps the tooth-ache, helps the phthisicks, dropsy and fluxes, and is an admirable remedy for ulcers in the reins and bladder, to be used as common drink: the herb is in its prime in *May*.

Strawberry water cools, quenches thirst, clarifies the blood, breaks the stone, helps all inward inflammations, especially those in the reins, bladder and passages of the urine; it strengthens the liver and helps the yellow jaundice.

The distilled water of *Dog grass*, or *Couch grass*, as some call it, cleanses the reins gallantly, and provokes urine, opens obstructions of the liver and spleen, and kills worms.

Black Cherry water provokes urine, helps the dropsy. It is usually given in diseases of the brain, as convulsions, falling-sickness, palsy and apoplexy.

Betony is in its prime in May, the distilled water thereof is very good for such as are pained in their heads, it prevails against the dropsy and all sorts of fevers, it succours the liver and spleen, and helps want of digestion and evil disposition of the body thence arising; it hastens travail in women with child, and is excellent against the bitings of venomous beasts.

Distil *Sage* whilst the flowers be on it, the water strengthens the brain, provokes the menses, helps nature much in all its actions.

Marjoram is in its prime in June, distilled water is excellent for such whose brains are too cold, it provokes urine, heats the womb, provokes the menses, strengthens the memory and helps the judgment, causes an able brain.

Distil *Camomel* water about the beginning of June. It eases the cholick and pains in the belly; it breaks the stone in the reins and bladder, provokes the menses, expels the dead child, and takes away pains in the head.

Fennel water strengthens the heart and brain; dilates the breast, the cough, provokes the menses, encreases milk in nurses, and if you wash your eyes with it, it clears the sight.

The *Hooves* of the fore feet of a Cow dried and taken any away, encrease milk in nurses, the smoke of them drives away mice. *Mizaldus*.

Calaminth water heats and cleanses the womb, provokes the menses, and eases the pains of the head, distil it in May.

The distilled water of *Rosemary flowers*, helps such as are troubled with the yellow Jaundice, Asthmas, it cleanses the blood, helps concoction, strengthens the brain and body exceedingly.

Water of the *flowers of Lilies* of the *valley*, strengthens the brain and all the senses.

The water of *Cowslip flowers* helps the palsey; takes away pains in the head, the vertigo and megrim, and is exceedingly good for pregnant women.

The eyes being washed every morning with *Eyebright* water, most strangely clears and strengthens the sight.

Maidenhair distilled in May, the water cleanses both liver and lungs, clarifies the blood, and breaks the stone.

Hyssop water cleanses the lungs of flegm, helps coughs and Asthmas, distil it in August.

The water of *Hore-hound*, helps the cough and straitness of the breast; it strengthens the breast, lungs and stomach, and liver, distil it in June.

Carduus water succours the head, strengthens the memory, helps such as are troubled with vertigoes and quartan agues, it provokes sweat, strengthens the heart, and all other fevers of choler. It is in its prime in May and June.

Scabious water helps pleurises and pains, and pricking in the sides; Aposthumes, coughs, pestilences, and straitness of the breast.

Water of *Flower-de-luce* is very profitable in dropsies, an ounce being drank continually every morning and evening; as also pains and torments in the bowels.

Bawm water distilled in May, restores memory, it quickens all the senses, strengthens the brain, heart, and stomach, causes a merry mind and a sweet breath.

The water of *Comfrey* solders broken bones, being drank, helps ruptures, outwardly it stops the bleeding of wounds, they being washed with it.

Wormwood water distilled cold, about the end of May, heats and strengthens the stomach, helps concoction, stays vomiting, kills worms in the stomach and bowels, it mitigates the pains in the teeth, and is profitably given in fevers of choler.

Mint water strengthens the stomach, helps concoction and stays vomiting, distil it in the latter end of May, or beginning of June, as the year is in forwardness or backwardness, observe that in all the rest.

Chervil water distilled about the end of May, helps ruptures, breaks the stone, dissolves congealed blood, strengthens the heart and stomach.

The water of *Mother of Time* strengthens the brain and stomach, gets a man a good stomach to his victuals, provoke urine and the menses, heats the womb. It is in its prime about the end of June.

The water of *Marigold flowers* is appropriated to most cold diseases of the head, eyes, and stomach: they are in their vigour when the Sun is in the Lion.

The distilled water of *Centaury* comforts a cold stomach, helps in fever of choler, it kills worms, and provokes appetite.

Maudlin and Costmary water distilled in May or June, strengthens the liver, helps the yellow jaundice, opens obstructions, and helps the dropsy.

Water-cresses distilled in March, the water cleanses the blood, and provokes urine exceedingly, kills worms, outwardly mixed with honey, it clears the skin of morphew and sunburning.

Distil *Nettles* when they are in flower, the water helps coughs and pains in the bowels, provokes urine, and breaks the stone.

Saxifrage water provokes urine, expels wind, breaks the stone, cleanses the reins and bladder of gravel, distil them when they are in flower.

The water of *Pellitory of the Wall*, opens obstructions of the liver and spleen, by drinking an ounce of it every morning; it cleanses the reins and bladder, and eases the gripings of the bowels coming of wind. Distil it in the end of May, or beginning of June.

Cinquefoil water breaks the stone, cleanses the reins, and is of excellent use in putrified fevers. Distil it in May.

The water of Radishes breaks the stone, cleanses the reins and bladder, provokes the menses, and helps the yellow jaundice.

Elicampane water strengthens the stomach and lungs, provokes urine, and cleanses the passages of it from gravel.

Distil *Burnet* in May or June, the water breaks the stone, cleanses the passages of urine, and is exceeding profitable in pestilential times.

Mugwort water distilled in May, is excellent in coughs and diseases proceeding from stoppage of the menses, it warms the stomach, and helps the dropsy.

Distil *Penny-royal* when the flowers are upon it: the water heats the womb gallantly, provokes the menses, expels the afterbirth; cuts, and casts out thick and gross humours in the breast, eases pains in the bowels, and consumes flegm.

The water of *Lovage* distilled in May, eases pains in the head, and cures ulcers in the womb being washed with it; inwardly taken it expels wind, and breaks the stone.

The tops of *Hops* when they are young, being distilled, the water cleanses the blood of melancholy humours, and therefore helps scabs, itch, and leprosy, and such like diseases thence proceeding; it opens obstructions of the spleen, helps the rickets, and hypo-chondriac melancholy.

The water of *Borrage and Bugloss* distilled when their flowers are upon them, strengthens the heart and brain exceedingly, cleanses the blood, and takes away sadness, griefs and melancholy.

Dodder water cleanses the liver and spleen, helps the yellow jaundice.

Tamarisk water opens obstructions, and helps the hardness of the spleen, and strengthens it.

English Tobacco distilled, the water is excellently good for such as have dropsy, to drink an ounce or two every morning; it helps ulcers in the mouth, strengthens the lungs, and helps such as have asthmas.

The water of *Dwarf Elder*, hath the same effects.

Thus you have the virtues of enough of cold waters, the use of which is for mixtures of other medicines, whose operation is the same, for they are very seldom given alone. If you delight most in liquid medicines, having regard to the disease, and part of the body afflicted by it, these will furnish you with where withal to make them so as will please your pallate best.

COMPOUNDS, SPIRIT AND COMPOUND DISTILLED WATERS

Culpeper.] Before I begin these, I thought good to premise a few words. They are all hot in operation, and therefore not to be meddled with by people of hot constitutions when they are in health, for fear of fevers and adustion of blood, but for people of cold constitutions, as melancholy and flegmatic people. If they drink of them moderately now and then for recreation, due consideration being had to the part of the body which is weakest, they may do them good: yet in diseases of melancholy, neither strong waters nor sack is to be drank, for they make the humour thin, and then up to the head it flies, where it fills the brain with foolish and fearful imaginations.

2. Let all young people forbear them whilst they are in health, for their blood is usually hot enough without them.

3. Have regard to the season of the year, so shall you find them more beneficial in Summer than in Winter, because in summer the body is always coldest within, and digestion weakest, and that is the reason why men and women eat less in Summer than in Winter.

Thus much for people in health, which drink strong waters for recreation.

As for the medicinal use of them, it shall be shewed at the latter end of every receipt, only in general they are (due respect had to the humours afflicting, and part of the body afflicted) medicinal for diseases of cold and flegm, chilliness of the spirits, &c.

But that my countrymen may not be mistaken in this, I shall give them some symptoms of each complexion how a man may know when it exceeds its due limits.

Signs of choler abounding

Leanness of body, costiveness, hollow eyes, anger without a cause, a testy disposition, yellowness of the skin, bitterness in the throat, pricking pains in the head, the pulse swifter and stronger than ordinary, the urine higher coloured, thinner and brighter, troublesome sleeps, much dreaming of fire, lightning, anger, and fighting.

Signs of blood abounding

The veins are bigger (or at least they seem so) and fuller than ordinary; the skin is red, and as it were swollen; pricking pains in the sides, and about the temples, shortness of breath, head-ache, the pulse great and full, urine high coloured and thick, dreams of blood, &c.

Signs of melancholy abounding

Fearfulness without a cause, fearful and foolish imaginations, the skin rough and swarthy, leanness, want of sleep, frightful dreams, sourness in the throat, the pulse very weak, solitariness, thin clear urine, often sighing, &c.

Signs of flegm abounding

Sleepiness, dulness, slowness, heaviness, cowardliness, forgetfulness, much spitting, much superfluities at the nose, little appetite to meat and as bad digestion, the skin whiter, colder and smoother than it was want to be; the pulse slow and deep: the urine thick and low coloured: dreams of rain, floods, and water, &c.

These things thus premised, I come to the matter.
The first the College presents you with is

Spiritus et Aqua Absinthis minus Composita
Or, Spirit and water of Wormwood, the lesser composition

College.] Take of the leaves of dryed Wormwood two pounds, Annis seeds, half a pound: steep them in six gallons of small wine twenty four hours, then distil them in an Alembick, adding to every pound of the distilled water two ounces of the best Sugar.

Let the two first pound you draw out be called Spirit of Wormwood, those which follow, Wormwood water the lesser composition.

Culpeper.] I like this distinction of the College very well, because what is first stilled out, is far stronger than the rest, and therefore very fitting to be kept by itself: you may take which you please, according as the temperature of your body, either to heat or cold, and the season of year requires.

It hath the same virtues Wormwood hath, only fitter to be used by such whose bodies are chilled by age, and whose natural heat abates. You may search the herbs for the virtues, it heats the stomach, and helps digestion.

College.] After the same manner (only omitting the Annis seeds) is distilled spirit and water of Angelica, both Herb and Root, Bawm, Mints, Sage, &c. the Flowers of Rosemary, Clary, Clove-gilliflowers, &c. the seeds of Caraway, &c. Juniper-berries, Orange Pills, Lemons, Citrons, &c. Cinnamon, Nutmegs, &c.

Spiritus et Aqua Absynthii magis composita
Or spirit and water of Wormwood, the greater composition

College.] Take of common and Roman Wormwood, of each a pound; Sage, Mints, Bawm, of each two handfuls; the Roots of Galanga, Ginger, Calamus, Aromaticus, Elecampane, of each three drachms; Liquorice, an ounce, Raisins of the Sun stoned, three ounces, Annis seeds, and sweet Fennel seeds, of each three drachms; Cinnamon, Cloves, Nutmegs, of each two drachms; Cardamoms, Cubebs, of each one drachm: let the things be cut that are to be cut, and the things be bruised that are to be bruised, all of them infused in twenty four pints of Spanish wine, for twenty four hours, then, distilled in an Alembick, adding two ounces of white sugar to every pint of distilled water.

Let the first pint be called Spirit of Wormwood the greater composition.

Culpeper.] The opinion of Authors is, That it heats the stomach, and strengthens it and the lungs, expels wind, and helps digestion in ancient people.

Spiritus et Aqua Angelica magis composita
Or Spirit and water of Angelica, the greater composition

College.] Take of the leaves of Angelica eight ounces, of Carduus Benedictus six ounces, of Bawm and Sage, of each four ounces, Angelica seeds six ounces; sweet Fennel seeds nine ounces. Let the herbs, being dryed, and the seeds be grossly bruised, to which add of the species called Aromaticum Rosarum, and of the species called Diamoschu Dulce, of each an ounce and a half, infuse them two days in thirty two pints of Spanish Wine, then distil them with a gentle fire, and with every pound mix two ounces of sugar dissolved in Rose-water.

Let the three first pounds be called by the name of Spirit, the rest by the name of water.

Culpeper.] The chief end of composing this medicine, was to strengthen the heart and resist infection, and therefore is very wholesome in pestilential times, and for such as walk in stinking air.

I shall now quote you their former receipt in their former dispensatory.

Angelica water the greater composition

College.] Take of Angelica two pounds, Annis seed half a pound, Coriander and Caraway seeds, of each four ounces, Zedoary bruised, three ounces: steep them twenty four hours in six gallons of small wine, then draw out the spirit, and sweeten it with sugar.

Culpeper.] It comforts the heart, cherishes the vital spirits, resists the pestilence, and all corrupt airs, which indeed are the natural causes of epidemical diseases, the sick may take a spoonful of it in any convenient cordial, and such as are in health, and have bodies either cold by nature, or cooled by age, may take as much either in the morning fasting, or a little before meat.

Spiritus Lavendula compositus Matthiæ
Or compound spirit of Lavender. Matthias

College.] Take of Lavender flowers one gallon, to which pour three gallons of the best spirits of wine, let them stand together in the sun six days, then distil them with an Alembick with this refrigeratory.

Take of the flowers of Sage, Rosemary, and Bettony, of each one handful; the flowers of Borrage, Bugloss, Lilies of the Valley, Cowslips, of each two handfuls: let the flowers be newly and seasonably gathered, being infused in one gallon of the best spirits of wine, and mingled with the foregoing spirit of Lavender flowers, adding the leaves of Bawm, Feather-few, and Orange tree fresh gathered; the flowers of Stœchas and Orange tree, May berries, of each one ounce. After convenient digestion distil it again, after which add Citron pills the outward bark, Peony seed husked, of each six drams, cinnamon, Mace, Nutmegs, Cardamoms, Cubebs, yellow Sanders, of each half an ounce, Wood of Aloes one dram, the best Jujubes, the stones being taken out, half a pound, digest them six weeks, then strain it and filter it, and add to it prepared Pearls two drams, Emeralds prepared a scruple, Ambergrease, Musk, Saffron, of each half a scruple, red Roses dryed, red Sanders, of each half an ounce, yellow Sanders, Citron Pills, dryed, of each one dram. Let the species being tyed up in a rag, be hung into the aforementioned spirit.

Culpeper.] I could wish the Apothecaries would desire to be certified by the College.

1. Whether the gallon of Lavender flowers must be filled by heap, or by strike. 2. Next, whether the flowers must be pressed

down in the measure or not. 3. How much must be drawn off in the first distillation. 4. Where they should get Orange leaves and flowers fresh gathered. 5. What they mean by *convenient digestion*. 6. Where you shall find Borrage, Bugloss, and Cowslips, flowering together, that so you may have them all fresh according to their prescript, the one flowering in the latter end of April, and beginning of May, the other in the end of June, and beginning of July. 7. If they can make a shift to make it, how, or which way the virtues of it will countervail the one half of the charge and cost, to leave the pains and trouble out.

Spiritus Castorii
Or Spirit of Castoreum

College.] Take of fresh Castoreum four ounces, Lavender flower an ounce, the tops of Sage and Rosemary, of each half an ounce, Cinnamon six drams, Mace, Cloves, of each two drachms, spirits of Wine rectified, six pounds, digest them in a phial filled only to the third part, close stopped with cork and bladder in warm ashes for two days, then distilled in Balneo Mariæ, and the distilled water kept close stopped.

Culpeper.] By reason of its heat it is no ways fit to be taken alone, but mixed with other convenient medicines appropriated to the diseases you would give it for, it resists poison, and helps such as are bitten by venomous beasts: it causes speedy delivery to women in travail, and casteth out the Placenta: it helps the fits of the mother, lethargies and convulsions, being mixed with white wine, and dropped into the ears, it helps deafness; if stopping be the cause of it, the dose to be given inwardly is between one dram, and half a dram, according to the strength and age of the patient.

Aqua Petasitidis composita
Or compound water of Butter-bur

College.] Take of the fresh roots of Butter-bur bruised, one pound and a half, the roots of Angelica and Masterwort, of each half a pound, steep them in ten pints of strong Ale, then distil them till the change of the taste gives a testimony that the strength is drawn out.

Culpeper.] This water is very effectual being mixed with other convenient cordials, for such as have pestilential fevers: also a spoonful taken in the morning, may prove a good preservative in pestilential times: it helps the fits of the mother, and such as are short winded, and being taken inwardly, dries up the moisture of such sores as are hard to be cured.

Aqua Raphani Composita
Or Compound water of Radishes

College.] Take of the leaves of both sorts of Scurvy-grass, of each six pound, having bruised them, press the juice out of them, with which mix of the juice of brook-lime, and Water-cresses, of each one pound and a half, of the best white wine, eight pounds, twelve whole Lemons, pills and all, fresh Briony roots four pound, the roots of wild Radishes two pound, Captain Winter's Cinnamon half a pound, Nutmegs four ounces, steep them altogether, and then distil them.

Culpeper.] I fancy it not, and so I leave it; I suppose they intended it for purgation of women in child-bed.

Aqua Peoniæ Composita
Or Compound water of Peony

College.] Take of the flowers of Lilies of the Valley, one pound: infuse them in four gallons of Spanish wine so long till the following flowers may be had fresh.

Take of the fore-named flowers half a pound, Peony flowers four ounces: steep them together fourteen days, then distil them in *Balneo Mariæ* till they be dry: in the distilled liquor infuse again male Peony roots gathered in due time, two ounces and a half, white Dittany, long Birthwort, of each half an ounce, the leaves of Misselto of the Oak, and Rue, of each two handfuls, Peony seeds husked, ten drams, Rue seeds three drams and a half, Castoreum two scruples, Cubebs, Mace, of each two drachms, Cinnamon an ounce and a half, Squills prepared, three drachms, Rosemary flowers six pugils, Arabian Stæchas, Lavender, of each four pugils, the flowers of Betony, Clove-gilliflowers, and Cowslips, of each eight pugils, then adding four pound of the juice of black Cherries, distil it in a glass till it be dry.

Aqua Bezoartica
Or Bezoar Water

College.] Take of the leaves of Celandine, roots and all, three handfuls and a half, Rue two handfuls, Scordium four handfuls, Dittany of Crete, Carduus, of each one handful and a half, Zedoary and Angelica roots, of each three drams, Citrons and Lemon pills, of each six drams, Clove-gilliflowers one ounce and a half, Red Rose, Centaury the less, of each two drams, Cinnamon, Cloves, of each three drams, Venice Treacle three ounces, Mithridates one ounce and a half, Camphire two scruples, Troches of Vipers two ounces, Mace two drams, Wood of Aloes half an ounce, Yellow Sanders one dram and a half, Carduus seeds one ounce, Citron seeds six drams, let them be cut and infused in spirits of Wine, and Malaga Wine, of each three pound and a half, Vinegar of Clove-gilliflowers, Juice of Lemons, of each one pound, and distilled in a glass still in *Balneo Mariæ*, after it is half distilled off, the residue may be strained through a linen cloath, and be reduced to the thickness of Honey, and called the Bezoartic extract.

Culpeper.] Extracts have the same virtues with the waters they are made from, only the different form is to please the palates of such whose fancy loathes any one particular form.

This Bezoar water strengthens the heart, arteries, and vital spirits. It provokes sweat, and is exceeding good in pestilential fevers, in health it withstands melancholy and consumptions, and makes a merry, blithe, chearful creature. Of the extract you may take ten grains at a time, or somewhat more, if your body be not feverish, half a spoonful of water is sufficient at a time, and that mixed with other cordials or medicines appropriated to the disease that troubles you.

Aqua et Spiritus Lambricorum, magistralis
Or Water and Spirit of Earthworms

College.] Take of Earthworms well cleansed, three pound, Snails, with shells on their backs cleansed, two gallons, beat them in a mortar, and put them into a convenient vessel, adding stinging Nettles, roots and all, six handfuls, wild Angelica, four handfuls, brank Ursine, seven handfuls, Agrimony, Bettony, of each three handfuls, Rue one handful, common Wormwood two handfuls, Rosemary flowers six ounces, Dock roots ten ounces, the roots of Sorrel five ounces, Turmerick, the inner bark of Barberries, of each four ounces, Fenugreek seeds two ounces, Cloves three ounces, Hart's-horn, Ivory in gross powder, of each four ounces, Saffron three drams, small spirits of Wine four gallons and a half, after twenty-four hours infusion, distil them in an alembick. Let the four first pounds be reserved for spirit, the rest for water.

Culpeper.] 'Tis a mess altogether, it may be they intended it for a universal medicine.

Aqua Gentianæ compositæ
Or Gentian Water compound

College.] Take of Gentain roots sliced, one pound and a half, the leaves and flowers of Centaury the less, of each four ounces, steep them eight days in twelve pounds of white Wine, then distil them in an alembick.

Culpeper.] It conduces to preservation from ill air, and pestilential fevers: it opens obstructions of the liver, and helps such as they say are liver-grown; it eases pains in the stomach, helps digestion, and eases such as have pains in their bones by ill lodging abroad in the cold, it provokes appetite, and is exceeding good for the yellow jaundice, as also for prickings or stitches in the sides: it provokes the menses, and expels both birth and placenta: it is naught for pregnant women. If there be no fever, you may take a spoonful by itself; if there be, you may, if you please, mix it with some cooler medicine appropriated to the same use you would give it for.

Aqua Gilbertii
Or Gilbert's Water

College.] Take of Scabious, Burnet, Dragons, Bawm, Angelica, Pimpernel, with purple flowers, Tormentil, roots and all, of each two handfuls, let all of them, being rightly gathered and prepared, be steeped in four gallons of Canary Wine, still off three gallons in an alembick, to which add three ounces of each of the cordial flowers, Clove-gilliflowers six ounces, Saffron half an ounce, Turmerick two ounces, Galanga, Bazil seeds, of each one dram, Citron pills one ounce, the seed of Citrons and Carduus, Cloves of each five ounces, Hart's-horn four ounces, steep them twenty four hours and then distil them in *Balneo Mariæ*: to the distilled water add Pearls prepared, an ounce and a half, red Coral, Crabs eyes, white Amber, of each two drams, Crabs claws, six drams, Bezoar, Ambergrease, of each two scruples, steep them six weeks in the sun, in a vessel well stopped, often shaking it, then filter it, (you may keep the powders for Spicord. temp.) by mixing twelve ounces of Sugar candy, with six ounces of red Rose-water, and four ounces of spirit of Cinnamon with it.

Culpeper.] I suppose this was invented for a cordial to strengthen the heart, to relieve languishing nature. It is exceeding dear. I forbear the dose, they that have money enough to make it themselves, cannot want time to study both the virtues and dose. I would have gentlemen to be studious.

Aqua cordialis frigida Saxeniæ

College.] Take of the juice of Borrage, Bugloss, Bawm, Bistort, Tormentil, Scordium, Vervain, sharp-pointed Dock, Sorrel, Goat's Rue, Mirrhis, Blue Bottle great and small, Roses, Marigolds,

Lemon, Citrons, of each three ounces, white Wine Vinegar one pound, Purslain seeds two ounces, Citron and Carduus seeds, of each half an ounce, Water Lily flowers two ounces, the flowers of Borrage, Bugloss, Violets, Clove-gilliflowers, of each one ounce, Diatrion Sentalon six drams: let all of them, being rightly prepared, be infused three days, then distilled in a glass still: to the distilled Liquor add earth of Lemnos, Siletia, and Samos, of each one ounce and an half, Pearls prepared with the juice of Citrons, three drams, mix them, and keep them together.

Culpeper.] It mightily cools the blood, and therefore profitable in fevers, and all diseases proceeding of heat of blood; it provokes sleep. You may take half an ounce at a time, or two drams if the party be weak.

Aqua Theriacalis
Or Treacle Water

College.] Take of the juice of green Walnuts, four pounds, the juice of Rue three pounds, juice of Carduus, Marigolds, and Bawm, of each two pounds, green Petasitis roots one pound and a half, the roots of Burs one pound, Angelica and Master-wort, of each half a pound, the leaves of Scordium four handfuls, old Venice Treacle, Mithridates, of each eight ounces, Canary Wine twelve pounds, Vinegar six pounds, juice of Lemons two pounds, digest them two days, either in Horse-dung, or in a bath, the vessel being close shut, then distil them in sand; in the distillation you may make a Theriacal extraction.

Culpeper.] This water is exceeding good in all fevers, especially pestilential; it expels venomous humours by sweat; it strengthens the heart and vitals; it is an admirable counter-poison, special good for such as have the plague, or are poisoned, or bitten by venomous beasts, and expels virulent humours from such as have the venereal disease. If you desire to know more virtues of it, see the virtues of Venice Treacle. The dose is from a spoonful to an ounce.

Aqua Brioniæ composita
Or Briony Water compound

College.] Take of the juice of Briony roots, four pounds, the leaves of Rue and Mugwort, of each two pounds, dryed Savin three handfuls, Featherfew, Nep, Pennyroyal, of each two handfuls, Bazil, Dittany, of Crete, of each one handful and a half, Orange pills four ounces, Myrrh two ounces, Castoreum one ounce, Canary Wine twelve pounds, digest them four days in a convenient vessel, then still them in *Balneo Mariæ*. About the middle of the distillation strain it out, and make an Hysterical extraction of the residue.

Culpeper.] A spoonful of it taken, eases the fits of the mother in women that have them; it potently expels the afterbirth, and clears the body of what a midwife by heedlessness or accident hath left behind; it cleanses the womb exceedingly, and for that I fancy it much, take not above a tasterful at a time, and then in the morning fasting, for it is of a purging quality, and let pregnant women forbear it.

Aqua Imperialis
Or Imperial Water

College.] Take of dried Citron, and Orange pills, Nutmegs, Cloves, Cinnamon, of each two ounces, the roots of Cypress, Orris, Florentine, Calamus Aromaticus, of each one ounce, Zedoary Galanga, Ginger, of each half an ounce, the tops of Lavender and Rosemary, of each two handfuls, the leaves of Bay, Marjoram, Bawm, Mints, Sage, Thyme, of each one handful, the flowers of white and Damask Roses fresh, of each half a handful, Rosewater four pounds, white Wine eight pounds, let all of them be bruised and infused twenty four hours, then distil them according to art.

Culpeper.] You must distil it in a bath, and not in sand. It comforts and strengthens the heart against faintings and swoonings, and is held to be a preservative against consumptions and apoplexies. You may take half a spoonful at a time.

Aqua Mirabilis

College.] Take of Cloves, Galanga, Cubebs, Mace, Cardamoms, Nutmegs, Ginger, of each one dram, Juice of Celandine half a pound, spirits of Wine one pound, white Wine three pounds, infuse them twenty-four hours, and draw off two pounds with an alembick.

Culpeper.] The simples also of this, regard the stomach, and therefore the water heats cold stomachs, besides authors say it preserves from apoplexies, and restores lost speech.

Aqua Protheriacalis

College.] Take of Scordium, Scabius, Carduus, Goat's Rue, of each two handfuls, Citron and Orange pills, of each two ounces, the seeds of Citrons, Carduus, Hartwort, Treacle Mustard, of each one ounce, the flowers of Marigolds and Rosemary, of each one handful, cut them, and bruise them grossly, then infuse them in four pounds of white Wine, and two pounds of Carduus water, in a glass, close stopped, and set it in the sun or bath for a fortnight, often shaking it, then distil it in *Balneo Mariæ*. Let the two first pounds be kept by themselves for use, and the remainder of the distillation by itself. Lastly, mix one ounce of Julep of Alexandria, and a spoonful of Cinnamon water with each pound.

Culpeper.] *Aqua Protheriacalis*, signifies a water for Treacle, so then if you put Diascoridum to it, it is a water for Diascoridum; well then, we will take it for a general water for all physick.

Aqua Caponis
Or Capon Water

College.] Take a Capon the guts being pulled out, cut in pieces, the fat being taken away, boiled in a sufficient quantity of spring-water in a close vessel, take of this broth three pounds. Borrage and Violet-water, of each a pound and a half, white Wine one pound, red rose leaves two drams and an half, the flowers of Borrage, Violets and Bugloss, of each one dram, pieces of bread, hot out of the oven, half a pound, Cinnamon bruised, half an ounce, distil it in a glass still according to art.

Culpeper.] The simples are most of them appropriated to the heart, and in truth the composition greatly nourishes and strengthens such as are in consumptions, and restores lost strength, either by fevers or other sickness. It is a sovereign remedy for hectic fevers, and Marasmos, which is nothing else but a consumption coming from them. Let such as are subject to these diseases, hold it for a jewel.

Aqua Limacum Magistr.
Or Water of Snails

College.] Take of the juice of Ground Ivy, Colt's-foot, Scabious, Lungwort, of each one pound and a half, the juice of Purslain, Plantain, Ambrosia, Paul's Bettony, of each a pound, Hog's blood, white Wine, of each four pounds, Garden Snails, two pounds, dried Tobacco leaves eight, powder of Liquorice two ounces, of Elecampane half an ounce, of Orris an ounce, Cotton seeds an ounce and a half, the greater cold seeds, Annis seeds of each six drams, Saffron one dram, the flowers of red Roses, six pugils, of Violets and Borrage, of each four pugils, steep them three days warm, and then distil them in a glass still, in sand.

Culpeper.] It purges the lungs of flegm and helps consumptions there. If you should happen to live where no better nor readier medicine can be gotten, you may use this.

Aqua Scordii composita
Or Compound Water of Scordium

College.] Take of the juice of Goat's Rue, Sorrel, Scordium, Citrons, of each one pound, London Treacle, half a pound, steep it three days, and distil it in sand.

Culpeper.] A tasterful taken in the morning, preserves from ill airs.

Aqua Mariæ

College.] Take of Sugar Candy a pound, Canary Wine six ounces, Rose Water four ounces; boil it well into a Syrup, and add to it Imperial water two pounds, Ambergreese, Musk, of each eighteen grains, Saffron fifteen grains, yellow Sanders infused in Imperial water, two drams; make a clear water of it.

Aqua Papaveries composita
Or Poppy Water compound

College.] Take of red Poppies four pounds, sprinkle them with white Wine two pounds, then distil them in a common still, let the distilled water be poured upon fresh flowers and repeated three times; to which distilled water add two Nutmegs sliced, red Poppy flowers a pugil, Sugar two ounces, set it in the sun to give it a pleasing sharpness; if the sharpness be more than you would have it, put some of the same water to it which was not set in the sun.

Aqua Juglandium composita
Or Walnut Water compound

College.] Take of green Walnuts a pound and an half, Radish roots one pound, green Asarabacca six ounces, Radish seeds, six ounces. Let all of them, being bruised, be steeped in three pounds of white Wine for three days, then distilled in a leaden still till they be dry.

TINCTURES
Tinctura Croci
Or Tincture of Saffron

College.] Take two drams of Saffron, eight ounces of Treacle water, digest them six days, then strain it.

Culpeper.] See the virtues of Treacle water, and then know that this strengthens the heart something more, and keeps melancholy vapours thence by drinking a spoonful of it every morning.

Tinctura Castorii
Or Tincture of Castoreum

College.] Take of Castoreum in powder half an ounce, spirit of Castoreum half a pound, digest them ten days cold, strain it, and keep the Liquor for Tincture.

Culpeper.] A learned invention! 'Tis something more prevalent than the spirit.

Tinctura Fragroram
Or Tincture of Strawberries

College.] Take of ripe Wood-strawberries two pounds, put them in a phial, and put so much small spirits of Wine to them, that it may overtop them the thickness of four fingers, stop the vessel close, and set it in the sun two days, then strain it, and press it but gently; pour this spirit to as many fresh Strawberries, repeat this six times, at last keep the clear liquor for your use.

Culpeper.] A fine thing for Gentlemen that have nothing else to do with their money, and it will have a lovely look to please their eyes.

Tinctura Scordii
Or Tincture of Scordium

College.] Take of the leaves of Scordium gathered in a dry time, half a pound, digest them in six pounds of small spirits of Wine, in a vessel well stopped, for three days, press them out gently, and repeat the infusion three times, and keep the clarified liquor for use.

So is made Tincture of Celandine, Restharrow, and Rosa-solis.

Culpeper.] See the herbs for the virtues, and then take notice that these are better for cold stomachs, old bodies.

Tinctura Theriacalis vulgo Aqua Theriacalis Ludg. per infus.
Or Tincture of Treacle

College.] Take of Canary Wine often times distilled, Vinegar in which half an ounce of Rue seeds have been boiled, two pounds choice treacle, the best Mithridate, of each half a pound; mix them and set them in the sun, or heat of a bath, digest them, and keep the water for use.

Tinctura Cinnamoni, vulgo, Aqua Clareta Cinnam.
Or Tincture of Cinnamon

College.] Take of bruised Cinnamon two ounces, rectified spirits of Wine two pounds, infuse them four days in a large glass stopped with cork and bladder, shake it twice a day, then dissolve half a pound of Sugar Candy by itself in two pounds of Rose Water, mix both liquors, into which hang a nodule containing, Ambergris half a scruple, Musk four grains.

Tinctura Viridis
Or a green Tincture

College.] Take of Verdigris, half an ounce, Auripigmentum six drams, Alum three drams, boil them in a pound of white Wine till half be consumed, adding, after it is cold, the water of red Roses, and Nightshade, of each six ounces.

Culpeper.] This was made to cleanse ulcers, but I fancy it not.

Aqua Aluminosa Magistralis

College.] Take of Plantain and red Rose water, of each a pound, roch Alum and Sublimatum, of each two drams; let the Alum and Sublimatum, being in powder, boil in the waters, in a vessel with a narrow mouth till half be consumed, when it has stood five days, strain it.

PHYSICAL WINES

Vinum Absynthitis
Or Wormwood Wine

College.] Take a handful of dried Wormwood, for every gallon of Wine, stop it in a vessel close, and so let it remain in steep: so is prepared wine of Rosemary flowers, and Eye-bright.

Culpeper.] It helps cold stomachs, breaks wind, helps the wind cholic, strengthens the stomach, kills worms, and helps the green sickness.

Rosemary-flower Wine, is made after the same manner. It is good against all cold diseases of the head, consumes flegm, strengthens the gums and teeth.

Eye-bright Wine is made after the same manner. It wonderfully clears the sight being drank, and revives the sight of elderly men. A cup of it in the morning is worth a pair of spectacles.

All other Wines are prepared in the same manner.

The best way of taking any of these Wines is, to drink a draught of them every morning. You may, if you find your body old or cold, make Wine of any other herb, the virtues of which you desire; and make it and take it in the same manner.

Vinum Cerassorum Nigrorum
Or Wine of Black Cherries

College.] Take a gallon of Black Cherries, keep it in a vessel close stopped till it begin to work, then filter it, and an ounce of Sugar being added to every pound, let it pass through Hippocrates' sleeve, and keep in a vessel close stopped for use.

Vinum Helleboratum
Or Helleborated Wine

College.] Take of white Hellebore cut small, four ounces, Spanish Wine two pounds, steep it in the sun in a phial close stopped, in the dog days, or other hot weather.

Vinum Rubellum

College.] Take of Stibium, in powder, one ounce, Cloves sliced two drams, Claret Wine two pounds, keep it in a phial close shut.

Vinum Benedictum

College.] Take of Crocus Metallorum, in powder, one ounce, Mace one dram, Spanish Wine one pound and an half, steep it.

Vinum Antimoniale
Or Antimonial Wine

College.] Take of Regulus of Antimony, in powder, four ounces, steep it in three pounds of white Wine in a glass well stopped, after the first shaking let the Regulus settle.

Culpeper.] These last mentioned are vomits, and vomits are fitting medicines for but a few, the mouth being ordained to take in nourishment, not to cast out excrements, and to regulate a man's body in vomiting; and doses of vomits require a deeper study in physic, than I doubt the generality of people yet have; I omit it therefore at this time, not because I grudge it my country, but because I would not willingly have them do themselves a mischief. I shall shortly teach them in what diseases vomits may be used, and then, and not till then, the use of vomits.

Vinum Scilliticum
Or Wine of Squills

College.] Take of a white Squill of the mountains, gathered about the rising of the dog star, cut it in thin pieces, and dried for a month, one pound, put it in a glass bottle, and pour to it eight pounds of French Wine, and when it hath stood so four days, take out the Squill.

The virtues of this are the same with Vinegar of Squills, only it is hotter.

PHYSICAL VINEGARS
Acetum distillatum
Or distilled Vinegar

College.] Fill a glass or stone alembick with the best Vinegar to the third part, separate the flegm with a gentle fire, then increase the fire by degrees, and perform the work.

Acetum Rosarum
Or Rose Vinegar

College.] Take of red Rose buds, gathered in a dry time, the whites cut off, dried in the shade three or four days, one pound, Vinegar eight sextaries, set them in the sun forty days, then strain out the Roses, and repeat the infusion with fresh ones.

After the same manner is made Vinegar of Elder flowers, Rosemary flowers, and Clove-gilliflowers.

Culpeper.] For the virtues of all Vinegars, take this one only observation, They carry the same virtues with the flowers whereof they are made, only as we said of Wines, that they were better for cold bodies then the bare simples whereof they are made; so are Vinegars for hot bodies. Besides, Vinegars are often, nay, most commonly used externally, viz. to bathe the place, then look amongst the simples, and see what place of the body the simple is appropriated to, and you cannot but know both what Vinegar to use, and to what place to apply it.

Acetum Scilliticum
Or Vinegar of Squils

College.] Take of that part of the Squill which is between the outward bark and the bottom, cut in thin slices, and placed thirty or forty days in the sun or some remiss heat, then a pound of them (being cut small with a knife made of ivory or some white wood) being put in a vessel, and six pounds of Vinegar put to them; set the vessel, being close stopped, in the sun thirty or forty days, afterwards strain it, and keep it for use.

Culpeper.] A little of this medicine being taken in the morning fasting, and walking half an hour after, preserves the body in health, to extreme old age, (as *Sanius* tried, who using no other medicine but this, lived in perfect health till one hundred and seventeen years of age) it makes the digestion good, a long wind, a clear voice, an acute sight, a good colour, it suffers no offensive thing to remain in the body, neither wind, flegm, choler, melancholy, dung, nor urine, but brings them forth; it brings forth filth though it lie in the bones, it takes away salt and sour belchings, though a man be never so licentious in diet, he shall feel no harm. It hath cured such as have the phthisic, that have been given over by all Physicians. It cures such as have the falling sickness, gouts, and diseases and swellings of the joints. It takes away the hardness of the liver and spleen. We should never have done if we should reckon up the particular benefits of this medicine. Therefore we commend it as a wholesome medicine for soundness of body, preservation of health, and vigour of mind. Thus *Galen*.

Acetum Theriacale, Norimberg
Or Treacle Vinegar

College.] Take of the roots of Celandine the greater, one ounce and a half: the roots of Angelica, Masterwort, Gentian, Bistort, Valerian, Burnet, white Dittany, Elecampane, Zedoary, of each one dram, of Plantain the greater one dram and a half, the leaves of Mousear, Sage, Scabious, Scordium, Dittany of Crete, Carduus, of each half an handful, barks and seeds of Citrons, of each half a dram, Bole Amoniac one dram, Saffron three drams, of these let the Saffron, Hart's-horn, Dittany, and Bole, be tied up in a rag, and steeped with the things before mentioned, in five pints of Vinegar, for certain days by a temperate heat in a glass well stopped, strain it, and add six drams of the best Treacle to it, shake it together, and keep it for your use.

Acetum Theriacale
Or Treacle Vinegar

College.] Add to the description of Treacle water, Clove-gilli-flowers two ounces, Lavender flowers an ounce and a half, Rose, and Elder flower Vinegar, of each four pounds, digest it without boiling, three days, then strain it through Hippocrates' sleeve.

Culpeper.] See Treacle Water for the virtues, only this is more cool, a little more fantastical.

DECOCTIONS

Decoctum commune pro clystere
Or a common Decoction for a Clyster.

College.] Take of Mallows, Violets, Pellitory, Beets, and Mercury, Chamomel flowers, of each one handful, sweet Fennel seeds half an ounce, Linseeds two drams, boil them in a sufficient quantity of common water to a pound.

Culpeper.] This is the common decoction for all clysters, according to the quality of the humour abounding, so you may add what Simples, or Syrups, or Electuaries you please; only half a score Linseeds, and a handful of Chamomel flowers are added.

Decoctum Epythimi
Or a Decoction of Epithimum

College.] Take of Myrobalans, Chebs, and Inds, of each half an ounce, Stœchas, Raisins of the sun stoned, Epithimum, Senna, of each one ounce, Fumitory half an ounce, Maudlin five drams, Polipodium, six drams, Turbith half an ounce, Whey made with Goat's milk, or Heifer's milk four pounds, let them all boil to two pounds, the Epithimum excepted, which boil but a second or two, then take it from the fire, and add black Hellebore one dram and an half, Agerick half a dram, Sal. Gem. one dram and an half, steep them ten hours, then press it strongly out.

Culpeper.] It purges melancholy, as also choler, it resists madness, and all diseases coming of melancholy, and therefore let melancholy people esteem it as a jewel.

Decoctum Sennæ Gereonis
Or a Decoction of Senna

College.] Take of Senna two ounces, Pollipodium half an ounce, Ginger one dram, Raisins of the sun stoned two ounces, Sebestens,

Prunes, of each twelve, the flowers of Borrage, Violets, Roses, and Rosemary, of each two drams, boil them in four pounds of water till half be consumed.

Culpeper.] It is a common Decoction for any purge, by adding other simples or compounds to it, according to the quality of the humour you would have purged, yet, in itself, it chiefly purges melancholy.

Decoctum Pectorale
Or a Pectoral Decoction

College.] Take of Raisins of the sun stoned, an ounce, Sebestens, Jujubes, of each fifteen, Dates six, Figs four, French Barley one ounce, Liquorice half an ounce, Maiden-hair, Hyssop, Scabious, Colt's-foot, of each one handful, boil them in three pounds of water till two remain.

Culpeper.] The medicine is chiefly appropriated to the lungs, and therefore causes a clear voice, a long wind, resists coughs, hoarseness, asthmas, &c. You may drink a quarter of a pint of it every morning, without keeping to any diet, for it purges not.

I shall quote some Syrups fitting to be mixed with it, when I come to the Syrups.

Decoctum Trumaticum

College.] Take of Agrimony, Mugwort, wild Angelica, St. John's Wort, Mousear, of each two handfuls, Wormwood half a handful, Southernwood, Bettony, Bugloss, Comfrey the greater and lesser, roots and all, Avens, both sorts of Plantain, Sanicle, Tormentil with the roots, the buds of Barberries and Oak, of each a handful, all these being gathered in May and June and diligently dried, let them be cut and put up in skins or papers against the time of use, then take of the forenamed herbs three handfuls, boil them in four pounds of conduit water and two pounds of white Wine gently till half be consumed, strain it, and a pound of Honey being added to it, let it be scummed and kept for use.

Culpeper.] If sight of a medicine will do you good, this is as like to do it as any I know.

SYRUPS

ALTERING SYRUPS

Culpeper.] Reader, before we begin with the particular Syrups, I think good to advertise thee of these few things, which concern the nature, making, and use of Syrups in general. 1. A Syrup is a medicine of a liquid body, compounded of Decoction, Infusion, or Juice, with Sugar or Honey, and brought by the heat of the fire, into the thickness of Honey. 2. Because all Honey is not of a thickness, understand new Honey, which of all other is thinnest. 3. The reason why Decoctions, Infusions, Juices, are thus used, is, Because thereby, First, They will keep the longer. Secondly, They will taste the better. 4. In boiling Syrups have a great care of their just consistence, for if you boil them too much they will candy, if too little, they will sour.

All simple Syrups have the virtues of the simples they are made of, and are far more convenient for weak people, and delicate stomachs.

Syrupus de Absinthio simplex
Or Syrup of Wormwood simple

College.] Take of the clarified Juice of common Wormwood, clarified Sugar, of each four pounds, make it into a Syrup according to art. After the same manner, are prepared simple Syrups of Betony, Borrage, Bugloss, Carduus, Chamomel, Succory, Endive, Hedge-mustard, Strawberries, Fumitory, Ground Ivy, St. John's Wort, Hops, Mercury, Mousear, Plantain, Apples, Purslain, Rasberries, Sage, Scabious, Scordium, Houseleek, Colt's-foot, Paul's Bettony, and other Juices not sour.

Culpeper.] See the simples, and then you may easily know both their virtues, and also that they are pleasanter and fitter for delicate stomachs when they are made into Syrups.

Syrupus de Absinthio Compositus
Or Syrup of Wormwood compound

College.] Take of common Wormwood meanly dry, half a pound, red Roses two ounces, Indian Spikenard three drams, old white Wine, juice of Quinces, of each two pounds and an half, steep them a whole day in an earthen vessel, then boil them gently, and strain it, and by adding two pounds of sugar, boil it into a Syrup according to art.

Culpeper.] *Mesue* is followed verbatim in this; and the receipt is appropriated to cold and flegmatic stomachs, and it is an admirable remedy for it, for it strengthens both stomach and liver, as also the instruments of concoction, a spoonful taken in the morning, is admirable for such as have a weak digestion, it provokes an appetite to one's victuals, it prevails against the yellow jaundice, breaks wind, purges humours by urine.

Syrupus de Acetosus simplex
Or Syrup of Vinegar simple

College.] Take of clear Water four pounds, white Sugar five pounds, boil them in a glazed vessel over a gentle fire, scumming it till half the water be consumed, then by putting in two pounds of white Wine Vinegar by degrees, perfect the Syrup.

Culpeper.] That is, only melt the Sugar with the Vinegar over the fire, scum it, but boil it not.

Syrupus Acetosus simplicior
Or Syrup of Vinegar more simple

College.] Take of white Sugar five pounds, white Wine Vinegar two pounds, by melting it in a bath, make it into a Syrup.

Culpeper.] Of these two Syrups let every one use which he finds by experience to be best; the difference is but little. They both of them cut flegm, as also tough, hard viscous humours in the stomach; they cool the body, quench thirst, provoke urine, and prepare the stomach before the taking of a vomit. If you take it as a preparative for an emetic, take half an ounce of it when you go to bed the night before you intend it to operate, it will work the easier, but if for any of the foregoing occasions, take it with a liquorice stick.

Syrupus Acetosus compositus
Or Syrup of Vinegar compound

College.] Take of the roots of Smallage, Fennel, Endive, of each three ounces, the seeds of Annis, Smallage, Fennel, of each one ounce, of Endive half an ounce, clear Water six pounds, boil it gently in an earthen vessel till half the water be consumed, then strain and clarify it, and with three pounds of Sugar, and a pound and a half of white Wine Vinegar, boil it into a Syrup.

Culpeper.] This in my opinion is a gallant Syrup for such whose bodies are stuffed either with flegm, or tough humours, for it opens obstructions or stoppings both of the stomach, liver, spleen, and reins; it cuts and brings away tough flegm and choler, and is therefore a special remedy for such as have a stuffing at their stomach.

Syrupus de Agno Casto
Or Syrup of Agnus Castus

College.] Take of the seeds of Rue and Hemp, of each half a dram, of Endive, Lettice, Purslain, Gourds, Melons, of each two drams, of Fleawort half an ounce, of Agnus Castus four ounces, the flowers of Water Lilies, the leaves of Mints, of each half a handful, decoction of seeds of Lentils, and Coriander seeds, of each half an ounce, three pounds of the decoction, boil them all over a gentle fire till two pounds be consumed, add to the residue, being strained, two ounces of juice of Lemons, a pound and a half of white sugar, make it into a Syrup according to art.

Culpeper.] A pretty Syrup, and good for little.

Syrupus de Althæa
Or Syrup of Marsh-mallows

College.] Take of roots of Marsh-mallows, two ounces, the roots of Grass Asparagus, Liquorice, Raisins of the Sun stoned, of each half an ounce, the tops of Mallows, Marsh-mallows, Pellitory of the Wall, Burnet, Plantain, Maiden-hair white and black, of each a handful, red Cicers an ounce, of the four greater and four lesser cold seeds, of each three drams, boil them in six pounds of clear Water till four remain, which being strained, boil into a syrup with four pounds of white sugar.

Culpeper.] It is a fine cooling, opening, slipery Syrup, and chiefly commendable for the cholic, stone, or gravel, in the kidneys or bladder.

Syrupus de Ammoniaca
Or Syrup of Ammoniacum

College.] Take of Maudlin and Cetrach, of each four handfuls, common Wormwood an ounce, the roots of Succory, Sparagus, bark of Caper roots, of each two ounces, after due preparation steep them twenty-four hours in three ounces of white Wine, Radish and Fumitory water, of each two pounds, then boil it away to one pound eight ounces, let it settle, in four ounces of which, whilst it is warm, dissolve by itself Gum Ammoniacum, first dissolved in white Wine Vinegar, two ounces, boil the rest with a pound and an half of white sugar into a Syrup, adding the mixtures of the Gum at the end.

Culpeper.] It cools the liver, and opens obstructions both of it and the spleen, helps old surfeits, and such like diseases, as scabs, itch, leprosy, and what else proceed from the liver over heated. You may take an ounce at a time.

Syrupus de Artemisia
Or Syrup of Mugwort

College.] Take of Mugwort two handfuls, Pennyroyal, Calaminth, Origanum, Bawm, Arsmart, Dittany of Crete, Savin, Marjoram,

Germander, St. John's Wort, Camepitis, Featherfew with the flowers, Centaury the less, Rue, Bettony, Bugloss, of each a handful, the roots of Fennel, Smallage, Parsley, Sparagus, Bruscus, Saxifrage, Elecampane, Cypress, Madder, Orris, Peony, of each an ounce, Juniper Berries, the seeds of Lovage, Parsley, Smallage, Annis, Nigella, Carpobalsamum or Cubebs, Costus, Cassia Lignea, Cardamoms, Calamus Aromaticus, the roots of Asarabacca, Pellitory of Spain, Valerian, of each half an ounce, being cleansed, cut, and bruised, let them be infused twenty-four hours in fourteen pounds of clear water, and boiled till half be consumed, being taken off from the fire, and rubbed between your hands whilst it is warm, strain it, and with honey and sugar, of each two pounds, sharp Vinegar four ounces, boil it to a Syrup, and perfume it with Cinnamon and Spikenard, of each three drams.

Culpeper.] It helps the passion of the matrix, and retains it in its place, it dissolves the coldness, wind, and pains thereof, it strengthens the nerves, opens the pores, corrects the blood, it corrects and provokes the menses. You may take a spoonful of it at a time.

Syrupus de Betonica compositus
Or Syrup of Bettony compound

College.] Take of Bettony three handfuls, Marjoram four handfuls and a half, Thyme, red Roses, of each a handful, Violets, Stœchas, Sage, of each half a handful, the seeds of Fennel, Annis, and Ammi, of each half an ounce, the roots of Peons, Polypodium, and Fennel, of each five drams, boil them in six pounds of river water, to three pounds, strain it, and add juice of Bettony two pounds, sugar three pounds and a half, make it into a Syrup.

Culpeper.] It helps diseases coming of cold, both in the head and stomach, as also such as come of wind, vertigos, madness; it concocts melancholy, it provokes the menses, and so doth the simple Syrup more than the compound.

Syrupus Byzantinus, simple

College.] Take of the Juice of the leaves of Endive and Smallage, of each two pounds, of Hops and Bugloss, of each one pound, boil them together and scum them, and to the clarified liquor, add four pounds of white sugar, to as much of the juices, and with a gentle fire boil it to a Syrup.

Syrupus Byzantinus, compound

College.] Take of the Juices so ordered as in the former, four pounds, in which boil red Roses, two ounces, Liquorice half an ounce, the seeds of Annis, Fennel, and Smallage, of each three drams, Spikenard two drams, strain it, and to the three pounds remaining, add two pounds of Vinegar, four pounds of Sugar, make it into a syrup according to art.

Culpeper.] They both of them (viz. both Simple and Compound) open stoppings of the stomach, liver, and spleen, help the rickets in children, cut and bring away tough flegm, and help the yellow jaundice. You may take them with a Liquorice stick, or take a spoonful in the morning fasting.

Syrupus Botryos
Or Syrup of Oak of Jerusalem

College.] Take of Oak of Jerusalem, Hedge-mustard, Nettles, of each two handfuls, Colt's-foot, one handful and a half, boil them in a sufficient quantity of clear water till half be consumed; to two pounds of the Decoction, add two pounds of the Juice of Turnips baked in an oven in a close pot, and with three pounds of white sugar, boil it into a Syrup.

Culpeper.] This Syrup was composed against coughs, shortness of breath, and other the like infirmities of the breast proceeding of cold, for which (if you can get it) you may take it with a Liquorice stick.

Syrupus Capillorum Veneris
Or Syrup of Maiden-hair

College.] Take of Liquorice two ounces, Maiden-hair five ounces, steep them a natural day in four pounds of warm water, then after gentle boiling, and strong straining, with a pound and a half of fine sugar make it into a Syrup.

Culpeper.] It opens stoppings of the stomach, strengthens the lungs, and helps the infirmities of them. This may be taken also either with a Liquorice stick, or mixed with the Pectoral Decoction like Syrup of Coltsfoot.

Syrupus Cardiacus, vel Julepum Cardiacum
Or a Cordial Syrup

College.] Take of Rhenish Wine two pounds, Rose Water two ounces and a half, Cloves two scruples, Cinnamon half a dram,

Ginger, two scruples, Sugar three ounces and a half, boil it to the consistence of a Julep, adding Ambergris three grains, Musk one grain.

Culpeper.] If you would have this Julep keep long, you may put in more sugar, and yet if close stopped, it will not easily corrupt because it is made up only of Wine, indeed the wisest way is to order the quantity of sugar according to the palate of him that takes it. It restores such as are in consumptions, comforts the heart, cherishes the drooping spirits, and is of an opening quality, thereby carrying away those vapours which might otherwise annoy the brain and heart. You may take an ounce at a time, or two if you please.

Syrupus infusionis florum Cariophillorum
Or Syrup of Clove-gilliflowers

College.] Take a pound of Clove-gilliflowers, the whites being cut off, infuse them a whole night in two pounds of water, then with four pounds of sugar melted in it, make it into a Syrup without boiling.

Culpeper.] This Syrup is a fine temperate Syrup: it strengthens the heart, liver, and stomach; it refreshes the vital spirits, and is a good cordial in fevers; and usually mixed with other cordials, you can hardly err in taking it, it is so harmless a Syrup.

Syrupus de Cinnamomo
Or Syrup of Cinnamon

College.] Take of Cinnamon grossly bruised, four ounces, steep it in white Wine, and small Cinnamon Water, of each half a pound, three days, in a glass, by a gentle heat; strain it, and with a pound and a half of sugar, boil it gently to a Syrup.

Culpeper.] It refreshes the vital spirits exceedingly, and cheers both heart and stomach languishing through cold, it helps digestion exceedingly, and strengthens the whole body. You may take a spoonful at a time in a cordial.

College.] Thus also you may conveniently prepare Syrups (but only with white Wine,) of Annis seeds, sweet Fennel seeds, Cloves, Nutmegs, Ginger, &c.

Syrupus Acetositatis Citriorum
Or Syrup of Juice of Citrons

College.] Take of the Juice of Citrons, strained without expression, and cleansed, a pound, Sugar two pounds, make it into a Syrup like Syrup of Clove-gilliflowers.

Culpeper.] It prevails against all diseases proceeding from choler, or heat of blood, fevers, both pestilential, and not pestilential: it resists poison, cools the blood, quenches thirst, cures the vertigo, or dizziness in the head.

College.] After the same manner is made Syrups of Grapes, Oranges, Barberries, Cherries, Quinces, Lemons, Wood-sorrel, Mulberries, Sorrel, English Currants, and other sour Juices.

Culpeper.] If you look the simples you may see the virtues of them: they all cool and comfort the heart, and strengthen the stomach, Syrup of Quinces stays vomiting, so doth all Syrup of Grapes.

Syrupus Corticum Citriorum
Or Syrup of Citron Pills

College.] Take of fresh yellow Citron Pills five ounces, the berries of Chermes, or the juice of them brought over to us two drams, Spring Water four pounds, steep them all night, boil them till half be consumed, taking off the scum, strain it, and with two pounds and a half of sugar boil it into a Syrup: let half of it be without Musk, but perfume the other half with three grains of Musk tied up in a rag.

Culpeper.] It strengthens the stomach, resists poison, strengthens the heart, and resists the passions thereof, palpitation, faintings, swoonings; it strengthens the vital spirits, restores such as are in consumptions, and hectic fevers, and strengthens nature much. You may take a spoonful at a time.

Syrupus e Coralliis simplex
Or Syrup of Coral simple

College.] Take of red Coral in very fine powder four ounces, dissolve it in clarified juice of Barberries in the heat of a bath, a pound, in a glass well stopped with wax and cork, a digestion being made three or four days, pour off what is dissolved, put in fresh clarified juice, and proceed as before, repeat this so often till all the coral be dissolved; lastly, to one pound of this juice add a pound and a half of sugar, and boil it to a Syrup gently.

Syrupus e Coralliis compositus
Or Syrup of Coral compound

College.] Take of red Coral six ounces, in very fine powder, and levigated upon a marble, add of clarified juice of Lemons, the flegm being drawn off in a bath, sixteen ounces, clarified juice of Barberries, eight ounces, sharp white Wine Vinegar, and juice of Wood-sorrel, of each six ounces, mix them together, and put them in a glass stopped with cork and bladder, shaking it every day till it have digested eight days in a bath, or horse dung, then filter it, of which take a pound and a half, juice of Quinces half a pound, sugar of Roses twelve ounces, make them into a Syrup in a bath, adding Syrup of Clove-gilliflowers sixteen ounces, keep it for use, omitting the half dram of Ambergris, and four grains of Musk till the physician command it.

Culpeper.] Syrup of Coral both simple and compound, restore such as are in consumptions, are of a gallant cooling nature, especially the last, and very cordial, good for hectic fevers, it stops fluxes, the running of the reins, and the Fluor Albus, helps such as spit blood, and such as have the falling-sickness, it stays the menses. Half a spoonful in the morning is enough.

Syrupus Cydoniorum
Or Syrup of Quinces

College.] Take of the Juice of Quinces clarified six pounds, boil it over a gentle fire till half of it be consumed, scumming it, adding red Wine three pounds, white sugar four pounds, boil it into a Syrup, to be perfumed with a dram and a half of Cinnamon, Cloves and Ginger, of each two scruples.

Culpeper.] It strengthens the heart and stomach, stays looseness and vomiting, relieves languishing nature: for looseness, take a spoonful of it before meat, for vomiting after meat, for both, as also for the rest, in the morning.

Syrupus de Erysimo
Or Syrup of Hedge-mustard

College.] Take of Hedge-mustard, fresh, six handfuls, the roots of Elecampane, Colt's-foot, Liquorice, of each two ounces, Borrage, Succory, Maiden-hair, of each a handful and a half, the cordial flowers, Rosemary and Bettony, of each half a handful, Annis seeds half an ounce, Raisins of the sun stoned, two ounces, let all of them, being prepared according to art, be boiled in a sufficient quantity of Barley Water and Hydromel, with six ounces of juice of Hedge-mustard to two pounds and a half, the which, with three pounds of sugar, boil it into a Syrup according to art.

Culpeper.] It was invented against cold afflictions of the breast and lungs, as asthmas, hoarseness, &c. You may take it either with a Liquorice stick, or which is better, mix an ounce of it with three or four ounces of Pectoral Decoction, and drink it off warm in the morning.

Syrupus de Fumaria
Or Syrup of Fumitory

College.] Take of Endive, common Wormwood, Hops, Dodder, Hart's-tongue, of each a handful, Epithimum an ounce and a half, boil them in four pounds of water till half be consumed, strain it, and add the juice of Fumitory a pound and a half, of Borrage and Bugloss, of each half a pound, white sugar four pounds, make them into a Syrup according to art.

Culpeper.] The receipt is a pretty concoctor of melancholy, and therefore a rational help for diseases arising thence, both internal and external; it helps diseases of the skin, as Leprosies, Cancers, Warts, Corns, Itch, Tetters, Ringworms, Scabs, &c. and it is the better to be liked, because of its gentleness. It helps surfeits exceedingly, cleanses, cools, and strengthens the liver, and causes it to make good blood, and good blood cannot make bad flesh. I commend this receipt to those whose bodies are subject to scabs and itch. If you please you may take two ounces by itself every morning.

Syrupus de Glycyrrhiza
Or Syrup of Liquorice

College.] Take of green Liquorice, scraped and bruised, two ounces, white Maiden-hair an ounce, dryed Hyssop half an ounce, steep these in four pounds of hot water, after twenty-four hours, boil it till half be consumed, strain it, and clarify it, and with Honey, Penids, and Sugar, of each eight ounces, make it into a Syrup, adding, before it be perfectly boiled, red Rose Water six ounces.

Culpeper.] It cleanses the breast and lungs, and helps continual coughs and pleurisies. You may take it with a Liquorice stick, or add an ounce of it or more to the Pectoral Decoction.

Syrupus Granatorum cum Aceto; vulgo, Oxysaccharum simplex
Or Syrup of Pomegranates with Vinegar

College.] Take of white sugar a pound and a half, juice of Pomegranates eight ounces, white Wine Vinegar four ounces, boil it gently into a Syrup.

Culpeper.] Look the virtues of Pomegranates among the simples.

Syrupus de Hyssopo
Or Syrup of Hyssop

College.] Take eight pounds of Spring Water, half an ounce of Barley, boil it about half an hour, then add the Roots of Smallage, Parsley, Fennel, Liquorice, of each ten drams, Jujubes, Sebestens, of each fifteen, Raisins of the sun stoned, an ounce and a half, Figs, Dates, of each ten, the seeds of Mallows and Quinces, Gum Tragacanth tied up in a rag, of each three drams, Hyssop meanly dryed, ten drams, Maiden-hair six drams, boil them together, yet so, that the roots may precede the fruits, the fruits the seeds, and the seeds the herbs, about a quarter of an hour; at last, five pounds of water being consumed, boil the other three (being first strained and clarified) into a Syrup with two pounds and a half of sugar.

Culpeper.] It mightily strengthens the breast and lungs, causes long wind, clears the voice, is a good remedy against coughs. Use it like the Syrup of Liquorice.

Syrupus Ivæ arthriticæ, sive Chamæpityos
Or Syrup of Chamepitys

College.] Take of Chamepitys, two handfuls, Sage, Rosemary, Poley Mountain, Origanum, Calaminth, wild Mints, Pennyroyal, Hyssop, Thyme, Rue, garden and wild, Bettony, Mother of Thyme, of each a handful, the roots of Acorns, Birthwort long and round, Briony, Dittany, Gentian, Hog's Fennel, Valerian, of each half an ounce, the roots of Smallage, Asparagus, Fennel, Parsley, Bruscus, of each an ounce, Pellitory of Spain, an ounce and a half, Stœchas, the seeds of Annis, Ammi, Caraway, Fennel, Lovage, Hartwort, of each three drams, Raisins of the sun two ounces, boil them in ten pounds of water to four, to which add honey and sugar, of each two pounds, make it into a Syrup to be perfumed with Sugar, Nutmegs, and Cubebs, of each three drams.

Syrupus Jujubinus
Or Syrup of Jujubes

College.] Take of Jujubes, Violets, five drams, Maiden-hair, Liquorice, French Barley, of each an ounce, the seeds of Mallows five drams, the seeds of white Poppies, Melons, Lettice, (seeds of Quinces and Gum Tragacanth tied up in a rag) of each three drams, boil them in six pounds of rain or spring water till half be consumed, strain it, and with two pounds of sugar make it into a Syrup.

Culpeper.] It is a fine cooling Syrup, very available in coughs, hoarseness, and pleurisies, ulcers of the lungs and bladder, as also in all inflammations whatsoever. You may take a spoonful of it once in three or four hours, or if you please take it with a Liquorice stick.

Syrupus de Meconio, sive Diacodium
Or Syrup of Meconium, or Diacodium

College.] Take of white Poppy heads with their seeds, gathered a little after the flowers are fallen off, and kept three days, eight ounces, black Poppy heads (so ordered) six ounces, rain Water eight pounds, steep them twenty-four hours, then boil and press them gently, boil it to three pounds, and with twenty-four ounces of sugar boil it into a Syrup according to art.

Syrupus de Meconio compositus
Or Syrup of Meconium compound

College.] Take of white and black Poppy heads with their seeds, fifty drams, Maiden-hair fifteen drams, Jujubes thirty, the seeds of Lettice, forty drams, of Mallows and Quinces tied up in a rag, a dram and a half, Liquorice five drams, water eight pounds, boil it according to art, strain it, and to three pounds of Decoction add Sugar and Penids, of each one pound, make it into a Syrup.

Culpeper.] *Meconium* is nothing else but the juice of English Poppies boiled till it be thick. It prevails against dry coughs, phthisicks, hot and sharp gnawing rheums, and provokes sleep. It is an usual fashion for nurses when they have heated their milk by exercise or strong liquor (no marvel then if their children be froward) then run for Syrup of Poppies, to make their young ones sleep. I would fain have that fashion left, therefore I forbear the dose; let nurses keep their own bodies temperate, and their children will sleep well enough, never fear.

Syrupus Melissophylli
Or Syrup of Bawm

College.] Take of the Bark of Bugloss roots, an ounce, the roots of white Dittany, Cinquefoil, Scorzonera, of each half an ounce, the leaves of Bawm, Scabious, Devil's-bit, the flowers of both sorts of Bugloss, and Rosemary, of each a handful, the seeds of Sorrel, Citrons, Fennel, Carduus, Bazil, of each three drams, boil them in four pounds of water till half be consumed, strain it, and add three pounds of white sugar, juice of Bawm and Rose Water, of each half a pound, boil them to a Syrup, the which perfume with Cinnamon and yellow Sanders, of each half an ounce.

Culpeper.] It is an excellent cordial, and strengthens the heart, breast, and stomach, it resists melancholy, revives the spirits, is given with good success in fevers, it strengthens the memory, and relieves languishing nature. You may take a spoonfull of it at a time.

Syrupus de Mentha
Or Syrup of Mints

College.] Take of the juices of Quinces sweet and between sweet and sour, the juice of Pomegranates sweet, between sweet and sour, and sour, of each a pound and a half, dried Mints half a pound, red Roses two ounces, let them lie in steep one day, then boil it half away, and with four pounds of sugar boil it into a Syrup according to art, perfume it not unless the Physicians command.

Culpeper.] The Syrup is in quality binding, yet it comforts the stomach much, helps digestion, stays vomiting, and is as excellent a remedy against sour or offensive belchings, as any is in the Dispensatory. Take a spoonful of it after meat.

Syrupus de Mucilaginibus
Or Syrup of Mussilages

College.] Take of the seeds of Marsh-mallows, Mallows, Quinces, of each an ounce, Gum Tragacanth three drams, let these infuse six hours in warm Decoction of Mallows, white Poppy seeds, and Winter Cherries, then press out the Mussilage to an ounce and an half, with which, and three ounces of the aforesaid Decoction, and two ounces of sugar, make a Syrup according to art.

Culpeper.] A spoonful taken by itself, or in any convenient liquor, is excellent for any sharp corroding humours be they in what part of the body soever, phthisicks, bloody-flux, stone in the reins or bladder, or ulcers there: it is excellent good for such as have taken purges that are too strong for their bodies, for by its slippery nature it helps corrosions, and by its cooling helps inflammations.

Syrupus Myrtinus
Or Syrup of Myrtles

College.] Take of Myrtle Berries two ounces and an half, Sanders white and red, Sumach, Balaustines, Barberry stones, red Roses, of each an ounce and a half, Medlars half a pound, bruise them in eight pounds of water to four, strain it, and add juice of Quinces and sour Pomegranates, of each six ounces, then with three pounds of sugar, boil it into a Syrup.

Culpeper.] The Syrup is of a very binding, yet comforting nature, it helps such as spit blood, all fluxes of the belly, or corrosions of the internal parts, it strengthens the retentive faculty, and stops immoderate flux of menses. A spoonful at a time is the dose.

Syrupus Florum Nymphæ simplex
Or Syrup of Water-Lily flowers, simple

College.] Take of the whitest of white Water-Lily flowers, a pound, steep them in three pounds of warm water six or seven hours, let them boil a little, and strain them out, put in the same weight of flowers again the second and third time, when you have strained it the last time, add its weight of sugar to it, and boil it to a Syrup.

Syrupus Florum Nymphæ compositus
Or Syrup of Water-Lily flowers compound

College.] Take of white Water-Lily flowers half a pound, Violets two ounces, Lettice two handfuls, the seeds of Lettice, Purslain, and Gourds, of each half an ounce, boil them in four pounds of clear water till one be consumed, strain it, and add half a pound of red Rose water, white sugar four pounds, boil it into a Syrup according to art.

Culpeper.] They are both fine cooling Syrups, allay the heat of choler, and provoke sleep, they cool the body, both head, heart, liver, reins, and matrix, and therefore are profitable for hot diseases in either, you may take an ounce of it at a time when your stomach is empty.

Syrupus de Papavere Erratico, sive Rubro
Or Syrup of Erratic Poppies

College.] Take of the fresh flowers of red Poppies two pounds, steep them in four pounds of warm spring water, the next day strain it, and boil it into a Syrup with its equal weight in sugar.

Culpeper.] The Syrup cools the blood, helps surfeits, and may safely be given in frenzies, fevers, and hot agues.

Syrupus de Pilosella
Or Syrup of Mousear

College.] Take of Mousear three handfuls, the roots of Lady's-mantle an ounce and an half, the roots of Comfrey the greater,

Madder, white Dittany, Tormentil, Bistort, of each an ounce, the leaves of Wintergreen, Horsetail, Ground Ivy, Plantain, Adder's Tongue, Strawberries, St. John's Wort with the flowers, Golden Rod, Agrimony, Bettony, Burnet, Avens, Cinquefoil the greater, red Coleworts, Balaustines, red Roses, of each a handful, boil them gently in six pounds of Plantain Water to three, then strain it strongly, and when it is settled, add Gum Tragacanth, the seeds of Fleawort, Marsh-mallows and Quinces, made into a Mussilage by themselves in Strawberry and Bettony Water, of each three ounces, white sugar two pounds, boil it to the thickness of honey.

Culpeper.] It is drying and healing, and therefore good for ruptures.

Syrupus infusionis florum Pæoniæ
Or Syrup of the infusion of Peony flowers

College.] It is prepared in the same manner as Syrup of Clove-gilliflowers.

Syrupus de Pæonia compositus
Or Syrup of Peony compound

College.] Take of the Roots of both sorts of Peony taken up at the full Moon, cut in slices, and steeped in white Wine a whole day, of each an ounce and an half, Contra Yerva half an ounce, Siler Mountain six drams, Elk's Claws an ounce, Rosemary with the flowers on, one handful, Bettony, Hyssop, Origanum, Chame-pitys, Rue, of each three drams, Wood of Aloes, Cloves, Carda-moms the less, of each two drams, Ginger, Spikenard, of each a dram, Stœchas, Nutmegs, of each two drams and an half, boil them after one day's warm digestion, in a sufficient quantity of distilled water of Peony roots, to four pounds, in which (being strained through *Hippocrates*' sleeve) put four pounds and an half of white sugar, and boil it to a Syrup.

Culpeper.] It helps the falling-sickness, and convulsions.

Syrupus de Pomis aiterans
Or Syrup of Apples

College.] Take four pounds of the juice of sweet scented Apples, the juice of Bugloss, garden and wild, of Violet leaves, Rose Water, of each a pound, boil them together, and clarify them, and with six pounds of pure sugar, boil it into a Syrup according to art.

Culpeper.] It is a fine cooling Syrup for such whose stomachs are overpressed with heat, and may safely be given in fevers, for it rather loosens than binds: it breeds good blood, and is profitable in hectic fevers, and for such as are troubled with palpitation of the heart, it quenches thirst admirably in fevers, and stays hiccoughs. You may take an ounce of it at a time in the morning, or when you need.

Syrupus de Prasio
Or Syrup of Horehound

College.] Take of white Horehound fresh, two ounces, Liquorice, Polipodium of the Oak, Fennel, and Smallage roots, of each half an ounce, white Maiden-hair, Origanum, Hyssop, Calaminth, Thyme, Savory, Scabious, Colt's-foot, of each six drams, the seeds of Annis and Cotton, of each three drams, Raisins of the sun stoned two ounces, fat Figs ten, boil them in eight pounds of Hydromel till half be consumed, boil the Decoction into a Syrup with honey and sugar, of each two pounds, and perfume it with an ounce of the roots of Orris Florentine.

Culpeper.] It is appropriated to the breast and lungs, and is a fine cleanser to purge them from thick and putrified flegm, it helps phthisicks and coughs, and diseases subject to old men, and cold natures. Take it with a Liquorice stick.

Syrupus de quinq. Radicibus
Or Syrup of the five opening Roots

College.] Take of the roots of Smallage, Fennel, Parsley, Bruscus, Sparagus of each two ounces, spring Water, six pounds, boil away the third part, and make a Syrup with the rest according to art, with three pounds of sugar, adding eight ounces of white Wine Vinegar, towards the latter end.

Culpeper.] It cleanses and opens very well, is profitable against obstructions, provokes urine, cleanses the body of flegm, and is safely and profitably given in the beginning of fevers. An ounce at a time upon an empty stomach is a good dose.

Syrupus Raphani
Or Syrup of Radishes

College.] Take of garden and wild Radish roots, of each an ounce, the roots of white Saxifrage, Lovage, Bruscus, Eringo, Rest-harrow, Parsley, Fennel, of each half an ounce, the leaves of Bettony, Burnet, Pennyroyal, Nettles, Water-cresses, Samphire, Maiden-hair, of each one handful, Winter Cherries, Jujubes, of each ten, the seeds of Bazil, Bur, Parsley of Macedonia, Hartwort, Carraway, Carrots, Gromwell, the bark of the root of Bay-tree, of each two drams, Raisins of the sun stoned, Liquorice, of each six drams, boil them in twelve pounds of water to eight, strain it, and with four pounds of sugar, and two pounds of honey, make it into a Syrup, and perfume it with an ounce of Cinnamon, and half an ounce of Nutmegs.

Culpeper.] A tedious long medicine for the stone.

Syrupus Regius, alias Julapium Alexandrinum
Or Julep of Alexandria

College.] Boil four pounds of Rose-water, and one pound of white Sugar into a Julep. Julep of Roses is made with Damask Rose water, in the very same manner.

Culpeper.] Two fine cooling drinks in the heat of summer.

Syrupus de Rosis siccis
Or Syrup of dried Roses

College.] Make four pounds of spring water hot, in which infuse a pound of dried Roses, by some at a time, press them out and with two pounds of sugar, boil it into a Syrup according to art.

Culpeper.] Syrup of dried Roses, strengthens the heart, comforts the spirits, binds the body, helps fluxes, and corrosions, or gnawings of the bowels, it strengthens the stomach, and stays vomiting. You may take an ounce at a time, before meat, if for fluxes; after meat if for vomiting.

Syrupus Scabiosæ
Or Syrup of Scabious

College.] Take of the roots of Elecampane, and Polypodium of the Oak, of each two ounces, Raisins of the sun stoned an ounce, Sebestens twenty, Colt's-foot, Lungwort, Savory, Calaminth, of each a handful and an half, Liquorice, Spanish Tobacco, of each half an ounce, the seeds of Nettles and Cotton, of each three drams, boil them all (the roots being infused in white Wine the day before) in a sufficient quantity of Wine and Water to eight ounces, strain it, and adding four ounces of the Juice of Scabious, and ten ounces of sugar, boil it to a Syrup, adding to it twenty drops of oil of sulphur.

Culpeper.] It is a cleansing Syrup appropriated to the breast and lungs, when you perceive them oppressed by flegm, crudites, or stoppings, your remedy is to take now and then a spoonful of this Syrup, it is taken also with good success by such as are itchy, or scabby.

Syrupus de Scolopendrio
Or Syrup of Hart's-tongue

College.] Take of Hart's-tongue three handfuls, Polypodium of the Oak, the roots of both sorts of Bugloss, bark of the roots of Capers and Tamerisk, of each two ounces, Hops, Dodder, Maidenhair, Bawm, of each two handfuls, boil them in nine pounds of Spring water to five, and strain it, and with four pounds of white sugar, make it into a Syrup according to art.

Culpeper.] It helps the stoppings of melancholy, opens obstructions of the liver and spleen, and is profitable against splenetic evils, and therefore is a choice remedy for the disease which the vulgar call the rickets, or liver-grown. A spoonful in a morning is a precious remedy for children troubled with that disease. Men that are troubled with the spleen, which is known by pain and hardness in their left side, may take three or four spoonfuls, they shall find this one receipt worth the price of the whole book.

Syrupus de Stœchade
Or Syrup of Stœchas

College.] Take of Stœchas flowers four ounces, Rosemary flowers half an ounce, Thyme, Calaminth, Origanum, of each an ounce and an half, Sage, Bettony, of each half an ounce, the seeds of Rue, Peony, and Fennel, of each three drams, spring water ten pounds, boil it till half be consumed, and with honey and sugar, of each two pounds, boil it into a Syrup, which perfume with Cinnamon, Ginger, and Calmus Aromaticus, of each two drams tied up in a rag.

Syrupus de Symphyto
Or Syrup of Comfrey

College.] Take of roots and tops of Comfrey, the greater and lesser, of each three handfuls, red Roses, Bettony, Plantain, Burnet, Knot grass, Scabious, Colt's foot, of each two handfuls, press the juice out of them all, being green and bruised, boil it, scum it, and strain it, add its weight of sugar to it that it may be made into a Syrup, according to art.

Culpeper.] The Syrup is excellent for all inward wounds and bruises, excoriations, vomitings, spittings, or evacuation of blood, it unites broken bones, helps ruptures, and stops the menses. You cannot err in taking of it.

Syrupus Violarum
Or Syrup of Violets

College.] Take of Violet flowers fresh and picked, a pound, clear water made boiling hot, two pounds, shut them up close together into a new glazed pot, a whole day, then press them hard out, and in two pounds of the liquor dissolve four pounds and three ounces of white sugar, take away the scum, and so make it into a Syrup without boiling. Syrup of the juice of Violets, is made with its double weight of sugar, like the former.

Culpeper.] This syrup cools and moistens, and that very gently, it corrects the sharpness of choler, and gives ease in hot vices of the breast, it quenches thirst in acute fevers, and resist the heat of the disease; it comforts hot stomachs exceedingly, cools the liver and heart, and resists putrefaction, pestilence, and poison.

College.] Julep of Violets is made of the water of Violet flowers and sugar, like Julep of Roses.

Culpeper.] It is cooling and pleasant.

PURGING SYRUPS

Syrupus de Cichorio cum Rhubarbaro
Or Syrup of Succory with Rhubarb

College.] Take of whole Barley, the roots of Smallage, Fennel, and Sparagus, of each two ounces, Succory, Dandelyon, Endive, smooth Sow-thistles, of each two handfuls, Lettuce, Liverwort, Fumitory, tops of Hops, of each one handful, Maiden-hair, white and black, Cetrachs, Liquorice, winter Cherries, Dodder, of each six drams, to boil these take sixteen pounds of spring water, strain the liquor, and boil in it six pounds of white sugar, adding towards the end six ounces of Rhubarb, six drams of Spikenard, bound up in a thin slack rag the which crush often in boiling, and so make it into a Syrup according to art.

Culpeper.] It cleanses the body of venemous humours, as boils, carbuncles, and the like; it prevails against pestilential fevers, it strengthens the heart and nutritive virtue, purges by stool and urine, it makes a man have a good stomach to his meat, and provokes sleep. But by my author's leave, I never accounted purges to be proper physic in pestilential fevers; this I believe, the Syrup cleanses the liver well, and is exceeding good for such as are troubled with hypocondriac melancholy. The strong may take two ounces at a time, the weak, one, or you may mix an ounce of it with the Decoction of Senna.

Syrupus de Epithymo
Or Syrup of Epithimum

College.] Take of Epithimum twenty drams, Mirobalans, Citron, and Indian of each fifteen drams, Emblicks, Belloricks, Polypodium, Liquorice, Agrick, Thyme, Calaminth, Bugloss, Stœchas of each six drams, Dodder, Fumitory, of each ten drams, red Roses, Annis-seeds and sweet Fennel seeds of each two drams and an half, sweet Prunes ten, Raisins of the sun stoned four ounces, Tamarinds two ounces and an half, after twenty-four hours infusion in ten pints of spring water, boil it away to six, then take it from the fire and strain it, and with five pounds of fine sugar boil it into Syrup according to art.

Culpeper.] It is best to put in the Dodder, Stœchas and Agarick, towards the latter end of the Decoction. It purges melancholy, and other humours, it strengthens the stomach and liver, cleanses the body of adduct choler and adduct blood, as also of salt humours, and helps diseases proceeding from these, as scabs, itch, tetters, ringworms, leprosy, &c. A man may take two ounces at a time, or add one ounce to the Decoction of Epithimum.

Syrupus e Floribus Persicorum
Or Syrup of Peach-flowers

College.] Take of fresh Peach-flowers a pound, steep them a whole day in three pounds of warm water, then boil a little and strain it out, repeat this infusion five times in the same liquor, in three pounds of which dissolve two pounds and an half of sugar and boil it into a Syrup.

Culpeper.] It is a gentle purger of choler, and may be given even in fevers to draw away the sharp choleric humours.

Syrupus de Pomis purgans
Or Syrup of Apples purging

College.] Take of the juice of sweet smelling Apples two pounds, the juice of Borrage and Bugloss of each one pound and an half, Senna two ounces, Annis seeds half an ounce, Saffron one dram; let the Senna be steeped in the juices twenty-four hours, and after a boil or two strain it, and with two pounds of white sugar boil it to a Syrup according to art, the saffron being tied up in a rag, and often crushed in the boiling.

Culpeper.] The Syrup is a cooling purge, and tends to rectify the distempers of the blood, it purges choler and melancholy, and therefore must needs be effectual both in yellow and black jaundice, madness, scurf, leprosy, and scabs, it is very gentle. The dose is from one ounce to three, according as the body is in age and strength. An ounce of it in the morning is excellent for such children as break out in scabs.

Syrupus de Pomis magistralis
Or Syrup of Apples magisterial

College.] Take of the Juice and Water of Apples of each a pound and an half, the Juice and Water of Borrage and Bugloss of each nine ounces, Senna half a pound, Annis seeds, and sweet Fennel seeds, of each three drams, Epithimum of Crete, two ounces, Agarick, Rhubarb, of each half an ounce, Ginger, Mace, of each four scruples, Cinnamon two scruples, Saffron half a dram, infuse the Rhubarb and Cinnamon apart by itself, in white Wine and Juice of Apples, of each two ounces, let all the rest, the Saffron excepted, be steeped in the Waters above mentioned, and the next day put in the juices, which being boiled, scummed, and strained, then with four ounces of white sugar boil it into a Syrup, crushing the saffron in it being tied up in a linen rag, the infusion of the Rhubarb being added at the latter end.

Culpeper.] Out of doubt this is a gallant Syrup to purge choler and melancholy, and to resist madness.

Syrupus de Rhubarbaro
Or Syrup of Rhubarb

College.] Take of the best Rhubarb and Senna of each two ounces and an half, Violet flowers a handful, Cinnamon one dram and an half, Ginger half a dram, Bettony, Succory and Bugloss Water of each one pound and an half, let them be mixed together warm all night, and in the morning strained and boiled into a Syrup, with two pounds of white sugar, adding towards the end four ounces of Syrup of Roses.

Culpeper.] It cleanses choler and melancholy very gently, and is therefore fit for children, old people, and weak bodies. You may add an ounce of it to the Decoction of Epithimum or to the Decoction of Senna.

Syrupus Rosaceus solutivus
Or Syrup of Roses solutive

College.] Take of Spring Water boiling hot four pounds, Damask Rose leaves fresh, as many as the water will contain; let them remain twelve hours in infusion, close stopped; then press them out and put in fresh Rose leaves; do so nine times in the same liquor, encreasing the quantity of the Roses as the liquor encreases, which will be almost by the third part every time: Take six parts of this liquor, and with four parts of white sugar, boil it to a Syrup according to art.

Culpeper.] It loosens the belly, and gently brings out choler and flegm, but leaves a binding quality behind it.

Syrupus e succo Rosarum
Or Syrup of the Juice of Roses

College.] It is prepared without steeping, only with the juice of Damask Roses pressed out, and clarified, and an equal proportion of sugar added to it.

Culpeper.] This is like the other.

Syrupus Rosaceus solutivus cum Agarico
Or Syrup of Roses solutive with Agarick

College.] Take of Agarick cut thin an ounce, Ginger two drams, Sal. Gem. one dram, Polipodium bruised two ounces, sprinkle them with white Wine and steep them two days over warm ashes, in a pound and an half of the infusion of Damask Roses prescribed before, and with one pound of sugar boil it into a Syrup according to art.

Culpeper.] It purges flegm from the head, relieves the senses oppressed by it, provokes the menses, purges the stomach and liver, and provokes urine.

Syrupus Rosaceus solutivus cum Helleboro
Or Syrup of Roses solutive with Hellebore

College.] Take of the bark of all the Myrobalans, of each four ounces, bruise them grossly, and steep them twenty-four hours in twelve pounds of the infusion of Roses before spoken, Senna, Epithimum, Polypodium of the Oak, of each four ounces, Cloves an ounce, Citron seeds, Liquorice, of each four ounces, the bark of black Hellebore roots six drams, let the fourth part of the liquor gently exhale, strain it, and with five pounds of sugar, and sixteen drams of Rhubarb tied up in a linen rag, make it into a Syrup according to art.

Culpeper.] The Syrup, rightly used, purges melancholy, resists madness.

Syrupus Rosaceus solutivus cum Senna
Or Syrup of Roses solutive with Senna

College.] Take of Senna six ounces, Caraway, and sweet Fennel seeds, of each three drams, sprinkle them with white Wine, and infuse them two days in three pounds of the infusion of Roses aforesaid, then strain it, and with two pounds of sugar boil it into a Syrup.

Culpeper.] It purges the body of choler and melancholy, and expels the relics a disease hath left behind it; the dose is from one ounce to two, you may take it in a Decoction of Senna, it leaves a binding quality behind it.

Syrupus de Spina Cervina
Or Syrup of Purging Thorn

College.] Take of the berries of Purging Thorn, gathered in September, as many as you will, bruise them in a stone mortar, and press out the juice, let the fourth part of it evaporate away in a bath, then to two pounds of it add sixteen ounces of white sugar, boil it into a Syrup, which perfume with Mastich, Cinnamon, Nutmegs, Anniseeds in fine powder, of each three drams.

SYRUPS MADE WITH VINEGAR AND HONEY
Mel Anthosatum
Or Honey of Rosemary Flowers

College.] Take of fresh Rosemary flowers a pound, clarified Honey three pounds, mix them in a glass with a narrow mouth, set them in the sun, keep them for use.

Culpeper.] It hath the same virtues with Rosemary flowers, to which I refer you, only by reason of the Honey it may be somewhat cleansing.

Mel Helleboratum
Or Honey Helleborated

College.] Take of white Hellebore roots bruised a pound, clear Water fourteen pounds, after three days infusions, boil it till half be consumed, then strain it diligently, and with three pounds of Honey, boil it to the thickness of Honey.

Mel Mercuriale
Or Honey of Mercury

College.] Boil three pounds of the juice of Mercury, with two pounds of Honey to the thickness of Honey.

Culpeper.] It is used as an emollient in clysters.

Mel Mororum, vel Diamoron
Or Honey of Mulberries

College.] Take of the juice of Mulberries and Blackberries, before they be ripe, gathered before the sun be up, of each a pound and a half, Honey two pounds, boil them to their due thickness.

Culpeper.] It is vulgarly known to be good for sore mouths, as also to cool inflammations there.

Mel Nuceum, alias Diacarion et Dianucum
Or Honey of Nuts

College.] Take of the juice of the outward bark of green Walnuts, gathered in the dog days two pounds, boil it gently till it be thick, and with one pound of Honey, boil it to the thickness of Honey.

Culpeper.] It is a good preservative in pestilential times, a spoonful being taken as soon as you are up.

Mel Passalatum
Or Honey of Raisins

College.] Take of Raisins of the sun cleansed from the stones two pounds, steep them in six pounds of warm water, the next day boil it half away, and press it strongly, and with two pounds of Honey, let the expressed liquor boil to its thickness.

Culpeper.] It is a pretty pleasing medicine for such as are in consumptions, and are bound in body.

Mel Rosatum commune, sive Foliatum
Or common Honey of Roses

College.] Take of red Roses not quite open two pounds, Honey six pounds, set them in the sun according to art.

Mel Rosatum Colatum

Or Honey of Roses strained

College.] Take of the best clarified Honey ten pounds, juice of fresh red Roses one pound, set it handsomely over the fire, and when it begins to boil, put in four pounds of fresh red Roses, the whites being cut off; the juice being consumed by boiling and stirring, strain it and keep it for use.

Culpeper.] They are both used for diseases in the mouth.

Mel Rosatum solutivum

Or Honey of Roses solutive

College.] Take of the often infusion of Damask Roses five pounds, Honey rightly clarified four pounds, boil it to the thickness of Honey.

Culpeper.] It is used as a laxative in clysters, and some use it to cleanse wounds.

College.] After the same manner is prepared Honey of the infusion of red Roses.

Mel scilliticum

Or Honey of Squils

College.] Take one Squil full of juice, cut in bits, and put it in a glass vessel, the mouth close stopped, and covered with a skin, set in the sun forty days, to wit, twenty before and after the rising of the dog star, then open the vessel, and take the juice which lies at the bottom, and preserve it with the best Honey.

College.] Honey of Violets is prepared like as Honey of Roses.

Oxymel, simple

College.] Take of the best Honey four pounds, clear Water and white Wine Vinegar, of each two pounds, boil them in an earthen vessel, taking the scum off with a wooden scummer, till it be come to the consistence of a Syrup.

Culpeper.] It cuts flegm, and it is a good preparative against a vomit.

Oxymel compound

College.] Take of the Bark of the Root of Fennel, Smallage, Parsley, Bruscus, Asparagus, of each two ounces, the seeds of Fennel, Smallage, Parsley, Annis, of each one ounce, steep them all (the roots being first cleansed and the seeds bruised) in six pounds of clear Water and a pound and a half of Wine Vinegar, the next day boil it to the consumption of the third part, boil the rest being strained, with three pounds of Honey into a liquid Syrup according to art.

Culpeper.] First having bruised the roots and seeds, boil them in the water till half be consumed, then strain it and add the Honey, and when it is almost boiled enough, add the Vinegar.

Oxymel Helleboratum
Or Oxymel Helleborated

College.] Take of Rue, Thyme, Dittany of Crete, Hyssop, Pennyroyal, Horehound, Carduus, the roots of Celtick, Spikenard without leaves, the inner bark of Elders, of each a handful, Mountain Calaminth two pugils, the seeds of Annis, Fennel, Bazil, Roman Nettles, Dill, of each two drams, the roots of Angelica, Marsh-mallows, Aron, Squills prepared, Birthwort, long, round, and climbing, Turbith, English Orris, Costus, Polypodium, Lemon pills, of each an ounce, the strings of black Hellebore, Spurge, Agerick, added at the end of the Decoction, of each two drams, the bark of white Hellebore half an ounce, let all of them being dried and bruised, be digested in a glass, or glazed vessel close stopped, in the heat of the sun, or of a furnace, Posca, made of equal parts of Water and Vinegar, eight pounds, Sapa two ounces, three days being expired, boil it little more than half away, strain it, pressing it gently, and add to the liquor a pound and a half of Honey Roses, wherein two ounces of Citron pills have been infused, boil it to the thickness of Honey, and perfume it with Cloves, Saffron, Ginger, Galanga, Mace, of each a dram.

Oxymel Julianizans

College.] Take of the Bark of Caper roots, the roots of Orris, Fennel, Parsley, Bruscus, Chicory, Sparagus, Cypress, of each half an ounce, the leaves of Harts-tongue, Schænanth, Tamarisk, of each half a handful, sweet Fennel seed half an ounce, infuse them in three pounds of Posca, which is something sour, afterwards boil it till half be consumed, strain it, and with Honey and sugar clarified, of each half a pound, boil it to the thickness of Honey.

Culpeper.] This medicine is very opening, very good against Hypocondriac melancholy, and as fit a medicine as can be for that disease in children called the Rickets.

College.] Oxymel of Squills simple, is made of three pounds of clarified Honey; Vinegar of Squills two pounds, boil them according to art.

Culpeper.] It cuts and divides humours that are tough and viscous, and therefore helps the stomach and bowels afflicted by such humours, and sour belchings. If you take but a spoonful in the morning, an able body will think enough.

Oxymel Scilliticum compositus
Or Oxymel of Squills compound

College.] Take of Origanum, dried Hyssop, Thyme, Lovage, Cardamoms the less, Stœchas, of each five drams, boil them in three pounds of Water to one, strain it and with two pounds of Honey, Honey of Raisins half a pound, juice of Briony five ounces, Vinegar of Squills a pound and a half, boil it, and scum it according to art.

Culpeper.] This is good against the falling-sickness, Megrim, Head-ache, Vertigo, or swimming in the head, and if these be occasioned by the stomach as many times they are, it helps the lungs obstructed by humour, and is good for women not well cleansed after labour, it opens the passage of the womb.

Syrup of Purslain. Mesue

College.] Take of the seeds of Purslain grossly bruised, half a pound, of the juice of Endive, boiled and clarified, two pounds, Sugar two pounds, Vinegar nine ounces, infuse the seeds in the juice of Endive twenty-four hours, afterwards boil it half away with a gentle fire, then strain it, and boil it with the sugar to the consistence of a Syrup, adding the Vinegar towards the latter end of the decoction.

Culpeper.] It is a pretty cooling Syrup, fit for any hot disease incident to the stomach, reins, bladder, matrix, or liver; it thickens flegm, cools the blood, and provokes sleep. You may take an ounce of it at a time when you have occasion.

Compound Syrup of Colt's-foot. Renod

College.] Take six handfuls of green Colt's-foot, two handfuls of Maiden-hair, one handful of Hyssop and two ounces of Liquorice, boil them in four pints, either of rain or spring water till the fourth part be consumed, then strain it, and clarify it, to which add three pounds of white sugar, boil it to the perfect consistence of a Syrup.

Culpeper.] The composition is appropriated to the lungs, and therefore helps the infirmities, weaknesses, or failings thereof, as want of voice, difficulty of breathing, coughs, hoarseness, catarrhs,

&c. The way of taking it is with a Liquorice-stick, or if you please, you may add an ounce of it to the Pectoral Decoction before mentioned.

Syrup of Poppies, the lesser composition

College.] Take of the heads of white Poppies and black, when both of them are green, of each six ounces, the seeds of Lettice, the flowers of Violets, of each one ounce, boil them in eight pints of water till the virtue is out of the heads; then strain them, and with four pounds of sugar boil the liquor to a Syrup.

Syrup of Poppies, the greater composition

College.] Take of the heads of both white and black Poppies, seeds and all, of each fifty drams, Maiden-hair, fifteen drams, Liquorice, five drams, Jujubes, thirty by number, Lettice seeds, forty drams, of the seeds of Mallows and Quinces, (tied up in a thin linen cloth) of each one dram and an half, boil these in eight pints of water till five pints be consumed, when you have strained out the three pints remaining, add to them, Penids and white sugar, of each a pound, boil them into a Syrup according to art.

Culpeper.] All these former Syrups of Poppies provoke sleep, but in that, I desire they may be used with a great deal of caution and wariness: such as these are not fit to be given in the beginning of fevers, nor to such whose bodies are costive, yet to such as are troubled with hot, sharp rheums, you may safely give them. The last is appropriated to the lungs. It prevails against dry coughs, phthisicks, hot and sharp gnawing rheums, and provokes sleep. It is an usual fashion for nurses when they have heated their milk by exercise or strong liquor then run for Syrup of Poppies to make their young ones sleep. I would fain have that fashion left off, therefore I forbear the dose. Let nurses keep their own bodies temperate, and their children will sleep well enough.

Syrup of Eupatorium (or Maudlin). Mesue

College.] Take of the Roots of Smallage, Fennel, and Succory, of each two ounces, Liquorice, Schænanth, Dodder, Wormwood, Roses, of each six drams, Maiden-hair, Bedeguar, or instead thereof, the roots of Carduus Mariæ, Suchaha or instead thereof the roots of Avens, the flowers or roots of Bugloss, Annis seeds, sweet Fennel seeds, Ageratum, or Maudlin, of each five drams, Rhubarb, Mastich, of each three drams, Spikenard, Indian leaf, or instead of it put Roman spike, of each two drams, boil them in eight pints of

Water till the third part be consumed, then strain the Decoction, and with four pounds of sugar, clarified juice of Smallage and Endive, of each half a pound, boil it into a Syrup.

Culpeper.] It amends infirmities of the liver coming of cold, opens obstructions, helps the dropsy, and evil state of the body; it extenuates gross humours, strengthens the liver, provokes urine, and is a present succour for hypocondriac melancholy. You may take an ounce at a time in the morning, it opens but purges not.

Honey of Emblicks. Augustanus

College.] Take fifty Emblick Myrobalans, bruise them and boil them in three pints of water till two be consumed, strain it, and with the like weight of Honey, boil it into a Syrup.

Culpeper.] It is a fine gentle purger both of flegm and melancholy: it strengthens the brain and nerves, and senses both internal and external, helps tremblings of the heart, stays vomiting, provokes appetite. You may take a spoonful at a time.

ROB, OR SAPA: AND JUICES

Culpeper.] 1. Rob, or Sapa, is the juice of a fruit, made thick by the heat either of the sun, or the fire, that it is capable of being kept safe from putrefaction. 2. Its use was first invented for diseases in the mouth. 3. It is usually made, in respect of body, somewhat thicker than new Honey. 4. It may be kept about a year, little more or less.

Rob sive Sapa, simplex
Or Simple Rob, or Sapa

College.] Take of Wine newly pressed from white and ripe Grapes, boil it over a gentle fire to the thickness of Honey.

Culpeper.] Whenever you read the word Rob, or Sapa throughout the Dispensatory, simply quoted in any medicine without any relation of what it should be made, this is that you ought to use.

Rob de Barberis
Or Rob of Barberries

College.] Take of the juice of Barberries strained as much as you will, boil it by itself (or else by adding half a pound of sugar to each pound of juice) to the thickness of Honey.

Culpeper.] It quenches thirst, closes the mouth of the stomach, thereby staying vomiting, and belching, it strengthens stomachs weakened by heat, and procures appetite. Of any of these Robs you may take a little on the point of a knife when you need.

Rob de Cerasis
Or Rob of Cherries

College.] Take of the juice of red Cherries somewhat sowerish, as much as you will, and with half their weight in sugar boil them like the former.

Culpeper.] See the virtue of Cherries, and there you have a method to keep them all the year.

Rob de Cornis
Or Rob of Cornels

College.] Take of the juice of Cornels two pounds, sugar a pound and an half; boil it according to art.

Culpeper.] Of these Cornel trees are two sorts, male and female, the fruit of the male Cornel, or Cornelian Cherry is here to be used. The fruit of male Cornel, binds exceedingly, and therefore good in fluxes, and the immoderate flowing of the menses.

Rob Cydoniorum
Or Rob of Quinces

College.] Take of the clarified juice of Quinces, boil it till two parts be consumed and with its equal weight in sugar boil it into a Rob.

Miva vel Gelatina Eorundem
Or Jelly of Quinces

College.] Take of the juice of Quinces clarified twelve pounds, boil it half away, and add to the remainder, old white Wine five pounds, consume the third part over a gentle fire, taking away the scum (all you ought) let the rest settle, and strain it, and with three pounds of sugar boil it according to art.

Culpeper.] Both are good for weak and indisposed stomachs.

College.] Rob of sour Plums is made as Rob of Quinces, the use of sugar is indifferent in them both.

Rob of English Currants is made in the same manner, let the juice be clarified.

Culpeper.] The virtues are the same with Rob of Barberries.

Rob Baccarum Sambuci
Or Rob of Elder Berries

College.] Take of the juice of Elder Berries, and make it thick with the help of a gentle fire, either by itself, or a quarter of its weight in sugar being added.

Culpeper.] Both Rob of Elder Berries, and Dwarf-Elder, are excellent for such whose bodies are inclining to dropsies, neither let them neglect nor despise it. They may take the quantity of a nutmeg each morning, it will gently purge the watery humour.

College.] In the same manner is made Rob of Dwarf-Elder, Junipers, and Paul's Betony, only in the last, the sugar and juice must be equal in weight.

Succus Glycyrrhizæ simplex
Or Juice of Liquorice simple

College.] Infuse Liquorice Roots cleansed and gently bruised, three days in Spring Water, so much that it may over-top the roots the breadth of three fingers, then boil it a little, and press it hard out, and boil the liquor with a gentle fire to its due thickness.

Culpeper.] It is vulgarly known to be good against coughs, colds, &c. and a strengthener of the lungs.

Succus Glycyrrhizæ compositus
Or Juice of Liquorice compound

College.] Take of the water of tender Oak leaves, of Scabious, of each four pounds, English Liquorice scraped and bruised two pounds, boil them by degrees till they be soft, then press out the liquor strongly in a press, to which add three pounds of juice of Hyssop, and dry it away in the sun in a broad earthen vessel.

Culpeper.] The virtues are the same with the former.

Succus Pronorum Sylvestrum
Or Juice of Sloes, called Acacia

College.] Take of Sloes hardly ripe, press out the juice, and make it thick in a bath.

Culpeper.] It stops fluxes, and procures appetite.

College.] So are the Juices of Wormwood, Maudlin, and Fumitory made thick, to wit, the herbs bruised while they be tender, and the juice pressed out and after it be clarified, boil over the fire to its just thickness.

LOHOCH, OR ECLEGMATA

Culpeper.] Because this word also is understood but by few, we will first explain what it is. 1. The word *Lohoch* is an Arabick word, called in Greek *Eclegma*, in Latin *Linctus*, and signifies a thing to be licked up. 2. It is in respect of body, something thicker than a Syrup, and not so thick as an electuary. 3. Its use was against the roughness of the windpipe, diseases, and inflammations of the lungs, difficulty of breathing, colds, coughs, &c. 4. Its manner of reception is with a Liquorice stick, bruised at the end, to take up some and retain it in the mouth, till it melt of its own accord.

Lohoch de Farfara
Or Lohoch of Coltsfoot

College.] Take of Colts-foot roots cleansed eight ounces, Marsh-mallow roots four ounces cleansed, boil them in a sufficient quantity of water, and press the pulp out through a sieve, dissolve this again in the Decoction, and let it boil once or twice, then take it from the fire, and add two pounds of white sugar, Honey of Raisins fourteen ounces, juice of Liquorice two drams and an half, stir them stoutly with a wooden pestle, mean season sprinkle in Saffron and Cloves, of each a scruple, Cinnamon and Mace, of each two scruples, make them into a Lohoch according to art.

Culpeper.] It was invented for the cough.

Lohoch de Papavere
Or Lohoch of Poppies

College.] Take white Poppy seeds twenty four drams, sweet Almonds blanched in Rose Water, Pine-nuts cleansed, Gum Arabick and Tragacanth, of each ten drams, juice of Liquorice an ounce, Starch three drams, the seeds of Lettuce, Purslain, Quinces, of each half an ounce, Saffron a dram, Penids four ounces, Syrup of Meconium three pounds, make it into a Lohoch according to art.

Culpeper.] It helps salt, sharp and thin distillations upon the lungs, it allays the fury of such sharp humours, which occasion both roughness of the throat, want of sleep, and fevers; it is excellent for such as are troubled with pleurises to take now and then a little of it.

Lohoch e Passulis
Or Lohoch of Raisins

College.] Take of male Peony roots, Liquorice, of each half an ounce, Hyssop, Bawm, Hart's-tongue, or Cetrach, of each half a handful, boil them in Spring Water, and press them strongly, and by adding a pound of Raisins bruised, boil it again, pressing it through a linen cloth, then with a pound of white sugar, make it into a Lohoch according to art.

Culpeper.] It is very good against coughs, consumptions of the lungs, and other vices of the breast, and is usually given to children for such diseases, as also for convulsions, and falling-sickness.

Lohoch e Pino
Or Lohoch of Pinenuts

College.] Take of Pine-nuts, fifteen drams, sweet Almonds, Hazel Nuts gently roasted, Gum Arabick and Tragacanth, powder and juice of Liquorice, white Starch, Maiden-hair, Orris roots, of each two drams, the pulp of Dates seventeen drams, bitter Almonds one dram and an half, Honey of Raisins, white Sugar-candy, fresh Butter, of each two ounces, Honey one pound and an half, dissolve the Gums in so much Decoction of Maiden-hair as is sufficient; let the rest be mixed over a gentle fire, and stirred, that so it may be made into a Lohoch.

Culpeper.] The medicine is excellent for continual coughs, and difficulty of breathing, it succours such as are asthmatic, for it cuts and atenuates tough humours in the breast.

Lohoch de Portulaca
Or Lohoch of Purslain

College.] Take of the strained Juice of Purslain two pounds, Troches of *Terra Lemnia* two drams, Troches of Amber, Gum Arabic, Dragon's-blood of each one dram, *Lapis Hematilis*, the wool of a Hare toasted, of each two scruples, white Sugar one pound, mix them together, that so you may make a Lohoch of them.

Culpeper.] The medicine is so binding that it is better let alone than taken, unless in inward bruises when men spit blood, then you may safely take a little of it.

Lohoch e Pulmone Vulpis
Or Lohoch of Fox Lungs

College.] Take of Fox Lungs rightly prepared, juice of Liquorice, Maiden-hair, Annis-seeds, sweet Fennel seeds, of each equal parts, Sugar dissolved in Colt's-foot, and Scabious Water, and boiled into a Syrup, three times their weight; the rest being in fine powder, let them be put to it and strongly stirred together, that it may be made into a Lohoch according to art.

Culpeper.] It cleanses and unites ulcers in the lungs and breast, and is a present remedy in phthisicks.

Lohoch sanum et Expertum
Or a sound and well experienced Lohoch

College.] Take of dried Hyssop and Calaminth, of each half an ounce, Jujubes, Sebestens, the stones being taken out, fifteen Raisins of the Sun stoned, fat Figs, Dates, of each two ounces, Linseed, Fenugreek seed, of each five drams, Maiden-hair one handful, Annis-seeds, sweet Fennel seeds, Orris Roots cut, Liquorice, Cinnamon, of each an ounce, boil them according to art in four pounds of clear water till half be consumed, and with two pounds of Penids boil it into a Syrup, afterwards cut and bruise very small Pine-nuts five drams, sweet Almonds blanched, Liquorice, Gum Tragacanth and Arabick, white Starch of each three drams, let these be put into the Syrup when it is off the fire, and stir it about swiftly with a wooden pestle till it look white.

Culpeper.] It succors the breast, lungs, throat, oppressed by cold, it restores the voice lost by reason of cold, and attenuates thick and gross humours in the breast and throat.

Lohoch Scilliticum
Or Lohoch of Squils

College.] Take three drams of a Squil baked in paste, Orris Roots two drams, Hyssop, Hore-hound, of each one dram, Saffron, Myrrh, of each half a dram, Honey two ounces and an half, bruise the Squil, after it is baked, in a stone mortar, and after it hath boiled a walm or two with the Honey, put in the rest of the things in powder, diligently stirring it, and make it into a Lohoch according to art.

Eclegma of Squils. Mesue

College.] Take of the juice of Squils and Honey, both of them clarified, of each two pounds, boil them together according to art to the consistence of Honey.

Culpeper.] For the virtues of it see Vinegar of Squils, and Oximel of Squils, only this is more mild, and not so harsh to the throat, because it hath no Vinegar in it, and therefore is far more fitting for *Asthmaes*, and such as are troubled with difficulty of breathing, it cuts and carries away humours from the breast, be they thick or thin, and wonderfully helps indigestion of victuals, and eases pains in the breast, and for this, I quote the authority of *Galen*.

Lohoch of Coleworts. Gordonius

College.] Take one pound of the juice of Coleworts, clarified Saffron three drams, clarified Honey, and Sugar, of each half a pound, make of them a Lohoch according to art.

Culpeper.] It helps hoarseness, and loss of voice, eases surfeits and head-ache coming of drunkenness, and opens obstructions of the liver and spleen, and therefore is good for that disease in children called the rickets.

PRESERVED ROOTS, STALKS, BARKS, FLOWERS, FRUITS

College.] Take of Eringo Roots as many as you will, cleanse them without and within, the pith being taken out, steep them two days in clear water, shifting the water sometimes, then dry them with a cloth, then take their equal weight in white Sugar, and as much Rose-water as will make it into a Syrup, which being almost boiled, put in the roots, and let them boil until the moisture be consumed, and let it be brought to the due body of a Syrup. Not much unlike to this are preserved the roots of Acorus, Angelica, Borrage, Bugloss, Succory, Elecampane, Burnet, Satyrion, Sicers, Comfrey the greater, Ginger, Zedoary. Take of the stalks of Artichokes, not too ripe, as many as you will, and (*contrary to the roots*) take only the pith of these, and preserve them with their equal weight in sugar, like the former. So is prepared the stalks of Angelica, Burs, Lettuce, &c. before they be too ripe. Take of fresh Orange pills as many as you will, take away the exterior yellowness, and steep them in spring water three days at the least, often renewing the water, then preserve them like the former. In like manner are Lemon and Citron pills preserved. Preserve the flowers of Citrons, Oranges, Borrage, Primroses, with Sugar, according to art. Take of Apricots as many as you will, take away the outer skin and the stones, and mix them with their like weight in sugar, after four hours take them out, and boil the Sugar without any other Liquor, then put them in again, and boil them a little. Other Fruits may be preserved in the same manner, or at least not much unlike to it, as whole Barberries, Cherries, Cornels, Citrons, Quinces, Peaches, common Apples, the five sorts of Myrobalans, Hazel Nuts, Walnuts, Nutmegs, Raisins of the Sun, Pepper brought green from India, Plums, garden and wild Pears, Grapes. Pulps are also preserved, as Barberries, Cassia Fistula, Citrons, Cinosbatus, Quinces, and Sloes, &c. Take of Barberries as many as you will, boil them in spring water till they are tender, then having pulped them through a sieve, that they are free from the stones, boil it again in an earthen vessel over a gentle fire, often stirring them for fear of burning, till the watery humour be consumed, then mix ten pounds of sugar with six pounds of this pulp, boil it to its due thickness. Broom buds are also preserved, but with brine and vinegar, and so are Olives and Capers. Lastly, Amongst the Barks, Cinnamon, amongst the flowers, Roses, and Marigolds, amongst the fruits, Almonds, Cloves, Pine-nuts, and Fistick-nuts, are said to be preserved but with this difference, they are encrusted with dry sugar, and are more called confects than preserves.

CONSERVES AND SUGARS

College.] Conserves of the herbs of Wormwood, Sorrel, Woodsorrel, the flowers of Oranges, Borrage, Bugloss, Bettony, Marigolds, the Tops of Carduus, the Flowers of Centaury the less, Clove-gilliflowers, Germander, Succory, the Leaves of Scurvygrass, the flowers of Comfrey the greater, Citratiæ, Cinosbati, the roots of Spurge, herbs and flowers of Eye-bright, the tops of Fumitory, Goat's-rue, the flowers of Broom not quite open, Hyssop, Lavender, white Lilies, Lilies of the Valley, Marjoram, Mallows, the tops of Bawm, the leaves of Mints, the flowers of Water Lilies, red Poppies, Peony, Peaches, Primroses, Roses, the leaves of Rue, the flowers of Sage, Elder, Scabious, the leaves of Scordium, the flowers of Limetree, Coltsfoot, Violets, with all these are conserves made with their treble proportion of white sugar; yet note, that all of them must not be mixed alike, some of them must be cut, beaten, and gently boiled, some neither cut, beaten nor boiled, and some admit but one of them, which every artist in his trade may find out by this premonition and avoid error.

SUGARS

Diacodium Solidum, sive Tabulatum

College.] Take of white Poppy heads, meanly ripe, and newly gathered, twenty, steep them in three pounds of warm spring water, and the next day boil them until the virtue is out, then strain out the liquor, and with a sufficient quantity of good sugar, boil it according to art, that you may make it up into Lozenges.

Culpeper.] The virtues are the same with the common Diacodium, viz. to provoke sleep, and help thin rheums in the head, coughs, and roughness of the throat, and may easily be carried about in one's pocket.

Saccharum tabulatum simplex, et perlatum
Or Lozenges of Sugar both simple and pearled

College.] The first is made by pouring the sugar upon a marble, after a sufficient boiling in half its weight in Damask Rose Water: And the latter by adding to every pound of the former towards the latter end of the decoction, Pearls, prepared and bruised, half an ounce, with eight or ten leaves of gold.

Culpeper.] It is naturally cooling, appropriated to the heart, it restores lost strength, takes away burning fevers, and false imaginations, (I mean that with Pearls, for that without Pearls is ridiculous) it hath the same virtues Pearls have.

Saccharum Tabulatum compositum
Or Lozenges of Sugar compound

College.] Take of choice Rhubarb four scruples, Agarick Trochiscated, Corallins, burnt Hart's-horn, Dittany of Crete, Wormseed and Sorrel seed, of each a scruple, Cinnamon, Zedoary, Cloves, Saffron, of each half a scruple, white Sugar a pound, dissolved in four ounces of Wormwood Water, Wormwood Wine, an ounce, Cinnamon Water a spoonful, with the forenamed powders make it into Lozenges according to art.

Culpeper.] The title shews you the virtues of it.

Saccharum Penidium
Or Sugar Penids

College.] Are prepared of sugar dissolved in spring water by a gentle fire, and the whites of Eggs diligently beaten, and clarified once, and again whilst it is boiling, then strain it and boil it gently again, till it rise up in great bubbles, and being chewed it stick not to your teeth, then pour it upon a marble, anointed with oil of Almonds, (let the bubbles first sink, after it is removed from the fire) bring back the outsides of it to the middle till it look like Larch rosin, then, your hands being rubbed with white starch, you may draw it into threads either short or long, thick or thin, and let it cool in what form you please.

Culpeper.] I remember country people were wont to take them for coughs, and they are sometimes used in other compositions.

Confectio de Thure
Or Confection of Frankincense

College.] Take Coriander seeds prepared half an ounce, Nutmegs, white Frankincense, of each three drams, Liquorice, Mastich, of each two drams, Cubebs, Hart's-horn prepared, of each one dram, conserve of Red roses an ounce, white Sugar as much as is sufficient to make it into mean bits.

Culpeper.] I cannot boast much of the rarity nor virtues of this receipt.

Saccharum Rosatum
Or Sugar of Roses

College.] Take of red Rose leaves, the whites being cut off, and speedily dried in the sun an ounce, white Sugar a pound, melt the Sugar in Rose-water and juice of Roses of each two ounces which being consumed by degrees, put in the Rose leaves in powder, mix them, put it upon a marble, and make it into Lozenges according to art.

Culpeper.] As for the virtues of this, it strengthens weak stomachs, weak hearts, and weak brains, restores such as are in consumptions, restores lost strength, stays fluxes, eases pains in the head, ears and eyes, helps spitting, vomiting, and urining of blood; it is a fine commodity for a man in a consumption to carry about with him, and eat now and then a bit.

SPECIES, OR POWDERS
Aromaticum Caryophyllatum

College.] Take of Cloves seven drams, Mace, Zedoary, Galanga the less, yellow Sanders, Troches, Diarrhodon, Cinnamon, wood of Aloes, Indian Spikenard, long Pepper, Cardamoms the less, of each a dram, Red Roses four ounces, Gallia Moschata, Liquorice, of each two drams, of Indian leaf, Cubebs of each two scruples, beat them all diligently into powder.

Culpeper.] This powder strengthens the heart and stomach, helps digestion, expels wind, stays vomiting, and cleanses the stomach of putrified humors.

Aromaticum Rosatum

College.] Take of Red Roses exungulated fifteen drams, Liquorice seven drams, wood of Aloes, yellow Sanders, of each three drams, Cinnamon five drams, Cloves, Mace, of each two drams and an half, Gum Arabic and Tragacanth, of each eight scruples, Nutmegs, Cardamoms the less, Galanga of each one dram, Indian Spikenard two scruples, make it into a powder to be kept in a glass for use.

Culpeper.] It strengthens the brain, heart and stomach, and all such internal members as help towards decoction, it helps digestion, consumes the watery excrements of the bowels, strengthens such as are pined away by reason of the violence of a disease, and restores such as are in consumption.

Pulvus ex chelus Cancrorum compositus
Or Powder of Crab's claws compound

College.] Take of Pearls prepared, Crab's eyes, red Coral, white Amber Hart's-horn, oriential Bezoar, of each half an ounce, powder of the black tops of Crab's claws, the weight of them all, beat them into powder, which may be made into balls with jelly, and the skins which our vipers have cast off, warily dried and kept for use.

Culpeper.] This is that powder they ordinarily call *Gascoigns* powder, there are divers receipts of it, of which this is none of the worst, four, or five, or six grains is excellently good in a fever to be taken in any cordial, for it cheers the heart and vital spirits exceedingly, and makes them impregnable.

Species Cordiales Temperatæ

College.] Take of wood of Aloes, Spodium of each a dram, Cinnamon, Cloves, bone of a Stag's-heart, the roots of Angelica, Avens, and Tormentil, of each a dram and an half, Pearls prepared six drams, raw Silk toasted, both sorts of Coral of each two drams, Jacinth, Emerald, Samphire, of each half a dram, Saffron a scruple, the leaves of gold and silver, of each ten, make them into powder according to art.

Culpeper.] It is a great cordial, a great strengthener of the heart, and brain.

Diacalaminthe Simple

College.] Take of Mountain Calaminth, Pennyroyal, Origanum, the seeds of Macedonian Parsley, common Parsley, and Hartwort, of each two drams, the seeds of Smallage, the tops of Thyme of each half an ounce, the seeds of Lovage, black Pepper, of each an ounce, make them into powder according to art.

Culpeper.] It heats and comforts cold bodies, cuts thick and gross flegm, provokes urine and the menses. I confess this differs something from *Galen*, but is better for our bodies in my opinion than his. It expels wind exceedingly, you may take half a dram of the powder at a time. There is nothing surer than that all their powders will keep better in Electuaries than they will in powders, and into such a body, you may make it with two pound and an half of white sugar dissolved in rose water.

Diacalamintha compound

College.] Take of Diacalamintha simple, half an ounce, the leaves of Horehound, Marjoram, Bawm, Mugwort, Savin dried, of each a dram, Cypress roots, the seeds of Maddir and Rue, Mace, Cinnamon, of each two scruples, beat them and mix them diligently into a powder according to art.

Culpeper.] This seems to be more appropriated to the feminine gender than the former, viz. to bring down the terms, to bring away the birth, and after-birth, to purge them after labour, yet it is dangerous for pregnant women.

Dianisum

College.] Take of Annis seeds two ounces and an half, Liquorice, Mastich, of each an ounce, the seeds of Caraway, Fennel, Galanga, Mace, Ginger, Cinnamon, of each five drams, the three sorts of Pepper, Cassia Lignea, mountain Calaminth, Pellitory of Spain, of each two drams, Cardamoms the greater, Cloves, Cubebs, Indian Spikenard, Saffron, of each a dram and an half, make them into powder.

Culpeper.] It is chiefly appropriated to the stomach, and helps the cold infirmities thereof, raw, flegm, wind, continual coughs, and other such diseases coming of cold. You may safely take a dram of the electuary at a time. You may make an electuary of it with its treble weight of clarified Honey.

Pulvis Radicum Ari compositus
Or Powder of Aron Roots compound

College.] Take of Aron Roots two ounces, of common Water Flag, and Burnet, of each one ounce, Crab's eyes, half an ounce,

Cinnamon three drams, salt of Wormwood, and Juniper, of each one dram, make them into powder.

Culpeper.] And when you have done tell me what it is good for.

Diaireos simple

College.] Take of Orris roots half an ounce, Sugar-candy, Diatragacanthum frigidum, of each two drams, make them into powder.

Culpeper.] I do not mean the Diatragacanthum frigidum, for that is in powder before. It comforts the breast, is good in colds, coughs, and hoarseness. You may mix it with any pectoral Syrups which are appropriated to the same diseases, and so take it with a Liquorice stick.

Dialacca

College.] Take of Gum-lacca, prepared Rhubarb, Schænanth, of each three drams, Indian Spikenard, Mastich, the juice of Wormwood and Agrimony, made thick, the seeds of Smallage, Annis, Fennel, Ammi, Savin, bitter Almonds, Myrrh, Costus, or Zedoary, the roots of Maddir, Asarabacca, Birthwort long and round, Gentian, Saffron, Cinnamon, dried Hyssop, Cassia Lignea, Bdellium, of each a dram and an half, black Pepper, Ginger, of each a dram, make them into powder according to art.

Culpeper.] It strengthens the stomach and liver, opens obstructions, helps dropsies, yellow jaundice, provokes urine, breaks the stone in the reins and bladder. Half a dram is a moderate dose, if the patient be strong they may take a dram in white Wine. Let pregnant women forbear it.

Pulvis Cardiacus Magistralis

College.] Take of East Bezoar, bone of a Stag's-heart, of each a dram and an half, Magisterium, of white and red Coral, white Amber, Magisterium of Pearl, Hart's-horn, Ivory, Bole-amoniac, Earth of Germany, Samos and Lemnos, Elk's-claw, Tormentil roots, of each a dram, Wood of Aloes, Citron peels, the roots of Angelica and Zedoary, of each two scruples, leaves of Gold twenty, Ambergris one scruple, Musk six grains, mix them and make them into powder.

Culpeper.] It is too dear for a vulgar purse, yet a mighty cordial and great strengthener of the heart and vitals in fevers.

Diamargariton frigidum

College.] Take of the four greater cold seeds, the seeds of Purslain, white Poppies, Endive, Sorrel, Citrons, the three Sanders, Wood of Aloes, Ginger, red Roses exungulated, the flowers of Water-lilies, Bugloss, Violets, the berries of Mirtles, bone in a Stag's heart, Ivory, Contra yerva, Cinnamon of each one dram, both sorts of Coral, of each half a dram, Pearls three drams, Camphire six grains, make them into powder according to art. Observe that the four greater cold seeds, and the Poppy seeds, are not to be added before the powder be required by physician for use. Do so by the other powder in the composition of which these powders are used.

Culpeper.] Authors hold it to be restorative in consumptions, to help such as are in hectic fevers, to restore strength lost, to help coughs, asthmaes, and consumptions of the lungs, and restore such as have laboured long under languishing or pining diseases.

Diamoschu Dulce

Take of Saffron, Galanga, Zedoary, Wood of Aloes, Mace, of each two drams, Pearls, raw Silk toasted, white Amber, red Coral prepared, Gallia Moschata, Bazil, of each two drams and an half, Ginger, Cubebs, Long Pepper, of each a dram and an half, Nutmegs, Indian leaf or Cinnamon, Cloves, of each one dram, Musk two scruples, make them into powder according to art.

Culpeper.] It wonderfully helps cold afflictions of the brain, that come without a fever, melancholy and its attendants, viz. sadness without a cause, vertigo or diziness in the head, falling-sickness, palsies, resolution of the nerves, convulsions, heart-qualms, afflictions of the lungs, and difficulty of breathing. The dose of the powder is half a dram, or two scruples, or less; according to the age or strength of him or her that takes it. *Mesue* appoints it to be made into an electuary with clarified honey, and of the electuary, two drams is the dose. The time of taking it is, in the morning fasting.

Diamoschu Amarum

College.] Is prepared by adding to the forenamed Wormwood, dried Roses, of each three drams, Aloes half an ounce, Cinnamon two drams and an half, Castorium and Lovage, of each one dram, make them into powder.

Culpeper.] Besides the virtues of the former, it purges the stomach of putrified humours.

Specia Dianthus

College.] Take of Rosemary flowers an ounce, red Roses, Violets, Liquorice, of each six drams, Cloves, Indian Spikenard, Nutmegs, Galanga, Cinnamon, Ginger, Zedoary, Mace, Wood of Aloes, Cardamoms the less, the seeds of Dill and Anis, of each four scruples, make them into powder according to art.

Culpeper.] It strengthens the heart and helps the passions thereof, it causes a joyful and cheerful mind, and strengthens such as have been weakened by long sickness, it strengthens cold stomachs, and helps digestion notably. The dose is half a dram, you may make it into an electuary with honey, and take two drams of that at a time.

Diapendion

College.] Take of Penides two ounces, Pine-nuts, sweet Almonds blanched, white Poppy seeds, of each three drams and a scruple, (Cinnamon, Cloves, Ginger, which three being omitted, it is a Diapendion without spices) juice of Liquorice, Gum Tragacanth and Arabic, white Starch, the four greater cold seeds husked, of each a dram and an half, Camphire seven grains, make them into powder.

Culpeper.] It helps the vices of the breast, coughs, colds, hoarseness, and consumptions of the lungs, as also such as spit matter. You may mix it with any pectoral syrup, and take it with a Liquorice stick if you fancy the powder best, but if the electuary, you may take a dram of it upon a knife's point at any time when the cough comes.

Diarrhodon Abbatis

College.] Take of Sanders white and red, of each two drams and an half, Gum Tragacanth, Arabic, Ivory of each two scruples, Asarabacca roots, Mastich, Indian Spikenard, Cardamoms, Liquorice, Saffron, Wood of Aloes, Cloves, Gallia Moschata, Annis and sweet Fennel seeds, Cinnamon, Rhubarb, Bazil seeds, Barberry seeds, the seeds of Succory, Purslain, the four greater cold seeds cleansed, white Poppy seeds, of each a scruple, Pearls, bone of a Stag's-heart of each half a scruple, red Roses exungulated, one ounce and three drams, Camphire seven grains, make them into powder according to art.

Culpeper.] It cools the violent heat of the heart and stomach, as also of the liver, lungs, and spleen, eases pains in the body, and most infirmities coming to the body by reason of heat. The dose of the powder is half a dram, and two ounces of the electuary, into which with sugar dissolved in Rose-water you may make it.

Diospoliticum

College.] Take of Cummin seeds steeped in vinegar and dried, long Pepper, Rue leaves, of each an ounce, Nitre half an ounce, make them into powder.

Culpeper.] It is an admirable remedy for such whose meat is putrified in their stomachs, it helps cold stomachs, cold belchings and windy. You may take half a dram after meat, either in a spoonful of Muskadel, or in a Syrup of Mirtles or Quinces, or any Cordial Water whose effects is the same.

Species Diatragacanthi frigidi

College.] Take of Gum Tragacanth two ounces, Gum Arabic an ounce and two drams, white Starch half an ounce, Liquorice, the seeds of Melons and white Poppies, of each three drams, the seeds of Citruls, Cucumbers and Gourds, of each two drams, Penids three ounces, Camphire half a scruple, make of them a powder according to art. Also you may make an electuary of them with a sufficient quantity of Syrup of Violets, but have a care of what was told you before of the seeds.

Culpeper.] Make up into an electuary. It helps the faults of the breast and lungs coming of heat and dryness, it helps consumptions, leanness, inflammations of the sides, pleurises, &c. hot and dry coughs, roughness of the tongue and jaws.

Diatrion Piperion

College.] Take of the three sorts of Peppers, of each six drams and fifteen grains, Annis seeds, Thyme, Ginger, of each one dram, beat them into gross powder.

Culpeper.] It heats the stomach and expels wind. Half a dram in powder, or two drams in electuary (for so *Galen* who was author of it, appoints it to be made with clarified honey, a sufficient quantity) if age and strength permit, if not, half so much, is a sufficient dose, to be taken before meat, if to heat the stomach and help digestion; after meat, if to expel wind.

Diatrion Santalon

College.] Take of all the sorts of Sanders, red Roses, of each three drams, Rhubarb, Ivory, Juice of Liquorice, Purslain seeds, of each two drams and fifteen grains, white Starch, Gum Arabic, Tragacanth, the seeds of Melons, Cucumbers, Citruls, Gourds, Endive, of each a dram and an half, Camphire a scruple, make them into powder according to art.

Culpeper.] It is very profitable against the heat of the stomach and liver, besides, it wonderfully helps such as have the yellow jaundice, and consumptions of the lungs. You may safely take a dram of the powder, or two drams of the electuary in the morning fasting, for most of these powders will keep better by half in electuaries.

Pulvis Haly

College.] Take of white Poppy seeds ten drams, white Starch, Gum Arabic and Tragacanth, of each three drams, the seeds of Purslain, Marsh-mallows, Mallows, of each five drams, Cucumbers, Melons, Gourds, Citruls, Quinces of each seven drams, Ivory, Liquorice, of each three drams, Penids the weight of them all, make them into powder according to art.

Culpeper.] It is a gallant cool powder, fit for all hot imperfections of the breast and lungs, as consumptions, pleurisies, &c. Your best way is to make it into a soft electuary with Syrups of Violets, and take it as *Diatragacanthum frigidum*.

Lætificans

College.] Take the flowers of Clove-bazil, or the seeds thereof, Saffron, Zedoary, Wood of Aloes, Cloves, Citron pills, Galanga, Mace, Nutmegs, Styrax Calamitis, of each two drams and an half, Ivory, Annis seeds, Thyme, Epithimum, of each one dram, bone of a Stag's heart, Pearls, Camphire, of each half a dram, leaves of Gold and Silver, of each half a scruple, make it into powder according to art.

Culpeper.] It causes a merry heart, a good colour, helps digestion, and keeps back old age. You may mix half a dram of it to take at one time, or less if you please, in any cordial Syrup, or cordial electuary appropriated to the same uses.

Pulvis Saxonicus

College.] Take of the roots of both sorts of Angelica, Swallow-wort, garden Valerian, Polipodium of the Oak, Marsh-mallows, Nettles, of each half an ounce, the bark of German Mezereon, two drams, twenty grains of herb True-love, the leaves of the same, roots and all, thirty six, the roots being steeped in vinegar and dried, beat it all into powder.

Culpeper.] It seems to be as great an expeller of poison, and as great a preservative against it, and the pestilence, as one shall usually read of.

Rosate Novelle

College.] Take of red Roses, Liquorice, of each one ounce, one dram, two scruples, and an half, Cinnamon two drams, two scruples, and two grains, Cloves, Indian Spikenard, Ginger, Galanga, Nutmegs, Zedoary, Styrax, Calamitis, Cardamoms, Parsley seeds, of each one scruple eight grains, beat them into powder.

Culpeper.] It quenches thirst, and stays vomiting, and the author saith it helps hot and dry stomachs, as also heat and dryness of the heart, liver, and lungs, (yet is the powder itself hot,) it strengthens the vital spirits, takes away heart-qualms, it provokes sweat, and strengthens such as have laboured under long chronical diseases. You may take a dram of the electuary every morning, if with clarified Honey you please to make it into such a body.

Pulvus Thuraloes

College.] Take of Frankincense one dram, Aloes half a dram, beat them into powder.

Culpeper.] And when you have occasion to use it, mix so much of it with the white of an egg, (beat the white of the egg well first) as will make it of the thickness of Honey, then dip the wool of a Hare in it, and apply it to the sore or part that bleeds, binding it on.

Pulvis Hermidactylorum compositus
Or Powder of Hermodactils compound

College.] Take of men's bones burnt, Scammony, Hermodactils, Turbith, Sena, Sugar, of each equal parts, beat them into powder.

Pulvis Senæ compositus major
Or Powder of Sena the greater composition

College.] Take of the seeds of Annis, Carraway, Fennel, Cummin, Spikenard, Cinnamon, Galanga, of each half an ounce, Liquorice, Gromwell, of each an ounce, Sena, the weight of them all, beat it into powder.

Culpeper.] That this receipt is gallantly composed none can deny, and is an excellent purge for such whose bodies as are troubled with the wind cholic, or stoppage either of guts or kidneys, two drams taken in white Wine will work sufficiently with any ordinary body. Let weak men and children take less, keeping within doors, and warm.

Pulvis Senæ compositus minor

Or Powder of Sena, the lesser composition

College.] Take of Sena two ounces, Cremor Tartar half an ounce, Mace two scruples and an half, Ginger, Cinnamon, of each a dram and an half, Salgem one dram, beat it into powder according to art.

Culpeper.] This powder purges melancholy, and cleanses the head.

Diasenæ

College.] Take of Sena, Cremor Tartar, of each two ounces, Cloves, Cinnamon, Galanga, Ammi, of each two drams, Diacridium half an ounce, beat it into powder according to art.

Diaturbith with Rhubarb

College.] Take of Turbith, Hermodactils, of each an ounce, Rhubarb ten drams, Diacrydium half an ounce, Sanders red and white, Violets, Ginger, of each a dram and an half, Mastich, Annis seeds, Cinnamon, Saffron, of each half a dram, make it into powder.

Culpeper.] This also purges flegm and choler. Once more let me desire such as are unskilful in the rules of physic, not to meddle with purges of this nature (unless prescribed by a skilful Physician) lest they do themselves more mischief in half an hour, than they can remove in half a year.

The lesser cordial Powder. Fernelius

College.] Take of Hart's-horn, Unicorn's horn, Pearls, Ivory, of each six grains beat them into fine powder. If you mean to keep it, you may encrease the quantity analogically.

The greater cordial Powder. Fern

College.] Take of the roots of Tormentil, Dittany, Clove-gilli-flowers, Scabious, the seed of Sorrel, Coriander prepared, Citron, Carduus Benedictus, Endive, Rue, of each one dram, of the three sorts of Sanders, (white, red, and yellow,) Been, white and red (or if you cannot get them, take the roots of Avens and Tormentil, in their stead) Roman Doronicum, (a kind of wolf-bane) Cinnamon, Cardamoms, Saffron, the flowers of both sorts of Bugloss, (viz. Borrage and Bugloss,) red Roses, and Water-Lilies, Wood of Aloes, Mace, of each two scruples, Ivory, Spodium, bone of a Stag's-heart, red Coral, Pearls, Emerald, Jacinth, Granite of each one scruple, raw Silk torrified, (dried or roasted by the fire,) Bole-amoniac, Earth of Lemnos, of each half a dram, Camphire, Amber-gris, Musk, of each six grains, beat them into powder according to art, and with eight times their weight in white sugar, dissolved in Rose-water, you may make them into Lozenges, if you please.

Culpeper.] Both this and the former powder, are appropriated to the heart, (as the title shew) therefore they do strengthen that, and the vital spirit, and relieve languishing nature. All these are cordial Powders, and seldom above half a dram of them given at a time.

A Powder for such as are bruised by a fall
The Augustan Physicians

College.] Take of Terra sigillata, Sanguis Draconis, Mummy of each two drams, Spermaceti one dram, beat them into powder according to art.

Culpeper.] You must beat the rest into powder, and then add the Spermaceti to them afterwards, for if you put the Spermaceti and the rest all together and go to beat them in that fashion, you may as soon beat the mortar into powder, as the simples; indeed your best way is to beat them severally, and then mix them altogether, which being done, makes you a gallant medicine for the infirmities specified in the title, a dram of it taken in Muskadel and sweating after it.

Species Electuarii Dyacymini. Nicholaus

College.] Take of Cummin seeds infused a natural day in Vine-gar, one ounce and one scruple, Cinnamon, Cloves, of each two drams and an half, Galanga, Savory, Calaminth, of each one dram and two scruples, Ginger, black Pepper, of each two drams and five grains, the seeds of Lovage, and Ammi, (Bishop's-weed,) of each one dram and eighteen grains, long Pepper one dram, Spikenard, Nutmegs, Cardamoms, of each two scruples and an half, beat them and keep them diligently in powder for your use.

Culpeper.] It heats the stomach and bowels, expels wind ex-ceedingly, helps the wind cholic, helps digestion hindered by cold or wind, is an admirable remedy for wind in the bowels, and helps quartan agues. The powder is very hot, half a dram is enough to take at one time, and too much if the patient be feverish, you may take it in white Wine. It is in my opinion a fine composed powder.

Species Electuarii Diagalangæ. Mesue

College.] Take of Galanga, wood of Aloes, of each six drams, Cloves, Mace, seeds of Lovage of each two drams, Ginger, long and white Pepper, Cinnamon, Calamus Aromaticus of each a dram and an half, Calaminth, and Mints dried, Cardamoms the greater, Indian Spikenard, the seeds of Smallage, Annis, Fennel, Caraway, of each one dram, beat them into powder according to art. Also it may be made into an electuary with white sugar dissolved in Malaga wine, or twelve times the weight of it of clarified Honey.

Culpeper.] *Mesue* quotes it only as an electuary, which he saith prevails against wind, sour belchings, and indigestion, gross humours and cold afflictions of the stomach and liver. You may take half a dram of the powder at a time, or two of the electuary in the morning fasting, or an hour before meat. It helps digestion exceedingly, expels wind, and heats a cold stomach.

Species Electuarii Diamargariton Calidi. Avicenna

College.] Take of Pearls and Pellitory of the Wall, of each one dram, Ginger, Mastich, of each half an ounce, Doronicum, Zedoary, Smallage seeds, both sorts of Cardamoms, Nutmegs, Mace, of each two drams, Been of both sorts, (if they cannot be procured take the roots of Avens and Tormentil) black and long Pepper of each three drams, beat them into powder and keep them for your use.

Culpeper.] This (quoth *Avicenna*) is appropriated to women, and in them to diseases incident to their matrix; but his reasons I know not. It is cordial and heats the stomach.

Lithontribon Nicholaus, according to Fernelius

College.] Take of Spikenard, Ginger, Cinnamon, black Pepper, Cardamoms, Cloves, Mace, of each half a dram, Costus, Liquorice, Cypress, Tragacanth, Germander, of each two scruples, the seeds of Bishop's-weed, (Ammi), Smallage, Sparagus, Bazil, Nettles, Citrons, Saxifrage, Burnet, Caraway, Carrots, Fennel, Bruscus, Parsley of Macedonia, Burs, Seseli, (or Hartwort), Asarabacca, of each one dram, Lapis Spongiæ, Lyncis, Cancri, Judaici, of each one dram and an half, Goat's blood prepared an ounce and half, beat them all into powder according to art.

Culpeper.] It heats the stomach, and helps want of digestion coming through cold, it eases pains in the belly and loins, the Illiac passion, powerfully breaks the stone in the reins and bladder, it speedily helps the cholic, stranguary, and disury. The dose is from a dram to half a dram, take it either in white Wine, or decoction of herbs tending to the same purposes.

Pleres Arconticon. Nicholaus

College.] Take of Cinnamon, Cloves, Galanga, Wood of Aloes, Indian Spikenard, Nutmegs, Ginger, Spodium, Schœnanthus, Cypress, Roses, Violets of each one dram, Indian Leaf or Mace, Liquorice, Mastich, Styrax Calamitis, Marjoram, Costmary, or Water-mints, Bazil, Cardamoms, long and white Pepper, Myrtle berries, and Citron pills, of each half a dram and six grains, Pearls, Been white and red, (or, if they be wanting, take the roots of Avens and Tormentil in their stead) red Coral, torrified Silk, of each eighteen grains, Musk six grains, Camphire four grains, beat them into powder according to art, and with ten times their weight in sugar dissolved in Bawm water, you may make them into an electuary.

Culpeper.] It is exceedingly good for sad, melancholy, lumpish, pensive, grieving, vexing, pining, sighing, sobbing, fearful, careful spirits, it strengthens weak stomachs exceedingly, and help such as are prone to faintings and swoonings, it strengthens such as are weakened by violence of sickness, it helps bad memories, quickens all the senses, strengthens the brain and animal spirits, helps the falling-sickness, and succours such as are troubled with asthmas, or other cold afflictions of the lungs. It will keep best in an electuary, of which you may take a dram in the morning, or more, as age and strength requires.

A Preservative Powder against the Pestilence. Montagnam

College.] Take of all the Sanders, (white, red, and yellow,) the seeds of Bazil, of each an ounce and an half, Bole Amoniac, Cinnamon, of each an ounce, the roots of Dittany, Gentian, and Tormentil, of each two drams and an half, the seeds of Citron and Sorrel, of each two drams, Pearls Saphire, bone of a Stag's heart, of each one dram, beat them into powder according to art.

Culpeper.] The title tells you the virtue of it, besides, it cheers the vital spirits, and strengthens the heart. You may take half a dram every morning either by itself, or mixed with any other convenient composition, whether Syrup or Electuary.

Diaturbith the greater, without Rhubarb

College.] Take of the best Turbith an ounce, Diagridium, Ginger, of each half an ounce, Cinnamon, Cloves, of each two drams, Galanga, long Pepper, Mace, of each one dram, beat them into powder, and with eight ounces and five drams of white sugar dissolved in Succory Water, it may be made into an electuary.

Culpeper.] It purges flegm, being rightly administered by a skilful hand. I fancy it not.

A Powder for the Worms

College.] Take of Wormseed, four ounces, Sena, one ounce, Coriander seeds prepared, Hart's-horn, of each half a dram, Rhubarb half an ounce, dried Rue, two drams, beat them into powder.

Culpeper.] I like this powder very well; the quantity (or to write more scholastically, the dose) must be regulated according to the age of the patient, even from ten grains to a dram, and the manner of taking it by their palate. It is something purging.

ELECTUARIES

Antidotus Analeptica

College.] Take of red Roses, Liquorice of each two drams and five grains, Gum Arabic and Tragacanth, of each two drams and two scruples, Sanders white and red, each four scruples, juice of Liquorice, white Starch, the seeds of white Poppies, Purslain, Lettuce, and Endive, of each three drams, the four greater cold seeds husked, of Quinces, Mallows, Cotton, Violets, Pine-nuts, fistic Nuts, sweet Almonds, pulp of Sebestens, of each two drams, Cloves, Spodium, Cinnamon, of each one dram, Saffron five grains, Penids half an ounce, being beaten, make them all into a soft electuary with three times their weight in Syrup of Violets.

Culpeper.] It restores consumptions, and hectic fevers, lost strength, it nourishes much, and restores radical moisture, opens the pores, resists choler, takes away coughs, quenches thirst, and resists fevers. You may take an ounce in a day, by a dram at a time, if you please.

Confectio Alkermes

College.] Take of the juice of Apples, Damask Rose-water, of each a pound and an half, in which infuse for twenty-four hours, raw Silk four ounces, strain it strongly, and add Syrup of the berries of Cherms brought over to us, two pounds, Sugar one pound, boil it to the thickness of Honey; then removing it from the fire whilst it is warm, add Ambergris cut small, half an ounce, which being well mingled, put in these things following in powder, Cinnamon, Wood of Aloes, of each six drams, Pearls prepared, two drams, Leaf-Gold a dram, Musk a scruple, make it up according to art.

Culpeper.] Questionless this is a great cordial, and a mighty strengthener of the heart, and vital spirits, a restorer of such as are in consumptions, a resister of pestilences and poison, a relief to languishing nature, it is given with good success in fevers, but give not too much of it at a time, lest it prove too hot for the body, and too heavy for the purse. You may mix ten grains of it with other convenient cordials to children, twenty or thirty to men.

Electuarium e Sassaphras

College.] Take of Sassafras two ounces, common Water three pounds, boil it to the consumption of the third part, adding, towards the end, Cinnamon bruised half an ounce, strain it, and with two pounds of white sugar, boil it to the thickness of a Syrup, putting in, in powder, Cinnamon, a dram, Nutmegs, half a scruple, Musk three grains, Ambergris, two and thirty grains, ten leaves of Gold, Spirit of Vitriol four drops, and so make it into an electuary according to art.

Culpeper.] It opens obstruction of the liver and spleen, helps cold rheums or defluxions from the head to the lungs, or teeth, or eyes, it is excellent in coughs, and other cold afflictions of the lungs and breast, it helps digestion, expels wind and the gravel of the kidneys, it provokes the menses, warms and dries up the moisture of the womb, which is many times the cause of barrenness, and is generally a helper of all diseases coming of cold, raw thin humours, you may take half a dram at a time in the morning.

Electuarium de Baccis Lauri
Or Electuary of Bay-berries

College.] Take of the leaves of dried Rue ten drams, the seeds of Ammi, Cummin, Lovage, Origanum, Nigella, Caraway, Carrots, Parsley, bitter Almonds, Pepper black and long, wild Mints,

Calamus Aromaticus, Bay-berries, Castorium of each two drams, Sagapenum half an ounce, Opopanax three drams, clarified Honey a pound and an half, the things to be beaten; being beaten, and the Gums dissolved in Wine, make it into an electuary according to art.

Culpeper.] It is exceeding good either in the cholic or Iliac passion, or any other disease of the bowels coming of cold or wind, it generally eases pains in the bowels. You may give a dram in the morning fasting, or half an ounce in a clyster, according as the disease is.

Diacapparit

College.] Take of Capers four ounces, Agrimony Roots, Nigella seeds, Squils, Asarabacca, Centaury, black Pepper, Smallage, Thyme of each an ounce, Honey three times their weight, make it into an electuary according to art.

Culpeper.] They say it helps infirmities of the spleen, and indeed the name seems to promise so much, it may be good for cold bodies, if they have strength of nature in them.

Diacinnamomum

College.] Take of Cinnamon fifteen drams, Cassia Lignea, Elecampane roots, of each half an ounce, Galanga, seven drams, Cloves, long Pepper, both sorts of Cardamoms, Ginger, Mace, Nutmegs, Wood of Aloes, of each three drams, Saffron, one dram, Sugar five drams, Musk two scruples, adding according to the prescript of the Physician, and by adding three pounds eight ounces of clarified Honey, boil it and make it into an electuary according to art.

Culpeper.] *Diacinnamomum*, or in plain English, *A composition of Cinnamon*, heats the stomach, causes digestion, provokes the menses, strengthens the stomach and other parts that distribute the nourishment of the body, a dram of it taken in the morning fasting, is good for ancient people and cold bodies, such as are subject to dropsies and diseases of flegm, or wind, for it comforts and strengthens nature much. If you take it to help digestion, take it an hour before meat, do so in all things of like quality.

Diacorallion

College.] Take of Coral white and red, Bole-amoniac, Dragon's-blood, of each one dram, Pearls half a dram, Wood of Aloes, red Roses, Gum Tragacanth, Cinnamon, of each two scruples, Sanders white and red, of each one scruple, with four times its weight in sugar dissolved in small Cinnamon Water, make it into an electuary, according to art.

Culpeper.] It comforts and strengthens the heart exceedingly, and restores such as are in consumptions, it is cooling, therefore good in hectic fevers, very binding, and therefore stops fluxes, neither do I know a better medicine in all the dispensatory for such as have a consumption accompanied with looseness. It stops the menses and Fluor Albus. Take but a dram at a time every morning, because of its binding quality, except you have a looseness, for then you may take so much two or three times a day.

Diacorum

College.] Take of the roots of Cicers, Acorus, or Calamus Aromaticus, Pine-nuts, of each a pound and a half, let the Cicers roots, being cleansed, cut, boiled, and pulped, be added to ten pounds of clarified honey, and boiled, (stirring it) to its just thickness, then being removed from the fire, add the Acorus roots beaten, the Pine-nuts cut, and these following in powder. Take of black Pepper an ounce, long Pepper, Cloves, Ginger, Mace, of each half an ounce, Nutmegs, Galanga, Cardamons, of each three drams, mix them with the roots and Honey into an electuary according to art.

Culpeper.] The electuary provokes lust, heats the brain, strengthens the nerves, quickens the senses, causes an acute wit, eases pains in the head, helps the falling-sickness and convulsions, coughs, catarrhs, and all diseases proceeding from coldness of the brain. Half a dram is enough to take at one time, because of its heat.

Peony is an herb of the *sun*, the roots of it cure the falling-sickness.

Diacydonium simple

College.] Take of the flesh of Quinces cut and boiled in fair water to a thickness, eight pounds, white sugar six pounds, boil it to its just thickness.

Diacydonium with Species

College.] Take of the juice of Quinces, Sugar, of each two pounds, white Wine Vinegar half a pound, added at the end of the decoction, it being gently boiled, and the scum taken away, add Ginger two ounces, white Pepper ten drams and two scruples, bruise them grossly, and boil it again to the thickness of Honey.

Diacydonium compound, Magisterial

College.] Take of white Sugar six pounds, Spring Water four pounds, clarify them well with the white of an egg, scumming them, then take of ripe Quinces cleansed from the rind and seeds, and cut in four quarters, eight pounds, boil them in the foregoing Syrup till they be tender, then strain the Syrup through a linen cloth, *vocata Anglice*, Boulter; boil them again to a jelly, adding four ounces of white wine Vinegar towards the end; remove it from the fire, and whilst it is warm put in these following species in powder, Ginger an ounce, white Pepper, Cinnamon, Nutmegs, of each two drams, keep it for use.

Culpeper.] The virtues of all these three are, they comfort the stomach, help digestion, stays vomiting, belchings, &c. stop fluxes and the menses. They are all harmless, you may take the quantity of a nutmeg of them at a time, before meat to help digestion and fluxes, after meat to stay vomiting, in the morning for the rest.

Confectio de Hyacintho

College.] Take of Jacinth, red Coral, Bole-amoniac, Earth of Lemnos, of each half an ounce, the berries of Chermes, the Roots of Tormentil and Dittany, the seeds of Citrons, Sorrel, and Purslain, Saffron, Myrrh, red Roses exungulated, all the sorts of Sanders, bone of a Stag's heart, Hart's-horn, Ivory prepared, of each four scruples, Samphire, Emerald, Topaz, Pearls, raw Silk, leaves of Gold and Silver, of each two scruples, Camphire, Musk, Ambergris, of each five grains, with Syrup of Lemons make it into a confection according to art.

Culpeper.] It is a great cordial and cool, exceeding good in acute fevers and pestilences, it mightily strengthens and cherishes the heart. Never above half a dram is given at a time.

Antidotum Hæmagogum

College.] Take of Lupines husked two drams, black Pepper five scruples and six grains, Liquorice four scruples, long Birthwort, Mugwort, Cassia Lignea, Macedonian Parsley seed, Pellitory of Spain, Rue seed, Spikenard, Myrrh, Pennyroyal, of each two scruples and fourteen grains, the seeds of Smallage, Savin, of each two scruples and thirteen grains, Centaury the greater, Cretish Carrots, Nigella, Caraway, Annis, Cloves, Alum, of each two scruples, Bay leaves one scruple, one half scruple, and three grains,

Schænanth one scruple and thirteen grains, Asarabacca, Calamus Aromaticus, Amomum, Centaury the less, the seed of Orrach, Peony, Fennel, of each one scruple and six grains, wood of Aloes, a scruple and fourteen grains, Cypress, Elecampane, Ginger, Cappar roots, Cummin, Orobus, of each one scruple, all of them being beaten into very fine powder, let them be made into an electuary according to art, with four times their weight in sugar, let it stand one month before you use it.

Culpeper.] It provokes the menses, brings away both birth and after-birth, the dead child, purges such as are not sufficiently purged after travail, it provokes urine, breaks the stone in the bladder, helps the stranguary, disury, iskury, &c. helps indigestion, the cholic, opens any stoppings in the body, it heats the stomach, purges the liver and spleen, consumes wind, stays vomiting, but let it not be taken by pregnant women, nor such people as have the hemorrhoids. The dose is from one dram to two drams.

Diasatyrion

College.] Take of Satyrion roots three ounces, Dates, bitter Almonds, Indian Nuts, Pine nuts, Festick nuts, green Ginger, Eringo roots preserved, of each one ounce, Ginger, Cloves, Galanga, Pepper long and black, of each three drams, Ambergris one scruple, Musk two scruples, Penins four ounces, Cinnamon, Saffron, of each half an ounce, Malaga Wine three ounces, Nutmegs, Mace, Grains of Paradise, of each two drams, Ash-tree keys, the belly and loins of Scinks, Borax, Benjamin, of each three drams, wood of Aloes, Cardamoms, of each two drams, the seeds of Nettles and Onions, the roots of Avens, of each a dram and a half, with two pounds and an half of Syrup of green Ginger, make them into an electuary according to art.

Electuarium Diaspermaton

College.] Take of the four greater and lesser cold seeds, the seeds of Asparagus, Burnet, Bazil, Parsley, Winter Cherries, of each two drams, Gromwell, Juice of Liquorice, of each three drams, Cinnamon, Mace, of each one dram, with eight times their weight in white Sugar dissolved in Marsh-mallows water, make it into an electuary according to art.

Culpeper.] It breaks the stone, and provokes urine. Men may take half an ounce at a time, and children half so much, in water of any herb or roots, &c. (or decoction of them) that break the stone.

Micleta

College.] Take of the barks of all the Myrobalans torrified, of each two drams and an half, the seeds of Water-cresses, Cummin, Annis, Fennel, Ammi, Caraway, of each a dram and an half, bruise the seeds and sprinkle them with sharp white wine Vinegar, then beat them into powder, and add the Mirobalans, and these things that follow, Spodium, Balaustines, Sumach, Mastich, Gum Arabic, of each one dram and fifteen grains, mix them together, and with ten ounces of Syrup of Myrtles, make them into an electuary according to art.

Culpeper.] It gently eases the bowels of the wind cholic, wringing of the bowels, infirmities of the spleen, it stops fluxes, the hemorrhoids, as also the menses.

Electuarium Pectorale
Or a Pectoral Electuary

College.] Take of the juice of Liquorice, sweet Almonds, Hazel-Nuts, of each half an ounce, Pine-nuts an ounce, Hysop, Maiden-hair, Orris, Nettle seeds, round Birthwort, of each a dram and an half, black Pepper, the seeds of Water-cresses, the roots of Elecampane, of each half a dram, Honey fourteen ounces, make them into an electuary according to art.

Culpeper.] It strengthens the stomach and lungs, and helps the vices thereof. Take it with a Liquorice stick.

Theriaca Diatessaron

College.] Take of Gentain, Bay-berries, Myrrh, round Birthwort, of each two ounces, Honey two pounds, make them into an electuary according to art.

Culpeper.] This is a gallant electuary. It wonderfully helps cold infirmities of the brain, as convulsions, falling-sickness, dead palsies, shaking palsies, &c. As also the stomach, as pains there, wind, want of digestion, as also stoppings of the liver, dropsies, it resists the pestilence and poison, and helps the bitings of venomous beasts. The dose is from half a dram to two drams, according to the age and strength of the patient, as also the strength of the diseases: you may take it either in the morning, or when urgent occasion calls for it.

Diascordium

College.] Take of Cinnamon, Cassia Lignea, of each half an ounce, Scordium, an ounce, Dittany of Crete, Tormentil, Bistort,

Galbanum, Gum Arabic, of each half an ounce, Opium one dram and an half, Sorrel seeds one dram and a half, Gentain half an ounce, Bole-amoniac an ounce and an half, Earth of Lemnos half an ounce, long Pepper, Ginger, of each two drams, clarified Honey two pounds and an half, Sugar of Roses one pound, Canary Wine ten ounces, make them into an electuary according to art.

Culpeper.] It is a well composed electuary, something appropriated to the nature of women, for it provokes the menses, hastens labour, helps their usual sickness at the time of their lying in; I know nothing better, it stops fluxes, mightily strengthens the heart and stomach, neither is so hot but it may safely be given to weak people, and besides provokes sleep. It may safely be given to young children ten grains at a time, ancient people may take a dram or more. It is given as an excellent cordial in such fevers as are accompanied with want of sleep.

Mithridate

College.] Take of Myrrh, Saffron, Agarick, Ginger, Cinnamon, Spikenard, Frankincense, Treacle, Mustard seeds, of each ten drams, the seeds of Hartwort, Opobalsamum, or oil of Nutmegs by expression, Schenanth, Stœchas, Costus, Galbanum, Turpentine, long Pepper, Castorium, juice of Hypocistis, Styrax, Calamitis, Opopanax, Indian leaf, or for want of it Mace, of each an ounce, Cassia Lignea, Poley Mountain, white Pepper, Scordium, the seeds of Carrots of Crete, Carpobalsamum or Cubebs, Troch, Cypheos, Bdelium, of each seven drams, Celtic Spikenard, Gum Arabic, Macedonian Parsley seeds, Opium, Cardamoms the less, Fennel seed, Gentian, red Rose leaves, Dittany of Crete, of each five drams, Annis seeds, Asarabacca, Orris Acorus, the greater Valerian, Sagapen, of each three drams, Meum Acacia, the bellies of Scinks, the tops of St. John's Wort, of each two drams and an half, Malaga Wine, so much as is sufficient to dissolve the juices and gums, clarified Honey the treble weight of all, the wine excepted, make them into an electuary according to art.

Culpeper.] It is good against poison and such as have done themselves wrong by taking filthy medicines, it provokes sweat, it helps continual waterings of the stomach, ulcers in the body, consumptions, weakness of the limbs, rids the body of cold humours, and diseases coming of cold, it remedies cold infirmities of the brain, and stopping of the passage of the senses, (viz. hearing, seeing, smelling, &c.) by cold, it expels wind, helps the cholic, provokes appetite to one's victuals, it helps ulcers in the bladder, if *Galen* say true, as also difficulty of urine, it casts out the dead child, and helps such women as cannot conceive by reason of cold, it is an admirable remedy for melancholy, and all diseases of the body coming through cold, it would fill a whole sheet of paper to reckon them all up particularly. You may take a scruple or half a dram in the morning, and follow your business, two drams will make you sweat, yea one dram if your body be weak, for then two drams may be dangerous because of its heat.

Phylonium Persicum

College.] Take of white Pepper, the seeds of white Henbane, of each two drams, Opium, Earth of Lemnos, of each ten drams, Lap, Hematitus, Saffron, of each five drams, Castorium, Indian Spikenard, Euphorbium prepared, Pellitory of Spain, Pearls, Amber, Zedoary, Elecampane, Troch, Ramach, of each a dram, Camphire a scruple, with their treble weight in Honey of Roses, make it into an electuary according to art.

Culpeper.] It stops blood flowing from any part of the body, the immoderate flowing of the menses, the hemorrhoids in men, spitting of blood, bloody fluxes, and is profitable for such women as are subject to miscarry. See the next receipt.

Phylonium Romanum

College.] Take of white Pepper, white Henbane seeds, of each five drams, Opium two drams and an half, Cassia Lignea a dram and an half, the seeds of Smallage a dram, Parsley of Macedonia, Fennel, Carrots of Crete, of each two scruples and five grains, Saffron a scruple and an half, Indian Spikenard, Pellitory of Spain, Zedoary fifteen grains, Cinnamon a dram and an half, Euphorbium prepared, Myrtle Castorium, of each a dram with their treble weight in clarified Honey, make it into an electuary.

Electuarium de Ovo
Or electuary of Eggs

College.] Take a Hen's Egg new laid, and the white being taken out by a small hole, fill up the void place with Saffron, leaving the yolk in, then the hole being stopped, roast it in ashes till the shell begin to look black, take diligent heed the Saffron burn not, for then is the whole medicine spoiled, then the matter being taken out dry, if so that it may be beaten into powder and add to it as much powder of white Mustard seed as it weighs. Then take the roots of white Dittany and Tormentil, of each two drams, Myrrh, Hart's-horn, Petasitis roots, of each one dram, the roots of Angelica and Burnet, Juniper Berries, Zedoary, Camphire of each half an ounce, mix them all together in a mortar, then add Venice Treacle the weight of them all, stir them about with a pestle three hours together, putting in so much Syrup of Lemons, as is enough to make it into an electuary according to art.

Culpeper.] A dram of it given at a time, is as great a help in a pestilential fever as a man shall usually read of in a Galenist. It provokes sweat, and then you shall be taught how to use yourself. If years do not permit, give not so much.

Theriaca Andromachi
Or Venice Treacle

College.] Take of Troches of Squils forty-eight drams, Troches of Vipers, long Pepper, Opium of Thebes, Magma, Hedycroi dried, of each twenty-four drams, red Roses exungulated, Orris, Illirick, juice of Liquorice, the seeds of sweet Navew, Scordium, Opobalsamum, Cinnamon, Agerick, of each twelve drams, Myrrh, Costus, or Zedoary, Saffron, Cassia Lignea, Indian Spikenard, Schenanth, Pepper white and black, Olibanum, Dittany of Crete, Rhapontic, Stœchas, Horehound, Macedonian Parsley seed, Calaminth, Cypress, Turpentine, the roots of Cinquefoyl and Ginger, of each six drams, Poley Mountain, Chamepitis, Celtic Spikenard, Amomus, Styrax Calamitis, the roots of Meum, the tops of Germander, the roots of Rhapontic Earth of Lemnos, Indian Leaf, Chalcitis burnt, or instead thereof Roman Vitriol burnt, Gentian roots, Gum Arabic, the juice of Hypositis, Carpobalsamum or Nutmegs, or Cubebs, the seeds of Annis, Cardamoms, Fennel, Hartwort, Acacia, or instead thereof the juice of Sloes made thick, the seeds of Treacle Mustard, and Ammi, the tops of St. John's Wort, Sagapen, of each four drams, Castorium, the roots of long Birthwort, Bitumen, Judaicum, Carrot seed, Opopanax, Centaury the less, Galbanum, of each two drams, Canary Wine enough to dissolve what is to be dissolved, Honey the treble weight of the dry species, make them into an Electuary according to art.

Culpeper.] It resists poison, and the bitings of venomous beasts, inveterate headaches, vertigo, deafness, the falling-sickness, astonishment, apoplexies, dulness of sight, want of voice, asthmaes, old and new coughs, such as spit or vomit blood, such as can hardly spit or breathe, coldness of the stomach, wind, the cholic, and illiac passion, the yellow jaundice, hardness of the spleen, stone in the reins and bladder, difficulty of urine, ulcers in the bladder, fevers, dropsies, leprosies, it provokes the menses, brings forth birth and after-birth, helps pains in the joints, it helps not only the body, but also the mind, as vain fears, melancholy, &c. and is a good remedy in pestilential fevers. You may take half a dram and go about your business, and it will do you good if you have occasion to go in ill airs, or in pestilent times, if you shall sweat under it, as your best way is, if your body be not in health, then take one dram, or between one and two, or less than one, according as age and strength is, if you cannot take this or any other sweating medicine by itself, mix it with a little Carduus or Dragon's water, or Angelica water, which in my opinion is the best of the three.

Theriacca Londinensis
Or London Treacle

College.] Take of Hart's-horn two ounces, the seeds of Citrons, Sorrel, Peony, Bazil, of each one ounce, Scordium, Coralliana, of each six drams, the roots of Angelica, Tormentil, Peony, the leaves of Dittany, Bay-berries, Juniper-berries, of each half an ounce, the flowers of Rosemary, Marigolds, Clove Gilliflowers, the tops of Saint John's Wort, Nutmegs, Saffron, of each three drams, the Roots of Gentian, Zedoary, Ginger, Mace, Myrrh, the leaves of Scabious, Devil's-bit, Carduus, of each two drams, Cloves, Opium, of each a dram, Malaga Wine as much as is sufficient, with their treble weight in Honey, mix them according to art.

Culpeper.] The receipt is a pretty cordial, resists the pestilence, and is a good antidote in pestilential times, it resists poison, strengthens cold stomachs, helps digestion, crudities of the stomach. A man may safely take two drams of it in a morning, and let him fear no harm.

Diacrocuma

College.] Take of Saffron, Asarabacca roots, the seeds of Parsley, Carrots, Annis, Smallage, of each half an ounce, Rhubarb, the roots of Meum, Indian Spikenard, of each six drams, Cassia Lignea, Costus, Myrrh, Schenanth, Cubebs, Madder roots, the juices of Maudlin, and Wormwood made thick, Opobalsamum, or oil of Nutmegs, of each two drams, Cinnamon, Calamus Aromaticus, of each a dram and an half, Scordium, Cetrach, juice of Liquorice, of each two drams and an half, Tragacanth a dram, with eight times their weight in white sugar, dissolved in Endive water, and clarified, make it into an electuary, according to art.

Culpeper.] It is exceeding good against cold diseases of the stomach, liver, or spleen, corruption of humours and putrefaction of meat in the stomach, ill favoured colour of the body, dropsies, cold faults in the reins and bladder, provokes urine. Take a dram in the morning.

PURGING ELECTUARIES

Benedicta Laxativa

College.] Take of choice Turbith ten drams, Diacridium, bark of Spurge Roots prepared, Hermodactils, Red Roses, of each five drams, Cloves, Spikenard, Ginger, Saffron, long Pepper, Amomus, or for want of it Calamus Aromaticus, Cardamoms the less, the seeds of Smallage, Parsley, Fennel, Asparagus, Bruscus, Saxifrage, Gromwell, Caraway, sal. gem. Galanga, Mace, of each a dram, with their treble weight of clarified Honey: make them into an electuary according to art. Also you may keep the species itself in your shops.

Culpeper.] It purges flegm, chiefly from the joints, also it purges the reins and bladder.

Caryocostinum

College.] Take of Cloves, Costus, or Zedoary, Ginger, Cummin, of each two drams, Hermodactils, Diacridium, of each half an ounce: with their double weight of Honey clarified in white wine, make them into an electuary according to art.

Culpeper.] Authors say it purges hot rheums, and takes away inflammations in wounds. I assure you the electuary works violently, and may safely be given in clysters, and so you may give two or three drams at a time, if the patient be strong. For taken otherwise it would kill a horse *cum privilegio*.

Cassia Extracta pro Clysteribus
Or Cassia extracted for Clysters

College.] Take of the leaves of Violets, Mallows, Beets, Mercury, Pellitory of the Wall, Violet flowers, of each a handful, boil them in a sufficient quantity of water, the benefit of which let the Cassia be extracted, and the canes washed; then take of this Cassia so drawn, and boil it to its consistence, a pound, Sugar a pound and a half, boil them to the form of an electuary according to art.

Culpeper.] You may take it in white Wine; it is good for gentle bodies, for if your body be hard to work upon, perhaps it will not work at all; it purges the reins gallantly, and cools them, thereby preventing the stone, and other diseases caused by their heat.

Electuarium Amarum Magistrale majus
Or the greater bitter Electuary

College.] Take of Agarick, Turbith, Species Hiera Simplex, Rhubarb, of each one dram, choice Aloes unwashed two drams, Ginger, Crystal of Tartar, of each two scruples, Orris, Florentine, sweet Fennel seeds, of each a scruple, Syrup of Roses solutive as much as is sufficient to make it into an electuary according to art.

Electuarium Amarum minus
Or the lesser bitter Electuary

College.] Take of Epithimum half an ounce, the roots of Angelica three drams, of Gentian, Zedoary, Acorus, of each two drams, Cinnamon one dram and an half, Cloves, Mace, Nutmegs, Saffron, of each one dram, Aloes six ounces, with Syrup of Fumitory, Scabious and Sugar so much as is sufficient to make it into a soft electuary.

Culpeper.] Both these purge choler, the former flegm, and this melancholy, the former works strongest, and this strengthens most, and is good for such whose brains are annoyed. You may take half an ounce of the former, if your body be any thing strong, in white Wine, if very strong an ounce, a reasonable body may take an ounce of the latter, the weak less. I would not have the unskilful too busy about purges without advice of a physician.

Diacassia with Manna

College.] Take of Damask Prunes two ounces, Violet flowers a handful and an half, Spring Water a pound and an half, boil it according to art till half be consumed, strain it, and dissolve in the decoction six ounces of Cassia newly drawn, sugar of Violets, Syrup of Violets, of each four ounces, Pulp of Tamarinds an ounce, Sugar Candy an ounce and an half, Manna two ounces, mix them, and make them into an electuary according to art.

Culpeper.] It is a fine cool purge for such as are bound in the body, for it works gently, and without trouble, it purges choler, and may safely be given in fevers coming of choler: but in such cases, if the body be much bound, the best way is first to administer a clyster, and then the next morning an ounce of this will cool the body, and keep it in due temper.

Cassia extracta sine soliis Senæ
Or Cassia extracted without the leaves of Sena

College.] Take twelve Prunes, Violet flowers a handful, French Barley, the seed of Annis, and bastard Saffron, Polypodium of the Oak, of each five drams, Maiden-hair, Thyme, Epithimum, of each half a handful, Raisins of the Sun stoned half an ounce, sweet Fennel seeds two drams, the seeds of Purslain, and Mallows, of each three drams, Liquorice half an ounce, boil them in a sufficient quantity of water, strain them and dissolve in the decoction, pulp of Cassia two pounds, of Tamarinds an ounce, Cinnamon three drams, Sugar a pound, boil it into the form of an electuary.

Cassia extracta cum soliis Senæ
Or Cassia extracted with the leaves of Sena

College.] Take of the former receipt two pounds, Sena in powder two ounces, mix them according to art.

Culpeper.] This is also a fine cool gentle purge, cleansing the bowels of choler and melancholy without any griping, very fit for feverish bodies, and yet the former is gentler than this. They both cleanse and cool the reins; a reasonable body may take an ounce and an half of the former, and an ounce of the latter in white Wine, if they keep the house, or their bodies be oppressed with melancholy, let them take half the quantity in four ounces of decoction of Epithimum.

Diacarthamum

College.] Take of Diatragacanthum frigidum, half an ounce, pulp of preserved Quinces an ounce, the inside of the seeds of Bastard Saffron half an ounce, Ginger two drams, Diacrydium beaten by itself three drams, Turbith, six drams, Manna two ounces, Honey of Roses solutive, Sugar Candy, of each an ounce, Hermodactils half an ounce, Sugar ten ounces and an half, make of them a liquid electuary according to art.

Diaphænicon

College.] Take of the pulp of Dates boiled in Hydromel, Penids, of each half a pound, sweet Almonds blanched, three ounces and an half, to all of them being bruised and mixed, add clarified Honey two pounds, boil them a little, and then strew in Ginger, long Pepper, Mace, Cinnamon, Rue leaves, the seeds of Fennel and

Carrots, of each two drams, Turbith four ounces, Diacridium an ounce and an half, make of them an electuary according to art.

Culpeper.] I cannot believe this is so profitable in fevers taken downwards as authors say, for it is a very violent purge.

Diaprunum Lenitive

College.] Take one hundred Damask Prunes, boil them in water till they be soft, then pulp them, and in the liquor they were boiled in, boil gently one of Violet flowers, strain it, and with two pounds of sugar boil it to a Syrup, then add half a pound of the aforesaid pulp, the pulp of Cassia, and Tamarinds, of each one ounce, then mix with it these powders following: Sanders white and red, Spodium, Rhubarb, of each three drams, red Roses, Violets, the seeds of Purslain, Succory, Barberries, Gum Tragacanth, Liquorice, Cinnamon, of each two drams, the four greater cold seeds, of each one dram, make it into an electuary according to art.

Culpeper.] It may safely, and is with good success, given in acute, burning, and all other fevers, for it cools much, and loosens the body gently: it is good in agues, hectic fevers, and Mirasmos. You may take an ounce of it at a time, at night when you go to bed, three hours after a light supper, neither need you keep your chamber next day, unless the weather be very cold, or your body very tender.

Diaprunum solutive

College.] Take of Diaprunum Lenitive whilst it is warm, four pounds, Scammony prepared two ounce and five drams, mix them into an electuary according to art.

Seeing the dose of Scammony is increased according to the author in this medicine, you may use a less weight of Scammony if you please.

Catholicon

College.] Take of the pulp of Cassia and Tamarinds, the leaves of Sena, of each two ounces, Polypodium, Violets, Rhubarb, of each one ounce, Annis seeds, Penids, Sugar Candy, Liquorice, the seeds of Gourds, Citruls, Cucumbers, Melons, of each two drams, the things to be bruised being bruised, take of fresh Polypodium three ounces, sweet Fennel seeds six drams, boil them in four pounds of water till the third part be consumed, strain it, and with two pounds of sugar, boil the decoction to the thickness of a Syrup; then with the pulps and powder make it into an electuary according to art.

Culpeper.] It is a fine cooling purge for any part of the body, and very gentle, it may be given (an ounce, or half an ounce at a time, according to the strength of the patient) in acute, or peracute diseases, for it gently loosens the belly, and adds strength, it helps infirmities of the liver and spleen, gouts of all sorts, quotidian, tertian, and quartan agues, as also head-aches. It is usually given in clysters. If you like to take it inwardly, you may take an ounce at night going to bed; in the morning drink a draught of hot posset drink and go about your business.

Electuarium de Citro Solutivum
Or Electuary of Citrons, solutive

College.] Take of Citron pills preserved, conserves of the flowers of Violets and Bugloss, Diatragacanthum frigidum, Diacrydium, of each half an ounce, Turbith five drams, Ginger half a dram, Sena six drams, sweet Fennel seeds one dram, white sugar dissolved in Rose-water, and boiled according to art, ten ounces, make a solid electuary according to art.

Culpeper.] Here are some things very cordial, others purge violently, both put together, make a composition no way pleasing to me; therefore I account it a pretty receipt, good for nothing.

Electuarium Elescoph

College.] Take of Diacrydium, Turbith, of each six drams, Cloves, Cinnamon, Ginger, Myrobalans, Emblicks, Nutmegs, Polypodium, of each two drams and an half, Sugar six ounces, clarified Honey ten ounces, make it into an electuary according to art.

Culpeper.] It purges choler and flegm, and wind from all parts of the body, helps pains of the joints and sides, the cholic, it cleanses the reins and bladder, yet I advise you not to take too much of it at a time, for it works pretty violently, let half an ounce be the most, for such whose bodies are strong, always remembering that you had better ten times take too little, than once too much; you may take it in white wine, and keep yourself warm. If you would have my opinion of it, I do not like it.

Confectio Hamech

College.] Take of the bark of Citron, Myrobalans two ounces, Myrobalans, Chebs and blacks, Violets, Colocynthis, Polypodium of the Oak, of each one ounce and an half, Wormwood, Thyme, of each half an ounce, the seeds of Annis, and Fennel, the flowers of red Roses of each three drams, let all of them being bruised, be infused one day in six pounds of Whey, then boiled till half be consumed, rubbed with your hands and pressed out: to the decoction add juice of Fumitory, pulp of Prunes, and Raisins of the Sun, of each half a pound, white Sugar, clarified Honey, of each one pound, boil it to the thickness of Honey, strewing in towards the end. Agarick trochiscated, Sena of each two ounces, Rhubarb one ounce and an half, Epithimum one ounce, Diacrydium six drams, Cinnamon half an ounce, Ginger two drams, the seeds of Fumitory and Annis, Spikenard, of each one dram, make it into an electuary according to art.

Culpeper.] The receipt is chiefly appropriated as a purge for melancholy and salt flegm, and diseases thence arising, as scabs, itch, leprosies, cancers, infirmities of the skin, it purges adust humours, and is good against madness, melancholy, forgetfulness, vertigo. It purges very violently, and is not safe given alone. I would advise the unskilful not to meddle with it inwardly. You may give half an ounce of it in clysters, in melancholy diseases, which commonly have astringency a constant companion with them.

Electuarium Lenitivum
Or Lenitive Electuary

College.] Take of Raisins of the Sun stoned, Polypodium of the Oak, Sena, of each two ounces, Mercury one handful and an half, Jujubes, Sebestens, of each twenty, Maidenhair, Violets, French Barley, of each one handful, Damask Prunes stoned, Tamarinds of each six drams, Liquorice half an ounce, boil them in ten pounds of water till two parts of the three be consumed; strain it, and dissolve in the decoction, pulp of Cassia, Tamarinds, and fresh Prunes, Sugar of Violets, of each six ounces, Sugar two pounds, at last add powder of Sena leaves, one ounce and an half, Annis seeds in powder, two drams to each pound of electuary, and so bring it into the form of an electuary according to art.

Culpeper.] It gently opens and molifies the bowels, brings forth choler, flegm, and melancholy, and that without trouble, it is cooling, and therefore is profitable in pleurisies, and for wounded people. A man of reasonable strength may take an ounce of it going to bed, which will work next morning.

Electuarium Passulatum

College.] Take of fresh Polypodium roots three ounces, fresh Marsh-mallow roots, Sena, of each two ounces, Annis seeds two drams, steep them in a glazed vessel, in a sufficient quantity of spring water, boil them according to art; strain it and with pulp of Raisins of the Sun half a pound, white Sugar, Manna, of each four ounces, boil it to the thickness of a Cydoniate, and renew it four times a year.

Culpeper.] It gently purges both choler and melancholy, cleanses the reins and bladder, and therefore is good for the stone and gravel in the kidneys.

Electuarium e succo Rosarum
Or Electuary of the Juice of Roses

College.] Take of Sugar, the juice of red Roses clarified, of each a pound and four ounces, the three sorts of Sanders of each six drams, Spodium three drams, Diacydonium twelve drams, Camphire a scruple, let the juice be boiled with the sugar to its just thickness, then add the rest in powder, and so make it into an electuary according to art.

Culpeper.] It purges choler, and is good in tertian agues, and diseases of the joints, it purges violently, therefore let it be warily given.

Hiera Picra simple

College.] Take of Cinnamon, Xylobalsamum, or wood of Aloes, the roots of Asarabacca, Spikenard, Mastich, Saffron, of each six drams, Aloes not washed twelve ounces and an half, clarified Honey four pounds and three ounces, mix them into an electuary according to art. Also you may keep the species by itself in your shops.

Culpeper.] It is an excellent remedy for vicious juices which lie furring the tunicle of the stomach, and such idle fancies and symptoms which the brain suffers thereby, whereby some think they see, others that they hear strange things, especially when they are in bed, and between sleeping and waking; besides this, it very gently purges the belly, and helps such women as are not sufficiently purged after their travail.

Hiera with Agarick

College.] Take of species Hiera, simple without Aloes, Agarick trochiscated, of each half an ounce, Aloes not washed one ounce, clarified Honey six ounces, mix it, and make it into an electuary according to art.

Culpeper.] Look but to the virtues of Agarick and add them to the virtues of the former receipt, so is the business done without any further trouble.

Hiera Logadii

College.] Take of Coloquintida, Polypodium, of each two drams, Euphorbium, Poley mountain, the seeds of Spurge, of each one dram and an half, and six grains, Wormwood, Myrrh, of each one dram and twelve grains, Centaury the less, Agarick, Gum Ammoniacum, Indian leaf or Mace, Spikenard, Squills prepared, Diacrydium of each one dram, Aloes, Thyme Hermander, Cassia Lignea, Bdellum, Horehound, of each one scruple and fourteen grains, Cinnamon, Oppopanax, Castorium, long Birthwort, the three sorts of Pepper, Sagapen, Saffron, Parsley of each two drams, Hellebore black and white, of each six grains, clarified Honey a pound and a half, mix them, and make of them an electuary according to art. Let the species be kept dry in your shops.

Culpeper.] It takes away by the roots daily evils coming of melancholy, falling-sickness, vertigo, convulsions, megrim, leprosies, and many other infirmities; for my part I should be loth to take it inwardly unless upon desperate occasions, or in clysters. It may well take away diseases by the roots, if it takes away life and all.

Hiera Diacolocynthidos

College.] Take of Colocynthis, Agarick, Germander, white Horehound, Stœchas, of each ten drams, Opopanax, Sagapen, Parsley seeds, round Birthwort roots, white Pepper of each five drams, Spikenard, Cinnamon, Myrrh, Indian leaf or Mace, Saffron, of each four drams, bruise the Gums in a mortar, sift the rest, and with three pounds of clarified honey, three ounces, and five drams, make it into an electuary according to art.

Culpeper.] It helps the falling-sickness, madness, and the pain in the head called Kephalalgia, pains in the breast and stomach whether they come by sickness or bruises, pains in the loins or back-bone, hardness of womens breasts, putrefaction of meat in the stomach, and sour belchings. It is but used seldom and therefore hard to be gotten.

Triphera the greater

College.] Take of Myrobalans, Chebs, Bellericks, Inds and Emblicks, Nutmegs, of each five drams, Water-cress seeds, Asarabacca roots, Persian Origanum, or else Dittany of Crete, black Pepper, Olibanum, Ammi, Ginger, Tamarisk, Indian Nard, Squinanth, Cypress roots of each half an ounce, filings of steel prepared with Vinegar twenty drams, let the Myrobalans be roasted with fresh butter, let the rest, being powdered, be sprinkled with oil of sweet Almonds, then add Musk one dram, and with their treble weight in Honey, make it into an electuary according to art.

Culpeper.] It helps the immoderate flowing of the menses in women, and the hæmorrhoids in men, it helps weakness of the stomach, and restores colour lost, it frees the body from crude humours, and strengthens the bladder, helps melancholy, and rectifies the distempers of the spleen. You may take a dram in the morning, or two if your body be any thing strong.

Triphera solutive

College.] Take of Diacrydium, ten drams, Turbith, an ounce and an half, Cardamoms the less, Cloves, Cinnamon, Honey, of each three drams, yellow Sanders, Liquorice, sweet Fennel seeds, of each half an ounce, Acorns, Schœnanth, of each a dram, red Roses, Citron pills preserved, of each three drams, Violets two drams, Penids four ounces, white Sugar half a pound, Honey clarified in juice of Apples one pound, make an electuary according to art.

Culpeper.] The Diacrydium and Turbith, are a couple of untoward purges, the rest are all cordials.

Athanasia Mithridatis. Galen

College.] Take of Cinnamon, Cassia, Schœnanth, of each an ounce and an half, Saffron, Myrrh, of each one ounce, Costus, Spignel, (Meum,) Acorus, (Water-flag perhaps they mean. See the root in the Catalogue of Simples,) Agarick, Scordium, Carrots, Parsley, of each half an ounce, white Pepper eleven grains, Honey so much as is sufficient to make it into an electuary according to art.

Culpeper.] It prevails against poison, and the bitings of venomous beasts, and helps such whose meat putrifies in their stomach, stays vomiting of blood, helps old coughs, and cold diseases in the liver, spleen, bladder, and matrix. The dose is half a dram.

Electuarium scoriaferri. Rhasis

College.] Take of the flakes of Iron infused in Vinegar seven days and dried, three drams, Indian Spikenard, Schœnanth, Cypress, Ginger, Pepper, Bishop's weed, Frankincense, of each half an ounce, Myrobalans, Indian Bellericks, and Emblicks, Honey boiled with the decoction of Emblicks, sixteen ounces, mix them together, and make of them an electuary.

Culpeper.] The medicine heats the spleen gently, purges melancholy, eases pains in the stomach and spleen, and strengthens digestion. People that are strong may take half an ounce in the morning fasting, and weak people three drams. It is a good remedy for pains and hardness of the spleen.

Confectio Humain. Mesua

College.] Take of Eyebright two ounces, Fennel seeds five drams, Cloves, Cinnamon, Cubebs, long Pepper, Mace, of each one dram, beat them all into powder, and with clarified Honey one pound, in which boil juice of Fennel one ounce, juice of Celandine and Rue, of each half an ounce, and with the powders make it up into an electuary.

Culpeper.] It is chiefly appropriated to the brain and heart, quickens the senses, especially the sight, and resists the pestilence. You may take half a dram if your body be hot, a dram if cold, in the morning fasting.

Diaireos Solomonis. Nich.

College.] Take of Orris roots one ounce, Pennyroyal, Hyssop, Liquorice, of each six drams, Tragacanth, white Starch, bitter Almonds, Pine-nuts, Cinnamon, Ginger, Pepper, of each three drams, fat Figs, the pulp of Raisins of the Sun, and Dates, of each three drams and an half, Styrax, Calamitis two drams and an half, Sugar dissolved in Hyssop water, and clarified Honey, of each twice the weight of all the rest, make them into an electuary according to art.

Culpeper.] The electuary is chiefly appropriated to the lungs, and helps cold infirmities of them, as asthmaes, coughs, difficulty of breathing, &c. You may take it with a Liquorice stick, or on the point of a knife, a little of it at a time, and often.

Diasaiyrion. Nich.

College.] Take of the roots of Satyrion fresh and sound, garden Parsnips, Eringo, Pine-nuts, Indian Nuts, or, if Indian Nuts be wanting, take the double quantity of Pine-nuts, Fistic-nuts, of each one ounce and an half, Cloves, Ginger, the seeds of Annis, Rocket, Ash Keys, of each five drams, Cinnamon, the tails and loins of Scincus, the seeds of Bulbus Nettles, of each two drams and an half, Musk seven grains, of the best sugar dissolved in Malaga Wine, three pounds, make it into an electuary according to art.

Culpeper.] It helps weakness of the reins and bladder, and such as make water with difficulty, it provokes lust exceedingly, and speedily helps such as are impotent in the acts of *Venus*. You may take two drams or more at a time.

Matthiolus's *great antidote against Poison and Pestilence*

College.] Take of Rhubarb, Rhapontic, Valerian roots, the roots of Acorus, or Calamus Aromaticus, Cypress, Cinquefoyl, Tormentil, round Birthwort, male Peony, Elecampane, Costus, Illirick, Orris, white Chamelion, or Avens, of each three drams, the Roots of Galanga, Masterwort, white Dictamni, Angelica, Yarrow, Filli-pendula or Dropwort, Zedoary, Ginger, of each two drams, Rose-mary, Gentian, Devil's-bit, of each two drams and an half, the seeds of Citrons, and Agnus Castus, the berries of Kermes, the seeds of Ash-tree, Sorrel, wild Parsnips, Navew, Nigella, Peony the male, Bazil, Hedge Mustard, (Irio) Treacle Mustard, Fennel, Bishop's-weed, of each two drams, the berries of Bay, Juniper, and Ivy, Sarsaparilla, (or for want of it the double weight of Cubebs,) Cubebs, of each one dram and an half, the leaves of Scordium, Germander, Chamepitys, Centaury the less, Stœchas, Celtic Spikenard, Calaminth, Rue, Mints, Betony, Vervain, Scabious, Carduus Benedictus, Bawm, of each one dram and an half, Dittany of Crete three drams, Marjoram, St. John's Wort, Schœnanth, Horehound, Goats Rue, Savin, Burnet, of each two drams, Figs, Walnuts, Fistic-nuts, of each three ounces, Emblicks, Myrobalans half an ounce, the flowers of Violets, Borrage, Bugloss, Roses, Lavender, Sage, Rosemary, of each four scruples, Saffron three drams, Cassia Lignea, ten drams, Cloves, Nutmegs, Mace, of each two drams and an half, black Pepper, long Pepper, all the three sorts of Sanders, wood of Aloes, of each one dram and an half, Hart's-horn half an ounce, Unicorn's-horn, or in its stead, Bezoar stone, one dram, bone in a Stag's heart, Ivory, Stag's pizzle, Cas-toreum, of each four scruples, Earth of Lemnos three drams, Opium one dram and an half, Orient Pearls, Emeralds, Jacinth, red Coral, of each one dram and an half, Camphire two drams, Gum Arabic, Mastich, Frankincense, Styrax, Turpentine, Sagapenum, Opopanax, Laserpitium, or Myrrh, of each two drams and an half, Musk, Amber-gris, of each one dram, oil of Vitriol half an ounce, species cordiales temperatæ, Diamargariton, Diamoscu, Diambra, Electuarij de Gem-mis, Troches of Camphire, of Squills, of each two drams and an half, Troches of Vipers two ounces, the juice of Sorrel, Sow Thistles, Scordium, Vipers Bugloss, Borrage, Bawm, of each half a pound, Hypocistis two drams, of the best Treacle and Mithridate, of each six ounces, old Wine three pounds, of the best Sugar, or choice

Honey eight pounds six ounces. These being all chosen and prepared with diligence and art, let them be made into an electuary just as Treacle or Mithridate is.

Culpeper.] The title shews you the scope of the author in compiling it. I believe it is excellent for those uses. The dose of this is from a scruple to four scruples, or a dram and an half. It provokes sweating abundantly, and in this or any other sweating medicine, order your body thus: Take it in bed, and cover yourself warm, in your sweating, drink posset-drink as hot as you can, if it be for a fever, boil Sorrel and red Sage in posset-drink, sweat an hour or two if your strength will bear it, then the chamber being kept very warm, shift yourself all but your head, about which (your cap which you sweat in being kept on) wrap a hot napkin, which will be a means to repel the vapours back. This I hold the best method for sweating in fevers and pestilences, in which this electuary is very good. I am very loth to leave out this medicine, which if it were stretched out, and cut in thongs, would reach round the world.

Requies. Nicholaus

College.] Take of red Rose leaves, the whites being cut off, blue Violets, of each three drams, Opium of Thebes, dissolved in Wine, the seeds of white Henbane, Poppies white and black, the roots of Mandrakes, the seeds of Endive, Purslain, garden Lettuce, Psyllium, Spodium, Gum Tragacanth, of each two scruples and five grains, Nutmegs, Cinnamon, Ginger, of each a dram and an half, Sanders, yellow, white, and red, of each a dram and an half, Sugar three times their weight, dissolved in Rose-water: mix them together, and make of them an electuary according to art.

Culpeper.] I like not the receipt taken inwardly.

Electuarium Reginæ Coloniens

College.] Take of the seeds of Saxifrage and Gromwell, juice of Liquorice, of each half an ounce, the seeds of Caraway, Annis, Smallage, Fennel, Parsley of Macedonia, Broom, Carrots, Bruscus, Asparagus, Lovage, Cummin, Juniper, Rue, Siler Mountain, the seeds of Acorus, Pennyroyal, Cinquefoyl, Bayberries, of each two drams, Indian Spikenard, Schœnanth, Amber, Valerian, Hog's Fennel, Lapis Lincis, of each a dram and an half, Galanga, Ginger, Turbith, of each two drams, Sena an ounce, Goat's blood prepared half an ounce, mix them together: first beat them into powder, then make them into an electuary according to art, with three times their weight in Sugar dissolved in white Wine.

Culpeper.] It is an excellent remedy for the stone and wind cholic, a dram of it taken every morning. I assure such as are troubled with such diseases, I commend it to them as a jewel.

PILLS

Culpeper.] Pills in Greek are called, *Katopotia*, in Latin, *Pilulæ*: which signifies little balls, because they are made up in such a form, that they may be the better swallowed down, by reason of the offensiveness of their taste.

Pilulæ de Agarico
Or Pills of Agarick

College.] Take of Agarick three drams, our own blue Orris roots, Mastich, Horehound, of each one dram, Turbith five drams, Species Hiera Picra half an ounce, Colocynthis, Sarcocol, of each two drams, Myrrh one dram, Sapa as much as is sufficient to make it into a mass according to art.

Culpeper.] It was invented to cleanse the breast and lungs of flegm, it works pretty strongly. Half a dram at a time (keeping yourself warm,) cannot well do you harm, unless your body be very weak.

Pilulæ Aggregativæ

College.] Take of Citron, Myrobalans, Rhubarb, of each half an ounce, juice of Agrimony and Wormwood made thick, of each two drams, Diagridium five drams, Agarick, Colocynthis, Polypodium of each two drams, Turbith, Aloes, of each six drams, Mastich, red Roses, Sal. Gem. Epithymum, Annis, Ginger, of each a dram, with Syrup of Damask Roses, make it into a mass according to art.

Culpeper.] It purges the head of choler, flegm and melancholy, and that stoutly: it is good against quotidian agues, and faults in the stomach and liver, yet because it is well corrected if you take but half a dram at a time, and keep yourself warm, I suppose you may take it without danger.

Pilulæ Alæphanginæ

College.] Take of Cinnamon, Cloves, Cardamoms the less, Nutmegs, Mace, Calamus Aromaticus, Carpobalsamum, or Juniper berries, Squinanth, Wood of Aloes, yellow Sanders, red Roses dried, Wormwood, of each half an ounce, let the tincture be taken out of these, being grossly bruised in spirit of Wine, the vessel being close stopped; in three pounds of this tincture, being strained, dissolve Aloes one pound, which being dissolved, add Mastich, Myrrh, of each half an ounce, Saffron two drams, Balsam of Peru one dram, the superfluous liquor being consumed, either over hot ashes, or a bath, bring it into a mass of pills.

Culpeper.] It cleanses both stomach and brain of gross and putri-fied humours, and sets the senses free when they are thereby troubled, it cleanses the brain offended by ill humours, wind, &c. helps vertigo and head-aches, and strengthens the brain exceed-ingly, helps concoction, and strengthens the stomach, one dram taken at night going to bed, will work gently next day: if the party be weak, you may give less, if strong more. If you take but half a dram, you may go abroad the next day: but if you take a dram, you may keep the house; there can be no harm in that.

Pilulæ de Aloe Lota
Or Pills of washed Aloes

College.] Take of Aloes washed with juice of red Roses, one ounce, Agarick three drams, Mastich two drams, Diamoscu Dulce half a dram, Syrup of Damask-roses, so much as is sufficient to make it into a mass according to art.

Culpeper.] It purges both brain, stomach, bowels, and eyes of putrified humours, and also strengthens them. Use these as the succeeding.

Aloe Rosata

College.] Take of Aloes in powder four ounces, juice of Damask Roses clarified one pound, mix them and digest them in the sun, or in a bath, till the superfluous liquor be drawn off, digest it, and evaporate it four times over, and keep the mass.

Culpeper.] It is a gallant gentle purger of choler, frees the sto-mach from superfluous humours, opens stoppings, and other in-firmities of the body proceeding from choler and flegm, as yellow jaundice, &c. and strengthens the body exceedingly. Take a scruple, or half a dram at night going to bed, you may walk abroad, for it will hardly work till next day in the afternoon.

Pilulæ Aureæ

College.] Take of Aloes, Diacrydium, of each five drams, red Roses, Smallage seeds, of each two drams and an half, the seeds of Annis and Fennel, of each one dram and an half, Mastich, Saffron,

Troch, Alhandal, of each one dram, with a sufficient quantity of Honey Roses, make it into a mass according to art.

Culpeper.] They are held to purge the head, to quicken the senses, especially the sight, and to expel wind from the bowels, but works something harshly. Half a dram is the utmost dose, keep the fire, take them in the morning, and sleep after them, they will work before noon.

Pilulæ Cochiæ, the greater

College.] Take of Species, Hiera Picra, ten drams, Troch, Alhandal, three drams and an half, Diacrydium two drams and an half, Turbith, Stœchas, of each five drams, with a sufficient quantity of Syrup of Stœchas, make it into a mass, according to art.

Culpeper.] It is held to purge the head, but it is but a dogged purge at best, and must be given only to strong bodies, and but half a dram at a time, and yet with great care.

Pilulæ Cochiæ, the less

College.] Take of Aloes, Scammony, Colocynthis, of each one ounce, with equal parts of Syrup of Wormwood, and of purging thorn, make it into a mass according to art.

Pilulæ de Cynoglosso
Or Pills of Hound's-tongue

College.] Take of the Roots of Hound's-tongue dried, white Henbane seed, Opium prepared, of each half an ounce, Myrrh six drams, Olibanum five drams, Saffron, Castoreum, Styrax, Calamitis, of each one dram and an half, with Syrup of Stœchas, make it into a mass.

Culpeper.] It stays hot rheums that fall down upon the lungs, therefore is good in phthisics, also it mitigates pain, a scruple is enough to take at a time going to bed, and too much if your body be weak: have a care of opiates for fear they make you sleep your last.

Pilulæ ex Duobus
Or Pills of two things

College.] Take of Colocynthis, and Scamony, of each one ounce, oil of Cloves as much as is sufficient to malax them well, then with a little Syrup of purging Thorn, make it into a mass.

Pilulæ de Eupatorio
Or Pills of Eupatorium

College.] Take of the juice of Maudlin, and Wormwood made thick, Citron, Myrobalans, of each three drams, Rhubarb three drams and an half, Mastich one dram, Aloes five drams, Saffron half a dram, Syrup of the juice of Endive, as much as is sufficient to make it into a mass.

Culpeper.] It is a gallant gentle purge, and strengthening, fitted for such bodies as are much weakened by disease or choler. The author appropriates it to such as have tertian agues, the yellow jaundice, obstructions or stoppings of the liver; half a dram taken at night going to bed, will work with an ordinary body, the next day by noon.

Pilulæ Fætidæ
Or Stinking Pills

College.] Take of Aloes, Colocynthis, Ammoniacum, Sagapen, Myrrh, Rue-seeds, Epithymum, of each five drams, Scamony three drams, the roots of Turbith half an ounce, the roots of Spurge the less prepared, Hermodactils of each two drams, Ginger one dram and an half, Spikenard, Cinnamon, Saffron, Castoreum, of each one dram, Euphorbium prepared two scruples, dissolve the Gums in juice of Leeks, and with Syrup made with the juice of Leeks and Sugar, make it into a mass.

Culpeper.] They purge gross and raw flegm, and diseases thereof arising; gouts of all sorts, pains in the back-bone, and other joints: it is good against leprosies, and other such like infirmities of the skin. I fancy not the receipt much.

Pilulæ de Hermodactilis
Or Pills of Hermodactils

College.] Take of Sagapen six drams, Opopanax three drams, melt them in warm juice of Coleworts, so much as is sufficient, then strain it through a convenient rag, afterwards boil it to a mean thickness, then take of Hermodactils, Aloes, Citron, Myrobalans, Turbith, Coloquintida, soft Bdellium, of each six drams, Euphorbium prepared, the seeds of Rue and Smallage, Castoreum, Sarcocol of each three drams, Saffron one dram and an half, with the Syrup of the juice of Coleworts made with honey, make it into a mass according to art.

Culpeper.] They are good against the gout, and other cold

afflictions of the joints. These are more moderate by half than *Pilulæ Fœtidæ*, and appropriated to the same diseases.

Pilulæ de Hiera cum Agarico
Or Pills of Hiera with Agarick

College.] Take of Species Hiera Picra, Agarick, of each half an ounce, Aloes one ounce, Honey Roses so much as is sufficient to make it into a mass according to art.

Pilulæ Imperiales
Or Imperial Pills

College.] Take of Aloes two ounces, Rhubarb one ounce and an half, Agarick, Sena, of each one ounce, Cinnamon three drams, Ginger two drams, Nutmegs, Cloves, Spikenard, Mastich, of each one dram, with Syrup of Violets, make it into a mass according to art.

Culpeper.] It cleanses the body of mixt humours, and strengthens the stomach exceedingly, as also the bowels, liver, and natural spirits: it is good for cold natures, and cheers the spirits. The dose is a scruple or half a dram, taken at night.

Pilulæ de Lapide Lazuli
Or Pills of Lapis Lazuli

College.] Take of Lapis Lazuli in powder and well washed, five drams, Epithymum, Polypodium, Agarick, of each an ounce, Scamony, black Hellebore roots, Sal. Gem. of each two drams and an half, Cloves, Annis seeds, of each half an ounce, Species Hiera simple fifteen drams, with Syrup of the juice of Fumitory, make it into a mass according to art.

Culpeper.] It purges melancholy very violently.

Pilulæ Macri

College.] Take of Aloes two ounces, Mastich half an ounce, dried Marjoram two drams, Salt of Wormwood one dram, make them all, being in powder, into a mass according to art with juice of Coleworts and Sugar, so much as is sufficient.

Culpeper.] It strengthens both stomach and brain, especially the nerves and muscles, and eases them of such humours as afflict them, and hinder the motion of the body, they open obstructions of the liver and spleen, and takes away diseases thence coming.

Pilulæ Mastichinæ
Or Mastich Pills

College.] Take of Mastich two ounces, Aloes four ounces, Agarick, Species Hiera simple, of each one ounce and an half, with Syrup of Wormwood, make it into a mass according to art.

Culpeper.] They purge very gently, but strengthen much, both head, brain, eyes, belly, and reins.

Pilulæ Mechoacanæ
Or Pills of Mechoacan

College.] Take of Mechoacan roots half an ounce, Turbith three drams, the leaves of Spurge steeped in Vinegar and dried, the seeds of Walwort, Agarick trochiscated, of each two drams, Spurge roots prepared, Mastich, of each one dram and an half, Mace, Cinnamon, Sal. Gem. of each two scruples, beat them into powder, and with white Wine, bring them into a mass. When it is dry, beat it into powder, and with Syrup made with the juice of Orris roots and sugar, make it the second time into a mass for pills.

Culpeper.] They purge flegm very violently.

Pilulæ de Opopanace
Or Pills of Opopanax

College.] Take of Opopanax, Sagapen, Bdellium, Ammoniacum, Hermodactils, Coloquintida, of each five drams, Saffron, Castoreum, Myrrh, Ginger, white Pepper, Cassia Lignea, Citron, Myrobalans, of each one dram, Scamony two drams, Turbith half an ounce, Aloes an ounce and an half, the Gums being dissolved in clarified juice of Coleworts, with Syrup of the juice of Coleworts, make them into a mass according to art.

Culpeper.] It helps tremblings, palsies, gouts of all sorts, cleanses the joints, and is helpful for such as are troubled with cold afflictions of the nerves. It works violently.

Pilulæ Rudii

College.] Take of Coloquintida six drams, Agarick, Scamony, the roots of black Hellebore, and Turbith, of each half an ounce, Aloes one ounce, Diarrhodon Abbatis half an ounce, let all of them (the Diarrh. Abbatis excepted) be grossly bruised, and infused eight days in the best spirits of Wine in a vessel close stopped, in the sun, so that the liquor may swim at top the breadth of six fingers: afterwards infuse the Diarrhodon Abbatis in the same manner four days in Aqua vitæ, then having strained and pressed them hard, mix them both together, casting the dross away, and draw off the moisture in a glass Alembick, and let the thick matter remain in a mass.

Culpeper.] It cleanses both head and body of choler, flegm, and melancholy: it must not be taken in any great quantity, half a dram is sufficient for the strongest body.

Pilulæ Russi

College.] Take of Aloes two ounces, Myrrh one ounce, Saffron half an ounce, with Syrup of the juice of Lemons, make it into a mass according to art.

Culpeper.] A scruple taken at night going to bed, is an excellent preservative in pestilential times; also they cleanse the body of such humours as are gotten by surfeits, they strengthen the heart, and weak stomachs, and work so easily that you need not fear following your business the next day.

Pilulæ sine Quibus
Or Pills without which——

College.] Take of washed Aloes fourteen drams, Scammony prepared six drams, Agarick, Rhubarb, Sena, of each half an ounce, Wormwood, red Roses exungulated, Violet flowers, Dodder, Mastich, of each one dram, salt of Wormwood, of each half a dram, with Syrup of the juice of Fennel made with Honey, make it into a mass according to art.

Culpeper.] It purges flegm, choler, and melancholy from the head, makes the sight and hearing good, and gives ease to a burdened brain.

Pilulæ Stomachiæ
Or Stomach Pills

College.] Take of Aloes six drams, Mastich, red Roses, of each two drams, with Syrup of Wormwood, make it into a mass according to art.

Culpeper.] They cleanse and strengthen the stomach, they cleanse but gently, strengthen much, help digestion.

Pilulæ Stomachiæ cum Gummi
Or Stomach Pills with Gums

College.] Take of Aloes an ounce, Sena five drams, Gum Amoniacum dissolved in Elder-flower Vinegar half an ounce, Mastich, Myrrh, of each a dram and an half, Saffron, salt of Wormwood, of each half a dram, with Syrup of purging Thorn, make it into a mass according to art.

Culpeper.] They work more strongly than the former.

Pilulæ e Styrace
Or Pills of Styrax

College.] Take of Styrax Calamitis, Olibanum, Myrrh, juice of Liquorice, Opium, of each half an ounce, with Syrup of white Poppies, make it into a mass according to art.

Culpeper.] They help such as are troubled with defluxion of rheum, coughs, and provoke sleep to such as cannot sleep for coughing.

Pilulæ de Succino
Or Pills of Amber

College.] Take of white Amber, Mastich, of each two drams, Aloes five drams, Agaric a dram and an half, long Birthwort half a dram, with Syrup of Wormwood make it into a mass.

Culpeper.] It amends the evil state of a woman's body, strengthens conception, and takes away what hinders it; it gently purges choler and flegm, and leaves a binding, strengthening quality behind it.

Pilulæ ex Tribus
Or Pills of three things

College.] Take of Mastich two ounces, Aloes four ounces, Agarick, Hiera simple, of each an ounce and an half, Rhubarb two ounces, Cinnamon two drams, with Syrup of Succory, make it into a mass according to art.

Culpeper.] They gently purge choler, and help diseases thence arising, as itch, scabs, wheals, &c. They strengthen the stomach and liver, and open obstructions, as also help the yellow jaundice.

Pilulæ Turpeti Aureæ

College.] Take of Turbith two ounces, Aloes an ounce and an half, Citron Myrobalans ten drams, red Roses, Mastich, of each

six drams, Saffron three drams, beat them all into powder, and with
Syrup of Wormwood bring them into a mass.

Culpeper.] They purge choler and flegm, and that with as much
gentleness as can be desired; also they strengthen the stomach and
liver, and help digestion.

Laudanum

College.] Take of Thebane Opium extracted in spirit of Wine,
one ounce, Saffron alike extracted, a dram and an half, Castorium
one dram: let them be taken in tincture of half an ounce of species
Diambræ newly made in spirit of Wine, add to them Ambergris,
Musk, of each six grains, oil of Nutmegs ten drops, evaporate the
moisture away in a bath, and leave the mass.

Culpeper.] It was invented (and a gallant invention it is) to
mitigate violent pains, stop the fumes that trouble the brain in
fevers, (but beware of Opiates in the beginning of fevers) to provoke
sleep, take not above two grains of it at a time, going to bed; if
that provoke not sleep, the next night you may make bold with
three. Have a care how you be too busy with such medicines, lest
you make a man sleep to doom's-day.

Nepenthes Opiatum

College.] Take of tincture of Opium made first with distilled
Vinegar, then with spirit of Wine, Saffron extracted in spirit of
Wine, of each an ounce, salt of Pearl and Coral, of each half an
ounce, tincture of species Diambræ seven drams, Ambergris one
dram: bring them into the form of Pills by the gentle heat of a bath.

Culpeper.] The operation is like the former.

Pilulæ Assaireth. Avicenna

College.] Take of Species Hiera Picra Galeni one ounce, Mastich,
Citron, Myrobalans, of each half an ounce, Aloes two ounces, the
Syrup of Stœchas as much as is sufficient, make of them a mass
according to art.

Culpeper.] It purges choler and flegm, and strengthens the whole
body exceedingly, being very precious for such whose bodies are
weakened by surfeits, or ill diet, to take half a dram or a scruple at
night going to bed.

Pills of Bdellium. Mesue

College.] Take of Bdellium ten drams, Myrobalans, Bellericks,
Emblicks, and Blacks, of each five drams, flakes of Iron, Leek

seeds, of each three drams, Choncula Veneris burnt, Coral burnt, Amber, of each a dram and an half, Pearls half an ounce, dissolve the Bdellium in juice of Leeks and with so much Syrup of juice of Leeks as is sufficient, make it into a mass according to art.

Culpeper.] Both this and the former are seldom used, and therefore are hardly to be had.

Pills of Rhubarb. Mesue

College.] Take of choice Rhubarb three drams, Citron Myrobalans, Trochisci Diarrhodon, of each three drams and an half, juice of Liquorice, and juice of Wormwood, Mastich, of each one dram, the seeds of Smallage and Fennel, of each half a dram, Species Hiera Picra simp. Galeni, ten drams, with juice of Fennel not clarified, and Honey so much as is sufficient, make it into a mass.

Culpeper.] It purges choler, opens obstructions of the liver, helps the yellow jaundice, and dropsies in the beginning, strengthens the stomach and lungs.

Pilulæ Arabica. Nicholaus

College.] Take of the best Aloes four ounces, Briony roots, Myrobalans, Citrons, Chebs, Indian Bellerick, and Emblick, Mastich, Diagrydium, Asarabacca, Roses, of each an ounce, Castorium three drams, Saffron one dram, with Syrup of Wormwood, make it into a mass according to art.

Culpeper.] It helps such women as are not sufficiently purged in their labour, helps to bring away what a careless midwife hath left behind, purges the head, helps headache, megrim, vertigo, and purges the stomach of vicious humours.

Pilulæ Arthriticæ. Nicholaus

College.] Take of Hermodactils, Turbith, Agarick, of each half an ounce, Cassia Lignea, Indian Spikenard, Cloves, Xylobalsamum, or Wood of Aloes, Carpobalsamum or Cubebs, Mace, Galanga, Ginger, Mastich, Assafœtida, the seeds of Annis, Fennel, Saxifrage, Sparagus, Bruscus, Roses, Gromwell, Sal. Gem. of each two drams, Scammony one ounce, of the best Aloes, the weight of them all, juice of Chamepitys made thick with sugar, so much as is sufficient: or Syrup of the juice of the same, so much as is sufficient to make it into a mass.

Culpeper.] It helps the gout, and other pains in the joints, comforts and strengthens both brain and stomach, and consumes diseases whose original comes of flegm.

Pilulæ Cochiæ with Helebore

College.] Take of the powder of the Pills before prescribed, the powder of the bark of the roots of black Hellebore, one ounce: make it into a mass with Syrup of Stœchas according to art.

Pills of Fumitory. Avicenna

College.] Take of Myrobalans, Citrons, Chebs, and Indian Diagrydium, of each five drams, Aloes seven drams; let all of them being bruised, be thrice moistened with juice of Fumitory, and thrice suffered to dry, then brought into a mass with Syrup of Fumitory.

Culpeper.] It purges melancholy. Be not too busy with it I beseech you.

Pilulæ Indæ. Mesue *out of* Haly

College.] Take of Indian Myrobalans, black Hellebore, Polypodium of the Oak, of each five drams, Epithymum, Stœchas, of each six drams, Agarick, Lapis Lazuli often washed troches Alhandal, Sal Indi, of each half an ounce, juice of Maudlin made thick, Indian Spikenard, of each two drams, Cloves one dram, Species Hiera Picra simplex Galeni, twelve drams, with juice of Smallage make it into a mass according to art.

Culpeper.] It wonderfully prevails against afflictions coming of melancholy, cancers which are not ulcerated, leprosy, evils of the mind coming of melancholy, as sadness, fear, &c. quartan agues, jaundice, pains and infirmities of the spleen.

Pilulæ Lucis Majores. Mesue

College.] Take of Roses, Violets, Wormwood, Colocynthis, Turbith, Cubebs, Calamus Aromaticus, Nutmegs, Indian Spikenard, Epithimum, Carpobalsamum, or instead thereof, Cardamoms, Xylabalsamum, or Wood of Aloes, the seeds of Seseli or Hartwort, Rue, Annis, Fennel and Smallage, Schænanthus, Mastich, Asarabacca roots, Cloves, Cinnamon, Cassia Lignea, Saffron, Mace, of each two drams, Myrobalans, Citrons, Chebuls, Indian Bellerick, and Emblick, Rhubarb, of each half an ounce, Agarick, Sena, of each five drams, Aloes Succotrina, the weight of them all: with Syrup of the juice of Fennel make it into a mass according to art.

Culpeper.] It purges mixt humours from the head, and clears it of such excrements as hinder the sight.

Pills of Spurge. Fernelius

College.] Take of the bark of the roots of Spurge the less, steeped twenty-four hours in Vinegar and juice of Purslain, two drams, grains of Palma Christi torrified, by number, forty, Citron Myrobalans one dram and an half, Germander, Chamepitys, Spikenard, Cinnamon, of each two scruples, being beaten into fine powder with an ounce of Gum Tragacanth dissolved in Rose Water, and Syrup of Roses so much as is sufficient, let it be made into a mass.

Pills of Euphorbium. Mesue

College.] Take of Euphorbium, Colocynthis, Agarick, Bdellium, Sagapenum, of each two drams, Aloes five drams, with Syrup made of the juice of Leeks, make it into a mass.

Culpeper.] The Pills are exceeding good for dropsies, pains in the loins, and gouts coming of a moist cause. Take not above half a dram at a time and keep the house.

Pilulæ Scribonii

College.] Take of Sagapen, and Myrrh, of each two drams, Opium, Cardamoms, Castorium, of each one dram, white Pepper half a dram, Sapa so much as is sufficient to make it into a mass according to art.

Culpeper.] It is appropriated to such as have phthisicks, and such as spit blood, but ought to be newly made, a scruple is sufficient taken going to bed.

TROCHES

Trochisci de Absinthio
Or Troches of Wormwood

College.] Take of red Roses, Wormwood leaves, Annis seeds, of each two drams, juice of Maudlin made thick, the roots of Asarabacca, Rhubarb, Spikenard, Smallage seeds, bitter Almonds, Mastich, Mace, of each one dram, juice of Succory so much as is sufficient to make it into troches according to art.

Culpeper.] They strengthen the stomach exceedingly, open obstructions, or stoppings of the belly and bowels: strengthen digestion, open the passages of the liver, help the yellow jaundice, and consume watery superfluities of the body. They are somewhat bitter, and seldom taken alone; if your pallate affect bitter things, you may take a dram of them in the morning. They cleanse the body of choler, but purge not, or not to any purpose.

Agaricus Trochiscatus
Or Agarick Trochiscated

College.] Take of Agarick sifted and powdered, three ounces, steep it in a sufficient quantity of white Wine, in which two drams of ginger have been infused, and make it into troches.

Trochisci Albi. Rhasis
Or white Troches

College.] Take of Ceruss washed in Rosewater ten drams, Sarcocol three drams, white Starch two drams, Gum Arabic and Tragacanth, of each one dram, Camphire half a dram, either with Rosewater, or women's milk, or make it into troches according to art.

Trochisci Alexiterii

College.] Take of Zedoary roots, powder of Crab's Claws, of each one dram, and an half, the outward Citron preserved and dried, Angelica seeds, Pills, of each one dram, Bole-amoniac half a dram, with their treble weight in sugar make them into powder, and with a sufficient quantity of Mussilage of Gum Tragacanth, made into treacle water distilled, make it into paste, of which make troches.

Culpeper.] This preserves the body from ill airs, and epidemical diseases, as the pestilence, small pox, &c. and strengthens the heart exceedingly, eating now and then a little: you may safely keep any troches in your pocket, for the drier you keep them, the better they are.

Trochisci Alhandal

College.] Take of Coloquintida freed from the seeds and cut small, and rubbed with an ounce of oil of Roses, then beaten into fine powder, ten ounces, Gum Arabic, Tragacanth, Bdellium, of each six drams. Steep the Gums three or four days in a sufficient quantity of Rose-water till they be melted, then with the aforesaid pulp, and part of the said mussilage, let them be dried in the

shadow, then beaten again, and with the rest of the mussilage, make
it up again, dry them and keep them for use.

Culpeper.] They are too violent for a vulgar use.

Trochisci Aliptæ Moschatæ

College.] Take of Labdanum bruised three ounces, Styrax Calamitis one ounce and an half, Benjamin one ounce, Wood of Aloes
two drams, Ambergris one dram, Camphire half a dram, Musk
half a scruple, with a sufficient quantity of Rose-water, make it
into troches according to art.

Culpeper.] It is singularly good for such as are asthmatic, and
can hardly fetch their breath; as also for young children, whose
throat is so narrow that they can hardly swallow down their milk.

Trochisci Alkekengi
Or Troches of Winter-cherries

College.] Take of Winter Cherries three drams, Gum Arabic,
Tragacanth, Olibanum, Dragon's-blood, Pine-nuts, bitter Almonds,
white Styrax, juice of Liquorice, Bole ammoniac, white Poppy
seeds, of each six drams, the seeds of Melons, Cucumbers, Citruls,
Gourds, of each three drams and an half, the seeds of Smallage and
white Henbane, Amber, Earth of Lemnos, Opium, of each two
drams, with juice of fresh Winter-Cherries, make them into troches
according to art.

Culpeper.] They potently provoke urine, and break the stone.
Mix them with other medicine of that nature, half a dram at a time,
or a dram if age permit.

Trochisci Bechici aloi, vel, Rotulæ pectorales
Or, Pectoral Rolls

College.] Take of white Sugar one pound, white Sugar Candy,
Penids, of each four ounces, Orris Florentine one ounce, Liquorice
six drams, white Starch one ounce and an half, with a sufficient
quantity of mussilage of Gum Tragacanth made in Rose Water,
make them into small troches. You may add four grains of Ambergris, and three grains of Musk to them, if occasion serve.

Trochisci Bechici nigri

College.] Take of juice of Liquorice, white Sugar, of each one
dram, Gum Tragacanth, sweet Almonds blanched, of each six

drams, with a sufficient quantity of mussilage of Quince seeds, made thick with Rose Water. Make them into troches according to art.

Culpeper.] Both this and the former will melt in ones mouth, and in that manner to be used by such as are troubled with coughs, cold, hoarseness, or want of voice. The former is most in use, but in my opinion, the latter is most effectual.

Trochisci de Barberis
Or, Troches of Barberries

College.] Take of juice of Barberries, and Liquorice made thick, Spodium, Purslain seeds, of each three drams, red Roses, six drams, Indian Spikenard, Saffron, white Starch, Gum Tragacanth, of each a dram, Citrul seeds cleansed three drams and an half, Camphire half a dram; with Manna dissolved in juice of Barberries, make them into troches according to art.

Culpeper.] They wonderfully cool the heat of the liver, reins, and bladder, breast, and stomach, and stop looseness, cools the heat of fevers.

Trochisci de Camphora
Or, Troches of Camphire

College.] Take of Camphire half a dram, Saffron two drams, white Starch three drams, red Roses, Gum Arabic, and Tragacanth, Ivory, of each half an ounce, the seeds of Cucumbers husked, of Purslain, Liquorice, of each an ounce, with mussilage of the seeds of Fleawort, drawn in Rose-water, make them into troches.

Culpeper.] It is exceeding good in burning fevers, heat of blood and choler, together with hot distempers of the stomach and liver, and extreme thirst coming thereby, also it is good against the yellow jaundice phthisics, and hectic fevers.

Trochisci de Capparibus
Or, Troches of Capers

College.] Take of the bark of Caper roots, the seeds of Agnus Castus, of each six drams, Ammoniacum half an ounce, the seeds of Water Cresses and Nigella, the leaves of Calaminth and Rue, the roots of Acorus and long Birthwort, the juice of Maudlin made thick, bitter Almonds, of each two drams, Hart's-tongue, the roots of round Cypress, Madder, Gum Lac. of each one dram: being bruised let them be made into troches according to art, with Ammoniacum dissolved in Vinegar, and boiled to the thickness of Honey.

Culpeper.] They open stoppings of the liver and spleen, and help diseases thereof coming; as rickets, hypochondriac melancholy, &c. Men may take a dram, children a scruple in the morning.

Trochisci de Carabe
Or, Troches of Amber

College.] Take of Amber an ounce, Hart's-horn burnt, Gum Arabic burnt, red Coral burnt, Tragacanth, Acacia, Hypocistis, Balaustines, Mastich, Gum Lacca washed, black Poppy seeds roasted, of each two drams and two scruples, Frankincense, Saffron, Opium, of each two drams, with a sufficient quantity of mussilage of the seeds of Fleawort drawn in Plantain Water, make them into troches according to art.

Culpeper.] They were invented to stop fluxes of blood in any part of the body, the menses, the hæmorrhoids or piles; they also help ulcers in the breast and lungs. The dose is from ten grains to a scruple.

Trochisci Cypheos, for Mithridate

College.] Take of pulp of Raisins of the Sun, Cypress, Turpentine, of each three ounces, Myrrh, Squinanth, of each an ounce and an half, Cinnamon half an ounce, Calamus Aromaticus nine drams, the roots of round Cypress, and Indian Spikenard, Cassia Lignea, Juniper berries, Bdellium, Aspalthus or Wood of Aloes, two drams and an half, Saffron one dram, clarified Honey as much as is sufficient, Canary Wine a little: let the Myrrh and Bdellium be ground in a mortar with the wine, to the thickness of liquid Honey, then add the Turpentine, then the pulp of Raisins, then the powders: at last with the Honey, let them all be made into troches.

Culpeper.] It is excellently good against inward ulcers in what part of the body soever they be. It is chiefly used in compositions, as Treacle and Mithridate.

Trochisci de Eupatorio
Or Troches of Maudlin

College.] Take of the juice of Maudlin made thick, Manna, of each an ounce, red Roses half an ounce, Spodium three drams and an half, Spikenard three drams, Rhubarb, Asarabacca roots, Annis seeds, of each two drams. Let the Nard, Annis seeds, and Roses be beaten together, the Spodium, Asarabacca, and Rhubarb by themselves, then mix the Manna and juice of Maudlin in a mortar, add the powders, and with new juice make it into troches.

Culpeper.] Obstructions, or stoppings, and swelling above nature, both of the liver and spleen, are cured by the inward taking of these troches, and diseases thereof coming, as yellow and black jaundice, the beginning of dropsies, &c.

Troches of Gallia Moschata

College.] Take of Wood of Aloes five drams, Ambergris three drams, Musk one dram, with mussilage of Gum Tragacanth made in Rose Water, make it into troches according to art.

Culpeper.] They strengthen the brain and heart, and by consequence both vital and animal spirits, and cause a sweet breath. They are of an extreme price, therefore I pass by the dose.

Trochisci Gordonii

College.] Take of the four greater cold seeds husked, the seeds of white Poppies, Mallows, Cotton, Purslain, Quinces, Mirtles, Gum Tragacanth, and Arabic, Fistic-nuts, Pine-nuts, Sugar-candy, Penids, Liquorice, French-barley, mussilage of Fleawort seeds, sweet Almonds blanched, of each two drams, Bole-ammoniac, Dragon's-blood, Spodium, red Roses, Myrrh, of each half an ounce, with a sufficient quantity of Hydromel, make it into troches according to art.

Culpeper.] They are held to be very good in ulcers of the bladder, and all other inward ulcers whatsoever, and ease fevers coming thereby, being of a fine cooling, slippery heating nature.

Trochisci Hedichroi (Galen) *for Treacle*

College.] Take of Aspalthus, or yellow Sanders, the leaves of Mastich, the roots of Asarabacca, of each two drams, Rhupontic, Castus, Calamus Aromaticus, Wood of Aloes, Cinnamon, Squinanth, Opobalsamum or oil of Nutmegs by expression, of each three drams, Cassia Lignea, Indian Leaf or Mace, Indian Spikenard, Myrrh, Saffron, of each six drams, Amomus, or Cardamoms the less, an ounce and an half, Mastich a dram, Canary Wine as much as is sufficient. Let the Myrrh be dissolved in the wine, then add the Mastich and Saffron well beaten, then the Opobalsamum, then the rest in powder, and with the wine, make them up into troches, and dry them gently.

Culpeper.] They are very seldom or never used but in other compositions, yet naturally they heat cold stomachs, help digestion, strengthen the heart and brain.

Trochisci Hysterici

College.] Take of Asafœtida, Galbanum, of each two drams and an half, Myrrh two drams, Castoreum a dram and an half, the roots of Asarabacca and long Birthwort, the leaves of Savin, Featherfew, Nep, of each one dram, Dittany half a dram, with either the juice or decoction of Rue, make it into troches according to art.

Culpeper.] These are applied to the fœminine gender, help fits of the mother, expel both birth and after-birth, cleanse women after labour, and expel the relics of a careless midwife.

Trochisci de Ligno Aloes
Or Troches of Wood of Aloes

College.] Take of Wood of Aloes, red Roses, of each two drams, Mastich, Cinnamon, Cloves, Indian Spikenard, Nutmegs, Parsnip seed, Cardamoms the greater and lesser, Cubebs, Gallia Moschata, Citron Pills, Mace, of each one dram and an half, Ambergris, Musk, of each half a scruple, with Honey of Raisins make it into troches.

Culpeper.] It strengthens the heart, stomach, and liver, takes away heart-qualms, faintings, and stinking breath, and resists the dropsy.

Trochisci e Mirrha
Or Troches of Myrrh

College.] Take of Myrrh three drams, the Meal of Lupines five drams, Madder roots, the leaves of Rue, wild Mints, Dittany of Crete, Cummin seeds, Asafœtida, Sagapen, Opopanax, of each two drams, dissolve the Gums in Wine wherein Mugwort hath been boiled, or else Juniper-berries, then add the rest, and with juice of Mugwort, make it into troches according to art.

Culpeper.] They provoke the menses, and that with great ease to such as have them come down with pain. Take a dram of them beaten into powder, in a spoonful or two of Syrup of Mugwort, or any other composition tending to the same purpose.

Sief de Plumbo
Or Sief of Lead

College.] Take of Lead burnt and washed, Brass burnt, Antimony, Tutty washed, Gum Arabic and Tragacanth of each an ounce, Opium half a dram, with Rose-water, make them, being beaten and sifted, into troches.

Trochisci Polyidæ Androm

College.] Take of Pomegranate flowers twelve drams, Roach Album three drams, Frankincense, Myrrh, of each half an ounce, Chalcanthum two drams, Bull's gall six drams, Aloes an ounce, with austere Wine, or juice of Nightshade or Plantain, make them into troches according to art.

Culpeper.] They are very good they say, being outwardly applied, both in green wounds and ulcers. I fancy them not.

Trochisci de Rhubarbaro
Or Troches of Rhubarb

College.] Take of Rhubarb ten drams, juice of Maudlin made thick, bitter Almonds, of each half an ounce, red Roses three drams, the roots of Asarabacca, Madder, Indian Spikenard, the leaves of Wormwood, the seeds of Annis and Smallage, of each one dram, with Wine in which Wormwood hath been boiled, make them into troches according to art.

Culpeper.] They gently cleanse the liver, help the yellow jaundice, and other diseases coming of choler and stoppage of the liver.

Trochisci de Santalis
Or Troches of Sanders

College.] Take of the three Sanders, of each one ounce, the seeds of Cucumbers, Gourds, Citruls, Purslain, Spodium, of each half an ounce, red Roses seven drams, juice of Barberries six drams, Bole-ammoniac half an ounce, Camphire one dram, with Purslain Water make it into troches.

Culpeper.] The virtues are the same with troches of Spodium, both of them harmless.

Trochisci da Scilla ad Theriacam
Or Troches of Squils, for Treacle

College.] Take a Squil gathered about the beginning of July, of a middle bigness, and the hard part to which the small roots stick, wrap it up in paste, and bake it in an oven, till the paste be dry, and the Squil tender, which you may know by piercing it with a wooden skewer, or a bodkin, then take it out and bruise it in a mortar, adding to every pound of the Squil, eight ounces of white Orobus, or red Cicers in powder, then make it into troches, of the weight of two drams a piece, (your hands being anointed with Oil of Roses) dry them on the top of the house, opening towards the South, in the shadow, often turning them till they be well dry, then keep them in a pewter or glass vessel.

Troches of Spodium

College.] Take of red Roses twelve drams, Spodium ten drams, Sorrel seed six drams, the seeds of Purslain and Coriander, steeped in Vinegar and dried, pulp of Sumach, of each two drams and an half, white Starch roasted, Balaustines, Barberries, of each two drams, Gum Arabic, roasted one dram and an half, with juice of unripe Grapes, make it into troches.

Culpeper.] They are of a fine cooling binding nature, excellent in fevers coming of choler, especially if they be accompanied with a looseness, they also quench thirst.

Trochisci de terra Lemnia
Or Troches of Earth of Lemnos

College.] Take of Earth of Lemnos, Bole-ammoniac, Acacia, Hypocystis, Gum Arabic toasted, Dragon's blood, white Starch, red Roses, Rose seeds, Lap. Hematitis, red Coral, Amber, Balaustines, Spodium, Purslain seeds a little toasted, Olibanum, Hart's-horn burnt, Cypress Nuts, Saffron of each two drams, black Poppy seeds, Tragacanth, Pearls, of each one dram and an half, Opium prepared one dram, with juice of Plantain, make it into troches.

Sief de Thure
Or Sief of Frankincense

College.] Take of Frankincense, Lap. Calaminaris, Pompholix, of each ten drams, Cyrus forty drams, Gum Arabic, Opium, of each six drams, with fair water make it into balls: dry them and keep them for use.

Trochisci e Violis solutivi
Or Troches of Violets solutive

College.] Take of Violet flowers meanly dry, six drams, Turbith one ounce and an half, juice of Liquorice, Scammony, Manna, of each two drams, with Syrup of Violets, make it into troches.

Culpeper.] They are not worth talking of, much less worth cost, the cost and labour of making.

Trochisci de Vipera ad Theriacum
Or Troches of Vipers, for Treacle

College.] Take of the flesh of Vipers, the skin, entrails, head, fat, and tail being taken away, boiled in water with Dill, and a little salt, eight ounces, white bread twice baked, grated and sifted, two ounces, make it into troches, your hands being anointed with Opobalsamum, or Oil of Nutmegs by expression, dry them upon a sieve turned the bottom upwards in an open place, often turning them till they are well dried, then put them in a glass or stone pot glazed, stopped close, they will keep a year, yet is it far better to make Treacle, not long after you have made them.

Culpeper.] They expel poison, and are excellently good, by a certain sympathetical virtue, for such as are bitten by an adder.

Trochisci de Agno Casto
Or Troches of Agnus Castus

College.] Take of the seeds of Agnus Castus, Lettuce, red Rose flowers, Balaustins, of each a dram, Ivory, white Amber, Bole-ammoniac washed in Knotgrass Water two drams, Plantain seeds four scruples, Sassafras two scruples, with mussilage of Quince seeds, extracted in water of Water-lily flowers, let them be made into troches.

Culpeper.] Very pretty troches and good for little.

Trochisci Alexiterii. Renodæus

College.] Take of the roots of Gentian, Tormentil, Orris Floren-tine, Zedoary, of each two drams, Cinnamon, Cloves, Mace, of each half a dram, Angelica roots three drams, Coriander seeds pre-pared, Roses, of each one dram, dried Citron pills two drams, beat them all into powder, and with juice of Liquorice softened in Hippocras, six ounces, make them into soft paste, which you may form into either troches or small rolls, which you please.

Culpeper.] It preserves and strengthens the heart exceedingly, helps faintings and failings of the vital spirits, resists poison and the pestilence, and is an excellent medicine for such to carry about them whose occasions are to travel in pestilential places and corrupt air, only taking a very small quantity now and then.

Troches of Annis seed. Mesue

College.] Take of Annis seeds, the juice of Maudlin made thick, of each two drams, the seeds of Dill, Spikenard, Mastich, Indian leaf or Mace, the leaves of Wormwood, Asarabacca, Smallage, bitter Almonds, of each half a dram, Aloes two drams, juice of Wormwood so much as is sufficient to make it into troches according to art.

Culpeper.] They open obstructions of the liver, and that very gently, and therefore diseases coming thereof, help quartan agues. You can scarce do amiss in taking them if they please but your palate.

Trochisci Diarhodon. Mesue

College.] Take of the flowers of red Roses six drams, Spikenard, Wood of Aloes, of each two drams, Liquorice three drams, Spodium one dram, Saffron half a dram, Mastich two drams, make them up into troches with white Wine according to art.

Culpeper.] They wonderfully ease fevers coming of flegm, as quotidian fevers, agues, *epiatos*, &c. pains in the belly.

Trochisci de Lacca. Mesue

College.] Take of Gum Lacca cleansed, the juice of Liquorice, Maudlin, Wormwood, and Barberries, all made thick, Rhubarb, long Birthwort, Costus, Asarabacca, bitter Almonds, Madder, Annis, Smallage, Schænanth, of each one dram, with the decoction of Birthwort, Schænanth, or the juice of Maudlin, or Wormwood, make them into troches according to art.

Culpeper.] It helps stoppings of the liver and spleen, and fevers thence coming, it expels wind, purges by urine, and resists dropsies.

Pastilli Adronis. Galen

College.] Take of Pomegranate flowers ten drams, Copperas twelve drams, unripe Galls, Birthwort, Frankincense, of each an ounce, Alum, Myrrh, of each half an ounce, Misy two drams, with eighteen ounces of austere Wine, make it into troches according to art.

Culpeper.] This also is appropriated to wounds, ulcers, and fistulas, it clears the ears, and represses all excrescences of flesh, cleanses the filth of the bones.

Trochisci Musæ. Galen

College.] Take of Alum, Aloes, Copperas, Myrrh, of each six drams, Crocomagma, Saffron, of each three drams, Pomegranate flowers half an ounce, Wine and Honey, of each so much as is sufficient to make it up into troches according to art.

Culpeper.] Their use is the same with the former.

Crocomagma of Damocrates. Galen

College.] Take of Saffron an hundred drams, red Roses, Myrrh, of each fifty drams, white Starch, Gum, of each thirty drams, Wine, so much as is sufficient to make it into troches.

Culpeper.] It is very expulsive, heats and strengthens the heart and stomach.

Trochisci Ramich. Mesue

College.] Take of the juice of Sorrel sixteen ounces, red Rose Leaves, an ounce, Myrtle Berries two ounces, boil them a little together, and strain them, add to the decoction, Galls well beaten, three ounces, boil them again a little, then put in these following things, in fine powder: take of red Roses an ounce, yellow Sanders, ten drams, Gum Arabic an ounce and an half, Sumach, Spodium, of each an ounce, Myrtle berries four ounces, Wood of Aloes, Cloves, Mace, Nutmegs, of each half an ounce, sour Grapes seven drams, mix them all together, and let them dry upon a stone, and grind them again into powder, and make them into small troches with one dram of Camphire, and so much Rose Water as is sufficient, and perfume them with fifteen grams of Musk.

Culpeper. They strengthen the stomach, heart, and liver, as also the bowels, they help the cholic, and fluxes of blood, as also bleeding at the nose if you snuff up the powder of them, disburden the body of salt, fretting, choleric humours. You may carry them about you, and take them at your pleasure.

Troches of Roses. Mesue

College.] Take of red Roses half an ounce, Wood of Aloes two drams, Mastich, a dram and an half, Roman Wormwood, Cinnamon, Indian Spikenard, Cassia Lignea, Schœnanth, of each one dram, old Wine, and decoction of the five opening roots, so much as is sufficient to make it into troches according to art.

Culpeper.] They help pains in the stomach, and indigestion, the illiac passion, hectic fevers, and dropsies, in the beginning, and cause a good colour.

Trochisci Diacorallion. Galen

College.] Take of Bole-ammoniac, red Coral, of each an ounce, Balaustines, Terra Lemnia, white Starch, of each half an ounce, Hypocistis, the seeds of Henbane, Opium, of each two drams, juice of Plantain so much as is sufficient to make them into troches according to art.

Culpeper.] These also stop blood, help the bloody flux, stop the menses, and are a great help to such whose stomachs loath their victuals. I fancy them not.

Trochisci Diaspermaton. Galen

College.] Take of the seeds of Smallage, and Bishop's weed, of each an ounce, Annis and Fennel seeds, of each half an ounce, Opium, Cassia Lignea, of each two drams, with rain water, make it into troches according to art.

Culpeper.] These also bind, ease pain, help the pleurisy.

Hæmoptoici Pastilli. Galen

College.] Take of white Starch, Balaustines, Earth of Samos, juice of Hypocystis, Gum, Saffron, Opium, of each two drams, with juice of Plantain, make them into troches according to art.

Culpeper.] The operation of this is like the former.

Troches of Agarick

College.] Take of choice Agarick three ounces, Sal. Gem. six drams, Ginger two drams, with Oxymel simplex, so much as is sufficient, make it into troches according to art.

OILS

SIMPLE OILS BY EXPRESSION

Oil of Sweet Almonds

College.] Take of Sweet Almonds not corrupted, as many as you will, cast the shells away, and blanch them, beat them in a stone mortar, beat them in a double vessel, and press out the oil without heat.

Culpeper.] It helps roughness and soreness of the throat and stomach, helps pleurisies, encreases seed, eases coughs and hectic fevers, by injection it helps such whose water scalds them; ulcers in the bladder, reins, and matrix. You may either take half an ounce of it by itself, or mix it with half an ounce of Syrup of Violets, and so take a spoonful at a time, still shaking them together when you take them: only take notice of this, if you take it inwardly, let it be new drawn, for it will be sour in three or four days.

Oil of bitter Almonds

College.] It is made like Oil of sweet Almonds, but that you need not blanch them, nor have such a care of heat in pressing out the oil.

Culpeper.] It opens stoppings, helps such as are deaf, being dropped into their ears, it helps the hardness of the nerves, and takes away spots in the face. It is seldom or never taken inwardly.

Oil of Hazel Nuts

College.] It is made of the Kernels, cleansed, bruised, and beat, and pressed like Oil of sweet Almonds.

Culpeper.] You must put them in a vessel (viz. a glass, or some such thing) and stop them close that the water come not to them when you put them into the bath. The oil is good for cold afflictions of the nerves, the gout in the joints, &c.

College.] So is Oil of Been, Oil of Nutmegs, and Oil of Mace drawn.

Oleum Caryinum

College.] Is prepared of Walnut Kernels, in like manner, save only that in the making of this sometimes is required dried, old, and rank Nuts.

Oleum Chrysomelinum

College.] Is prepared in the same manner of Apricots, so is also Oils of the Kernels of Cherry stones, Peaches, Pine-nuts, Fistic Nuts, Prunes, the seeds of Oranges, Hemp, Bastard Saffron, Citrons, Cucumbers, Gourds, Citruls, Dwarf Elder, Henbane, Lettuce, Flax, Melons, Poppy, Parsley, Radishes, Rape, Ricinum, Sesani, Mustard seed, and Grape stones.

Culpeper.] Because most of these Oils are out of use, I took not the pains to quote the virtues of them; if any wish to make them, let them look to the simples, and there they have them; if the simples be not to be found in this book, there are other plentiful medicines conducing to the cure of all usual diseases; which are—

Oil of Bays

College.] Take of Bay-berries, fresh and ripe, so many as you please, bruise them sufficiently, then boil them in a sufficient quantity of water till the Oil swim at top, which separate from the water, and keep for your use.

Culpeper.] It helps the cholic, and is a sovereign remedy for any diseases in any part of the body coming either of wind or cold.

College.] *Common Oil of Olives*, is pressed out of ripe olives, not out of the stones. Oil of Olives omphacine, is pressed out of unripe olives.

Oil of Yolks of Eggs

College.] Boil the yolks till they be hard, and bruise them with your hand or with a pestle and mortar; beat them in an earthen vessel glazed until they begin to froth, stirring them diligently that they burn not, being hot, put them in a linen bag, and sprinkle them with Aromatic Wine, and press out the oil according to art.

Culpeper.] It is profitable in fistulas, and malignant ulcers, it causes the hair to grow, it clears the skin, and takes away deformities thereof, viz. tetters, ringworms, morphew, scabs.

SIMPLE OILS BY INFUSION AND DECOCTION

Oil of Roses omphacine

College.] Take of red Roses before they be ripe, bruised in a stone mortar, four ounces, oil Omphacine one pound, set them in a hot sun, in a glass close stopped, a whole week, shaking them every day, then boil them gently in a bath, press them out, and put in others, use them in like manner, do so a third time: then keep the Oil upon a pound of juice of Roses.

Oil of Roses complete

Is made in the same manner, with sweet and ripe oil, often washed, and red Roses fully open, bruised, set in the sun, and boiled gently in a double vessel, only let the third infusion stand in the sun forty days, then keep the roses and oil together.

In the same manner is made Oil of Wormwood, of the tops of common Wormwood thrice repeated, four ounces, and three pounds of ripe oil; only, the last time put in four ounces of the juice of Wormwood, which evaporate away by gentle boiling.

Oil of Dill. Of the flowers and leaves of Dill four ounces, complete oil, one pound, thrice repeated.

Oil of Castoreum. Of one ounce of Castoreum oil one pound, Wine four ounces, which must be consumed with the heat of a bath.

Oil of Chamomel (which more than one call Holy) of complete oil, and fresh Chamomel flowers, the little white leaves taken away, cut, bruised, and the vessel covered with a thin linen cloth, set in the sun, pressed out, and three times repeated.

Oil of Wall-flowers, as oil of Dill.

Oil of Quinces. Of six parts of oil Omphacine, the meat and juice of Quinces one part, set them in the sun fifteen days in a glass, and afterwards boil them four hours in a double vessel, press them out, and renew them three times.

Oil of Elecampane. Of ripe oil, and the roots of Elecampane bruised, and their juice, of each one part, and of generous Wine half a part, which is to be evaporated away.

Oil of Euphorbium. Of six drams of Euphorbium, Oil of Wall-flowers, and sweet Wine, of each five ounces, boiling it in a double vessel till the Wine be consumed.

Oil of Ants. Of winged Ants infused in four times their weight of sweet oil, set in the sun in a glass forty days, and then strain it out.

Oil, or Balsam of St. John's Wort simple, is made of the oil of seeds beaten and pressed, and the flowers being added, and rightly set in the sun.

Oil of Jesmine, is made of the flowers of Jesmine, put in clear oil, and set in the sun and afterwards pressed out.

Oil of Orris, made of the roots of Orris Florentine one pound, purple Orris flowers half a pound: boil them in a double vessel in a sufficient quantity of decoction of Orris Florentine, and six pounds of sweet oil, putting fresh roots and flowers again and again; the former being cast away as in oil of Roses.

Oil of Earthworms, is made of half a pound of Earthworms washed in white Wine, ripe Oil two pounds, boiled in a double vessel with eight ounces of good white Wine till the Wine be consumed.

Oil of Marjoram is made with four ounces of the herb a little bruised, white Wine six ounces, ripe oil a pound, mixed together, let them be set in the sun repeated three times; at last boiled to the consumption of the Wine.

Oil of Mastich, is made of oil of Roses omphacine one pound, Mastich three ounces, Wine four ounces: boil them in a double vessel to the consumption of the Wine.

Oil of Melilot is made with the tops of the herb like oil of Chamomel.

Oil of Mints is made of the herb and oil omphacine, as oil of Roses.

Oil of Mirtles, is made of Mirtle berries bruised and sprinkled with sharp Wine one part, oil omphacine three parts; set it in the sun twenty-four days, and in the interim thrice renewed, boiled, and the berries pressed out.

Oil of Daffodils is made as oil of Roses.

Nard Oil is made of three ounces of Spikenard, sweet oil one pound and an half, sweet white Wine and clear water, of each two ounces and an half, boiled to the consumption of the moisture.

Oil of Water-lilies, is made of fresh white Water-lily flowers, one part, oil omphacine three parts, repeating the flowers as in oil of Roses.

Oil of Tobacco is made of the juice of Tobacco, and common oil, of each equal parts boiled in a bath.

Oil of Poppies, is made of the flowers, heads, and leaves of garden Poppies, and oil omphacine, as oil of Dill.

Oil of Poplars, is made of the buds of the Poplar tree three parts, rich white Wine four parts, sweet oil seven parts; first let the buds be bruised, then infused in the Wine and oil seven days, then boiled, then pressed out.

Oil of Rue, is made of the herb bruised, and ripe oil, like oil of Roses.

Oil of Savin is made in the same manner.

So also is Oil of Elder flowers made.

Oil of Scorpions, is made of thirty live Scorpions, caught when the sun is in the lion; oil of bitter Almonds two pounds, let them be set in the sun, and after forty days strained.

Oleum Cicyonium, is made of wild Cucumber roots, and their juice, of each equal parts; with twice as much ripe oil, boil it to the consumption of the juice.

Oil of Nightshade, is made of the berries of Nightshade ripe, and one part boiled in ripe oil, or oil of Roses three parts.

Oil of Styrax, is made of Styrax and sweet white Wine, of each one part, ripe oil four parts gently boiled till the Wine be consumed.

Oil of Violets, is made of oil omphacine, and Violet flowers, as oil of Roses.

Oil of Vervain, is made of the herb and oil, as oil of Mints.

Culpeper.] That most of these oils, if not all of them, are used only externally, is certain; and as certain that they retain the virtues of the simples whereof they are made, therefore the ingenious might help themselves.

COMPOUND OILS BY INFUSION AND DECOCTION

Oleum Benedictum
Or Blessed Oil

College.] Take of the roots of Carduus and Valerian, of each one ounce, the flowers of St. John's Wort two ounces, Wheat one ounce and an half, old Oil four ounces, Cypress Turpentine eight ounces, Frankincense in powder two ounces, infuse the roots and flowers, being bruised, in so much white Wine as is sufficient to cover them, after two days' infusion put in the Oil with the Wheat, bruised, boil them together till the Wine be consumed; then press it out, and add the Frankincense and Turpentine, then boil them a little, and keep it.

Culpeper.] It is appropriated to cleanse and consolidate wounds, especially in the head.

Oleum de Capparibus
Or, Oil of Capers

College.] Take of the bark of Caper roots an ounce, bark of Tamarisk, the leaves of the same, the seeds of Agnus Castus, Cetrach, or Spleenwort, Cypress roots, of each two drams, Rue one dram, oil of ripe Olives one pound, white Wine Vinegar, and white Wine, of each two ounces, cut them and steep them, and boil them (two days being elapsed) gently in a bath, then the Wine and Vinegar being consumed, strain it, and keep it.

Culpeper.] The oil is opening, and heating, absolutely appropriated to the spleen, hardness and pains thereof, and diseases coming of stoppings there, as hypocondriac melancholy, the rickets, &c.

Oil of Castoreum compound

College.] Take of Castoreum, Styrax Calamitis, Galbanum, Euphorbium, Opopanax, Cassia Lignea, Saffron, Carpobalsamum or Cubebs, Spikenard, Costus, of each two drams, Cypress, Squinanth, Pepper long and black, Savin, Pellitory of Spain, of each two drams and an half, ripe Oil four pounds, Spanish Wine two pounds, the five first excepted, let the rest be prepared as they ought to be, and gently boiled in the Oil and Wine, until the Wine be consumed, mean time the Galbanum, Opopanax, and Euphorbium beaten in fine powder, being dissolved in part of the Wine, and strained, let them be exquisitely mixed with it (while the oil is warm) by often stirring; the boiling being finished, put in the Styrax and Castoreum.

Culpeper.] The virtues are the same with the simple.

Oleum Castinum

College.] Take of the roots of bitter Castus two ounces, Cassia Lignea one ounce, the tops of Marjoram eight ounces, being bruised, steep them two days in twelve ounces of sweet white Wine; then with three pounds of sallad oil washed in white Wine, boil it in *Balneo Mariæ* till the Wine be consumed.

Culpeper.] It heats, opens obstructions, strengthens the nerves, and all nervous parts, as muscles, tendons, ligaments, the ventricle; besides these, it strengthens the liver, it keeps the hairs from turning grey, and gives a good colour to the body. I pray you take notice that this and the following oils, (till I give you warning to the contrary) are not made to eat.

Oleum Crocinum
Or, Oil of Saffron

College.] Take of Saffron, Calamus Aromaticus, of each one ounce, Myrrh, half an ounce, Cardamoms nine drams, steep them six days, (the Cardomoms excepted, which are not to be put in till the last day,) in nine ounces of Vinegar, the day after put in a pound and an half of washed oil, boil it gently according to art, till the Vinegar be consumed, then strain it.

Culpeper.] It helps pains in the nerves, and strengthens them, mollifies their hardness, helps pains in the matrix, and causes a good colour.

Oil of Euphorbium

College.] Take of Stavesacre, Sopewort, of each half an ounce, Pellitory of Spain six drams, dried Mountain Calamint one ounce and an half, Castus two drams, Castoreum five drams, being bruised, let them be three days steeped in three pounds and an half of Wine, boil them with a pound and an half of Oil of Wallflowers, adding half an ounce of Euphorbium, before the Wine be quite consumed, and so boil it according to art.

Culpeper.] It hath the same virtue, only something more effectual than the simple.

Oleum Excestrense
Or, Oil of Exeter

College.] Take of the leaves of Wormwood, Centaury the less, Eupatorium, Fennel, Hyssop, Bays, Marjoram, Bawm, Nep, Pennyroyal, Savin, Sage, Thyme, of each four ounces, Southernwood, Betony, Chamepitys, Lavender, of each six ounces, Rosemary one pound, the flowers of Chamomel, Broom, white Lilies, Elders, the seeds of Cummin, and Fenugreek, the roots of Hellebore black and white, the bark of Ash and Lemons, of each four ounces, Euphorbium, Mustard, Castoreum, Pellitory of Spain, of each an ounce, Oil sixteen pounds, Wine three pounds, the herbs, flowers, seeds, and Euphorbium being bruised, the roots, barks, and Castoreum cut, all of them infused twelve hours in the Wine and Oil, in a warm bath, then boiled with a gentle fire, to the consumption of the Wine and moisture, strain the Oil and keep it.

Culpeper.] Many people by catching bruises when they are young, come to feel it when they are old: others by catching cold, catch a lameness in their limbs, to both which I commend this sovereign oil to bathe their grieved members with.

Oleum Hirundinum
Or, Oil of Swallows

College.] Take of whole Swallows sixteen, Chamomel, Rue, Plantain the greater and lesser, Bay leaves, Pennyroyal, Dill, Hyssop, Rosemary, Sage, Saint John's Wort, Costmary, of each one handful, common Oil four pounds, Spanish Wine one pound, make it up according to art.

Culpeper.] Both this and the former are appropriated to old bruises and pains thereof coming, as also to sprains.

Oleum Hyperici compositum
Or, Oil of St. John's Wort compound

College.] Take of the tops of St. John's Wort four ounces, steep them three whole days in a pound of old Sallad Oil, in the heat either of a bath, or of the sun, then press them out, repeat the infusion the second or third time, then boil them till the wine be almost consumed, press them out, and by adding three ounces of Turpentine, and one scruple of Saffron, boil it a little and keep it.

Culpeper.] See the simple oil of St. John's Wort, than which this is stronger.

Oleum Hyperici magis compositum
Or, Oil of St. John's Wort more compound

College.] Take of white Wine three pounds, tops of St. John's Wort ripe and gently bruised, four handfuls, steep them two days in a glass, close stopped, boil them in a bath, and strain them strongly, repeat the infusion three times, having strained it the third time, add to every pound of decoction, old Oil four pounds, Turpentine six ounces, oil of Wormwood three ounces, Dittany, Gentian, Carduus, Tormentil, Carline, or Cordus Maria, Calamus Aromaticus, all of them bruised, of each two drams, Earth-worms often washed in white Wine two ounces, set it in the sun five or six weeks, then keep it close stopped.

Culpeper.] Besides the virtue of the simple oil of St. John's Wort, which this performs more effectually, it is an excellent remedy for old bruises, aches, and sprains.

Oleum Irinum
Or, Oil of Orris

College.] Take of the roots of Orris Florentine, three pounds four ounces, the flowers of purple Orris fifteen ounces, Cypress roots six ounces, of Elecampane three ounces, of Alkanet two ounces, Cinnamon, Spikenard, Benjamin, of each one ounce; let all of them, being bruised as they ought to be, be steeped in the sun, or other hot place, in fifteen pounds of old oil, and four pounds and an half of clear water, after the fourth day, boil them in *Balneo Mariæ*, the water being consumed, when it is cold, strain it and keep it.

Culpeper.] The effects are the same with the simple, only 'tis stronger.

Oleum Marjoranæ
Or, Oil of Marjoram

College.] Take of Marjoram four handfuls, Mother of Thyme two handfuls, the leaves and berries of Myrtles one handful, Southernwood, Water Mints, of each half an handful, being cut, bruised, and put in a glass, three pounds of Oil Omphacine being put to it, let it stand eight days in the Sun, or in a bath, close stopped, then strain it out, in the oil put in fresh simples, do so the third time, the oil may be perfected according to art.

Culpeper.] It helps weariness and diseases of the brain and nerves, coming of cold; it helps the dead palsy, the back (viz. the region along the back bone) being anointed with it; being snuffed up in the nose, it helps *Spasmus cynicus*, which is a wrying the mouth aside; it helps noise in the ears being dropped into them, it provokes the menses, and helps the biting of venomous beasts; it is a most gallant oil to strengthen the body, the back being anointed with it; strengthens the muscles, they being chafed with it; helps head-ache, the forehead being rubbed with it.

Moscholæum
Or, Oil of Musk

College.] Take two Nutmegs, Musk one dram, Indian leaf or Mace, Spikenard, Costus, Mastich, of each six drams, Styrax Calamitis, Cassia Lignea, Myrrh, Saffron, Cinnamon, Cloves, Carpobalsamum or Cubebs, Bdellium, of each two drams, pure Oil three pounds, Wine three ounces, bruise them as you ought to do, mix them, and let them boil easily, till the Wine be consumed, the Musk being mixed according to art after it is strained.

Culpeper.] It is exceeding good against all diseases of cold, especially those of the stomach, it helps diseases of the sides, they being anointed with it, the stranguary, cholic, and vices of the nerves, and afflictions of the reins.

Oleum Nardinum
Or, Oil of Nard

College.] Take of Spikenard three ounces, Marjoram two ounces, Wood of Aloes, Calamus Aromaticus, Elecampane, Cypress, Bay leaves, Indian leaf or Mace, Squinanth, Cardamoms, of each one ounce and a half, bruise them all grossly, and steep them in water and wine, of each fourteen ounces, Oil of Sesamin, or oil of Olives, four pounds and an half, for one day: then perfect the oil by boiling it gently in a double vessel.

Oleum Populeum. Nicholaus

College.] Take of fresh Poplar buds three pounds, Wine four pounds, common Oil seven pounds two ounces, beat the Poplar buds very well, then steep them seven days in the oil and wine, then boil them in a double vessel till the wine be consumed, (if you infuse fresh buds once or twice before you boil it, the medicine will be the stronger,) then press out the oil and keep it.

Culpeper.] It is a fine cool oil, but the ointment called by that name which follows hereafter is far better.

OINTMENTS MORE SIMPLE

Unguentum album
Or, white Ointment

College.] Take of Oil of Roses nine ounces, Ceruss washed in Rose-water and diligently sifted, three ounces, white Wax two ounces, after the wax is melted in the oil, put in the Ceruss, and make it into an ointment according to art, add two drams of Camphire, made into powder with a few drops of oil of sweet Almonds, so will it be camphorated.

Culpeper.] It is a fine cooling, drying ointment, eases pains, and itching in wounds and ulcers, and is an hundred times better with Camphire than without it.

Unguentum Egyptiacum

College.] Take of Verdigris finely powdered, five parts, Honey fourteen parts, sharp Vinegar seven parts, boil them to a just thickness, and a reddish colour.

Culpeper.] It cleanses filthy ulcers and fistulas forcibly, and not without pain, it takes away dead and proud flesh, and dries.

Unguentum Anodynum
Or, an Ointment to ease pain

College.] Take of Oil of white Lilies, six ounces, Oil of Dill, and Chamomel, of each two ounces, Oil of sweet Almonds one ounce, Duck's grease, and Hen's grease, of each two ounces, white Wax three ounces, mix them according to art.

Culpeper.] Its use is to assuage pains in any part of the body, especially such as come by inflammations, whether in wounds or tumours, and for that it is admirable.

Unguentum ex Apio
Or, Ointment of Smallage

College.] Take of the juice of Smallage one pound, Honey nine ounces, Wheat flower three ounces, boil them to a just thickness.

Culpeper.] It is a very fine, and very gentle cleanser of wounds and ulcers.

Liniment of Gum Elemi

College.] Take of Gum Elemi, Turpentine of the Fir-tree, of each one ounce and an half, old Sheep's Suet cleansed two ounces, old Hog's grease cleansed one ounce: mix them, and make them into an ointment according to art.

Culpeper.] It gently cleanses and fills up an ulcer with flesh, it being of a mild nature, and friendly to the body.

Unguentum Aureum

College.] Take of yellow Wax half a pound, common Oil two pounds, Turpentine two ounces, Pine Rozin, Colophonia, of each one ounce and an half, Frankincense, Mastich, of each one ounce, Saffron one dram, first melt the wax in the oil, then the Turpentine being added, let them boil together; having done boiling, put in the rest in fine powder, (let the Saffron be the last) and by diligent stirring, make them into an ointment according to art.

Basilicon, *the greater*

College.] Take of white Wax, Pine Rozin, Heifer's Suet, Greek Pitch, Turpentine, Olibanum, Myrrh, of each one ounce, Oil five ounces, powder the Olibanum and Myrrh, and the rest being melted, make it into an ointment according to art.

Basilicon, *the less*

College.] Take of yellow Wax, fat Rozin, Greek Pitch, of each half a pound, Oil nine ounces: mix them together, by melting them according to art.

Culpeper.] Both this and the former, heat, moisten, and digest, procure matter in wounds, I mean brings the filth or corrupted blood from green wounds: they cleanse and ease pain.

Ointment of Bdellium

College.] Take of Bdellium six drams, Euphorbium, Sagapen, of each four drams, Castoreum three drams, Wax fifteen drams, Oil of Elder or Wall-flowers, ten drams, the Bdellium, and Sagapen being dissolved in water of wild Rue, let the rest be united by the heat of a bath.

Unguentum de Calce
Or, Ointment of Chalk

College.] Take of Chalk washed, seven times at least, half a pound, Wax three ounces, Oil of Roses one pound, stir them all

together diligently in a leaden mortar, the wax being first melted
by a gentle fire in a sufficient quantity of the prescribed oil.

Culpeper.] It is exceeding good in burnings and scaldings.

Unguentum Dialthæ
Or, Ointment of Marsh-mallows

College.] Take of common Oil four pounds, mussilage of Marsh-
mallow roots, Linseed, and Fenugreek seed two pounds: boil them
together till the watry part of the mussilage be consumed, then add
Wax half a pound, Rozin three ounces, Turpentine an ounce, boil
them to the consistence of an ointment, but let the mussilage be
prepared of a pound of fresh roots bruised, and half a pound of each
of the seeds steeped, and boiled in eight pounds of spring water,
and then pressed out. *See the compound.*

Unguentum Diapompholygos

College.] Take of Oil of Nightshade sixteen ounces, white Wax,
washed, Ceruss, of each four drams, Lead burnt and washed,
Pompholix prepared, of each two ounces, pure Frankincense one
ounce: bring them into the form of an ointment according to art.

Culpeper.] This much differing from the former, you shall have
that inserted at latter end, and then you may use which you please.

Unguentum Enulatum
Or, Ointment of Elecampane

College.] Take of Elecampane roots boiled in Vinegar, bruised
and pulped, one pound, Turpentine washed in their decoction, new
Wax, of each two ounces, old Hog's grease salted ten ounces, old
oil four ounces, common salt one ounce, add the Turpentine to the
grease, wax, and oil, being melted, as also the pulp and salt being
finely powdered, and so make it into an ointment according to art.

Unguentum Enulatum cum Mercurio
Or, Ointment of Elecampane with Quicksilver

College.] Is made of the former ointment, by adding two ounces
of Quick-silver, killed by continual stirring, not only with spittle,
or juice of Lemons, but with all the Turpentine kept for that intent,
and part of the grease, in a stone mortar.

Culpeper.] My opinion of this ointment, is (briefly) this: It was

invented for the itch, without quick-silver it will do no good, with
quick-silver it may do harm.

Unguentum Laurinum commune
Or, Ointment of Bays common

College.] Take of Bay leaves bruised one pound, Bay berries
bruised half a pound, Cabbage leaves four ounces, Neat's-foot Oil
five pounds, Bullock's suet, two pounds, boil them together, and
strain them, that so it may be made into an ointment according to
art.

Unguentum de minie sive rubrum Camphora
Or, Ointment of red Lead

College.] Take of Oil of Roses one pound and an half, red Lead
three ounces, Litharge two ounces, Ceruss one ounce and an half,
Tutty three drams, Camphire two drams, Wax one ounce and an
half, make it into an ointment according to art, in a pestle and
mortar made of Lead.

Culpeper.] This ointment is as drying as a man shall usually read
of one, and withal cooling, therefore good for sores, and such as are
troubled with defluctions.

Unguentum e Nicotiona, seu Peto
Or, Ointment of Tobacco

College.] Take of Tobacco leaves bruised, two pounds, steep
them a whole night in red Wine, in the morning boil it in fresh
Hog's grease, diligently washed, one pound, till the Wine be consumed, strain it, and add half a pound of juice of Tobacco, Rozin
four ounces, boil it to the consumption of the juice, adding towards
the end, round Birthwort roots in powder, two ounces, new Wax
as much as is sufficient to make it into an ointment according to art.

Culpeper.] It would take a whole summer's day to write the
particular virtues of this ointment, and my poor *Genius* is too weak
to give it the hundredth part of its due praise. It cures tumours,
imposthumes, wounds, ulcers, gun-shot, stinging with nettles,
bees, wasps, hornets, venomous beasts, wounds made with poisoned
arrows, &c.

Unguentum Nutritum, seu Trifarmacum

College.] Take of Litharge of Gold finely powdered, half a
pound, Vinegar one pound, Oil of Roses two pounds, grind the

Litharge in a mortar, pouring to it sometimes Oil, sometimes Vinegar, till by continual stirring, the Vinegar do no more appear, and it come to a whitish ointment.

Culpeper.] It is of a cooling, drying nature, good for itching of wounds, and such like deformities of the skin.

Unguentum Ophthalmicum
Or, An Ointment for the Eyes

College.] Take of Bole-ammoniac washed in Rose water, one ounce, Lapis Calaminaris washed in Eyebright Water, Tutty prepared, of each two drams, Pearls in very fine powder half a dram, Camphire half a scruple, Opium five grains, fresh Butter washed in Plantain Water, as much as is sufficient to make it into an ointment according to art.

Culpeper.] It is exceeding good to stop hot rheums that fall down into the eyes, the eyelids being but anointed with it.

Unguentum ex Oxylapatho
Or, Ointment of sharp-pointed Dock

College.] Take of the roots of sharp-pointed Dock boiled in Vinegar until they be soft, and then pulped, Brimstone washed in juice of Lemons, of each one ounce and an half, Hog's grease often washed in juice of Scabious, half a pound, Unguentum Populeon washed in juice of Elecampane, half an ounce: make them into an ointment in a mortar.

Culpeper.] It is a wholesome, though troublesome medicine for scabs and itch.

Unguentum e Plumbo
Or, Ointment of Lead

College.] Take of Lead burnt according to art, Litharge, of each two ounces, Ceruss, Antimony, of each one ounce, Oil of Roses as much as is sufficient: make it into an ointment according to art.

Culpeper.] Take it one time with another, it will go neer to do more harm than good.

Unguentum Pomatum

College.] Take of fresh Hog's grease three pounds, fresh Sheep's suet nine ounces, Pomewater pared and cut, one pound and nine ounces, Damask Rose-water six ounces, the roots of Orris Florentine grossly bruised six drams, boil them in *Balneo Mariæ* till the

Apples be soft, then strain it, but press it not and keep it for use; then warm it a little again and wash it with fresh Rose-water, adding to each pound twelve drops of oil of *Lignum Rhodium*.

Culpeper.] Its general use is, to soften and supple the roughness of the skin, and take away the chops of the lips, hands, face, or other parts.

Unguentum Potabile

College.] Take of Butter without salt, a pound and an half, Spermaceti, Madder, Tormentil roots, Castoreum, of each half an ounce: boil them as you ought in a sufficient quantity of Wine, till the Wine be consumed, and become an ointment.

Culpeper.] I know not what to make of it.

Unguentum Resinum

College.] Take of Pine Rozin, or Rozin of the Pine-tree, of the purest Turpentine, yellow Wax washed, pure Oil, of each equal parts: melt them into an ointment according to art.

Culpeper.] It is as pretty a Cerecloth for a new sprain as most is, and cheap.

Unguentum Rosatum
Or, Ointment of Roses

College.] Take of fresh Hog's grease cleansed a pound, fresh red Roses half a pound, juice of the same three ounces, make it into an ointment according to art.

Culpeper.] It is of a fine cooling nature, exceeding useful in all gallings of the skin, and frettings, accompanied with choleric humours, angry pushes, tetters, ringworms, it mitigates diseases in the head coming of heat, as also the intemperate heat of the stomach and liver.

Desiccativum Rubrum
Or, a drying Red Ointment

College.] Take of the oil of Roses omphacine a pound, white Wax five ounces, which being melted and put in a leaden mortar, put in the Earth of Lemnos or Bole-ammoniac, Lapis Calaminaris, of each four ounces, Litharge of Gold, Ceruss, of each three ounces, Camphire one dram, make it into an ointment according to art.

Culpeper.] It binds and restrains fluxes of humours.

Unguentum e Solano
Or, Ointment of Nightshade

College.] Take of juice of Nightshade, Litharge washed, of each five ounces, Ceruss washed eight ounces, white Wax seven ounces, Frankincense in powder ten drams, oil of Roses often washed in water two pounds, make it into an ointment according to art.

Culpeper.] It was invented to take away inflammations from wounds, and to keep people from scratching of them when they are almost well.

Or, Ointment of Tutty

College.] Take of Tutty prepared two ounces, Lapis Calaminaris often burnt and quenched in Plantain Water an ounce, make them, being finely powdered, into an ointment, with a pound and an half of ointment of Roses.

Culpeper.] It is a cooling, drying ointment, appropriated to the eyes, to dry up hot and salt humours that flow down thither, the eyelids being anointed with it.

Valentia Scabiosæ

College.] Take of the juice of green Scabious, pressed out with a screw, and strained through a cloth, Hog's grease, of each as much as you will, heat the Hog's grease in a stone mortar, not grind it, putting in the juice by degrees for the more commodious mixture and tincture, afterwards set it in the sun in a convenient vessel, so as the juice may overtop the grease, nine days being passed, pour off the discoloured juice, and beat it again as before, putting in fresh juice, set it in the sun again five days, which being elapsed, beat it again, put in more juice, after fifteen days more, do so again, do so five times, after which, keep it in a glass, or glazed vessel.

Tapsivalentia

College.] Take of the juice of Mullen, Hog's grease, of each as much as you will, let the grease be cleansed and cut in pieces, and beat it with the juice, pressed and strained as you did the former ointment, then keep it in a convenient vessel nine or ten days, then beat it twice, once with fresh juice, until it be green, and the second time without juice beaten well, pouring off what is discoloured, and keep it for use.

Tapsimel

College.] Take of the juice of Celandine and Mullen, of each one part, clarified Honey, two parts, boil them by degrees till the juice be consumed, adding (the physician prescribing) Vitriol, burnt Alum, burnt Ink, and boil it again to an ointment according to art.

OINTMENTS MORE COMPOUND

Unguentum Agrippa

College.] Take of Briony roots two pounds, the roots of wild Cucumbers one pound, Squills half a pound, fresh English Orris roots, three ounces, the roots of male Fern, dwarf Elder, water Caltrops, or Aaron, of each two ounces, bruise them all, being fresh, and steep them six or seven days in four pounds of old oil, the whitest, not rank, then boil them and press them out, and in the oil melt fifteen ounces of white Wax, and make it into an ointment according to art.

Culpeper.] It purges exceedingly, and is good to anoint the bellies of such as have dropsies, and if there be any humour or flegm in any part of the body that you know not how to remove (provided the part be not too tender) you may anoint it with this; but yet be not too busy with it, for I tell you plainly it is not very safe.

Unguentum Amarum
Or, A bitter Ointment

College.] Take of Oil of Rue, Savin, Mints, Wormwood, bitter Almonds, of each one ounce and an half, juice of Peach flowers and leaves, and Wormwood, of each half an ounce, powder of Rue, Mints, Centaury the less, Gentian, Tormentil, of each one dram, the seeds of Coleworts, the pulp of Colocynthis, of each two drams, Aloes Hepatic, three drams, meal of Lupines half an ounce, Myrrh washed in Grass water a dram and an half, Bull's Gall an ounce and an half, with a sufficient quantity of juice of Lemons, and an ounce and an half of Wax, make it into an ointment according to art.

Unguentum Apostolorum
Or, Ointment of the Apostles

College.] Take of Turpentine, yellow Wax, Ammoniacum, of each fourteen drams, long Birthwort roots, Olibanum, Bdellium, of each six drams, Myrrh, Gilbanum, of each half an ounce, Opopanax, Verdigris, of each two drams, Litharge nine drams, Oil two pounds, Vinegar enough to dissolve the Gums, make it into an ointment according to art.

Culpeper.] It consumes corrupt and dead flesh, and makes flesh soft which is hard, it cleanses wounds, ulcers, and fistulas, and restores flesh where it is wanting.

Unguentum Catapsoras

College.] Take of Ceruss washed in Purslain water, then in Vinegar wherein wild Rhadish roots have been steeped and pressed out, Lapis Calaminaris, Chalcitis, of each six drams, burnt Lead, Goat's blood, of each half an ounce, Quick-silver sublimated an ounce, the juice of Houseleek, Nightshade, Plantain, of each two ounces, Hog's grease cleansed three pounds, Oil of Violets, Poppies, Mandrakes, of each an ounce: first let the sublimate and exungia, then the oils, juices, and powders, be mixed, and so made into an ointment according to art.

Unguentum Citrinum
Or, A Citron Ointment

College.] Take of Borax an ounce, Camphire a dram, white Coral half an ounce, Alum Plume an ounce, Umbilicus Marinus, Tragacanth, white Starch, of each three drams, Crystal, Dentalis Utalis, Olibanum, Niter, white Marble, of each two drams, Gersa Serpentaria an ounce, Ceruss six ounces, Hog's grease not salted, a pound and an half, Goat's suet prepared, an ounce and an half, Hen's fat two ounces and an half. Powder the things as you ought to do both together, and by themselves, melt the fats being cleansed in a stone vessel, and steep in them two Citrons of a mean bigness cut in bits, in a warm bath, after a whole week strain it, and put in the powders by degrees, amongst which let the Camphire and Borax be the last, stir them, and bring them into the form of an ointment.

Unguentum Martiatum

College.] Take of fresh Bay leaves three pounds, Garden Rue two pounds and an half, Marjoram two pounds, Mints a pound, Sage, Wormwood, Costmary, Bazil, of each half a pound, Sallad Oil twenty pounds, yellow Wax four pounds, Malaga Wine two pounds, of all of them being bruised, boiled, and pressed out as they ought, make an ointment according to art.

Culpeper.] It is a great strengthener of the head, it being anointed with it; as also of all the parts of the body, especially the nerves, muscles, and arteries.

Unguentum Mastichinum
Or, An Ointment of Mastich

College.] Take of the Oil of Mastich, Wormwood, and Nard, of each an ounce, Mastich, Mints, red Roses, red Coral, Cloves, Cinnamon, Wood of Aloes, Squinanth, of each a dram, wax as much as is sufficient to make it into an ointment according to art.

Culpeper.] This is like the former, and not a whit inferior to it; it strengthens the stomach being anointed with it, restores appetite and digestion. Before it was called a stomach ointment.

Unguentum Neapolitanum

College.] Take of Hog's grease washed in juice of Sage a pound, Quick-silver strained through leather, four ounces, oil of Bays, Chamomel, and Earthworms, of each two ounces, Spirit of Wine an ounce, yellow Wax two ounces, Turpentine washed in juice of Elecampane three ounces, powder of Chamepitys and Sage, of each two drams, make them into an ointment according to art.

Culpeper.] A learned art to spoil people: hundreds are bound to curse such ointments, and those that appoint them.

Unguentum Nervinum

College.] Take of Cowslips with the flowers, Sage, Chamepitys, Rosemary, Lavender, Bay with the berries, Chamomel, Rue, Smallage, Melilot with the flowers, Wormwood, of each a handful, Mints, Betony, Pennyroyal, Parsley, Centaury the less, St. John's Wort, of each a handful, oil of Sheep's or Bullock's feet, five pounds, oil of Spike half an ounce, Sheep's or Bullock's Suet, or the Marrow of either, two pounds: the herbs being bruised and boiled with the oil and suet, make it into an ointment according to art.

Culpeper.] It is appropriated to the nerves, and helps their infirmities coming of cold, as also old bruised, make use of it in dead palsies, chilliness or coldness of particular members, such as the arteries perform not their office to as they ought; for wind anoint your belly with it; for want of digestion, your stomach; for the cholic, your belly; for whatever disease in any part of the body comes of cold, esteem this as a jewel.

Unguentum Pectorale
Or, A Pectoral Ointment

College.] Take of fresh Butter washed in Violet Water six ounces, oil of Sweet Almonds four ounces, oil of Chamomel and Violets, white Wax, of each three ounces, Hen's and Duck's greese, of each two ounces, Orris roots two drams, Saffron half a dram. The two last being finely powdered, the rest melted and often washed in Barley or Hyssop water, make an ointment of them according to art.

Culpeper.] It strengthens the breast and stomach, eases the pains thereof, helps pleurises and consumptions of the lungs, the breast being anointed with it.

Unguentum Resumptivum

College.] Take of Hog's grease three ounces, the grease of Hens, Geese, and Ducks, of each two ounces, Oesipus half an ounce, oil of Violets, Chamomel, and Dill, fresh Butter a pound, white Wax six ounces, mussilage of Gum Tragacanth, Arabic, Quince seeds, Lin-seeds, Marsh-mallow roots, of each half an ounce. Let the mussilages be made in Rose water, and adding the rest, make it into an ointment according to art.

Culpeper.] It mightily molifies without any manifest heat, and is therefore a fit ointment for such as have agues, asthmas, hectic fevers, or consumptions. It is a good ointment to ease pains coming by inflammations of wounds or aposthumes, especially such as dryness accompanies, an infirmity wounded people are many times troubled with. In inward aposthumes, as pleurises, one of them to anoint the external region of the part, is very beneficial.

Unguentum Splanchnicum

College.] Take of Oil of Capers an ounce, oil of white Lillies, Chamomel, fresh Butter, juice of Briony and Sowbread, of each half an ounce, boil it to the consumption of the juice, add Ammoniacum dissolved in Vinegar, two drams and an half, Hen's grease, Oesypus, Marrow of a Calf's Leg, of each half an ounce, powder of the bark of the roots of Tamaris and Capers, Fern roots, Cetrach, of each a dram, the seeds of Agnus Castuus, and Broom, of each a scruple, with a sufficient quantity of Wax, make it into an ointment according to art.

Unguentum Splanchnicum Magistrale

College.] Take of the bark of Caper roots six drams, Briony roots, Orris Florentine, powder of sweet Fennel seeds, Ammoniacum dissolved in Vinegar, of each half an ounce, tops of Wormwood, Chamomel flowers, of each a dram, ointment of the juice and of flowers of Oranges, of each six drams, oil of Orris and Capers, of each an ounce and an half: the things which ought being powdered and sifted, the rest diligently mixed in a hot mortar, make it into an ointment according to art.

Culpeper.] Both these ointments are appropriated to the spleen, and eases the pains thereof, the sides being anointed with them. I fancy not the former.

Unguentum e Succis
Or, Ointment of Juices

College.] Take of the juice of Dwarf-Elder eight ounces, of Smallage and Parsley, of each four ounces, Wormwood and Orris, of each five ounces, common Oil half a pound, oil of white Lilies ten ounces, of Wormwood and Chamomel, of each six ounces, the fat of Ducks and Hens, of each two ounces, boil them together with a gentle fire till the juice be consumed, then strain it, and with seven ounces of white Wax, and a little white Wine Vinegar, make it into an ointment according to art.

See Unguentum ex Succis Aperitivis.

Unguentum Sumach

College.] Take of Sumach, unripe Galls, Myrtle berries, Balaustines, Pomegranate Pills, Acorn Cups, Cypress Nuts, Acacia, Mastich, of each ten drams, white Wax five ounces, oil of Roses often washed in Alum water, a pound and ten ounces, make a fine powder of the things you can, and steep them four whole days in juice of Medlars and Services, of each a sufficient quantity, then dry them by a gentle fire, and with the oil and wax boil it into an ointment.

Culpeper.] It is a gallant drying and binding ointment. Besides, the stomach anointed with it, stays vomiting, and the belly anointed with it stays looseness, if the fundament fall out, when you have put it up again anoint it with this ointment, and it will fall out no more. Do the like by the womb if that fall out.

Ointment of Marsh-mallows, compound. Nicholaus

College.] Take of Marsh-mallow roots two pounds, the seeds of
Flax and Fœnugreek, of each one pound, pulp of Squills half a
pound, Oil four pounds, Wax one pound, Turpentine, Gum of
Ivy, Galbanum, of each two ounces, Colophonia, Rozin, of each
half a pound. Let the roots be well washed and bruised, as also the
Linseed, Fœnugreek seed, and Squills, then steep them three days
in eight pints of water, the fourth day boil them a little upon the
fire, and draw out the mussilage, of which take two pounds, and
boil it with the oil to the consumption of the juice, afterwards add
the Wax, Rozin, and Colophonia, when they are melted, add the
Turpentine, afterwards the Galbanum and Gum of Ivy, dissolved
in Vinegar, boil them a little, and having removed them from the
fire, stir them till they are cold, that so they may be well incor-
porated.

Culpeper.] It heats and moistens, helps pains of the breast
coming of cold and pleurises, old aches, and stitches, and softens
hard swellings.

Unguentum Diapompholigos nihili. Nicholaus

College.] Take of Oil of Roses sixteen ounces, juice of Nightshade six ounces, let them boil to the consumption of the juice,
then add white Wax five ounces, Ceruss washed two ounces, Lead
burnt and washed, Pompholix prepared, pure Frankincense, of each
an ounce, let them be brought into the form of an ointment according to art.

Culpeper.] It cools and binds, drys, and stays fluxes, either of
blood or humours in wounds, and fills hollow ulcers with flesh.

Unguentum Refrigerans. Galenus
It is also called a Cerecloath

College.] Take of white Wax four ounces, Oil of Roses omphacine one pound, melt it in a double vessel, then pour it out into
another, by degrees putting in cold water, and often pouring it out
of one vessel into another, stirring it till it be white, last of all
wash it in Rose water, adding a little Rose Water, and Rose
Vinegar.

Culpeper.] It is a fine cooling thing, to cure inflammations in
wounds or tumours.

Unguentum e Succis Aperitivis primum. Fœsius

College.] Take of the juice of Smallage, Endive, Mints, Wormwood, common Parsley, Valerian, of each three ounces, oil of Wormwood and Mints, of each half a pound, yellow Wax three ounces, mix them together over the fire, and make of them an ointment.

Culpeper.] It opens stoppages of the stomach and spleen, eases the rickets, the breast and sides being anointed with it.

An Ointment for the Worms. Fœsius

College.] Take of oil of Rue, Savin, Mints, Wormwood, and bitter Almonds, of each an ounce and an half, juice of the flowers or leaves of Peaches, and Wormwood, of each half an ounce, powder of Rue, Mints, Gentian, Centaury the less, Tormentil, of each one dram, the seeds of Coleworts, the pulp of Colocynthis, of each two drams, Aloes Hepatic, three drams, the meal of Lupines half an ounce, Myrrh washed in grass water a dram and an half, Bull's Galls an ounce and an half, with juice of Lemons, so much as is sufficient, and an ounce and an half of Wax, make it into an ointment according to art.

Culpeper.] The belly being anointed with it kills the worms.

CERECLOATHS

Ceratum de Galbano
Or, Cerecloath of Galbanum

College.] Take of Galbanum prepared, an ounce and an half, Assafœtida half an ounce, Bdellium a dram, Myrrh two drams, Wax two ounces, Carrot seeds a scruple, Featherfew, Mugwort, of each half a dram, dissolve the Gums in Vinegar, and make it a cerecloath according to art.

Culpeper.] Being applied to the belly of a woman after labour, it cleanses her of any relicts accidently left behind, helps the fits of the mother, and other accidents incident to women in that case.

Ceratum Oesypatum

College.] Take of Oesypus ten ounces, Oil of Chamomel, and Orris, of each half a pound, yellow Wax two pounds, Rozin a pound, Mastich, Ammoniacum, Turpentine, of each an ounce,

Spikenard two drams and an half, Saffron a dram and an half, Styrax Calamitis half an ounce, make them into a cerecloath according to art.

Culpeper.] It molifies and digests hard swellings of the liver, spleen, womb, nerves, joints, and other parts of the body, and is a great easer of pain.

Ceratum Santalinum

College.] Take of red Sanders, ten drams, white and yellow Sanders, of each six drams, red Roses twelve drams, Bole-ammoniac seven drams, Spodium four drams, Camphire two drams, white Wax washed thirty drams, Oil of Roses omphacine six ounces: make it into a cerecloath according to art.

Culpeper.] It wonderfully helps hot infirmities of the stomach, liver, and other parts, being but applied to them.

PLAISTERS

Emplastrum ex Ammoniaco
Or, A Plaister of Ammoniacum

College.] Take of Ammoniacum, Bran well sifted, of each an ounce, Ointment of Marsh-mallows, Melilot plaister compound, roots of Briony, and Orris in powder, of each half an ounce, the fat of Ducks, Geese, and Hens, of each three drams, Bdellium, Galbanum, of each one dram and an half, Per-Rozin, Wax, of each five ounces, oil of Orris, Turpentine, of each half an ounce, boil the fats and oils with mussilage of Lin-seed, and Fenugreek seed, of each three ounces, to the consumption of the mussilage, strain it, and add the Wax, Rozin, and Turpentine, the ointment of Marsh-mallows with the plaister of Melilot; when it begins to be cold, put in the Ammoniacum, dissolved in Vinegar, then the Bdellium in powder, with the rest of the powders, and make it into a plaister according to art.

Culpeper.] It softens and assuages hard swellings, and scatters the humours offending, applied to the side it softens the hardness of the spleen, assuages pains thence arising.

Emplastrum e Baccus Lauri
Or, A Plaister of Bay-berries

College.] Take of Bay-berries husked, Turpentine, of each two ounces, Frankincense, Mastich, Myrrh, of each an ounce, Cypress,

Costus, of each half an ounce, Honey warmed and not scummed, four ounces: make it into a plaister according to art.

Culpeper.] It is an excellent plaister to ease any pains coming of cold or wind, in any part of the body, whether stomach, liver, belly, reins, or bladder. It is an excellent remedy for the cholic and wind in the bowels.

Emplastrum Barbarum Magnum

College.] Take of dry Pitch eight pounds, yellow Wax six pounds and eight ounces, Per-Rozin five pounds and four ounces, Bitumen, Judaicum, or Mummy, four pounds, Oil one pound and an half, Verdigris, Litharge, Ceruss, of each three ounces, Frankincense half a pound, Roach Alum not burnt, an ounce and an half, burnt, four ounces, Opopanax, scales of Brass, Galbanum, of each twelve drams, Aloes, Opium, Myrrh, of each half an ounce, Turpentine two pounds, juice of Mandrakes, or else dried bark of the root, six drams, Vinegar five pounds. Let the Litharge, Ceruss, and Oil, boil to the thickness of Honey, then incorporate with them the Pitch, being melted with Bitumen in powder; then add the rest, and boil them according to art, till the vinegar be consumed, and it stick not to your hands.

Culpeper.] It helps the bitings of men and beasts, eases inflammations of wounds, and helps infirmities of the joints, and gouts in the beginning.

Emplastrum de Betonica
Or, A Plaister of Betony

College.] Take of Betony, Burnet, Agrimony, Sage, Pennyroyal, Yarrow, Comfrey the greater, Clary, of each six ounces, Frankincense, Mastich, of each three drams, Orris, round Birthwort, of each six drams, white Wax, Turpentine, of each eight ounces, Per-Rozin six ounces, Gum Elemi, Oil of Fir, of each two ounces, white Wine three pounds: bruise the herbs, boil them in the Wine, then strain them, and add the rest, and make them into a plaister according to art.

Culpeper.] It is a good plaister to unite the skull when it is cracked, to draw out pieces of broken bones, and cover the bones with flesh. It draws filth from the bottom of deep ulcers, restores flesh lost, cleanses, digests, and drys.

Emplastrum Cæsarus

College.] Take of red Roses one ounce and an half, Bistort roots, Cypress Nuts, all the Sanders, Mints, Coriander seeds, of each three drams, Mastich half an ounce, Hypocistis, Acacia, Dragon's blood, Earth of Lemnos, Bole-ammoniac, red Coral, of each two drams, Turpentine washed in Plantain water four ounces, Oil of Roses three ounces, white Wax twelve ounces, Per-Rozin ten ounces, Pitch six ounces, the juice of Plantain, Houseleek, and Orpine, of each an ounce, the Wax, Rozin, and Pitch being melted together, add the Turpentine and Oil, then the Hypocistis and Acacia dissolved in the juices, at last the powders, and make it into a plaister according to art.

Culpeper.] It is of a fine, cool, binding, strengthening nature, excellently good to repel hot rheums or vapours that ascend up to the head, the hair being shaved off, and it applied to the crown.

Emplastrum Catagmaticum the first

College.] Take of juice of Marsh-mallow roots six ounces, bark of Ashtree roots, and their leaves, the roots of Comfrey the greater and smaller with their leaves, of each two ounces, Myrtle Berries an ounce and an half, the leaves of Willow, the tops of St. John's Wort, of each an handful and an half, having bruised them, boil them together in red Wine, and Smith's Water, of each two pound, till half be consumed, strain it, and add Oil of Myrtles, and Roses omphacine, of each one pound and an half, Goat's suet eight ounces, boil it again to the consumption of the decoction, strain it again, and add Litharge of Gold and Silver, red Lead, of each four ounces, yellow Wax one pound, Colophonia half a pound, boil it to the consistance of a plaister, then add Turpentine two ounces, Myrrh, Frankincense, Mastich, of each half an ounce, Bole-ammoniac, Earth of Lemnos, of each one ounce, stir them about well till they be boiled, and made into an emplaister according to art.

Catagmaticum the second

College.] Take of the roots of Comfrey the greater, Marsh-mallows, Misselto of the Oak, of each two ounces, Plantain, Chamepitys, St. John's Wort, of each a handful, boil them in equal parts of black Wine, and Smith's Water till half be consumed, strain it, and add mussilage of Quince seeds made in Tripe water, Oil of Mastich and Roses, of each four ounces, boil it to the consumption of the humidity, and having strained it, add Litharge of Gold four ounces, boil it to the consistence of an emplaister, then add yellow Wax four ounces, Turpentine three ounces, Colophonia six drams, Ship Pitch ten ounces, powders of Balaustines, Roses, Myrtles, Acacia, of each half an ounce, Mummy, Androsamum, Mastich, Amber, of each six drams, Bole-ammoniac fine flowers, Frankincense, of each twelve drams, Dragon's blood two ounces: make it into a plaister according to art.

Culpeper.] Both this and the former are binding and drying, the former rules will instruct you in the use.

Emplastrum Cephalicum
Or, A Cephalic Plaister

College.] Take of Rozin two ounces, black Pitch one ounce, Labdanum, Turpentine, flower of Beans, and Orobus, Dove's dung, of each half an ounce, Myrrh, Mastich, of each one dram and an half, Gum of Juniper, Nutmegs, of each two drams, dissolve the Myrrh and Labdanum in a hot mortar, and adding the rest, make it into a plaister according to art. If you will have it stronger, add the powders, Euphorbium, Pellitory of Spain, and black Pepper, of each two scruples.

Culpeper.] It is proper to strengthen the brain, and repel such vapours as annoy it, and those powders being added, it dries up the superfluous moisture thereof, and eases the eyes of hot scalding vapours that annoy them.

Emplastrum de Cerussa
Or, A Plaister of Ceruss

College.] Take of Ceruss in fine powder, white Wax, Sallad Oil, of each three ounces, add the Oil by degrees to the Ceruss, and boil it by continual stirring over a gentle fire, till it begin to swell, then add the Wax cut small by degrees, and boil it to its just consistence.

Culpeper.] It helps burns, dry scabs, and hot ulcers, and in general whatever sores abound with moisture.

Emplastrum ex Cicuta cum Ammoniaco
Or, A Plaister of Hemlock with Ammoniacum

College.] Take of the juice of Hemlock four ounces, Vinegar, of Squills, and Ammoniacum, of each eight ounces, dissolve the Gum in the juice and Vinegar, after a due infusion, then strain it into its just consistence according to art.

Culpeper.] I suppose it was invented to mitigate the extreme pains, and allay the inflammations of wounds, for which it is very good: let it not be applied to any principal part.

Emplastrum e crusta Panis
Or, A Plaister of a crust of Bread

College.] Take of Mastich, Mints, Spodium, red Coral, all the
Sanders, of each one dram, Oil of Mastich and Quinces, of each
one dram and an half, a crust of Bread toasted, and three times
steeped in red Rose Vinegar, and as often dried, Labdanum, of
each two ounces, Rozin four ounces, Styrax Calamitis half an
ounce, Barley meal five drams: make them into a plaister according
to art.

Culpeper.] I shall commend this for a good plaister to strengthen
the brain as any is in the Dispensatory, the hair being shaved off,
and it applied to the crown; also being applied to the stomach, it
strengthens it, helps digestion, stays vomiting and putrefaction of
the meat there.

Emplastrum e Cymino
Or, A Plaister of Cummin

College.] Take of Cummin-seed, Bay-berries, yellow Wax, of
each one pound, Per-Rozin two pounds, common Rozin three
pounds, Oil of Dill half a pound, mix them, and make them into a
plaister.

Culpeper.] It assuages swellings, takes away old aches coming of
bruises, and applied to the belly, is an excellent remedy for the wind
cholic. This I have often proved, and always with good success.

Emplastrum Diacalciteos

College.] Take of Hog's grease fresh and purged from the skins
two pounds, oil of Olives omphacine, Litharge of Gold beaten and
sifted, of each three pounds, white Vitriol burnt and purged four
ounces: let the Litharge, grease, and oil boil together with a gentle
fire, with a little Plantain water, always stirring it, to the consistence
of a plaister, into which (being removed from the fire) put in the
Vitriol and make it into a plaister according to art.

Culpeper.] It is a very drying, binding plaister, profitable in
green wounds to hinder putrefaction, as also in pestilential sores
after they are broken, and ruptures, and also in burnings and
scaldings.

Diachylon simple

College.] Take of mussilage of Linseed, Fenugreek seed, Marsh-
mallow roots, of each one pound, old Oil three pounds: boil it to the

consumption of the mussilage, strain it, and add Litharge of Gold
in fine powder, one pound and an half: boil them with a little water
over a gentle fire always stirring them to a just thickness.

Culpeper.] It is an exceeding good remedy for all swellings without pain, it softens hardness of the liver and spleen, it is very gentle.

Diachylon Ireatum

College.] Add one ounce of Orris in powder to every pound of
Diachylon simple.

Diachylon Magnum

College.] Take of mussilage of Raisins, fat Figs, Mastich, Mal-
low-roots, Linseeds, and Fenugreek-seeds, Bird-lime, the juice of
Orris and Squills, of each twelve drams and an half, Œsypus or oil
of Sheep's feet an ounce and an half, Oil of Orris, Chamomel, Dill,
of each eight ounces, litharge of Gold in fine powder one pound,
Turpentine three ounces, Per-Rozin, yellow Wax, of each two
ounces, boil the oil with the mussilages and juices to the consumption of the humidity, strain the oil from the faces, and by adding
the Litharge boil it to its consistence; then add the Rozin and Wax;
lastly, it being removed from the fire, add the Turpentine, Œsypus
and Birdlime, make of them a plaister by melting them according to
art.

Culpeper.] It dissolves hardness and inflammations.

Diachylon magnum cum Gummi

College.] Take of Bdellium, Sagapenum, Amoniacum, of each
two ounces, dissolved in Wine, and added to the mass of Diachylon magnum: first boil the gums being dissolved, to the thickness of Honey.

Culpeper.] This is the best to dissolve hard swellings of all the
three.

Diachylon compositum, sive Emplaistrum e Mussilaginibus
Or, A Plaister of Mussilages

College.] Take of mussilages of the middle bark of Elm, Marsh-
mallow roots, Linseed, and Fenugreek seed, of each four ounces
and an half, oil of Chamomel, Lilies, and Dill, of each an ounce
and an half, Ammoniacum, Galbanum, Sagapen, Opopanax, of
each half an ounce, new Wax twenty ounces, Turpentine two
ounces, Saffron two drams, dissolve the Gums in Wine, and make
it into a plaister according to art.

Culpeper.] It ripens swellings, and breaks them, and cleanses them when they are broken. It is of a most excellent ripening nature.

Emplaistrum Diaphænicon hot

College.] Take of yellow Wax two ounces, Per-Rozin, Pitch, of each four ounces, Oil of Roses and Nard, of each one ounce, melt them together, and add pulp of Dates made in Wine four ounces, flesh of Quinces boiled in red Wine an ounce, then the powders following: take of Bread twice baked, steeped in Wine and dried, two ounces, Mastich an ounce, Frankincense Wormwood, red Roses, Spikenard, of each two drams and an half, Wood of Aloes, Mace, Myrrh, washed Aloes, Acacia, Troches of Gallia Moschata, and Earth of Lemnos, Calamus Aromaticus, of each one dram, Labdanum three ounces, mix them and make them into a plaister according to art.

Culpeper.] It strengthens the stomach and liver exceedingly, helps fluxes, apply it to the places grieved.

Diaphænicon cold

College.] Take of Wax four ounces, Ship Pitch five ounces, Labdanum three ounces and an half, Turpentine an ounce and an half, Oil of Roses one ounce, melt these, and add pulp of Dates almost ripe, boiled in austere Wine four ounces, flesh of Quinces in like manner boiled, Bread twice baked often steeped in red Wine and dried, of each an ounce, Styrax Calamitis, Acacia, unripe Grapes, Balaustines, yellow Sanders, troches of Terra Lemnia, Myrrh, Wood of Aloes, of each half an ounce, Mastich, red Roses, of each an ounce and an half, austere Wine as much as is sufficient to dissolve the juices, make it into a plaister according to art.

Culpeper.] It strengthens the belly and liver, helps concoction in those parts, and distribution of humours, stays vomiting and fluxes.

Emplastrum Divinum
Or, A Divine Plaster

College.] Take of Loadstone four ounces, Ammoniacum three ounces and three drams, Bdellium two ounces, Galbanum, Myrrh, of each ten drams, Olibanum nine drams, Opopanax, Mastich, long Birthwort, Verdigris, of each an ounce, Litharge, common Oil, of each a pound and an half, new Wax eight ounces: let the Litharge in fine powder be boiled with the oil to a thickness, then add the Wax, which being melted, take it from the fire, add the Gums dissolved in Wine and Vinegar, strain it, then add the Myrrh, Mastich, Frankincense, Birthwort, and Loadstone in powder, last of all the Verdigris in powder, and make it into a plaster according to art.

Culpeper.] It is of a cleansing nature, exceeding good against malignant ulcers, it consumes corruption, engenders new flesh, and brings them to a scar.

Emplastrum Epispasticum

College.] Take of Mustard seed, Euphorbium, long Pepper, of each one dram and an half, Stavesacre, Pellitory of Spain of each two drams, Ammoniacum, Galbanum, Phellium, Sagapen, of each three drams, whole Cantharides five drams, Ship Pitch, Rozin, yellow Wax, of each six drams, Turpentine as much as is sufficient to make it into a plaster.

Culpeper.] Many people use to draw blisters in their necks for the tooth ache, or for rheums in their eyes; if they please to lay a plaster of this there, it will do it.

Emplastrum a nostratibus, Flos Unguentorum Dictum
Or, Flower of Ointments

College.] Take of Rozin, Per Rozin, yellow Wax, Sheep's Suet, of each half a pound, Olibanum four ounces, Turpentine two ounces and an half, Myrrh, Mastich, of each an ounce, Camphire two drams, white Wine half a pound, boil them into a plaster.

Culpeper.] I found this receipt in an old manuscript written in the year 1513, the quantity of the ingredients very little altered.

A Plaster of Gum Elemi

College.] Take of Gum Elemi three ounces, Per Rozin, Wax, Ammoniacum, of each two ounces, Turpentine three ounces and an half, Mallaga Wine so much as is sufficient: boil it to the consumption of the Wine, then add the Ammoniacum dissolved in Vinegar.

Culpeper.] The operation is the same with *Arceus* Liniment.

A Plaister of Lapis Calaminaris

College.] Take of Lapis Calaminaris prepared an ounce, Litharge two ounces, Ceruss half an ounce, Tutty a dram, Turpentine six drams, white Wax an ounce and an half, Stag's Suet two ounces,

Frankincense five drams, Mastich three drams, Myrrh two drams, Camphire a dram and an half, make it up according to art.

Emplastrum ad Herniam

College.] Take of Galls, Cypress Nuts, Pomegranate Pills, Balaustines, Acacia, the seeds of Plantain, Fleawort, Watercresses, Acorn Cups, Beans torrified, Birthwort long and round, Myrtles of each half an ounce. Let these be powdered, and steeped in Rose Vinegar four days, then torrified and dried, then take of Comfrey the greater and lesser, Horsetail, Woad, Cetrach, the roots of Osmond Royal, Fearn, of each an ounce, Frankincense, Myrrh, Aloes, Mastich, Mummy, of each two ounces, Bole-ammoniac washed in Vinegar, Lap, Calaminaris prepared, Litharge of Gold, Dragon's blood, of each three ounces, Ship Pitch two pounds, Turpentine six ounces, or as much as is sufficient to make it into a plaster according to art.

Culpeper.] The plaster is very binding and knitting, appropriated to ruptures or burstens, as the title of it specifies, it strengthens the reins and womb, stays abortion, it consolidates wounds, and helps all diseases coming of cold and moisture.

Emplastrum Hystericum

College.] Take of Bistort roots one pound, Wood of Aloes, yellow Sanders, Nutmegs, Barberry Kernels, Rose seeds, of each one ounce, Cinnamon, Cloves, Squinanth, Chamomel flowers, of each half an ounce, Frankincense, Mastich, Alipta Moschata, Gallia Moschata, Styrax Calamitis, of each one dram, Mosch half a dram, yellow Wax one pound and an half, Turpentine half a pound, Moschæleum four ounces, Labdanum four pounds, Ship Pitch three pounds: let the Labdanum and Turpentine be added to the Pitch and Wax, being melted, then the Styrax, lastly the rest in powder, and sifted, that they may be made into a plaster according to art.

Culpeper.] The plaster being applied to the navel, is a means to withstand the fits of the mother in such women as are subject to them, by retaining the womb in its place.

Emplastrum de Mastich
Or, A Plaster of Mastich

College.] Take of Mastich three ounces, Bole-ammoniac washed in black Wine, an ounce and an half, red Roses six drams, Ivory,

Myrtle Berries, red Coral, of each half an ounce, Turpentine, Colophonia, Tachamahacca, Labdanum, of each two ounces, yellow Wax half a pound, Oil of Myrtles four ounces: make it into a plaster according to art.

Culpeper.] It is a binding plaster, strengthens the stomach being applied to it, and helps such as loath their victuals, or cannot digest it, or retain it till it be digested.

Emplastrum de Meliloto Simplex
Or, A Plaster of Melilot simple

College.] Take of Rozin eight pounds, yellow Wax four pounds, Sheep's Suet two pounds: these being melted, add green Melilot cut small, five pounds: make it into a plaster according to art.

Emplastrum de Meliloto compositum
Or, A Plaster of Melilot compound

College.] Take of Melilot flowers six drams, Chamomel flowers, the seeds of Fenugreek, Bay berries husked, Marsh-mallow roots, the tops of Wormwood and Marjoram, of each three drams, the seeds of Smallage, Ammi, Cardamoms, the roots of Orris, Cypress, Spikenard, Cassia Lignea, of each one dram and an half, Bdellium five drams: beat them all into fine powder, the pulp of twelve Figs, and incorporate them with a pound and an half of Melilot plaster simple, Turpentine an ounce and an half, Ammoniacum dissolved in Hemlock Vinegar, three ounces, Styrax five drams, oil of Marjoram, and Nard, of each half an ounce, or a sufficient quantity, make it into a plaster with a hot mortar and pestle, without boiling.

Culpeper.] It mollifies the hardness of the stomach, liver, spleen, bowels, and other parts of the body: it wonderfully assuages pain, and eases hypochondriac melancholy, and the rickets.

Emplastrum de minio compositum
Or, A Plaster of red Lead compound

College.] Take of Oil of Roses omphacine twenty ounces, oil of Mastich two ounces, Suet of a Sheep and a Calf, of each half a pound, Litharge of Gold and Silver, red Lead, of each two ounces, a taster full of Wine: boil them by a gentle fire continually stirring it till it grow black, let the fire be hottest towards the latter end, then add Turpentine half a pound, Mastich two ounces, Gum Elemi one ounce, white Wax as much as is sufficient: boil them a little, and make them into a plaster according to art.

Culpeper.] It potently cures wounds, old maglignant ulcers, and is very drying.

Emplastrum de minio Simplicius
Or, A Plaster of red Lead simple

College.] Take of red Lead nine ounces, Oil of red Roses one pound and an half, white Wine Vinegar six ounces, boil it into the perfect body of a plaster. It is prepared without Vinegar, thus: take of red Lead one pound, Oil of Roses one pound and an half, Wax half a pound, make it into a plaster according to art.

Culpeper.] It is a fine cooling healing plaster, and very drying.

Emplastrum Metroproptoticon

College.] Take of Mastich one ounce and an half, Galbanum dissolved in red Wine and strained, six drams, Cypress Turpentine two drams, Cypress Nuts, Galls, of each one dram and an half, oil of Nutmegs by expression one dram, Musk two grains and an half, Pitch scraped off from old ships two drams and an half; beat the Galbanum, Pitch, Turpentine, and Mastich gently in a hot mortar and pestle, towards the end, adding the Oil of Nutmegs, then the rest in powder, last of all the Musk mixed with a little Oil of Mastich upon a marble, and by exact mixture make them into a plaster.

Emplastrum Nervinum

College.] Take of Oil of Chamomel and Roses, of each two ounces, of Mastich, Turpentine, and Linseeds, of each an ounce and an half, Turpentine boiled four ounces, Rosemary, Bettony, Horsetail, Centaury the less, of each a handful, Earth-worms washed and cleansed in Wine three ounces, tops of St. John's Wort a handful, Mastich, Gum Elemi, Madder roots, of each ten drams, Ship-pitch, Rozin of each an ounce and an half, Litharge of Gold and Silver, of each two ounces and an half, red Lead two ounces, Galbanum, Sagapen, Ammoniacum, of each three drams; boil the roots, herbs, and worms, in a pound and an half of Wine till half be consumed, then press them out, and boil the decoction again with the Oils, Suets, Litharge, and red Lead, to the consumption of the Wine: then add the Gums dissolved in Wine, afterwards the Turpentine, Rozin, Pitch, and Mastich, in powders and make them into a plaster according to art.

Culpeper.] It strengthens the brain and nerves, and then being applied to the back, down along the bone, it must needs add strength to the body.

Emplastrum Oxycroceum

College.] Take of Saffron, Ship-pitch, Colophonia, yellow Wax, of each four ounces, Turpentine, Galbanum, Ammoniacum, Myrrh, Olibanum, Mastich, of each one ounce and three drams. Let the Pitch and Colophonia be melted together, then add the Wax, then (it being removed from the fire) the Turpentine, afterwards the Gums dissolved in Vinegar, lastly the Saffron in powder, well mixed with Vinegar, and so make it into a plaster according to art.

Culpeper.] It is of a notable softening and discussing quality, helps broken bones, and any part molested with cold, old aches, stiffness of the limbs by reason of wounds, ulcers, fractures, or dislocations, and dissipates cold swellings.

Emplastrum Stephaniaion

College.] Take of Labdanum half an ounce, Styrax, Juniper Gum, of each two drams, Amber, Cypress, Turpentine, of each one dram, red Coral, Mastich, of each half a dram, the flowers of Sage, red Roses, the roots of Orris Florentine, of each one scruple, Rozin washed in Rose-water half an ounce, the Rozin, Labdanum, Juniper Gum, and Turpentine, being gently beaten in a hot mortar, with a hot pestle, sprinkling in a few drops of red Wine till they are in a body; then put in the powders, and by diligent stirring make them into an exact plaster.

Emplastrum Sticiticum

College.] Take of Oil of Olives six ounces, yellow Wax an ounce and an half, Litharge in powder four ounces and an half, Ammoniacum, Bdellium, of each half an ounce, Galbanum, Opopanax Oil of Bays, Lapis Calaminaris, both sorts of Birthwort, Myrrh, Frankincense, of each two drams, pure Turpentine an ounce. Let the Oil, Wax, and Litharge be boiled together till it stick not to your fingers, then the mass being removed from the fire and cooled a little, and the Gums dissolved in white Wine Vinegar, which evaporate away by boiling, strain it strongly, then add the powders, Turpentine, and Oil of Bays, that it may be made into a plaster according to art.

Culpeper.] It strengthens the nerves, draws out corruption, takes away pains and aches, and restores strength to members that have lost it: the last is most effectual.

Emplastrum Stomachicum Magistrale
Or, A Stomach Plaster

College.] Take of Mints, Wormwood, Stœchas, Bay leaves, of each a dram, Marjoram, red Roses, yellow Sanders, of each two drams, Calamus Aromaticus, Wood of Aloes, Lavender flowers, Nutmegs, Cubebs, Galanga, long Pepper, Mace, of each a dram, Mastich three drams, Cloves two drams and an half, Oil of Mints an ounce and an half, Oil of Nard an ounce, Oil of Spike a dram, Rozin, Wax, of each four ounces, Labdanum three ounces, Styrax half an ounce: make it into a plaster.

Culpeper.] Both this and the other of that name which you shall have by and by, strengthen the stomach exceedingly, help digestion and stay vomiting.

Emplastrum Ceroma, or, Ceroneum. Nich. Alex.

College.] Take of Pitch scraped from a Ship that hath been a long time at Sea, yellow Wax, of each seven drams, Sagapenum six drams, Ammoniacum, Turpentine, Colophonia, Saffron, of each four drams, Aloes, Olibanum, Myrrh, of each three drams, Styrax Calamitis, Mastich, Opopanax, Galbanum, Alum, the seeds of Fenugreek, of each two drams, the settlings or faces of liquid Styrax, Bdellium, of each one dram, Litharge half a dram.

Culpeper.] It is of a gentle emolient nature, prevails against stoppings of the stomach, coming of cold, hardness of the spleen, coldness of the liver and matrix.

Emplastrum Gratia Dei. Nich.
Or the Grace of God

College.] Take of Turpentine half a pound, Rozin one pound, white Wax four ounces, Mastich an ounce, fresh Betony, Vervain, and Burnet, of each one handful. Let the herbs, being bruised, be sufficiently boiled in white Wine, the liquor pressed out, in which let the Wax and Rozin be boiled to the consumption of the liquor: being taken from the fire, let the Turpentine be mixed with it; lastly the Mastich in powder, and so make of them a plaster according to art.

Culpeper.] It is excellent good in wounds and green ulcers, for it keeps back inflammations, cleanses and joins wounds, fills up ulcers with flesh.

Emplastrum de Janua, or of Betony. Nicholaus

College.] Take of the juice of Betony, Plantain, and Smallage, of each one pound, Wax, Pitch, Rozin, Turpentine, of each half a pound, boil the Wax and Rozin in the juices with a gentle fire, continually stirring them till the juice be consumed; then add the Turpentine and Pitch, continually stirring it till it be brought into the consistence of a plaster according to art.

Emplastrum Isis Epigoni. Galen

College.] Take of yellow Wax an hundred drams, Turpentine two hundred drams, scales of Copper, Verdigris, round Birthwort, Frankincense, Sal-ammoniac, Ammoniacum, burnt brass of each eight drams, burnt Alum six drams, Aloes, Myrrh, Galbanum, of each an ounce and a half, old Oil one pound, sharp Vinegar so much as is sufficient. Let the metals be dissolved in the sun with the Vinegar, then put in those things that may be melted, last of all the powders, and make them all into an emplaster.

Culpeper.] *Galen* appropriates it to the head, and ulcers there. I know no reason but why it may as well serve for other parts of the body.

A Plaster of Mastich. Nich. Alex.

College.] Take of Mastich, Ship Pitch, Sagapenum, Wax, of each six drams, Ammoniacum, Turpentine, Colophonia, Saffron, Aloes, Frankincense, Myrrh, of each three drams, Opopanax, Galbanum, Styrax, Calamitis, Alum, (Rondeletius appoints, and we for him) Bitumen, Fenugreek, of each two drams, the feces of Liquid Styrax, Bdellium, Litharge, of each half a dram. Let the Litharge, being beaten into powder, be boiled in a sufficient quantity of water; then add the pitch, which being melted, add the Wax and Ammoniacum, afterwards let the Sagapenum, Opopanax, and Galbanum be put in; then the Styrax and Feces being mixed with the Turpentine, last of all the Colophonia, Mastich, Frankincense, Bdellium, Alum, Myrrh, and Fenugreek in powder: let them be made into a plaster.

Culpeper.] It strengthens the stomach, and helps digestion.

Emplastrum Nigrum. August.
Called in High Dutch *Stichstaster*

College.] Take of Colophonia, Rozin, Ship Pitch, white Wax, roman Vitriol, Ceruss, Olibanum, Myrrh, of each eight ounces,

Oil of roses seven ounces, Oil of Juniper Berries three ounces, Oil of Eggs two ounces, Oil of Spick one ounce, white Vitriol, red Coral, Mummy, of each two ounces, Earth of Lemnos, Mastich, Dragon's blood, of each one ounce, the fat of an Heron one ounce, the fat of Pimullus three ounces, Load stone prepared, two ounces, Earthworms prepared, Camphire, of each one ounce; make them into a plaster according to art.

Culpeper.] It is very good in green wounds and shootings.

A Key to
Galen's Method of Physic

The general use of physic

I SHALL desire thee, whoever thou art, that intendest the noble
(though too much abused) study of physic, to mind heedfully these
following rules; which being well understood, shew thee the Key
of *Galen* and *Hippocrates* their method of physic: he that useth their
method, and is not heedful of these rules, may soon cure one
disease, and cause another more desperate.

That thou mayest understand what I intend, it is to discover in a
general way of the manifest virtues of medicines.

I say of the *manifest* virtues, and qualities, viz. such as are obvious
to the senses, especially to the taste and smell: for it hath been the
practice of most Physicians, in these latter ages as well as ours, to
say, when they cannot give, nor are minded to study a reason, why
an herb, plant, &c. hath such an operation, or produces such an
effect in the body of man: It doth it by an hidden quality, for they
not minding the whole creation, as one united body, not knowing
what belongs to *astral influence*, not regarding that excellent harmony the only wise God hath made in a composition of contraries
(in the knowledge of which consists the whole ground and foundation of physic) are totally led astray by *Tradition*.

It is the manifest qualities of medicines that here I am to speak
to, and you may be pleased to behold it in this order.

> SECTION 1. *Of the Temperature of Medicines*
> SECTION 2. *Of the appropriation of Medicines*
> SECTION 3. *Of the Properties of Medicines*

SECTION I

Of the Temperature of Medicines

HERBS, plants, and other medicines manifestly operate, either by
heat, coldness, dryness, or moisture, for the world being composed

of so many qualities, they and only they can be found in the world, and the mixtures of them one with another.

But that they may appear as clear as the sun when he is upon the meridian, I shall treat of them severally, and in this order:

1. *Of Medicines temperate.*

2. *Of Medicines hot.*

3. *Of Medicines cold.*

4. *Of Medicines moist.*

5. *Of Medicines dry.*

Of Medicines Temperate

If the world be composed of extremes, then it acts by extremes, for as the man is, so is his work: therefore it is impossible that any medicine can be temperate, but may be reduced to heat, cold, dryness, or moisture, and must operate, (I mean such as operate by manifest quality) by one of these, because there is no other to operate by, and that there should be such a temperate mixture, so exquisitely of these qualities in any medicine, that one of them should not manifestly excel the other, I doubt it is a system too rare to find.

Thus then I conclude the matter to be, those Medicines are called temperate (not because they have excess of temperature at all in them) which can neither be said, to heat nor cool so much as will amount to the first degree of excess, for daily experience witnesses that they being added to medicines, change not their qualities, they make them neither hotter nor colder.

Their use. They are used in such diseases where there is no manifest distemper of the first qualities, viz. heat and cold, for example: In obstruction of the bowels, where cold medicines might make the obstruction greater, and hot medicines cause a fever.

In fevers of flegm, where the cause is cold and moist, and the effect hot and dry; in such, use temperate medicines which may neither encrease the fever by their heat, nor condensate the flegm by their coldness.

Besides, because contraries are taken away by their contraries, and every like maintained by its like, they are of great use, to preserve the constitution of the body temperate, and the body itself in strength and vigour, and may be used without danger, or fear of danger, by considering which part of the body is weak, and using such temperate medicines as are appropriated to that part.

Of Medicines hot

The care of the ancient Physicians was such that they did not labour to hide from, but impart to posterity, not only the temperature of medicines in general, but also their degrees in temperature, that so the distempered part may be brought to its temperature, and no further; for all things which are of a contrary temperature, conduce not to cure, but the strength of the contrariety must be observed, that so the medicine may be neither weaker nor stronger, than just to take away the distemper; for if the distemper be but meanly hot, and you apply a medicine cold in the fourth degree, it is true, you may soon remove that distemper of heat, and bring another of cold twice as bad. *Galen, de simp. med. facul. lib.* 3. *cap.* 12.

Then, secondly, not only the distemper itself, but also the part of the body distempered must be heeded; for if the head be distempered by heat, and you give such medicines as cool the heart or liver, you will bring another disease, and not cure the former.

The degrees then of temperature are to be diligently heeded, which antient physicians have concluded to be four in the qualities, viz. heat and cold, of each we shall speak a word or two severally.

Of Medicines hot in the first degree

Those are said to be hot in the first degree, which induce a moderate and natural heat to the body, and to the parts thereof, either cold by nature, or cooled by accident, by which natural heat is cherished when weak, or restored when wanting.

Effect 1. The first effect then of medicines hot in the first degree, is, by their sweat and temperate heat to reduce the body to its natural heat, as the fire doth the external parts in cold weather, unless the affliction of cold be so great that such mild medicines will not serve the turn.

Effect 2. The second effect is, the mitigation of pain arising from such a distemper, and indeed this effect hath other medicines, some that are cold, and some that are hotter than the first degree, they being rationally applied to the distemper. These medicines the Greeks call *Anodyna*, and shall be spoken of in their proper places. In this place let it suffice that medicines hot in the first degree, make the offending humours thin, and expel them by sweat, or insensible transpiration, and these of all others are most congruous or agreeable to the body of man, for there is no such equal temperature of heat and cold in a sound man, but heat exceeds, for we live by heat and moisture, and not by cold.

Medicines then which are hot in the first degree, are such as just correspond to the natural heat of our bodies; such as are hotter or colder, are more subject to do mischief, being administered by an unskilful hand, than these are, because of their contrariety to nature; whereas these are grateful to the body by their moderate heat.

Effect 3. Thirdly, these take away weariness, and help fevers, being outwardly applied, because they open the pores of the skin, and by their gentle heat prepare the humours, and take away those fuliginous vapours that are caused by fevers.

Discommodities.] Yet may discommodities arise by heedless giving even of these, which I would have young students in physic to be very careful in, lest they do more mischief than they are aware of, viz. it is possible by too much use of them, to consume not only what is inimical in the body, but also the substance itself, and the strength of the spirits, whence comes faintings, and sometimes death: besides, by applying them to the parts of the body they are not appropriated to, or by not heeding well the complexion of the patient, or the natural temper of the part of the body afflicted, for the heart is hot, but the brain temperate.

Effect 4. Lastly, medicines hot in the first degree, cherish heat in the internal parts, help concoction, breed good blood, and keep it good in temper, being bred.

Of Medicines hot in the second degree

These are something hotter than the natural temper of a man.

Use. Their use for such whose stomachs are filled with moisture, because their faculty is too hot and dry; they take away obstructions or stoppings, open the pores of the skin, but not in the same manner that such do as are hot in the first degree, for they do it without force, by a gentle heat, concocting, and expelling the humours, by strengthening and helping nature in the work; but these cut tough humours, and scatter them by their own force and power when nature cannot.

Of Medicines hot in the third degree

Those which attain the third degree of heat, have the same faculties with those before mentioned; but as they are hotter, so are they more powerful in their operations, for they are so powerful in heating and cutting, that if unadvisedly given they cause fevers.

Use. Their use is to cut tough and compacted humours, to provoke sweat abundantly; hence it comes to pass they all of them resist poison.

Of Medicines hot in the fourth degree

Those medicines obtain the highest degree of heat, which are so hot that they burn the body of a man, being outwardly applied to it, and cause inflammations, or raise blisters, as Crowfoot, Mustard-seed, Onions, &c. Of these more hereafter.

Of cooling Medicines

Physicians have also observed four degrees of coldness in medicines, which I shall briefly treat of in order.

Of Medicines cold in the first degree

Those medicines which are least cold of all, obtain the first degree of coldness; and I beseech you take notice of this, that seeing our bodies are nourished by heat, and we live by heat, therefore no cold medicines are friendly to the body, but what good they do our bodies, they do it by removing an unnatural heat, or the body heated above its natural temper.

The giving then of cold medicines to a man in his natural temper, the season of the year also being but moderately hot, extinguishes natural heat in the body of man.

Yet have these a necessary use in them too, though not so frequent as hot medicines have; and that may be the reason why an all wise God hath furnished us with far more hot herbs and plants, &c. than cold.

Use 1. Their use is first, in nourishment, that so the heat of food may be qualified, and made for a weak stomach to digest.

Use 2. Secondly, to restrain and assuage the heat of the bowels, and to cool the blood in fevers.

Therefore if the distemper of heat be but gentle, medicines cold in the first degree will suffice; also children, and such people whose stomachs are weak, are easily hurt by cold medicines.

Of Medicines cold in the second and third degree

Use 1. Such whose stomachs are strong, and livers hot, may easily bear such medicines as are cold in the second degree, and in cases of extremity find much help by them: as also by such as are cold in the third degree, the extremity of the disease considered, for by both these the unbridled heat of choler is assuaged.

Use 2. Also they are outwardly applied to hot swellings, due consideration being had, that if the inflammation be not great, use

CHAPTER I

Of Medicines appropriated to the head

By [*head*] is usually understood all that part of the body which is between the top of the crown, and the uppermost joint of the neck, yet are those medicines properly called *Cephalical*, which are appropriated to the brain, not to the eyes, ears, nor teeth; neither are those medicines which are proper to the ears, proper also to the eyes, therefore (my intent being to write as plain as I can) I shall subdivide this chapter into these parts.

Medicines appropriated:

> 1. *To the brain.*
>
> 2. *To the eyes.*
>
> 3. *To the mouth, and nostrils.*
>
> 4. *To the ears.*
>
> 5. *To the teeth.*

For what medicines are appropriated to an unruly tongue, is not in my power at present to determine.

Of Medicines appropriated to the brain

Before we treat of medicines appropriated to the brain, it is requisite that we describe what the nature and affection of the brain is.

The brain, which is the seat of apprehension, judgment, and memory, the original of sense and motion, is by nature temperate, and if so, then you will grant me that it may easily be afflicted both by heat and cold, and it is indeed more subject to affliction by either of them, than any other part of the body, for if it be afflicted by heat, sense and reason, it is immoderately moved, if by cold, they languish, and are dulled, to pass by other symptoms which invade the head, if the brain be altered from its proper temper.

Also this is peculiar to the brain, that it is delighted or offended by smells, sights, and sounds, but I shall meddle no further with these here, because they are not medicines.

Cephalical Medicines may be found out from the affections of the brain itself. The brain is usually oppressed with moisture in such afflictions; therefore give such medicines as very gently warm, cleanse, cut, and dry: but withal, let them be such as are appropriated to the head, such as physicians say (by an hidden quality) strengthen the brain.

Again, if you consider the situation of the brain, you shall find it placed in the highest part of the body, therefore it is easily afflicted with hot vapours: this punishes a man with watching and headache, as the former did with sottishness and sleepiness, in such cases use such *Cephalecs* as gently cool the brain.

To make *Cephalecs* of *Narcoticks*, or stupifying medicines, is not my intent, for I am confident they are inimical both to brain and senses. Of these, and such medicines as also purge the brain, I shall speak by and by. To return to my purpose.

Some Cephalics purge the brain, some heat it, some cool it, some strengthen it; but how they perform this office peculiarly to the brain, most physicians confess they could neither comprehend by reason, nor describe by precepts, only thus, they do it by an hidden quality, either by strengthening the brain, thereby descending it from diseases, or by a certain antipathy between them and the diseases incident to the brain.

Lastly, for the use of Cephalics, observe, if the brain be much afflicted, you cannot well strengthen it before you have purged it, neither can you well purge the brain before you have cleansed the rest of the body, it is so subject to receive the vapours up to it; give cooling Cephalics when the brain is too hot, and hot Cephalics when it is too cold.

Beware of using cooling medicines to the brain when the crisis of a disease is near: how that time may be known, I shall (God assisting me) instruct you hereafter; let it suffice now, that according as the disease afflicting your head is, so let your remedy be.

Of Medicines appropriated to the eyes

Take such medicines as are appropriated to the eyes under the name of (*Ocular Medicines*). I do it partly to avoid multiplicity of words, and partly to instruct my countrymen in the terms of art belonging to physic, (I would have called them [*Ophthalmics*] had not the word been troublesome to the reading, much more to the understanding of a countryman) as I even now called such medicines [*Cephalics*] as were appropriated to the brain.

Ocular medicines are two-fold, viz. such as are referred to the visive virtues, and such as are referred to the eyes themselves.

Such as strengthen the visive virtue or the optick nerves which convey it to the eyes (say Doctors) do it by an hidden virtue, into the reason which no man can dive, unless they should fetch it from the similitude of the substance. And yet they say a Goat's liver conduces much to make one see in the night, and they give this reason, because Goats see as well in the night as in the day. Yet is there no affinity in temperature nor substance between the liver and the eyes. However, Astrologers know well enough that all herbs, plants, &c. that are under the dominion of either sun or moon, and appropriated to the head, be they hot or cold they strengthen the visive virtue, as Eyebright, which is hot *Lunaria*, or Moonwort which is cold.

As for what appertains to the constitution of the eyes themselves, seeing they are exact in sense, they will not endure the least inconvenience, therefore such medicines as are outwardly applied to them (for such medicines as strengthen the visive virtues are always given inwardly) let them neither hurt by their hardness nor gnawing quality, nor be so tough that they should stick to them. Therefore let ocular medicines be neither in powders nor ointments, because oil itself is offensive to the eyes, and how pleasing powders are to them, you may perceive yourself by just going into the dust.

Medicines appropriated to the mouth and nose

Apply no stinking medicine to a disease in the nose, for such offend not only the nose, but also the brain; neither administer medicines of any ill taste to a disease in the mouth, for that subverts the stomach, because the tunicle of the mouth and of the stomach is the same: and because both mouth and nostrils are ways by which the brain is cleansed, therefore are they infected with such vices as need almost continual cleansing, and let the medicines you apply to them be either pleasant, or at least, not ingrateful.

Medicines appropriated to the ears

The ears are easily afflicted by cold, because they are always open, therefore they require hot medicines. And because they are of themselves very dry, therefore they require medicines which dry much.

Medicines appropriated to the teeth

Vehement heat, and vehement cold, are inimical to the teeth, but they are most of all offended by sharp and sour things, and the reason is, because they have neither skin nor flesh to cover them, they delight in such medicines as are cleansing and binding, because they are troubled with defluxions and rheums upon every light occasion; and that's the reason the common use of fat and sweet things, soon rots the teeth.

CHAPTER II

Of Medicines appropriated to the breast and lungs

The medicines appropriated to the breast and lungs, you shall find called all along by the name of [*pectorals*] that's the term Physicians give them, when you hear them talk of pectoral Syrups, pectoral robs, or pectoral Ointments.

They are divers, some of which regard the part afflicted, others the matter afflicting.

But although sometimes in ulcers of the lungs, we are forced to use binding medicines, to join the ulcer, yet are not these called pectorals, because binding medicines are extreme hurtful to the breast and lungs, both because they hinder one's fetching his breath, and also because they hinder the avoiding that flegm by which the breast is oppressed.

Such medicines are called pectorals, which are of a lenifying nature.

Besides, those which make thin matter thicker are of two sorts, *viz.* some are mild and gentle, which may safely be administered, be the matter hot or cold which offendeth; others are very cold, which are used only when the matter offending is sharp.

But because such medicines as conduce to the cure of the phthisics (which is an ulceration of the lungs, and the disease usually called, the consumption of the lungs,) are also reckoned in amongst pectorals, it is not amiss to speak a word or two of them.

In the cure of this disease are three things to be regarded.

1. *To cut and bring away the concreted blood.*
2. *To cherish and strengthen the lungs.*
3. *To conglutinate the ulcer.*

And indeed some particular simples will perform all these, and physicians confess it; which shews the wonderful mystery the all-wise God hath made in the creation, that one and the same simple should perform two contrary operations on the same part of the body; for the more a medicine cleanses, the more it conglutinates.

To conclude then, Pectoral Medicines are such as either cut and cleanse out the compacted humours from the arteries of the lungs, or make thin defluxions thick, or temper those that are sharp, help the roughness of the wind-pipe, or are generally lenitive and softening, being outwardly applied to the breast.

CHAPTER III

Of Medicines appropriated to the heart

These are they which are generally given under the notion of Cordials; take them under that name here.

The heart is the seat of the vital spirit, the fountain of life, the original of infused heat, and of the natural affections of man.

So then these two things are proper to the heart.

1. By its heat to cherish life throughout the body.

2. To add vigour to the affections.

And if these be proper to the heart, you will easily grant me, that it is the property of cordials to administer to the heart in these particulars.

Of Cordials, some cheer the mind, some strengthen the heart, and refresh the spirits thereof, being decayed.

Those which cheer the mind, are not one and the same; for as the heart is variously disturbed, either by anger, love, fear, hatred, sadness, &c., so such things as flatter lovers or appease the angry, or comfort the fearful, or please the hateful, may well be called cordials; for the heart, seeing it is placed in the middle between the brain and the liver, is wrought upon by reason, as well as by digestion, yet these, because they are not medicines, are beside my present scope.

And although it is true, that mirth, love, &c. are actions, or motions of the mind, not of the body; yet many have been induced to think such affections may be wrought in the body by medicines.

The heart is chiefly afflicted by too much heat, by poison, and by stinking vapours, and these are remedied by the second sort of cordials, and indeed chiefly belong to our present scope.

According to these three afflictions, *viz.*

1. *Excessive heat.*

2. *Poison.*

3. *Melancholy vapours.*

are three kinds of remedies which succour the afflicted heart.

Such as

1. *By their cooling nature mitigate the heat of fevers.*

2. *Resist poison.*

3. *Cherish the vital spirits when they languish.*

All these are called Cordials.

1. Such as cool the heart in fevers, yet is not every thing that cooleth cordial, for lead is colder than gold, yet is not lead cordial as gold is, some hold it cordial by a hidden quality, others by reason.

2. Such as resist poison; there is a two-fold resisting of poison.

1. *By an antipathy between the medicine and poison.*

2. *By a sympathy between the medicine and the heart.*

Of the first we shall speak anon, in a chapter by itself. The latter belongs to this chapter, and they are such medicines, whose nature is to strengthen the heart, and fortify it against the poison, as Rue, Angelica, &c. For as the operation of the former is upon the poison, which afflicteth the heart, so the operation of the latter is upon the heart afflicted by the poison.

To this class may be referred all such medicines as strengthen the heart either by astral influence, or by likeness of substance, if there be such a likeness in medicines, for a Bullock's heart is of like substance to man's, yet I question whether it be cordial or not.

3. And lastly, such as refresh the spirits, and make them lively and active, both because they are appropriated to the office, and also because they drive stinking and melancholy vapours from the heart, for as the animal spirit be refreshed by fragrant smells, and the natural spirits by spices, so are the vital spirits refreshed by all such medicines as keep back melancholy vapours from the heart, as Borrage, Bugloss, Rosemary, Citron Pills, the compositions of them, and many others, which this treatise will amply furnish you with.

CHAPTER IV

Of Medicines appropriated to the stomach

By stomach, I mean that ventricle which contains the food till it be concocted into chyle.

Medicines appropriated to the stomach are usually called stomachicals.

The infirmities usually incident to the stomach are three:

1. Appetite lost.

2. Digestion weakened.

3. The retentive faculty corrupted.

When the appetite is lost, the man feels no hunger when his body needs nourishment.

When digestion is weakened it is not able to concoct the meat received into the stomach, but it putrifies there.

When the retentive faculty is spoiled the stomach is not able to retain the food till it be digested, but either vomits it up again, or causes fluxes.

Such medicines then as remedy all these, are called stomachicals. And of them in order.

1. Such as provoke appetite are usually of a sharp or sourish taste, and yet withal of a grateful taste to the palate, for although loss of appetite may proceed from divers causes, as from choler in the stomach, or putrefied humours or the like, yet such things as purge this choler or humours, are properly called *Orecticks*, not stomachicals; the former strengthen appetite after these are expelled.

2. Such medicines help digestion as strengthen the stomach, either by convenient heat, or aromatic (viz. spicy) faculty, by hidden property, or congruity of nature.

3. The retentive faculty of the stomach is corrected by binding medicines, yet not by all binding medicines neither, for some of them are adverse to the stomach, but by such binding medicines as are appropriated to the stomach.

For the use of these.

Use 1. Use not such medicines as provoke appetite before you have cleansed the stomach of what hinders it.

Use 2. Such medicines as help digestion, give them a good time before meat that so they may pass to the bottom of the stomach, (for the digestive faculty lies there,) before the food come into it.

Use 3. Such as strengthen the retentive faculty, give them a little before meat, if to stay fluxes, a little after meat, if to stay vomiting.

CHAPTER V

Of Medicines appropriated to the liver

Be pleased to take these under the name of *Hepatics*, for that is the usual name physicians give them, and these also are of three sorts.

1. Some the liver is delighted in.
2. Others strengthen it.
3. Others help its vices.

The palate is the seat of taste, and its office is to judge what food is agreeable to the stomach, and what not, by that is both the quality and quantity of food for the stomach discerned: the very same office the *meseraik* veins perform to the liver.

Sometimes such food pleases the palate which the liver likes not (but not often) and therefore the *meseraik* veins refuse it, and that is the reason some few men fancy such food as makes them sick after the eating thereof.

1. The liver is delighted exceedingly with sweet things, draws them greedily, and digests them as swiftly, and that is the reason honey is so soon turned into choler.

2. Such medicines strengthen the liver, as (being appropriated to it) very gently bind, for seeing the office of the liver is to concoct, it needs some adstriction, that so both the heat and the humour to be concocted may be stayed, that so the one slip not away, nor the other be scattered.

Yet do not hepatical medicines require so great a binding faculty as stomachicals do, because the passages of the stomach are more open than those of the liver by which it either takes in chyle, or sends out blood to the rest of the body, therefore medicines that are very binding are hurtful to the liver, and either cause obstructions, or hinder the distribution of the blood, or both.

And thus much for the liver, the office of which is to concoct chyle, (which is a white substance the stomach digests the food into) into blood, and distributes it, by the veins, to every part of the body, whereby the body is nourished, and decaying flesh restored.

CHAPTER VI

Of Medicines appropriated to the spleen

In the breeding of blood, are three excrements most conspicuous, viz. *urine, choler*, and *melancholy*.

The proper seat of choler is in the gall.

The urine passeth down to the reins or kidneys, which is all one.

The spleen takes the thickest or melancholy blood to itself.

This excrement of blood is twofold: for either by excessive heat, it is addust, and this is that the Latins call *Atra Bilis*: or else it is thick and earthly of itself, and this properly is called melancholy humour.

Hence then is the nature of splenical medicines to be found out, and by these two is the spleen usually afflicted for *Atra bilis*, (I know not what distinct English name to give it) many times causes madness, and pure melancholy causeth obstructions of the bowels, and tumours, whereby the concoction of the blood is vitiated, and dropsies many times follow.

Medicines then peculiar to the spleen must needs be twofold also, some appropriated to *Atra bilis*, others to pure melancholy; but of purging either of them, I shall omit till I come to treat of purging in a chapter by itself.

1. Such medicines are splenical, which by cooling and moistening temper *Atra bilis*: let not these medicines be too cold neither, for there is no such heat in *Atra bilis* as there is in choler, and therefore it needs no such excessive cooling; amongst the number of these

are such as we mentioned amongst the cordials to repel melancholy vapours from the heart, such temper and assuage the malice of *Atra bilis*.

2. Those medicines are also splenical, by which melancholy humours are corrected and so prepared, that they may the more easily be evacuated: such medicines are cutting and opening, and they differ from hepaticals in this that they are no ways binding; for the spleen being no ways addicted to concoction, binding medicines do it harm, and not good.

3. Sometimes the spleen is not only obstructed, but also hardened by melancholy humours, and in such cases emolient medicines may be well called splenicals, not such as are taken inwardly, for they operate upon the stomach and bowels, but such as are outwardly applied to the region of the spleen.

And although sometimes medicines, are outwardly applied to hardness of the liver, yet they differ from splenicals, because they are binding, so are not splenicals.

CHAPTER VII

Of Medicines appropriated to the reins and bladder

The office of the reins is, to make a separation between the blood and the urine; to receive this urine thus separated from the blood, is the bladder ordained, which is of a sufficient bigness to contain it.

Both these parts of the body officiating about the urine, they are both usually afflicted by the vices of the urine.

1. *By stones.*
2. *By inflammation.*
3. *By thick humours.*

Medicines appropriated to the reins and bladder are usually called *Nephriticals*, and are threefold; some cool, others cut gross humours, and a third sort breaks the stone.

In the use of all these, take notice, that the constitution of the reins and bladder is such, that they abhor all binding medicines because they cause stoppage of urine.

Take notice, that the reins and bladder being subject to inflammations endure not very hot medicines.

Because the bladder is further remote from the centre of the body than the kidneys are, therefore it requires stronger medicines than the kidneys do, lest the strength of the medicine be spent before it be come to the part afflicted.

CHAPTER VIII

Of Medicines appropriated to the womb

These, physicians call *Hystericals*, and to avoid multiplicity of words, take them in this discourse under that notion.

Take notice that such medicines as provoke the menses, or stop them when they flow immoderately, are properly hystericals, but shall be spoken to by and by in a chapter by themselves.

As for the nature of the womb, it seems to be much like the nature of the brain and stomach, for experience teacheth that it is delighted with sweet and aromatical medicines, and flies from their contraries.

For example: a woman being troubled with the fits of the mother, which is drawing of the womb upward, apply sweet things, as Civet, or the like, to the place of conception, it draws it down again; but apply stinking things to the nose, as Assafœtida, or the like, it expels it from it, and sends it down to its proper place.

CHAPTER IX

Of Medicines appropriated to the joints

The joints are usually troubled with cephalic diseases, and then are to be cured by cephalic medicines.

Medicines appropriated to the joints, are called by the name *Arthritical* medicines.

The joints, seeing they are very nervous, require medicines which are of a heating and drying nature, with a gentle binding, and withal, such as by peculiar virtue are appropriated to them, and add strength to them. It is true, most cephalics do so, yet because the joints are more remote from the centre, they require stronger medicines.

For removing pains in the joints this is the method of proceeding.

Pain is either taken away or eased, for the true cure is to take away the cause of the pain, sometimes the vehemency of the pain is so great that you must be forced to use *Anodines* (for so physicians call such medicines as ease pain) before you can meddle with the cause, and this is usually when the part pained is inflamed, for those medicines which take away the cause of pain being very hot, if there be any inflammation in the part pained, you must abstain from them till the inflammation be taken away.

SECTION III

Of the propriety or operation of Medicines

CHAPTER I

Of Emolient Medicines

The various mixtures of heat, cold, dryness, and moisture in simples, must of necessity produce variety of faculties, and operations in them, which now we come to treat of, beginning first at emolients.

What is hard, and what is soft, most men know, but few are able to express. Phylosophers define that to be hard which yields not to touching, and soft to be the contrary. An emolient, or softening medicine is one which reduceth a hard substance to its proper temperature.

But to leave phylosophy, and keep to what the physicians describe hardness to be two-fold.

1. A distention or stretching of a part by too much fulness.

2. Thick humours which are destitute of heat, growing hard in that part of the body into which they flow.

So many properties then ought emolient medicines to have, viz. to moisten what is dry, to discuss what is stretched, to warm what is congealed by cold; yet properly, that only is said to mollify which reduceth a hard substance to its proper temperature.

Dryness and thickness of humours being the cause of hardness, emolient medicines must of necessity be hot and moist; and although you may peradventure find some of them dry in the second or third degrees, yet must this dryness be tempered and qualified with heat and moisture, for reason will tell you that dry medicines make hard parts harder.

Mollifying medicines are known, (1) by their taste, (2) by their feeling.

1. In taste, they are near unto sweat, but fat and oily; they are neither sharp, nor austere, nor sour, nor salt, neither do they manifest either binding, or vehement heat, or cold to be in them.

2. In feeling you can perceive no roughness, neither do they stick to your fingers like Birdlime, for they ought to penetrate the parts to be mollified, and therefore many times if occasion be, are cutting medicines mixed with them.

CHAPTER II

Of hardening Medicines

Galen in *Lib. 5 de Simple, Med. Facult., Cap.* 10 determines hardening medicines to be cold and moist, and he brings some arguments to prove it, against which other physicians contest.

I shall not here stand to quote the dispute, only take notice, that if softening medicines be hot and moist (as we shewed even now) then hardening medicines must needs be cold and dry, because they are contrary to them.

The universal course of nature will prove it, for dryness and moisture are passive qualities, neither can extremeties consist in moisture as you may know, if you do but consider that dryness is not attributed to the air, nor water, but to the fire, and earth.

2. The thing to be *congealed* must needs be moist, therefore the medicine *congealing* must of necessity be dry, for if cold be joined with dryness, it contracts the pores, that so the humours cannot be scattered.

Yet you must observe a difference between medicines drying, making thick, hardening, and congealing, of which differences, a few words will not do amiss.

1. Such medicines are said to dry, which draw out, or drink up the moisture, as a spunge drinks up water.

2. Such medicines are said to make thick, as do not consume the moisture, but add dryness to it, as you make syrups into a thick electuary by adding powders to them.

3. Such as congeal, neither draw out the moisture, nor make it thick by adding dryness to it, but contract it by vehement cold, as water is frozen into ice.

4. Hardness differs from all these, for the parts of the body swell, and are filled with flegmatic humours, or melancholy blood, which at last grows hard.

That you may clearly understand this, observe but these two things.

1. What it is which worketh.
2. What it worketh upon.

That which worketh is outwardly cold. That which is wrought upon, is a certain thickness and dryness, of humours, for if the humour were fluid as water is, it might properly be said to be congealed by cold, but not so properly hardened. Thus you see cold and dryness to be the cause of hardening. This hardening being so far from being useful, that it is obnoxious to the body of man. I pass it without more words. I suppose when *Galen* wrote of hardening medicines, he intended such as make thick, and therefore amongst them he reckons up Fleawort, Purslain, Houseleek, and the like, which assuage the heat of the humours in swellings, and stops subtil and sharp defluxions upon the lungs; but of these more anon.

CHAPTER III

Of Loosening Medicines

By loosening here, I do not mean purging, nor that which is opposite to astringency; but that which is opposite to stretching. I knew not suddenly what fitter English name to give it, than loosening or laxation, which latter is scarce English.

The members are distended or stretched divers ways, and ought to be loosened by as many, for they are stretched sometimes by dryness, sometimes by cold, sometimes by repletion or fullness, sometimes by swellings, and sometimes by some of these joined together. I avoid terms of art as much as I can, because it would profit my country but little, to give them the rules of physic in such English as they understand not.

I confess the opinion of ancient physicians hath been various about these loosening medicines. *Galen's* opinion was, that they might be referred either to moistening, or heating, or mollifying, or evacuating medicines, and therefore ought not to be referred to a chapter by themselves.

It is likely they may, and so may all other medicines be referred to heat, or coldness, or dryness, or moisture: but we speak not here of the particular properties of medicines, but of their joined properties, as they heat and moisten.

Others, they question how they can be distinguished from such as mollify, seeing such as are loosening, and such as are emolient, are both of them hot and moist.

To that, thus: stretching and loosening are ascribed to the moveable parts of the body, as to the muscles and their tendons, to the ligaments and *Membranæ*; but softness and hardness to such parts of the body as may be felt with the hand: I shall make clear by a similitude, Wax is softened, being hard, but Fiddle-strings are loosened being stretched. And if you say that the difference lying only in the parts of the body is no true difference, then take notice, that such medicines which loosen, are less hot, and more moistening, than such as soften, for they operate most by heat, these by moisture.

The truth is, I am of opinion the difference is not much, nay, scarce sensible, between emolient and loosening medicines; only I quoted this in a chapter by itself, not so much because some authors do, as because it conduceth to the increase of knowledge in physic, for want of which, this poor nation is almost spoiled.

The chief use of loosening medicines is in convulsions and cramps, and such like infirmities which cause distention or stretching.

They are known by the very same marks and tokens that emolient medicines are.

CHAPTER IV

Of drawing Medicines

The opinion of physicians is, concerning these, as it is concerning other medicines, viz. some draw by a manifest quality, some by a hidden, and so (quoth they) they draw to themselves both humours and thorns, or splinters that are gotten into the flesh; however this is certain, they are all of them hot, and of thin parts; hot because the nature of heat is to draw off thin parts that so they may penetrate to the humours that are to be drawn out.

Their use is various, *viz.*:

Use 1. That the bowels may be disburdened of corrupt humours.

2. Outwardly used, by them the offending humour (I should have said the peccant humour, had I written only to scholars,) is called from the internal parts of the body to the superfices.

3. By them the crisis of a disease is much helped forward.

4. They are exceedingly profitable to draw forth poison out of the body.

5. Parts of the body over cooled are cured by these medicines, viz. by applying them outwardly to the place, not only because they heat, but also because they draw the spirits by which life and heat are cherished, to the part of the body which is destitute of them: you cannot but know that many times parts of the body fall away in flesh, and their strength decays, as in some persons arms or legs, or the like, the usual reason is, because the vital spirit decays in those parts, to which use such plaisters or ointments as are attractive (which is the physical term for drawing medicines) for they do not only cherish the parts by their own proper heat, but draw the vital

and natural spirits thither, whereby they are both quickened and nourished.

They are known almost by the same tokens that attenuating medicines are, seeing heat; and thinness of parts is in them both, they differ only in respect of quantity, thinness of parts being most proper to attenuating medicines, but attractive medicines are hotter.

CHAPTER V

Of discussive Medicines

The nature of discussing (or sweating) medicines is almost the same with attractive, for there are no discussive medicines but are attractive, nor scarce any attractive medicine but is in some measure or other discussing. The difference then is only this; that discussive medicines are hotter than attractive, and therefore nothing else need be written of their nature.

Use. Their use may be known even from their very name; for diseases that come by repletion or fulness, are cured by evacuation or emptying; yet neither blood nor gross humours are to be expelled by sweating, or insensible transpiration (as they call it) but the one requires blood-letting, the other purgation, but *scrosus* or thin humours and filthy vapours, and such like superfluities, are to be expelled by sweat, and be wary in this too, for many of them work violently, and violent medicines are not rashly to be given.

Caution 2. Besides, swellings are sometimes made so hard by sweating medicines, that afterwards they can never be cured; for what is thin being by such medicines taken away, nothing but what is perfectly hard remains: If you fear such a thing, mix emolients with them.

Caution 3. Again, sometimes by using discussives, the humours offending (which physicians usually call the *peccant humours*) is driven to some more noble part of the body, or else it draws more than it discusseth; in such cases, concoct and attenuate the matter offending before you go about to discuss it.

From hence may easily be gathered at what time of the disease discussive medicines are to be used, viz. about the declining of the disease, although in diseases arising from heat of blood, we sometimes use them in the encrease and state of them.

They are known by the same marks and tokens attenuating medicines are, viz. by their burning and biting quality, they being very hot, and of thin parts, void of any biting quality, therefore they contract not the tongue in tasting of them.

CHAPTER VI

Of repelling Medicines

Repelling medicines are of contrary operation to these three last mentioned, viz. attenuating, drawing, and discussive medicines. It is true, there is but little difference between these three, some hold none at all; and if you will be so nice, you may oppose them thus. And so medicines making thick, correspond to attenuating medicines, or such as make thin, repelling medicines are opposed to such as draw, and such as retain the humours and make them tough, are opposite to such as discuss, some hold this niceness needless.

2. The sentence of authors about repulsive medicines is various.

For seeing an influxion may be caused many ways, a repulsive hath got as many definitions.

For such things as cool, bind, stop, and make thick, stay influxions, and therefore repulsives are by authors opposed, not only to attractives, but also to attenuating, and discussing medicines.

But properly such things are called repulsives, which do not only stay influxions, (for so do such medicines which stop and make thick) but such as drive the humours flowing to, or inherit in the place, to some other place.

The truth is, binding is inherent to repulsives, so is not coldness nor making thick: Yet such as are binding, cold and thin in operation, are most effectual.

Your taste will find repulsives to be, tart, or sharp, or austere, with a certain binding which contracts the tongue.

Use 1. Their use is manifold, as in hot tumours, head-aches, or the like.

Use 2. By these in fevers are the vapours driven from the head, Vinegar of Roses is notable.

Time of giving. They are most commodious in the beginning and encrease of a disease, for then influxions most prevail.

But seeing that in the cure of tumours there are two scopes, 1. That that which flows to it may be repelled. 2. That that which is already in it may be discussed; repulsives are most commodiously used in the beginning, discussives in the latter end.

In the middle you may mix them, with this proviso, that repulsives exceed in the beginning, discussives in the latter end.

Caution 1. If the matter offending be of a venomous quality, either abstain from repulsives altogether, or use purging first, lest the matter fly to the bowels and prove dangerous, especially if the bowels be weak.

2. Also forbear repulsives, if the pain be great.

3. Lastly, have a care lest by repulsives you contract the pores so much, that the matter cannot be removed by discussives.

CHAPTER VII

Of cleansing Medicines

Cleansing medicines can neither be defined by heat, nor coldness, because some of both sorts cleanse.

A cleansing medicine, then, is of a terrene quality, which takes away the filth with it, and carries it out.

Definition.] Here, to avoid confusion, a difference must be made between washing and cleansing.

A thing which washeth, carries away by fluxion, as a man washeth the dirt off from a thing.

A cleansing medicine by a certain roughness or nitrous quality, carries away the compacted filth with it.

This also is the difference between cleansing and discussing medicines, the one makes thick humours thin, and so scatters them, but a cleansing medicine takes the most tenacious humour along with it, without any alteration.

Besides, of cleansing medicines, some are of a gentler nature, some are more vehement.

These are not known one and the same way; for some are sweet, some salt, and some bitter.

The use of cleansing is external, as the use of purges are internal.

They are used to cleanse the sanies and other filth of ulcers, yea, and to consume and eat away the flesh itself, as burnt Alum, *precipitate*, &c.

When these must be used, not only the effects of the ulcers, but also the temperature of the body will tell you.

For if you see either a disease of fulness, which our physicians call [*Plethora*] or corrupted humours which they call [*Cacochyma*] you must empty the body of these, viz. fulness by bleeding, and corrupt humours, or evil state of the body, by purging before you use cleansing medicines to the ulcer, else your cure will never proceed prosperously.

CHAPTER VIII

Of Emplasters

By Emplasters, here, I do mean things glutinative, and they are quite contrary to things cleansing.

They are of a far more glutinous and tenacious substance.

They differ from things stopping because they do not stop the pores so much, as stick to them like Birdlime.

They have a certain glutinous heat, tempered both with coldness and moisture.

From these plasters take their names.

Their taste is either none at all, or not discernable whether hot or cold, but fat, insipid, or without taste, or sweet, and viscous in feeling.

Their use is to stop flowing of blood, and other fluxes, to cause suppuration, to continue the heat, that so tumours may be ripened.

Also they are mixed with other medicines, that they may the better be brought into the form of an emplaster, and may stick the better to the members.

CHAPTER IX

Of suppuring Medicines

These have a great affinity with emolients, like to them in temperature, only emolients are somewhat hotter.

Yet is there a difference as apparent as the sun when he is upon the meridian, and the use is manifest. For,

Emolients are to make hard things soft, but what suppures, rather makes a generation than an alteration of the humour.

Natural heat is the efficient cause of suppuration, neither can it be done by any external means.

Therefore such things are said to suppure, which by a gentle heat cherish the inbred heat of man.

This is done by such medicines which are not only temperate in heat, but also by a gentle viscosity, fill up or stop the pores, that so the heat of the part affected be not scattered.

For although such things as bind hinder the dissipation of the spirits, and internal heat, yet they retain not the moisture as suppuring medicines properly and especially do.

The heat then of suppuring medicines is like the internal heat of our bodies.

As things then very hot, are ingrateful either by biting, as Pepper, or bitterness: in suppuring medicines, no biting, no binding, no nitrous quality is perceived by the taste, (I shall give you better satisfaction both in this and others, by and by.)

For reason will tell a man, that such things hinder rather than help the work of nature in maturation.

Yet it follows not from hence, that all suppuring medicines are grateful to the taste, for many things grateful to the taste provokes vomiting, therefore why may not the contrary be?

The most frequent use of suppuration is, to ripen *Phlegmonæ*, a general term physicians give to all swellings proceeding of blood, because nature is very apt to help such cures, and physic is an art to help, not to hinder nature.

The time of use is usually in the height of the disease, when the flux is stayed, as also to ripen matter that it may be the easier purged away.

CHAPTER X

Of Medicines provoking urine

The causes by which urine is suppressed are many.

1. By too much drying, or sweating, it may be consumed.

2. By heat or inflammation of the reins or passages whereby it passes from the reins, it may be stopped by compression.

Urine is the thinnest part of blood, separated from the thickest part in the reins.

If then the blood be more thick and viscous than ordinary, it cannot easily be separated without cutting and cleansing medicines.

This is for certain, that blood can neither be separated nor distributed without heat.

Yet amongst diureticks are some cold things, as the four greater cold seeds, Winter-cherries, and the like.

Although this seem a wonder, yet it may be, and doth stand with truth.

For cool diureticks, though they further not the separation of the blood one jot, yet they cleanse and purge the passages of the urine.

Diureticks then are of two sorts:

1. Such as conduce to the separation of the blood.

2. Such as open the urinal passages.

The former are biting (and are known by their taste) very hot and cutting, whence they penetrate to the reins, and cut the gross humours there.

Bitter things, although they be very hot, and cut gross humours, yet are they of a more dry and terrene substance than is convenient to provoke urine.

Hence then we may safely gather, that bitter things are not so moist nor penetrating, as such as bite like Pepper.

CHAPTER XI

Of Medicines breeding flesh

There are many things diligently to be observed in the cures of wounds and ulcers, which incur and hinder that the cure cannot be speedily done, nor the separated parts reduced to their natural state.

Viz. fluxes of blood, inflammation, hardness, pain, and other things besides our present scope.

Our present scope is, to shew how the cavity of ulcers may be filled with flesh.

Such medicines are called *Sarcoticks*.

This, though it be the work of nature, yet it is helped forward with medicines, that the blood may be prepared, that it may the easier be turned into flesh.

These are not medicines which breed good blood, nor which correct the intemperature of the place afflicted, but which defend the blood, and the ulcer itself from corruption in breeding flesh.

For nature in breeding flesh produceth two sorts of excrements, viz. scrosus humours, and purulent dross.

Those medicines then which cleanse and consume, these by drying are said to breed flesh, because by their helps nature performs that office.

Also take notice that these medicines are not so drying that they should consume the blood also as well as the sanies, nor so cleansing that they should consume the flesh with the dross.

Let them not then exceed the first degree unless the ulcer be very moist.

Their difference are various, according to the part wounded, which ought to be restored with the same flesh.

The softer then, and tenderer the place is, the gentler let the medicines be.

CHAPTER XII

Of glutinative Medicines

That is the true cure of an ulcer which joins the mouth of it together.

That is a glutinative medicine, which couples together by drying and binding, the sides of an ulcer before brought together.

These require a greater drying faculty than the former, not only to consume what flows out, but what remains liquid in the flesh, for liquid flesh is more subject to flow abroad than stick to together.

The time of using them, any body may know without teaching, viz. when the ulcer is cleansed and filled with flesh, and such symptoms as hinder are taken away.

For many times ulcers must be kept open that the sanies, or fords that lie in them may be purged out, whereas of themselves they would heal before.

Only beware, lest by too much binding you cause pain in tender parts.

CHAPTER XIII

Of Medicines resisting poison

Such medicines are called *Alexiteria*, and *Alexipharmaca*, which resist poison.

Some of these resist poison by astral influence, and some physicians (though but few) can give a reason for it.

These they have sorted into three ranks:

1. Such as strengthen nature, that so it may tame the poison the easier.

2. Such as oppose the poison by a contrary quality.

3. Such as violently thrust it out of doors.

Such as strengthen nature against poison, either do it to the body universally, or else strengthen some particular part thereof.

For many times one particular part of the body is most afflicted by the poison, suppose the stomach, liver, brain, or any other part: such as cherish and strengthen those parts, being weakened, may be said to resist poison.

Such as strengthen the spirits, strengthen all the body.

Sometimes poisons kill by their quality, and then are they to be corrected by their contraries.

They which kill by cooling are to be remedied by heating, and the contrary; they which kill by corroding, are to be cured by lenitives, such as temper their acrimony.

Those which kill by induration, or coagulation, require cutting medicines.

Also because all poisons are in motion, neither stay they in one till they have seized and oppressed the fountain of life, therefore they have invented another faculty to stay their motion, viz. terrene and emplastic.

For they judge, if the poison light upon these medicines, they embrace them round with a viscous quality.

Also they say the ways and passages are stopped by such means, to hinder their proceeding; take *Terra Lemnia* for one.

Truly if these reasons be good, which I leave to future time to determine, it may be done for little cost.

Some are of opinion that the safest way is to expel the poison out of the body, so soon as may be, and that is done by vomit, or purge, or sweat.

You need not question the time, but do it as soon as may be; for there is no parlying with poison.

Let vomiting be the first, purging the next, and sweating the last. This is general. But, if thou dost but observe the nature and motion of the venom, that will be thy best instructor.

In the stomach it requires vomiting, in the blood and spirits, sweating, if the body be plethoric, bleeding, if full of evil humours, purging.

Lastly, The cure being ended, strengthen the parts afflicted.

CHAPTER XIV

Of purging Medicines

Much jarring hath been amongst physicians about purging medicines, namely, whether they draw the humours to them by a hidden quality, which in plain English is, they know not how; or whether they perform their office by manifest quality, viz. by heat, dryness, coldness, or moisture. It is not my present scope to enter the lists of a dispute about the business, neither seem it such an hidden thing to me that every like should draw its like, only to make the matter as plain as I can, I subdivide this chapter into these following parts.

1. *Cautions concerning purging.*
2. *Of the choice of purging medicines.*
3. *Of the time of taking them.*
4. *Of the correcting of them.*
5. *Of the manner of purging.*

Cautions concerning purging

In this, first consider diligently, and be exceeding cautious in it too, what the matter offending is, what part of the body is afflicted by it, and which is the best way to bring it out.

Only here, by the way, first, have a care of giving vomits, for they usually work more violently, and afflict the body more than purges do, therefore are not fit for weak bodies; be sure the matter offending lie in the tunicle of the stomach, else is a vomit given in vain.

Vomits are more dangerous for women than men, especially such as are either with child, or subject to the fits of the mother.

What medicine is appropriated to the purging of such a humour, for seeing the offending matter is not alike in all, the purging medicine ought not to be the same to all. I shall speak more of this anon. As also of the divers ways whereby medicines draw out or cast out humours, *viz.* by lenifying, cleansing, provoking nature to expulsion, and (which is stranger than the doctor's *hidden quality*) some purge by binding, but indeed, and in truth, such as are properly called purging medicines, which, besides these faculties, have gotten another, by which they draw or call out the humours from the most remote parts of the body, whether these do it by heat or by an hidden quality, physicians are scarce able to determine, it being very well known to modern physicians, though the ancients denied it, that many cold medicines purge.

There is this faculty in all the purges of *Galen's* model, (because he gives the whole *simple* which must needs consist of divers qualities, because the creation is made up of and consists by an harmony of contraries) there is (I say) this faculty in all purges of that nature, that they contain in them a substance which is inimical both to the stomach and bowels, and some are of opinion this doth good, namely, provokes nature the more to expulsion; the reason might be good if the foundation of it were so, for by this reason nature herself should purge, not the medicine, and a physician should help nature in her business and not hinder her. But to forbear being critical, this substance which I told you was inimical to the stomach, must be corrected in every purge.

Culpeper's Last Legacies

SELECT MEDICINAL APHORISMS AND RECEIPTS
FOR MANY DISEASES OUR FRAIL NATURES ARE
INCIDENT TO

1. *A general Caution*

LET such as love their heads or brains, either forbear such things as are obnoxious to the brain, as Garlick, Leeks, Onions, beware of surfeiting and drunkenness.

2. *To purge the Head*

The head is purged by Gargarisms, of which Mustard, in my opinion, is excellent, and therefore a spoonful of Mustard put into the mouth, is excellent for one that is troubled with the lethargy: also the head is purged by sneezing; but be sure if you would keep your brain clear, keep your stomach clean.

3. *For a rheum in the Head, and the Palsy*

Take a red Onion, and bruise it well, and boil it in a little Verjuice, and put thereto a little clarified honey, and a great spoonful of good Mustard, when it is well boiled, raise the sick upright, and let him receive the smell up his nose twice a day, whilst it is very hot.

4. *For a rheum in the Head*

Boil Pimpernel well in Wine, and drink a draught of the Wine in the evening, hot, but in the morning cold.

5. *Another*

Stew Onions in a close pot, and bathe the head and mouth, and nose therewith.

6. *For the falling off of the Hair*

Beat Linseeds very well, and mix them with Sallad-oil; and when you have well mixed them, anoint the head therewith, and in three or four times using it will help you.

7. *To purge the Head*

Chew the root of Pellitory of Spain, and chew it on both sides of thy mouth, and as the rheum falls down into thy mouth, spit it out, but retain the root there still, till you think the head is purged enough for that time.

FOR THE EYES, AND THEIR IMPEDIMENTS

8. *For Eyes that are blasted*

Only wear a piece of black Sarcenet before thy eyes, and meddle with no medicine; only forbear wine and strong drink.

9. *An excellent water to clear the Sight*

Take of Fennel, Eyebright, Roses, white, Celandine, Vervain and Rue, of each a handful, the liver of a Goat chopt small, infuse them well in Eyebright-water, then distil them in an alembic, and you shall have a water will clear the sight beyond comparison.

10. *For a hurt in the Eye with a stroke*

Take Agrimony, and bruise it very well, and temper it with white Wine, and the white of an egg: spread it pretty thick upon a cloth, like a plaster, and apply it to the outside of the eye-lid, and, although it be almost out, it will cure it.

11. *To draw rheum back from the Eyes*

Take an egg and roast it hard, then pull off the shell, and slit it in two, and apply it hot to the nape of the neck, and thou shalt find ease presently.

12. *For the web in the Eye*

Take the gall of a hare, and clarified honey, of each equal proportions: mix them together, and lay it to the web.

FOR THE EARS, AND THEIR IMPEDIMENTS

13. *For pain in the Ears*

Drop a little oil of sweet Almonds into the ear, and it easeth the pain instantly; (and yet oil of bitter Almonds is our doctor's common remedy.)

14. *For an imposthume in the Ear*

Boil some milk, and put it into a stone pot with a narrow mouth, and hold the sore ear over the pot whilst the milk is very hot, that the vapour of the milk may ascend into the ear: this is an often approved remedy to take away the pain, and break the imposthume.

FOR THE NOSE, AND ITS INFIRMITIES

15. *For Polypus; or a fleshy substance growing in the Nose*

Take the juice of Ivy, and make a tent with a little cotton, the which dip in the juice and put it up in the nostril.

16. *To cleanse the Nose*

Snuff up the juice of red Beet-root; it will cleanse not only the nose, but also the head; this is a singular remedy for such as are troubled with hard congealed stuff in their nostrils.

17. *For bleeding at the Nose*

Bind the arms and legs as hard as you can with a piece of tape-ribboning; that, perhaps, may call back the blood.

18. *For a Canker in the Nose*

Boil strong ale till it be thick, if the Canker be in the outside of the nose, spread it as a plaster, and apply it; if in the inside, make a tent of a linen rag, and put it up the nostril.

19. *Another for the Polypus*

The water of Adder's-tongue snuffed up the nose, is very good: but it were better, in my opinion, to keep a rag continually moistened with it in the nose.

20. *For bleeding at the Nose*

Take Amber and bruise into gross powder, put it upon a chafing-dish of coals, and receive the smoke up into the nose with a funnel.

21. *Another*

When no other means will stop the bleeding at the nose, it has been known that it hath been stopped by opening a vein in the ear.

OF THE MOUTH, AND ITS DISEASES

22. *A Caution*

Whosoever would keep their mouth, or tongue, or nose, or eyes, or ears, or teeth, from pain or infirmities, let them often use sneezing, and such gargarisms as they were instructed in a preceding chapter; for, indeed, most of the infirmities, if not all, which infest those parts, proceed from rheum.

23. *For extreme heat of the Mouth*

Take Rib-wort, and boil it in red Wine, and hold the decoction as warm in your mouth as you can endure it.

24. *For a Canker in the Mouth*

Wash the mouth often with Verjuice.

OF THE TEETH, AND THEIR MEDICINES

25. *A Caution*

If you will keep your teeth from rotting, or aching, wash your mouth continually every morning with juice of Lemons, and afterwards rub your teeth either with a Sage-leaf, or else with a little Nutmeg in powder; also wash your mouth with a little fair water after meats; for the only way to keep teeth sound, and free from pain, is to keep them clean.

26. *To keep Teeth white*

Dip a little piece of white cloth in Vinegar of Quinces, and rub your gums with it, for it is of a gallant binding quality, and not only makes the teeth white, but also strengthens the gums, fastens the teeth, and also causeth a sweet breath.

27. *To fasten the Teeth*

Seethe the roots of Vervain in old Wine, and wash your teeth often with them, and it will fasten them.

28. *For the Tooth-ache*

Take the inner rind of an Elder-tree, and bruise it, and put thereto a little Pepper, and make it into balls, and hold them between the teeth that ache.

OF THE GUMS, AND THEIR INFIRMITIES

29. *For a Scurvy in the gums*

Take Cloves, and boil them in Rose-water, then dry them, and beat them to powder, and rub the gums with the powder, and drink the decoction in the morning fasting an hour after it. Use red Rose-water, for that is the best.

30. *For rotting and consuming of the gums*

Take Sage-water, and wash your mouth with it every morning, and afterwards rub your mouth with a Sage-leaf.

OF THE FACE, AND ITS INFIRMITIES

31. *The Cause*

It is palpable, that the cause of redness and breaking out of the face, is a venomous matter, or filthy vapours ascending from the stomach towards the head; where meeting with a rheum or flegm thence descending, mix with it, and break out in the face. Therefore let the first intention of cure be to cleanse the stomach.

32. *Caution negative*

Let such as are troubled with red faces, abstain from salt meats, salt fish and herrings, drinking of strong beer, strong waters or Wine, Garlick, Onions, and Mustard.

33. *For a face full of red pimples*

Dissolve Camphire in Vinegar, and mix it, and the Vinegar with Celandine-water, and wash the face with it: this cured a maid in twenty days, that had been troubled with the infirmity half so many years.

34. *To take away the marks of the small pox*

Take the juice of Fennel, heat it luke-warm, and when the small Pox are well scabbed, anoint the face with it divers times in a day, three or four days together.

OF THE THROAT, AND ITS INFIRMITIES

35. *A caution*

Diseases in the throat, most commonly proceed of rheum descending from the head upon the *trachea arteria*, or wind-pipe; in such cases there is many times no other cure than first to purge the body of flegm, and then the head of rheum, as you were taught in the first chapter.

36. *For hoarseness*

Take of sugar so much as will fill a common taster, then put so much rectified spirit of Wine to it as will just wet it, eat this up at night going to bed; use this three or four times together.

37. *Another*

If the body be feverish, use the former medicine as before, only use Oil of sweet Almonds, or for want of it, the best Sallad-oil instead of spirit of Wine.

38. *Another*

Take Penny-royal, and seethe it in running water, and drink a good draught of the decoction at night going to bed, with a little sugar in it.

39. *For the Quinsey*

Take notice that bleeding is good in all inflammations, therefore in this.

It were very convenient that a syrup, and an ointment of Orpine were always ready in the house for such occasions; for I know no better remedy for the Quinsey, than to drink the one, and anoint the throat with the other.

OF WOMEN'S BREASTS, THEIR INFIRMITIES AND CURES

40. *For sore breasts*

Take a handful of Figs, and stamp them well till the kernels are broken, then temper them with a little fresh grease, and apply them to the breast as hot as the patient can endure; it will presently take away the anguish, and if the breast will break, it will break it, else it will cure it without breaking.

41. *An inward medicine for a sore Breast*

Let her drink either the juice or decoction of Vervain: it were fit that syrup were made of it to keep all the year.

OF THE STOMACH, AND ITS INFIRMITIES

42. *A caution*

Infirmities of the stomach usually proceed from surfeiting.

43. *Another*

Let such as have weak stomachs, avoid all sweet things, as honey, sugar, and the like; milk, cheese and all fat meats: let him not eat till he is hungry, nor drink before he is dry; let him avoid anger, sadness, much travel, and all fryed meats: let him not vomit by any means, nor eat when he is hot.

44. *For moisture of the Stomach*

Take a drachm of Galanga, in powder, every morning in a draught of that Wine you like best.

45. *For heat of the Stomach*

Swallow four or five grains of Mastich every night going to bed.

OF THE LIVER, AND ITS INFIRMITIES

46. *A caution*

If the liver be too hot, it usually proceeds from too much blood, and is known by redness of urine, the pulse is swift, the veins great and full, the spittle, mouth, and tongue, seem sweeter than they used to be: the cure is letting blood in the right arm.

47. *To cause the Liver well to digest*

Take Oil of Wormwood, and so much Mastich in powder as will make it into a poultice, lay it warm to your right side.

48. *A caution*

If the liver be stopped, the face will swell, and you shall be as sure to have a pain in your right side, as though you had it there already.

49. *For stoppage of the Liver*

Use Garden-thyme in all your drinks and broaths, it will prevent stoppages before they come, and cure them after they are come.

50. *For the liver*

The liver of a Hare dryed, and beaten into powder, cures all the diseases of the liver of man.

FINIS

General Index

A List of the Principal Diseases

Abortion (to prevent). Sage 344. Tansey 346.

Aches in the joints 388. Of Beans, 321.

Agues. Archangel 15. Buck's-horn-plantain 46. Camomile 54. Pellitory 190. Meadow-sweet 207.

— Dry. Maudlin 162. Lovage 153.

— Hot. Mallows 156, 431. Wild Tansey 252.

— Quartan. Fumitory 335. Cinquefoil 342.

Almonds of the Ears. Devil's-bit 346.

Anthony's Fire. Crab's-claws 80. Duck's-meat 93. Hawk-weed 126.

Appetite (to restore). Wild Marjoram 159. Masterwort 339.

Apoplexy. Lavender 146. Lily of the Valley 149.

Asthma 505. Woodbine 273. Lungwort 154.

Blood (to cleanse). Nettles 179, 400. Hops 339.

Bloody Flux. Amaranthus 12. Mallows 158. Blackberry 37. Brank Ursine 41. Clown's-wood 73.

Blows (black and blue, marks of). Daisies 328. Of Solomon's-seal 317.

Boils. Barberry 22. Cuckow-point 84. Wheat 270.

Bowels (obstructions of) 504. Stachea 348. Hops 348.

Brain (to strengthen) 468, 508. Rosemary 349. Nutmegs 350.

Bruises. Bishop's-weed 35. Chervil 65. Solomon's-seal 230.

Burns 527. Burdock 51. Hound's-tongue 138.

Cancers. Asarabacca 17. Briony 42. Yellow Water-flag 107. Cinquefoil 69.

Cankers. Dragons 94. Flower-de-luce 110. Winter-green 122.

Chest (diseases of). Sweet Marjoram 160.

Chilblains. Henbane 129.

Chin-Cough. Thyme 258.

Cholic. All-Heal 2. Dove's-foot 93. Mullein 174. Osmond Royal 101.

Chops of the hands, &c. Pomatum 530.

Colds. Nep 178. Juice of Liquorice 449.

Consumption 347, 410, 417, 456. Sweet Chervil 66. Plantain 199. Pine-nuts 350.

Convulsions 475. Down 94. Pansies 347.

Corns. Houseleek 137, 327. Willow 270.

Coughs. Angelica 11. Garlick 115. Hore-hound 135.

Cramp. Mugwort 173. Mullein 174. Sage 228.

Diabetes (an involuntary discharge of urine) 357.

Dimness of Sight. Pearl-trefoil 262. Vervain 264. Mellilot 163. Valerian 263.

Dizziness of the Head. Sweet Marjoram 160. Sow-fennel 104. Rosemary 219.

Dropsy. Elder 95, 312. Bay 351. Juniper 141. Flax-weed 108. Pellitory of the Wall 190.

Ears 585. Fig-Tree 106. Ale-hoof 7. Sow Thistle 244.

Eyes 585. Eyebright 100. Hawkweed 126. Wild Clary 71. Rattlegrass 211. Beets 28.

— (inflammations of). Violets 266. Anemone 13. Groundsel 122.

Faintings. Balm 21. Endive 97. Pennyroyal 192. Heart Trefoil 262.

Face 588. Beans 25.

Falling Sickness. Elk's Claws 358. Mallows 156. Masterwort 161.

Felons of the Finger. Amara Dulcis 1. True Love 133. Nailwort 178.

Fevers 484. Endive 97. Flea-wort 109. Master-wort 161. Marigolds 161.

— (Pestilential). Butter-bur 50. Elecampane 98. Clove-gilliflowers 117.

— (Putrid). Borage 39.

Fistulas 513. Bugle 47. Wintergreen 122. Cow-parsnips 187. Campion, Wild 56.

Fits. Wild Arrach 14.

Flux. Bistort 35. Flux-weed 110. Rhubarb of Pontus 318.

Fundament falling 337, 536. Duck's Meat 358.

Gout. Comfrey 75. Sciatica-cresses 81. Gout-wort 120. Elm 96.

Gravel. Asparagus 19. Butcher's-broom 44. Parsley-piert 186.

Gums. 588.

Head 500, 584. Cives 70. Feverfew 102. Flower-de-luce 110. Pellitory 190. Roses 215.

— Ache. Beets 28. Duck's-meat 93. Ivy 140. Privet 207.

— Bald. White-lilies 149. Wall-Rue 155, 584.

— Scabby. Fox-glove 112. Knapweed 143. Nep 178.

— Scald. White Lilies 149.

Heart (to strengthen). 403, 407, 410, 425, 472, 508.

— (palpitation of). Syrup of Apples 433.

Heart-Burn. Vine 347.

Hiccough. Mint 166.

Hoarseness. Fig-tree 106. Liquorice 150. Peach-tree 188.

Imposthumes 528. Barley 23. Chickweed 67. Dandelion 87.

Indigestion 461, 551. Avens 20. Ragwort 210. Samphire 231.

Inflammations. Arssmart 16. Sea Coleworts 53. Cinquefoil 69. Black Cresses 80.

— in the sides. Violets 349.

Infection (to preserve from). Scabious 237. Bay 24.

Itch. Black alder 9. Celandine 59. Stinking-gladwin 118. Juniper 141.

Jaundice. Agrimony 5. Ash 20. Carduus Benedict 57.

— Yellow. Wormwood 276. Barberries 321.

King's-evil. Wheat 270.

Leprosy. Nigella 353.

Lice (in the head, to kill). Stavesacre 353. Olibanum 353.

Liver 398. Sage 228. Strawberries 247. Maple-tree 159.

— (inflammation of). Wild Thyme 259.

— (obstructions of). Rhubarb 223, 318. Parsley 185. Columbines 74. Liverwort 151. Alexander 8.

— (to strengthen). Cleavers 72. Costmary 78. Dock 90. Hart's-tongue 124.

Looseness (to stop). Cloves 350.

Lungs. Lungwort 154. Water Agrimony 6. Nettles 179. Filipendula 106. Scabious 237.

— (inflammation of). Garden Rue 224, 344. Heart's-ease 124.

— (ulcers of). Money-wort 168. Horehound 339.

Measles. Tormentil 259. Saffron 227.

— (to drive out). Alkanet 3. Marigolds 161.

Melancholy 502. Melancholy-thistle 253. Germander 117. Viper's Bugloss 267, 333. Motherwort 171. Burnet 49. Dodder 91.

Memory (to strengthen). Olibanum 386. Sage 344.

Menses (to provoke) 352, 366, 382, 388. Bdellium 384. Marjoram 398.

— (to stop). 366, 374, 382, 427, 436. Tansy 252.

Milk (to increase in nurses). Fennel 334, 353. Viper's Bugloss 313.

Miscarriage (good against). Ladies' Mantle. Tansy 251.

Mouth. 587.

Nervous Complaints 521, 534. Privet 325.

— Head-ache. Lily of the Valley 149. Plantain 317.

Nose. 586.
— (bleeding at). Fluellin 111. House-leek 137. Periwinkle 195.

Pain in the Bowels 399. Mouse-ear 172. Of Marsh-mallows 156.
— in the Side. Chick-pease 68. Coral-wort 77. Gentian 115.
— in the Stomach 387. Rupture-wort 226. Spignel 245. Black-thorn 257.
Palsies 475, 497, 584. Cowslips 79. Juniper 141. Lavender 146.
Piles. Lesser Celandine 61. Coltsfoot 75. Stone-crop 249.
Pleurisies 463. Lohoch of Poppies 450.
Poison (to expel) 490. White Lilies 149, Master-wort 161. Rue 344.
Polypus 586. Polypody 201.
Purging. Flowers 377.
— Fruits 380.
— Herbs 374.
— Syrups 437.

Quinsey. Cudweed 78. Hyssop 134. Orpine 184. Ragwort 210. Black-berry 37.

Rickets. Fearn 313. Syrup of Hart's-tongue 436.
Ring-worm. Savine 234. Celandine 59. Barberry 22.
Ruptures. Rupture-wort 333. Thorough wax 258. Tormentil 259. Consolida major 311.

Scrophula. Celandine 311. Eringo 313.
Scurvy. Scurvygrass 238. Watercresses 82. Winter Rocket 214. Cuckoo Flower 147.
Scurf (or running tetters). Beech 32. Plantain 199.
Shingles. Plantain 342.
Shortness of Breath. Angelica 11. Calamint 53. Hyssop 134. Pellitory of the Wall 190.
Skin (to clear). Madder 154. Cuckow-points 309. Vervain 347.
Sleep (to procure). Poppy 203, 446. Lettuce 147.
Small Pox. Marigolds 161. Saffron 227.
Sore Breasts 590. Purslain 205. Quince 208.

Sore (continued)
— Eyes. Buck's-horn-plantain 46. Succory 248. Celandine 59. Loose-strife 151.
— Head. Garden Rue 224. Tormentil 259.
— Mouth. Blue-bottle 40. Birch 34. Golden Rod 119.
— Throat 589. Sanicle 231. Self-heal 239. Saracen's Confound 232.
Sprains 522, 530.
Spring Medicine. Lady's Thistle 254. Nettles 179.
Stings and Venomous Bites. Bazil 23. St. John's-wort 139. Bay 24. Eringo 99. Rocket 213.
Stomach 590. Mint 166. Lovage 153.
— (inflammations of). Wallnut-tree 268.
— (obstructions of) 456. Crosswort 82. Rhubarb 221, 499.
— (to strengthen) 357, 397. Gentian 115. Mustard 175. Roses 215. Wood Sorrel 243.
Stone 357. Ash 20. Bird's-foot 34. Broom 45. Burdock 51. Camomile 54. Parsley-piert 186.
Surfeits. Liverwort 151.
Sweat (to provoke) 366, 399, 469, 476, 491.
Swellings. Common Alder 10. Sea-Cole-worts 53. Chickweed 67.
— in the Throat. Water Caltrops 55. Devil's-bit 89. Stinking Gladwin 118.

Teeth (to draw without pain) 356.
— (to fasten). Mastich 355. Bistort 309. Silver-weed 326.
— (to whiten). Vine 347, 587.
Teething of Children 357.
Tooth-ache 588. Tobacco 250. Wild Tansy 252. Henbane 128.
Tumours 525, 528. Cives 70. Hemlock 127. Lesser Celandine 59. True Love 133.
— (hard). Misselto 167. Mallows 156.
— (hot). Water Lily 148.

Ulcers. Centaury 62. Coralwort 77. Bistort 35. Archangel 15. Alehoof 7.

Venereal Disease. Sope-wort 344.

Voice (to restore) 445, 452, 506.

Vomit. Antimonial Wine 415.

Vomiting (to stay) 435, 447. Lady's Mantle 145, 464, 473.

Warts. Buck's-horn 46. Houseleek 137. Poplar 202.

Wens. Turnsole 260. Fuller's Thistle 314.

Wheezing. Liquorice 150. Hyssop 134. Lungwort 154.

Whitlows. Nail-wort 178.

Wind 373, 466. Bishop's-weed 35. Carraway 58. Dill 88. Fennel 103. Hemp 128.

— in the Stomach. Lovage 153. Thyme 258. Mint 166. Rosemary 219. Garden Tansy 251.

Womb (cold infirmities of). Bay berries 351.

— (diseases of) 536. Wild Arrach 14. Feverfew 102.

— (inflammations of). Schœnanth 348.

Women's Diseases. Dog Mercury 164. Mosses 170. Mugwort 173, 326.

— in Labour. Cinnamon 321. Horehound 339. Penny-royal 343.

Worms 469. Dog's-grass 92. Wormwood 274. Calamint 53. Arssmart 16. Butter-bur 50. Centaury 62. Lavender-cotton 146.

Wounds. Adder's-tongue 4. Bifoil 33. Primroses 206. Burnet 49. One Blade 37. Bistort 35. Moonwort 169. Lupines 352.

— the Head. Shepherd's purse 240.